615.5

The Illustrated Encyclopedia
of
Body-Mind Disciplines

The Illustrated Encyclopedia
of
Body-Mind Disciplines

Nancy Allison, CMA
Editor

The Rosen Publishing Group, Inc.
New York

Published in 1999 by The Rosen Publishing Group, Inc.
29 East 21st Street, New York, NY 10010

Library of Congress Cataloging-in-Publication Data

Allison, Nancy
The illustrated encyclopedia of body-mind disciplines/Nancy Allison, editor
    p. cm.
    Includes bibliographical references and index
    ISBN 0-8239-2546-3
    1. Alternative medicine—Encyclopedias. 2. Mind and body therapies—Encyclopedias.
I. Allison, Nancy, 1954-
R733.I46 1998
615.5—dc21
                                                  98-24969
                                                    CIP

Manufactured in the United States of America

About the Editor

Nancy Allison, CMA, has always been interested in the role of movement in human society, its inner impulses and outer forms. This interest led her to pursue a career in dance. She performed during her childhood with the National Ballet of Washington, DC, and with Moscow's world-renowned Bolshoi Ballet during its 1963 American tour. She graduated with honors from Ohio University with a B.F.A. in Dance. While at Ohio University she augmented her study of dance with courses in philosophy and psychology. As a young professional dancer she joined the Theater of the Open Eye in New York City, founded by choreographer Jean Erdman and the late Joseph Campbell. Allison distinguished herself as the leading interpreter of Erdman's dance repertory from the 1940s and 1950s, producing the three-volume video archive *Dance and Myth: The World of Jean Erdman*.

Inspired by both Erdman and Campbell, Allison expanded her exploration of movement to include the body-mind relationship. She has studied hatha yoga, t'ai chi ch'üan, the Pilates Method, bioenergetics, authentic movement, and Laban movement analysis, in which she earned a degree as a certified movement analyst. A much sought after teacher, Allison has taught master classes and workshops throughout the United States. She currently resides in New York, where she teaches at the School of Education of New York University.

Acknowledgments

So many people have helped create this volume that it is probably impossible to name them all, but given this opportunity, I would like to try. I feel deeply indebted to Joseph Campbell, whose personal encouragement guided my early explorations into the world of body-mind and whose spirit and knowledge are a constant wellspring of inspiration to me. I also want to thank my husband, who believed in my ability to complete this project and nurtured both it and me with his constant love and support.

I am eternally grateful to all of the distinguished teachers, healers, and writers who contributed entries to this volume. Their dedication to their respective fields and their generous gifts of time and knowledge to this project have earned my undying respect and admiration. I believe they are, each in their own wonderfully unique way, helping to make this world a better place.

Certain writers and consultants have been particularly influential in my own development, and I want to acknowledge their gifts to me: T'ai chi master Sophia Delza, who passed away during the course of our work, taught me to follow the flow of the life force in its endless cycle from full to empty and back to full again; Ed Groff; Janet Hamburg; Clio Pavlantos and Jackie Hand, who taught me to recognize the endless permutations of that force through the language of Laban movement analysis; Nina Robinson, who introduced me to the thrill of liberating that force through bioenergetics; Lillo (Leela) Way, who taught me the true nature of a spiritual practice; Jane Magee and Jackie Hand, whose healing hands managed to untangle the knots into which I seem to want to endlessly entangle my body; and Dr.

Domenick Masiello, whose healing artistry has restored me and so many of my loved ones to a vibrant state of health. I am also indebted to Dr. Masiello for the many fine contributing writers he recommended to this project. In that regard I am also deeply indebted to Thomas Claire and Ken Frey.

There are also those who, while not contributing writers, were important to my ability to realize this project: Clifford Schulman, Jeff McMahon, Anne Johnson, Joanna Kosartes Vergoth, and Cynthia Reynolds, all of whom recommended contributing writers to the project; Romana Kryzanowska, who gave me my first teaching job in the body-mind arena at the Pilates Studio; Carol Walker and Steven Giordano, who encouraged me to expand and explore that skill and knowledge at SUNY Purchase; Miriam Roskin Berger, who has supported so many of my creative endeavors and gave me the opportunity to develop my teaching at New York University, and all of my students over the years who continually show me through their amazing transformations that my approach to this material is valuable and life-enhancing.

Finally, I would like to thank the staff at the Rosen Publishing Group, all of whom were extraordinarily helpful and supportive; especially Christine Slovey, who worked long and diligently to uphold cohesive reference standards while allowing each individual voice to be heard; Michael Isaac and Margaret Haerens, who each offered their own perspective and editing skills; Kim Sonsky, whose artistic talents created the cover design; Vera Amadzadeh, whose tireless photo research efforts brought such vivid visual expression to the ideas contained in the writing; and Olga Vega, whose layout and design expertise give such visual clarity and accessibility to the volume.

With such a huge task, spanning so many years, I'm sure there are others I have missed. Please forgive me and know that you have my deepest respect and gratitude.

—Nancy Allison, CMA, Editor

Contributors

Acupressure, Process Acupressure

Aminah Raheem, Ph.D. and Diplomate of Process Work, is a transpersonal psychologist, bodyworker, writer, and the originator of process acupressure, who has worked for many years with the integration of bodywork and consciousness. She was an adjunct faculty member of the Institute for Transpersonal Psychology for ten years.

Acupuncture

Robert J. Abramson, D.D.S, M.D., had a private dental practice for over a decade before earning his M.D. from the State University of New York and completing a bachelor's course in acupuncture at the College of Traditional Chinese Medicine in England. Dr. Abramson is currently a privately practicing acupuncturist in New York City.

Aikido

Clio Pavlantos, M.A., CMA, holds a master's degree in dance, a certificate in Laban movement studies, and a black belt in aikido. She has taught all three disciplines at colleges, universities, and private institutions. Dance and Laban movement analysis helped her in learning and teaching aikido, which she finds to have many of the rhythms and expressive qualities of dance.

Marvin Bookman has been involved in the martial arts for twenty years. He is certified as an aikido instructor by the United States Aikido Federation. In 1989, he founded Aikido of Greenwich Village. Currently, Bookman gives seminars and classes throughout the United States.

Alexander Technique

Diane Young, NASAT, is a certified teacher and trainer of the Alexander technique. She has a modern dance background, having choreographed and performed in New York City since 1983. She is on the faculty at SUNY Stony Brook in the music department and maintains a private practice in New York and Connecticut. She has written various journals on body-mind healing and has received a grant from the New York Cardiac Center to study and report on complementary medicine.

Art Therapy

Cathy Malchiodi, M.A., ATR, LPAT, LPCC, is the director of the Institute for the Arts and Health in Salt Lake City, Utah. She is the editor of *Art Therapy: Journal of the American Art Therapy Association* and the author of several books and articles on the topic of art therapy with trauma, child physical abuse, and medical applications. Ms. Malchiodi has lectured at many universities, agencies, and institutions throughout the United States, Canada, Europe, and Asia.

Aston-Patterning®

Allison Funk has been working in the fields of bodywork and movement education for twelve years. A licensed physical therapist assistant, she received her Aston-Patterning® certification in 1996 and is currently enrolled in the faculty training program at the Aston-Patterning Center in Lake Tahoe, Nevada. Funk owns a private Aston-Patterning practice in Winter Park, Colorado, where she uses her skills to assist a variety of clients.

Authentic Movement

Daphne Lowell is a professor at Hampshire College and the Five College

Dance Department. She is also codirector of the Hampshire College Program in contemplative dance.

Ayurvedic Medicine

Dr. Vasant Lad, BAMS (bachelor of ayurvedic medicine and surgery), MASc (master of ayurvedic science), is the founder, director, chairman of the board, and principal instructor of the Ayurvedic Institute in Albuquerque, New Mexico. He practiced and taught ayurveda in Pune, India, before coming to the United States and teaching at the Santa Fe College of Natural Medicine in 1981.

Bartenieff Fundamentals℠

Janet Hamburg, CMA, M.A., directs the dance division at the University of Kansas, Lawrence. She was a faculty member of the Laban/Bartenieff Institute of Movement Studies Certificate Extension Program in New Mexico. She has taught LMA classes internationally, and throughout the United States Hamburg's work with athletes has been featured on national television, including the program *Science World*.

Behavioral Vision Therapy

Dr. Joseph Shapiro is a behavioral optometrist with twenty-five years of experience. He is the director of the Center for Unlimited Vision in New York City. He received his doctor of optometry degree from the Massachusetts College of Optometry and did his intern and residency program in vision therapy at the University Optometric Center, State College of Optometry, State University of New York. He has taught rehabilitative optometry at six major hospitals in the New York metropolitan area. He is coauthor of *Out of Sight into Vision*, a consumer self-help book presenting new models of seeing and vision therapy.

Bioenergetics

Nina Robinson, ADTR, M.A., CMA, has been a dance/movement therapist since 1973. She has taught in the New York University dance therapy program, from which she received her master's degree. She is a member of the Academy of Dance Therapists Registered. She has integrated bioenergetics into her dance therapy work throughout her career. She began her many years of bioenergetic therapy with Alexander Lowen, M.D., from 1965 to 1967.

Biofeedback

Les Fehmi, Ph.D., organized and chaired the first national meeting of biofeedback researchers in 1968. He has a Ph.D. in physiological psychology from UCLA and has been recognized by the Association for Applied Physiopsychology and Biofeedback for his contributions to the development of applied physiopathology and biofeedback. He directs biofeedback centers in New York City and Princeton, New Jersey.

Body-Mind Centering®

Vera Orlock is an assistant professor of dance at Kansas State University and has taught at Indiana University, Bloomington, and the University of North Carolina, Charlotte. Her choreography has been recognized by grants from the Ohio Arts Council and the New York State Council on the Arts. She is on the faculty of the School for Body-Mind Centering® and is also a certified practitioner of structural integration, the work of Ida P. Rolf. Orlock is frequently a guest artist/teacher in Europe and the United States.

Bodynamics Analysis

Peter Bernhardt, MFCC, is director of the Clement Street Counseling Center Faculty at California Institute of Integral Studies in Somatics program, in San Francisco, California, and a founding member of the Bodynamics Institute, USA. He has led trainings and workshops throughout the United States and Europe, has twenty years' experience as a body psychotherapist, and is in private practice near Berkeley, California.

Bowen Technique

Oswald H. Rentsch is the principal and founder of the Bowen Therapy Academy of Australia, the official organization of Bowtech®. From 1974 to 1976 he studied under Thomas A. Bowen, who commissioned Rentsch to document and teach his original techniques. He has earned a diploma of osteopathy from the South Pacific Council of Natural Therapies, an honorary doctorate of massage therapy from the Australian Registrar of Massage Therapists, and a diploma of homeopathy ionization principles from the Australian Academy of Homeopathy. Oswald Rentsch has twenty-two years of experience with the Bowen technique and, together with his wife Elaine, has spent ten years as a Bowtech teacher.

Brain Gym®

Lark Carroll has been teaching Brain Gym in the Bay Area since 1986. She completed certification in educational kinesiology, neurolinguistic programming, acupressure massage, and Bowen Therapy. Additionally, she holds training in a variety of modalities, including CranioSacral therapy, Living Vision™, meditation, Chinese five-element theory, and nutritional approaches to health and balance.

Chiropractic

Dr. Trina Marx is a doctor of chiropractic with a degree in clinical nutrition, also specializing in exercise psychology and holistic treatments. In addition to her private practice, she is the chiropractor for the American Tap Dance Orchestra. Her volunteer work includes providing chiropractic services for the Gay Men's Health Crisis and for children born with addictions and HIV. She has also written *Body Almanac* and *Tap Dance*.

Connective Tissue Therapy℠

Jackie Hand, M.A., is a certified Laban movement analyst (CMA) and a registered movement therapist (RMT). She is a movement consultant and a dance specialist, performing movement retraining and bodywork. On the faculty at the Laban/Bartenieff Institute of Movement Studies, she integrates her years of dance training with her movement observation skills to educate clients in movement awareness and observation. She studied anatomy with Irene Dowd and Connective Tissue Therapy™ with Theresa Lamb. She has a holistic approach to movement and bodywork and is nationally certified in therapeutic massage and bodywork (NCTMB).

Contact Improvisation

Paul Langland is a dancer, singer, choreographer, and teacher. A longtime practitioner of contact and other improvisational dance forms, he often presents his own work, as well as performing with others. His work has been seen at Dance Theater Workshop, PS 122, Franklin Furnace, and Movement Research. Since 1983, he has been a core faculty member of New York University's Experimental Theater Wing.

Core Energetics

Pamela L. Chubbuck, Ph.D., LPC, is on the senior international teaching faculty of the Core Energetic Institute in New York City, where she is also director of faculty development. Dr. Chubbuck is the director of Core Energetics South and has worked personally and extensively with John C. Pierrakos, M.D., for more than twenty-five years. Dr. Chubbuck is the author of *Passages to Womanhood: Stories of Celebration for Young Women*, and numerous articles on the core energetics process.

coreSomatics®

Kay Miller is certified in the Rubenfeld synergy method and the Feldenkrais Method® and received her gestalt training in the three-year postgraduate program at the Gestalt Institute of Cleveland. She has served as consultant, staff, and/or workshop leader for the Pennsylvania Department of Education, the University of Pittsburgh, Carlow College, the University of West Virginia, Long Island University, the Gestalt Institute of Cleveland, and the Western Psychiatric Institute.

CORE Structural Integrative Therapy

George P. Kousaleos has been a licensed massage therapist specializing in structural integration and myofascial therapy since 1978. A graduate of Harvard University and the SOMA Institute of Neuromuscular Integration, he has practiced and taught in Germany, Greece, and throughout America. In 1990, he founded the CORE Institute School of Massage Therapy of Tallahassee, Florida, a state-licensed and nationally accredited program. He trains massage therapists in continuing education certification courses in CORE myofascial therapy and CORE structural integrative therapy. Kousaleos also served as the general manager of the British Olympic Sports Massage Therapy Team (1994–1996).

Gary N. Genna, LMT, is the founder and owner of the CORE Institute of Tennessee. A graduate of SUNY Cortland with a degree in biology and education, Genna has been an advanced instructor for the CORE Institute since 1989. He has presented at various state and international conferences and spent more than three years working as a neuromuscular therapist at St. Anthony's Hospital Sports Medicine and Orthopedic Rehabilitation Center in St. Petersburg, Florida. He has been both a massage therapist and a massage educator for more than twenty-five years, highlighted as the head coach for the British Olympic Sports Massage Team in 1995 and 1996.

CranioSacral Therapy

Kenneth I. Frey, PT, is director of the Institute of Physical Therapy, a private practice and clinical resource center in New York City.

Dance Therapy

Anne L. Wennerstrad is a dance/movement therapist, clinical social worker, and dance educator working in mental health and education. Currently she is coordinator of undergraduate dance education at New York University, where she teaches and advises students. She has presented and written on the arts in education and therapy. Her clinical work focuses on creative mind/body approaches to helping people with eating problems, anxiety, depression, and chronic mental illness. A former professional dancer, she is also on the staff of Career Transition for Dancers, a nonprofit counseling service.

Do-In

John Kozinski has taught do-in, traditional exercises, and healing through food and natural therapies throughout the United States and in Asia and South America. He offers seminars on do-in, traditional exercises, and the macrobiotic approach to health and healing at the Kushi Institute in Massachusetts, as well as in Connecticut and New York. He also has an active health counseling practice in which he recommends specific traditional foods, remedies, and natural lifestyle practices to foster healing and general well-being.

Drama Therapy

Professor Patricia Sternberg RDT/BCT (registered drama therapist/board certified trainer) is the chairperson of the Board of Examiners of the National Association for Drama Therapy. She is a full professor of the Department of Theater at Hunter College in New York and heads the developmental drama program there. She is a playwright with more than twenty-five plays produced and/or published and is the author of seven books, including *Sociodrama: Who's in Your Shoes?* (with Antonina Garcia). She is currently working on her eighth, *Theater for Conflict Resolution*. A well-known presenter and workshop leader, having presented both nationally and internationally, Sternberg is a practicing drama therapist and for the past ten years has worked with a variety of populations in both psychiatric and educational facilities.

Emotional-Kinesthetic Psychotherapy

Linda Marks has practiced body-centered psychotherapy with individuals, couples, and groups for twelve years. She has helped found and served on the Board of the Interface Business Association (1984), the Organization Transformation Network (1985), the Massachusetts Association of Body-Oriented Psychotherapy and Counseling Bodyworkers (1989), and the Somatics Community of the Association for Humanistic Psychology. In 1990 she founded the Institute for Emotional-Kinesthetic Psychotherapy. She has written a column on psychology for *Spirit of Change* magazine for the past ten years. She is the author of *Living with Vision: Reclaiming the Power of the Heart*.

Enneagram

Janet Levine is an author, educator, and organizer. She is founder of Learning and The Enneagram, an educational enterprise dedicated to spreading knowledge of the enneagram system and its applications in education and related fields. She has taught at Milton Academy, Massachusetts, for ten years. She is director of the National Educators Institute for Enneagram Studies at Milton Academy. She has presented her work on education and the enneagram at national conferences and many other venues.

Eurythmy

Beth Dunn-Fox was raised and educated in northern California, where she studied and performed ballet, character, and modern dance. A graduate of Eurythmy Spring Valley, she has toured throughout North America and Europe with their professional ensemble for twelve years. In addition to performing, she has also carried the finance and development work of Eurythmy Spring Valley over a number of years.

Eye Movement Desensitization and Reprocessing

Barbara A. Parrett, RN, M.S., is a nurse and psychotherapist who brings a holistic approach to her work with individuals and organizations. She has been thoroughly trained in EMDR and teaches this discipline to other therapists on an international scale, where she is in much demand as trainer and educator.

Feldenkrais Method®

Alan S. Questel is a founding member of Delman/Questel Associates, Inc., and is a Feldenkrais practitioner.

Feng Shui

Marilyn Saltzman is a feng shui practitioner. She studied feng shui with Nancy SantoPietro, a certified teacher trained by Master Lin Yun. In addition, she has studied Transcendental Meditation and reiki, and she is a certified rebirther and hypnotherapist. Saltzman has given lectures and workshops on feng shui throughout Virginia and Maryland.

Flower Remedies

Leslie J. Kaslof is an internationally recognized pioneer, researcher, writer, and educator in the field of holistic health, preventative medicine, and natural approaches to stress reduction. He has written numerous articles in professional and popular publications and has written many other works, including *Herb and Ailment Cross-Reference Chart,* the pioneering book *Wholistic Dimensions in Healing,* and *The Traditional Flower Remedies of Dr. Edward Bach: A Self-Help Guide.*

Focusing

Joan Klagsbrun, Ph.D., is a clinical psychologist practicing focusing-oriented psychotherapy in private practice in Boston, Massachusetts. A college professor and a certified focusing train-

er and coordinator, she has been practicing and teaching focusing for twenty years.

Hakomi Integrative Somatics

Pat Ogden, M.A., is a founding member of the Hakomi Institute, serves on its trainers' board, and is the originator and director of hakomi integrative somatics. Trained in a wide variety of somatic approaches, she is a structural integrator (Guild for Structural Integration) and serves on the faculty of Ergos Institute (founded by Peter Levine, specializing in healing the effects of trauma) and the Naropa Institute.

Halprin Life Art Process

Daria Halprin-Khalighi, M.A., CET, is the cofounder and director of the Tampala Institute. She maintains a private practice in Marin County and is a certified expressive arts therapist. She is the author of *Coming Alive: The Creative Expression Method.*

Hanna Somatic Education®

Eleanor Criswell Hanna, Ed.D., is professor of psychology and former chair of the psychology department, Sonoma State University, California. In 1975, she cofounded, with Thomas Hanna, the Novato Institute for Somatic Research and Training, Novato, California. She trained in somatic education with Thomas Hanna in his 1981 Australian training program; she has worked closely with him in the development of the field of somatics over the years. She is currently serving as president of the Somatics Society and editor of *Somatics.* A licensed psychologist, she maintains a private practice in psychotherapy, biofeedback, and somatic education. She is the author of *Biofeedback and Somatics.*

Herbal Medicine

Mark Blumenthal is the founder and executive director of the American Botanical Council (ABC), a leading nonprofit research and education organization in Austin, Texas. He also edits the quarterly magazine *HerbalGram*.

Holistic Health

Suzan Walter, MBA, is cofounder and current president of the American Holistic Health Association and past president of the American Holistic Medical Foundation. She is the creator and director of the *Global Health Calendar* on the Internet at HealthWorld Online (www.healthy.net). She also facilitates networking for speakers, practitioners, and health care associations within this Web site.

Homeopathy, Osteopathy

Domenick John Masiello, D.O., DHt, CSPOMM, has been a solo, office-based practitioner of traditional osteopathy and classical homeopathy in New York City since 1986. He was certified with special proficiency in osteopathic manipulative medicine and is also certified in homeotherapeutics. He has written the foreword to *Osteopathy: An Integrated Whole Body Therapy* and has been published in the *Journal of the American Institute of Homeopathy*.

Holotropic Breathwork™

Kylea Taylor, M.S., is a certified Holotropic Breathwork™ practitioner and has been working in the field of addiction recovery since 1970. She has studied with Christine and Stanislav Grof, M.D., Ph.D., since 1984 and is a member of the teaching staff of Grof Transpersonal Training. She is the author of *The Breathwork Experience: Exploration and Healing in Nonordinary States of Consciousness* and *The Ethics of Caring: Honoring the Web of Life in Our Professional Healing Relationships*. She has served as editor of the *Inner Door,* the newsletter of the Association for Holotropic Breathwork International.

Hydrotherapy

Douglas C. Lewis, ND, is a naturopathic physician in Seattle, Washington.

Hypnotherapy

Oscar A. Gillespie, Ph.D., is the president of NYSEPH, the New York Milton H. Erickson Society for Psychology and Hypnosis, and is on the faculty of its training program. He taught psychology at Fordham University and currently is in private practice in New York City.

Ideokenesis

Andre Bernard teaches ideokenesis, drawing upon his background in science and the performing arts. He studied chemical engineering at the University of South Carolina, where he took his B.S. degree in chemistry and mathematics. Pursuing a professional acting career, he appeared in more than a hundred theatrical productions. He also studied dance and toured extensively with the Charles Weidman Dance Theater. He studied Mabel Elsworth Todd's movement therapy techniques, the foundation of ideokenesis, with Barbara Clark. He has been a member of the faculty at New York University, teaching Todd's work, since 1966.

Infant Massage Therapy

Mindy Zlotnick has worked with parents and their families as a teacher since 1975. She holds an M.A. in special education and worked for many years with deaf children, communicating in sign language. She was trained in massage in 1987 and began communicating through touch in her practice with adults. She became a certified infant massage instructor in 1989, combining her love for teaching and her love of massage. Her practice includes teaching parents with healthy babies as well as parents with babies who are medically fragile or have developmental delays.

Integral Yoga

Reverend Kumari de Sachy, Ed.D., has been a student of Swami Satchidananda since 1980. In 1981, she became an integral yoga instructor and proceeded to teach at integral yoga institutes, colleges, universities, and prisons. In 1994, she was ordained as an integral yoga minister. For the past ten years, she and her husband have been living and serving as whole-time members at Satchidananda Ashram–Yogaville with the spiritual master Sri Swami Satchidananda. At Yogaville, she has taught English and French, in addition to serving as director of the Yogaville Summer Program for Children and Teens. She is also the editor of Integral Yoga Publications, which publishes Swami Satchidananda's books and the quarterly magazine *Integral Yoga*.

Interactive Guided Imagery

Martin Rossman, M.D., is a 1969 graduate of the University of Michigan Medical School and is board certified in acupuncture. He is the founder and director of the Collaborative Medicine Center in Mill Valley, California. As the codirector of the Academy for Guided Imagery in Mill Valley, he has taught clinical guided imagery to more than 9,000 health care professionals since 1982. He was a founding member of the Scientific Advisory Board of the Institute for the Advancement of Health. He has written numerous articles and publications and was a winner of the American Health Book Award in 1987.

Iyengar Yoga

Janet MacLeod teaches yoga full-time, offering ongoing classes in San Francisco and teaching workshops around the country. She is on the faculty of the Iyengar Yoga Institute of San Francisco teacher training program. She is a certified teacher at the intermediate level and continues to study in Pune with the Iyengar family on a regular basis.

Jin Shin Do® Bodymind Acupressure™

Iona Marsaa Teeguarden, M.A., is the originator of Jin Shin Do® Bodymind Acupressure™. She founded the Jin Shin Do Foundation and began offering JSD teacher training programs. She has written several books and articles on the practice of JSD.

Jin Shin Jyutsu® Physio-Philosophy

Ian Kraut is a practitioner of Jin Shin Jyutsu and a licensed massage therapist. He is a member of the staff at Jin Shin Jyutsu, Inc., in Scarsdale, Arizona. He has a B.A. in music from SUNY Binghamton and has studied Andean music in South America.

Journal Therapy

Kathleen Adams, M.A., LPC, is a licensed psychotherapist and the founder/director of the Center for Journal Therapy in Denver, Colorado, an organization dedicated to teaching the healing art of journal writing to individuals, groups, and mental health professionals. She has specialized in journal therapy since 1985 and is one of the pioneers in the field. She is the author of three books on the use of journal writing as a therapeutic tool.

Ju Jutsu, Karate

Stefan Nikander is a certified karate and ju jutsu instructor. Having taught soccer to children since the age of fifteen, he became certified as a soccer trainer in 1983. He is also a certified nursery school teacher and has worked professionally at schools and play centers since 1990. He is the vice chairman of the children's committee of the Swedish Budo Federation, a martial arts organization. His writing has appeared in various martial arts magazines in several countries, and he has written columns for Scandinavian newspapers on the subject of martial arts as a means to stop violence. He is currently training to become a personal trainer and massage therapist.

Kendo

Daniel T. Ebihara is the chairman of Ken Zen Institute Ltd. and a member of the board of directors of All United States Kendo Federation. He has written several articles about the martial arts for various periodicals and is an advanced student of karate, kendo, and judo.

Bruce Robertson Smith is a first-degree black belt in kendo, having studied martial arts in Japan with the Budo master Fushi Sensei. He has trained extensively in bodywork and structural integration and has done shamanic journeywork.

Kestenberg Movement Profile

Susan Loman is the director of a master's program in dance/movement therapy at Antioch New England Graduate School in Keene, New Hampshire, and the author of numerous articles on the KMP. She has given intensive courses on this material in Germany and Italy. She is the coeditor of a textbook on the KMP published in 1997.

Janet Kestenberg Amighi is an anthropologist who has done fieldwork in Iran and Bali. She is the author of *Zoroastrians in Iran: Assimilation, Conversion and Persistence.* She coteaches a course on the KMP with Susan Loman and is coeditor of a textbook on the KMP.

Kinetic Awareness

Ellen Saltonstall, M.A., MCKA, is a certified master teacher of kinetic awareness, a licensed massage therapist, and a teacher and practitioner of hatha yoga. She has taught at the New School, Columbia University, and Bard College and is currently is on the staff of the Mind/Body Medical Institute of St. Peters Hospital in New Brunswick, New Jersey.

J. Robin Powell, Ph.D., CSW, MCKA, is a certified master teacher of kinetic awareness and teaches at New York University and other institutions, as well as privately. She is a founding board member of the Kinetic Awareness Center, Inc., and teaches in the teacher training program.

Michelle Berne, M.A., MCKA, introduced the first university course in body/mind therapies while on the faculty of New York University, where she taught for twelve years. As a professional dancer and choreographer in New York, she presented original work with her own company and performed with others. She is a certified master teacher of kinetic awareness and currently teaches kinetic awareness, neuromuscular reeducation, and alignment in Los Angeles, California. She is also a celebration artist who choreographs and produces large-scale community art events for cities and nonprofit organizations across the country.

Kung-Fu Wu Su

Oswald Rivera is a senior instructor at Alan Lee's Chinese Kung-Fu Wu-Su Association. He has practiced Shaolin style kung-fu for twenty-four years. He is also the author of the novel *Fire and Rain* and the cookbook *Puerto Rican Cuisine in America.*

Laban Movement Analysis

Ed Groff, M.F.A., CMA, is currently director of graduate studies in the department of modern dance at the University of Utah. He has served on the faculties of Temple University, Hampshire College, Connecticut College, Tufts University, and Evergreen State College. He has taught in the certification programs in Laban Movement Analysis at schools and institutions in New York, Seattle, Salt Lake City, Columbus, Rotterdam, and Berlin. His choreography has been presented in the United States, Europe, and Asia.

Light Therapy

Dr. Brian J. Breiling is a licensed marriage, family, and child counselor and school psychologist. He is the co-editor and publisher of *Light Years Ahead: The Illustrated Guide to Full Spectrum and Colored Light in Mindbody Healing.* He is also the author of three chapters in this book on the professional and self-care applications of light therapy. For the last ten years, he successfully used flashing colored light stimulation through the eyes to aid his clients in uncovering and working through emotional traumas, depression, and pain, as well as to enhance learning and intellectual performance in adults and children.

Magnet Therapy

Dr. John Zimmerman earned his Ph.D. in biological psychology and neurosciences at the University of Colorado at Boulder in 1981. He is a member of the American Sleep Disorders Association and the North American Academy of Magnetic Therapy. Currently he serves as the laboratory director of the Washoe Sleep Disorders Center in Reno. Dr. Zimmerman is also the founder and president of the nonprofit organization called the Bio-Electro-Magnetics Institute (BEMI), which researches and provides resources on magnet therapy.

Martial Arts

Michael Maliszewski received his Ph.D. in psychology from the University of Chicago. He has held a number of positions at the University of Chicago and has conducted research and published in a variety of areas ranging from medicine to religious studies. He is currently a consultant in psychiatry at Massachusetts General Hospital and lecturer at Harvard Medical School. He has been involved in the study of martial arts and meditative traditions since 1970 and has studied throughout the United States and Asia. Included among his publications in the martial arts are the book *Spiritual Dimensions of the Martial Arts*, as well as articles that have appeared in the *Journal of Asian Martial Arts*, where he also serves as an associate editor.

Massage

Katie Scoville is a New York State-licensed massage therapist who practices Swedish massage, shiatsu, medical massage, and pregnancy massage. She has a private practice in

Manhattan, Studio of Massage Arts (SOMA), and also works with physical therapists. She is a shiatsu and clinic instructor at the Swedish Institute of Massage Therapy and Allied Health Sciences in New York City and a member of the American Massage Therapy Association. Katie holds a B.F.A. in dance and brings to her practice more than fifteen years of dance training and professional dance experience.

Medical Orgone Therapy

Dr. Peter Crist received his M.D. from the UCLA School of Medicine in 1977. Dr. Crist is a fellow of the American College of Orgonomy and has been its president since 1991. As a member of the ACO training faculty, he has been training medical orgonomists since 1982. He has authored clinical and theoretical articles as well as book reviews and is an assistant editor of the *Journal of Orgonomy*. Dr. Crist is also assistant clinical professor, Department of Psychiatry, UMDNJ-Robert Wood Johnson School of Medicine, New Brunswick, New Jersey. He has a private practice in Belle Mead, New Jersey.

Dr. Richard Schwartzman, D.O., graduated from the Philadelphia College of Osteopathic Medicine in 1966. He is a member of the faculty of Hahnemann University, an assistant clinical professor of psychiatry, and medical director of the Hahnemann University Correctional Mental Health Program. He is a fellow of the American College of Orgonomy, where he conducts the advanced training seminar. He is an assistant editor and contributing author of the *Journal of Orgonomy*. Dr. Schwartzman maintains a private practice in medical orgone therapy in Philadelphia.

Meditation

Eugene Taylor, Ph.D., is a lecturer on psychiatry, Harvard Medical School; executive faculty, Saybrook Institute; and director of the Cambridge Institute of Psychology and Religion.

Marilyn Schlitz, Ph.D., is a social anthropologist and director of research at the Institute of Noetic Sciences in Sausalito, California.

Meir Schneider Self-Healing Method

Carol Gallup works at the Center for Self-Healing in San Francisco, California.

Movement Pattern Analysis

Warren Lamb developed movement pattern analysis with Rudolf Laban. In 1950 Lamb joined Paton Lawrence & Co., management consultants, to apply the newly developed assessment method. He has been a professional dancer, a producer of plays, and a lecturer in the United Kingdom and United States. In 1952 he founded his own consultancy firm to use movement pattern analysis for top management teams worldwide. His publications include *Posture and Gesture, Management Behavior, Body Code*, and more than 100 journal articles.

Multi-Modal Expressive Arts Therapy

Susan Spaniol, Ed.D., ATR-BC, LMHC, is assistant professor in the Expressive Therapies Division of Lesley College. She received her Ed.D. at Boston University and is a board-certified art therapist and a licensed mental health counselor. She serves as associate editor of *Art Therapy: Journal of the American Art Therapy Association* and is an associate in psychiatry at Harvard Medical School.

Phillip Speiser, Ph.D., REAT, RDT, is director of Arts Across Cultures, Boston.

Speiser is a psychodrama, drama, and expressive arts educator/therapist who has been developing and implementing integrated arts programs since 1980. He is an adjunct professor at Lesley College in Cambridge, Massachusetts, and has taught and lectured extensively at training institutes and colleges throughout Scandinavia, Europe, Israel, and the United States. He is the former chairperson of Very Special Arts, Sweden, and the International Expressive Arts Therapy Association.

Mariagnese Cattaneo, Ph.D., ATR, LMHC, is a professor in the Expressive Therapies Division at Lesley College, Cambridge, Massachusetts. She is an expressive therapist and has trained expressive therapists for more than twenty-five years. Presently she is the coordinator of art therapy specialization and director of field training.

Muscular Therapy

Ben E. Benjamin holds a Ph.D. in sports medicine and education and is the founder and president of the Muscular Therapy Institute in Cambridge, Massachusetts. He is the author of the widely used books in the field: *Are You Tense?—The Benjamin System of Muscular Therapy, Sports Without Pain,* and *Listen to Your Pain—Understanding, Identifying, and Treating Pain.* He has been a regular contributor to the *Muscular Therapy Journal* since 1986. He has been in private practice for more than thirty-five years and has been teaching massage therapists in workshops internationally since 1973.

Mary Ann diRoberts, LICSW, CMT, is on the faculty of the Muscular Therapy Institute in Cambridge, Massachusetts.

Music Therapy

Adva Frank-Schwebel has been a music therapist for fifteen years. Her work in music therapy has included child psychology, group therapy, and private practice. She studied musicology and anthropology at the Hebrew University of Jerusalem, and classical guitar in Israel and London. She holds a master's degree in musicology from Bar Ilan University and teaches at the Institute for Art Therapy of David Yellin College in Jerusalem and at the Department of Music Therapy of Bar Ilan University.

Myofascial Trigger Point Therapy

Elliot Shratter has been practicing trigger point myotherapy since 1987. He is board certified by the National Association of Trigger Point Myotherapists Certification Board and the American Academy of Pain Management. He has served as president and journal editor of the National Association of Trigger Point Myotherapists and chairperson of the Trigger Point Myotherapists National Certification Board. He is currently in practice in Albuquerque, New Mexico, at Synergy Physical Therapy.

Naturopathic Medicine

Lauri M. Aesoph, ND, a graduate of Bastyr University, is a medical writer, editor, and educator. Over the past ten years, Dr. Aesoph's work has appeared in dozens of magazines and numerous books. She makes her home in Sioux Falls, South Dakota, with her husband and two sons.

Network Chiropractic

Donald Epstein, DCA, is a chiropractor and developer of network spinal analysis. He is the president of the Association for Network Chiropractic. He is also the author of several articles on the practice of this discipline.

Organismic Psychotherapy

Elliot Greene, M.A., is a counselor who has specialized in body psychotherapy for the past twenty-four years. His principal training has been in organismic body psychotherapy with Dr. Malcolm Brown and Katherine Ennis-Brown. He is also trained in bioenergetics, gestalt, and other related body-oriented methods. In addition, he is nationally certified as a massage therapist and served as president of the American Massage Therapy Association from 1990 to 1994. He has a private practice in Silver Springs, Maryland.

Orthomolecular Medicine

California freelance writer Martin Zucker has been writing for many years about health, nutrition, and preventive medicine. He is a former Associated Press foreign correspondent. He has written numerous published articles, coauthored five books, ghostwritten several others, and written many safety and environmental videos for the National Safety Council and other organizations. He has been a contributing editor to *Let's Live,* a leading health magazine, since 1978.

Pesso Boyden System Psychomotor

Albert Pesso cofounded Pesso Boyden system psychomotor (PBSP) psychotherapy with his life partner, Diane Boyden Pesso, in 1961. He is president of the Psychomotor Institute, Inc., Boston, Massachusetts, a nonprofit organization that promotes PBSP internationally. He has been supervisor of psychomotor therapy at the McLean Hospital in Belmont, Massachusetts; consultant in psychiatric research at the Boston Veterans Administration Hospital; and director of psychomotor therapy at the Pain Unit of the New England Rehabilitation Hospital. Albert Pesso is the author of *Movement in Psychotherapy* (1969) and *Experience in Action* (1973) and coeditor with John Crandell of *Moving Psychotherapy: Theory and Applications of Pesso Boyden System/ Psychomotor Psychology* (1991).

Pilates Method of Body Conditioning®

Leah Chaback, director of the Movement Center, is a certified Pilates instructor and teacher-trainer. She began studying the Pilates Method in 1986 at SUNY Purchase, New York. Ms. Chaback has trained and worked extensively with Romana Kryzanowska, disciple of Joseph Pilates and master teacher of his method for more than fifty years. After teaching the Pilates Method in New York City studios, she opened the Movement Center in 1990.

Poetry Therapy

Nicholas Mazza, Ph.D., is a professor at the School of Social Work at Florida State University. He is also editor of the *Journal of Poetry Therapy.* He has lectured and published extensively on the use of poetry and music in clinical practice.

Polarity Therapy

John Beaulieu, ND, Ph.D., is the author of the *Polarity Therapy Workbook* (1994).

Process Oriented Psychology

Dr. Joseph Goodbread is a longtime student and colleague of Arnold Mindell. He is a cofounder of the Research Society for Process Oriented Psychology in Zurich, of the Process Work Center of Portland, Oregon, and of the Global Process Institute in Portland. He is the author of *The Dreambody Toolkit: A Practical Introduction to the Philosophy, Goals and*

Practice of Process Oriented Psychology and *Radical Intercourse: How Inevitable Relationships Are Created by Dreaming*, a book on the dynamics of therapeutic relationships. He practices and teaches process work in Portland and throughout the world.

Psychodrama

Adam Blatner, M.D., is the author of several books and articles on the practice of psychodrama.

Psychoneuroimmunology

Leonard A. Wisneski, M.D., is a physician, board certified in internal medicine and in endocrinology and metabolism; he is also certified in acupuncture and homeopathy, which he has incorporated into his practice. Dr. Wisneski is a member of the board of directors of the Integral Health Foundation.

Leonard Sherp is a medical writer and reiki practitioner. Mr. Sherp is program director of the Integral Health Foundation.

Psychosynthesis

Richard Schaub, Ph.D., cofounded the New York Psychosynthesis Institute with Bonney Gulino Schaub, M.S., RN, CS. They have worked in every phase of mental health, alcohol and drug rehabilitation, and health care in careers that span thirty years. They teach internationally in the fields of psychotherapy, recovery, higher self-education, clinical imagery, and contemplation. They have published numerous professional articles, are associate editors of *Alternative Health Practitioner,* and are the authors of *Healing Addictions.*

Qigong

Kenneth S. Cohen, M.A., director of the Taoist Mountain Retreat in the Colorado Rocky Mountains, is an internationally renowned China scholar, qigong master, and health educator. He has been teaching qigong for more than twenty-five years and is helping to build a bridge between qigong and medical science. He was one of nine "exceptional healers" studied in the Menninger Clinic's Copper Wall Project, where he demonstrated unusual physiological control while practicing qigong. Cohen has written more than 150 articles and is the author of *The Way of Qigong.*

Radix

Erica Kelley has shared the growth of Radix since its inception in the late sixties, including its teaching, training, facilities, and administration in the United States and Europe. She maintains a part-time practice in Vancouver and administers Kelley/Radix and K/R Publications.

Rebirthing

Maureen Malone is the director of the New York Rebirthing Center.

Tony Lo Mastro is the director of the Philadelphia Rebirthing Center.

Reflexology

Laura Norman is a certified reflexologist and New York State-licensed massage practitioner. She is also author of *Feet First: A Guide to Foot Reflexology.* With a B.S. from Boston University and three master's degrees from Adelphi University, she originally embarked on a career in education. She discovered the potency of reflexology when she used it in her early work with hyperactive and emotionally dysfunctional children at Maimonides Institute in Brooklyn. She established the Laura Norman Method Reflexology Training Center in New York, offering

Reiki

Elaine J. Abrams is a reiki master instructor. In private practice in New York City since 1987, she brings her extensive experience with more than 800 clients and knowledge as a reiki instructor to her workshops. As founder of the Reiki Group, she provides a continuing support system for her practitioners.

Relaxation Response Technique

Richard Friedman, Ph.D., was a Professor of Psychiatry at the State University of New York, Stonybrook.

Herbert Benson, M.D., is the Mind/Body Medical Institute Associate Professor of Medicine, Harvard Medical School; Chief of the Division of Behavioral Medicine at the Beth Israel Deaconess Medical Center; and the founding president of the Mind/Body Medical Institute. A graduate of Wesleyan University and the Harvard Medical School, he is the author or co-author of more than 150 scientific publications and six books.

Patricia Myers is a research associate at the Mind/Body Medical Institute at the Beth Israel Deaconess Hospital, Harvard Medical School. Her areas of interest include the economics of behavioral medicine and the use of behavioral interventions in the treatment of pain.

Rolfing®

Allan Davidson was trained by Ida Rolf in Big Sur and San Francisco, California, in 1973-75. He has been Rolfing® and lecturing, teaching and writing about Rolfing ever since. In the 1980s, he cofounded the Chicago School for Advanced Bodywork, a pioneering clinic and forum for new ideas and technologies. He now codirects the Structural Therapy Institute, where he teaches bodywork problem-solving courses to health professionals. He is also trained in the hakomi method of body-centered psychotherapy and in CranioSacral therapy.

ROM Dance

Patricia Yu, M.A., co-creator of the ROM dance, is the director of the T'ai-Chi Center in Madison, Wisconsin. She originally learned t'ai chi ch'üan and tao kung meditation in 1970 with Master Liu Pei Ch'ung in the Republic of China. She continues to practice daily.

Rosen Method

Ivy Green is a professor of psychology, a certified Rosen method practitioner, a certified teacher of the Alexander technique, and a licensed massage therapist. Her book on the Rosen method, a psychospiritual bodywork, was published in 1998.

Rubenfeld Synergy Method

Ilana Rubenfeld, a pioneer in integrating bodywork with psychotherapy, has been an influential healer for the past thirty-five years. She originated the Rubenfeld synergy method in the early 1960s and started its professional training program in 1977. Formerly on the faculties of the NYU Graduate School of Social Work and New School for Social Research, she currently teaches at the Omega and Esalen Institutes and the Open Center.

Sandplay Therapy

Lois Carey, MSW, BCDSW, is a practitioner of sandplay therapy.

Sensory Awareness

Mary Alice Roche was cofounder with Charlotte Selver of the Sensory Awareness Foundation. She served as managing secretary until she retired in 1988 but continued as bulletin editor and archivist. She has a private practice and is a member of the Sensory Awareness Leaders Guild.

Shamanism

Hal Zina Bennett, Ph.D., is a long-time student of shamanism. He is also the author of twenty-five books, including ones on health (*The Well Body Book*, with Mike Samuels, M.D.), psychology (*The Holotropic Mind*, with Stan Grof, M.D.), and Native American spirituality (*Zuni Fetishes*). He is an adjunct faculty member at the Institute of Transpersonal Psychology, a private graduate school in Palo Alto, California. He is a frequent contributor to *Shaman's Drum* magazine and *Sacred Hoop*, published in England.

SHEN®

Richard Pavek is director of the SHEN Therapy Institute. It provides information regarding SHEN research, development, and certification procedures.

Shiatsu Massage, Therapeutic Touch

Thomas Claire is a licensed massage therapist and author of the authoritative book *Bodywork: What Type of Massage to Get—and How to Make the Most of It*. A graduate of the Swedish and Ohashi Institutes, he is a reiki master and a practitioner of Swedish massage, shiatsu, CranioSacral therapy, myofascial release, and therapeutic touch. His work has been featured in numerous publications, and he is a frequent guest on radio and television.

Skinner Release Technique

Joan Skinner is the originator of the Skinner release technique. She earned a B.A. from Bennington College and an M.A. from the University of Illinois. She is Professor Emeritus at the University of Washington and a member of the Martha Graham and Merce Cunningham Dance Companies.

Soma Neuromuscular Integration

Marcia W. Nolte, LMP, has a background in movement studies ranging from performance dance, as a professional ballet and modern dancer and teacher, to a variety of therapeutic modalities of movement. She has been in private practice of soma bodywork since 1979 and continues to explore with her clients the use of movement as medicine.

Karen L. Bolesky, M.A., CMHC, LMP, has been a mental health counselor since 1972 and a soma practitioner since 1985. Karen trained with Elisabeth Kübler-Ross, M.D., and Gregg Furth, Ph.D., in interpretation of spontaneous drawings as an aid to the creative process.

Somato-Respiratory Integration

Donald Epstein is a chiropractor and developer of network spinal analysis. He is the president of the Association for Network Chiropractic. He is also the author of several articles on the practice of this discipline.

Sounding

Don Campbell is an internationally renowned expert in music, sound, health, and learning. In 1988, he founded the Institute for Music, Health, and Education in Boulder, Colorado, and served as executive director until 1995. He has written several books on the relationship between music, health, and education and travels extensively teaching musicians, teachers, physicians, therapists, and trainers. Presently,

Mr. Campbell directs year-long study programs on the therapeutic and transformational uses of sound and music.

Spatial Dynamics℠

Jaimen McMillan is the originator of Spatial Dynamics. He has trained hundreds of students as movement specialists and has worked with a broad spectrum of clients ranging from Olympic athletes to severely handicapped children. He is the director of the Spatial Studies Institute, Inc., as well as the Spatial Dynamics Institute.

Swedish Massage

Janie McGee is a licensed massage therapist with a private practice in New York City for fifteen years. She is also a licensed staff physical therapist in a geriatric facility. She studied physical therapy at Long Island University and premedical studies at Hunter College.

Tae-Kwon-Do

Mark V. Wiley, an internationally renowned martial arts master and scholar, has been involved in the martial arts for twenty years. He has written the best-selling books *Filipino Martial Arts: Cabales Serrada Escrima* and *Filipino Martial Culture* and is the author of more than fifty articles on the martial arts which have appeared in leading martial arts magazines and journals. He currently serves as martial arts editor for the Charles E. Tuttle Publishing Company and associate editor for the *Journal of Asian Martial Arts*. He is the cofounder of talahib-marga, a contemporary, cross-cultural, martial-meditative discipline.

T'ai Chi Ch'üan

Sophia Delza was the first western woman master of t'ai chi ch'üan,
dancer, lecturer, and writer. She is credited as being the first Westerner to bring the martial art to the United States. She was the 1996 recipient of the Chinese Martial Arts Association's Lifetime Achievement Award. She died on June 27, 1996.

Tomatis Method

Dr. Billie Thompson, founder and director of Sound Listening & Learning Centers in Phoenix, Arizona, and Pasadena, California, received her Ph.D. from Arizona State University in 1979. Dr. Thompson was one of the pioneers who brought the Tomatis method to the United States. She edited the English translations of Tomatis's autobiography, *The Conscious Ear,* and his first book, *The Ear and Language.* She established the Phoenix Center in 1987 to provide both corrective and accelerated learning opportunities for individuals, corporations, and other organizations.

Traditional Chinese Medicine

Cindy Banker is a certified instructor and practitioner of Oriental bodywork therapy. She began her shiatsu training with Shizuko Yamamoto in 1976 and now uses both five-element shiatsu and Chinese herbal medicine in her private practice. She is currently the National Director of Education for the American Oriental Bodywork Therapy Association. She is an active member of the National Certification Commission for Acupuncture and Oriental medicine's task force, which is developing the first national certification exam for oriental bodywork therapy. She has been teaching shiatsu in complete training programs since 1983 and currently owns and teaches at the New England Center for Oriental Bodywork in Brookline, Massachusetts.

Trager Psychophysical Integration

Deane Juhan has been on staff at Esalen Institute since 1973 and a Trager practitioner there since 1978. He lectures on anatomy and physiology for bodyworkers and has recently published a major work on that subject, *Job's Body: A Handbook for Bodywork.* Deane is also an instructor at the Trager Institute.

Transcendental Meditation

Robert Roth is the author of the popular book *Transcendental Meditation,* which has now been translated into ten languages. Roth has lectured and taught TM for more than twenty-five years to tens of thousands of people in the United States, Canada, and throughout Europe. He is a senior advisor to the Maharishi Corporate Development Program, the nonprofit organization that teaches the TM program in business and industry, as well as a founder of the Institute for Fitness and Athletic Excellence, which offers the technique to amateur and professional athletes.

Tui Na

Gina Martin is a licensed massage therapist and chair of the Eastern Studies Department of the Swedish Institute School of Massage Therapy. She was chair of the New York State Board of Massage Therapy from 1994 to 1998 and is a current board member. Ms. Martin is recognized by the American Oriental Bodywork Therapy Association as a certified instructor in fine element style shiatsu. She has been featured in the magazine *First for Women* and is a contributing author to the *Reader's Digest Family Guide to Natural Medicine.* Her book *The Shiatsu Workbook* is an Eastern anatomy coloring book published by the Swedish Institute. She maintains a private practice in Eastern bodywork, specializing in shiatsu, tui na, and nuad bo ran.

Unergi

Ute Arnold is an artist and therapist in private practice and is the director of the UNERGI Center. She is a certified Rubenfeld synergy practitioner and trainer and holds degrees in art and design from Schaeffer School of Design, San Francisco, and Chelsea School of Art, London. She has been leading workshops and trainings since 1978 for centers in Scandinavia, France, Canada, and the United States.

Wellness

Brian Luke Seaward, Ph.D., is a faculty member of the University of Colorado. He is recognized internationally as a leading expert in the fields of stress management, mind-body-spirit healing, and human spirituality. Dr. Seaward is the author of the critically acclaimed collegiate textbook *Managing Stress: Principles and Strategies for Health and Wellbeing* and the popular bestseller, *Stand like Mountain, Flow like Water: Reflections on Stress and Human Spirituality.*

Yoga

Lillo (Leela) Way is certified by the Integral Yoga Institute to teach hatha yoga asana (poses), prenatal yoga, panayama (breathing practices), deep relaxation, chanting, and meditation. She is an actor and dancer and has been the director of her own dance company. Way taught at New York University for seven years. She also taught at Hunter College and was a visiting professor at

Princeton University. In addition to her private practice, she is currently on the faculty of the Integral Yoga Institute and the Soho Sanctuary in New York.

Zero Balancing®

Originator of Zero Balancing®, Dr. Fritz Smith has taught body energy work to hundreds of health care practitioners since 1973. He is an Osteopathic M.D., acupuncturist, and teacher. Dr. Smith is a pioneer in the blending of Eastern energy systems with Western science and bodywork. He is the author of *Inner Bridges: A Guide to Energy Movement and Body Structure.*

Staff Credits

Editors: Margaret Haerens, Michael Isaac, Jane Kelly Kosek, Christine Slovey
Photo Researcher: Vera Ahmadzadeh
Book Designer: Olga M. Vega
Production Designer: Christine Innamorato

Table of Contents

Introduction   *xxvi*

I. Alternative Health Models -- *1*
    Ayurvedic Medicine   5
    Holistic Health   7
    Homeopathy   10
    Naturopathic Medicine   15
    Shamanism   18
    Traditional Chinese Medicine   23
    Wellness   29

II. Skeletal Manipulation Methods -- *33*
    Chiropractic   37
    CranioSacral Therapy   40
    Network Chiropractic   43
    Osteopathy   45
    Zero Balancing®   50

III. Nutritional and Dietary Practices ----------------------------------- *53*
    Herbal Medicine   57
    Orthomolecular Medicine   60

IV. Mind/Body Medicine --- *64*
    Biofeedback Training   68
    Guided Imagery   71
    Hypnotherapy   73
    Interactive Guided Imagery   77
    Psychoneuroimmunology   78

V. Sensory Therapies --- *82*
    Aromatherapy   86
    Bates Method   88
    Behavioral Vision Therapy   90
    Eye Movement Desensitization and Reprocessing   94
    Flower Remedies   96
    Hydrotherapy   99
    Light Therapy   103
    Sounding   109
    Tomatis Method   111

VI. Subtle Energy Practices ——————————— *115*

Do-In	*118*
Feng Shui	*119*
Magnet Therapy	*124*
Polarity Therapy	*126*
Qigong	*129*
Reiki	*133*
SHEN®	*137*
Therapeutic Touch	*139*

VII. Massage ——————————————— *142*

Bowen Technique	*148*
Connective Tissue Therapy℠	*150*
CORE Structural Integrative Therapy	*152*
Infant Massage	*153*
Muscular Therapy	*157*
Myofascial Release	*158*
Myofascial Trigger Point Therapy	*160*
Reflexology	*163*
Rolfing®	*165*
Rosen Method	*168*
St. John Method of Neuromuscular Therapy	*172*
Swedish Massage	*174*

VIII. Acupuncture and Asian Bodywork ———— *177*

Acupressure	*180*
Acupuncture	*183*
Jin Shin Do® Bodymind Acupressure™	*187*
Jin Shin Jyutsu® Physio-Philosophy	*191*
Process Acupressure	*192*
Shiatsu	*194*
Tui Na	*197*

IX. Movement Therapy Methods ——————— *200*

Alexander Technique	*204*
Aston-Patterning®	*207*
Bartenieff Fundamentals℠	*210*
Body-Mind Centering®	*212*
Feldenkrais Method®	*215*
Hanna Somatic Education™	*218*
Hellerwork	*222*
Ideokinesis	*224*
Kinetic Awareness	*226*
Meir Schneider Self-Healing Method	*228*
Sensory Awareness	*231*

Soma Neuromuscular Integration   235
Somato Respiratory Integration   238
Trager Psychophysical Integration   239

X. Somatic Practices ——————————————————————— 244

Brain Gym®   247
Contact Improvisation   249
Continuum   252
Eurythmy   254
Gurdjieff Movements   256
Pilates Method of Body Conditioning™   260
ROM Dance   263
Skinner Releasing Technique   265
Spatial Dynamics℠   268
T'ai Chi Ch'üan   270

XI. Martial Arts ——————————————————————————— 274

Aikido   278
Capoeira   280
Ju-Jutsu   283
Judo   286
Karate   289
Kendo   293
Kung Fu Wu Su   297
Taekwondo   301

XII. Yoga ——————————————————————————————— 305

Integral Yoga   313
Iyengar Yoga   314
Kripalu Yoga   315

XIII. Meditation ————————————————————————— 317

Relaxation Response   322
Transcendental Meditation   324

XIV. Psycho-Physical Evaluation Frameworks ———— 327

Enneagram   329
Kestenberg Movement Profile   332
Laban Movement Analysis   335
Movement Pattern Analysis   338

XV. Expressive and Creative Arts Therapies ———— 341

Art Therapy   347

Authentic Movement   350
Dance Therapy   352
Drama Therapy   356
Halprin Life/Art Process   359
Journal Therapy   361
Multi-Modal Expressive Arts Therapy   363
Music Therapy   366
Poetry Therapy   370
Sandplay Therapy   374

XVI. Body-Oriented Psychotherapies _____ 378
Bioenergetics   382
Bodynamic Analysis   385
Core Energetics   387
coreSomatics®   391
Emotional-Kinesthetic Psychotherapy   392
Focusing   394
Gestalt Therapy   397
Hakomi Integrative Somatics   399
Holotropic Breathwork™   402
Medical Orgone Therapy   405
Organismic Body Psychotherapy   409
Pesso Boyden System Psychomotor   411
Process Oriented Psychology   415
Psychodrama   416
Psychosynthesis   419
Radix   421
Rebirthing   422
Rubenfeld Synergy Method   425
Unergi   428

Introduction

Body-mind is a term often seen in print and heard in conversation today. It is used frequently both in private discussions about disease and healing and in public forums on health care, where the value of alternative or complementary medicine is gaining recognition. Today, many educators are developing new methods that use the body-mind connection to help children learn how to live productive and creative lives in today's complex technological society. The phrase *body-mind* resonates through the halls of gymnasiums, physical conditioning studios, and in self-defense classes. It echoes in theaters, dance studios, and music practice rooms. What exactly is this concept that is exciting so many people and changing the way we heal, learn, work, and play?

Body-mind is a way of seeing and understanding the human organism. To see a human being in terms of body-mind is to see him or her as a totality wherein his or her physical, psychological, and spiritual aspects are all interrelated and reflective of one another. In other words, the body is not simply the material receptacle of the mind or spirit, it is the medium through which we experience, each in a unique and individual way, the unfolding, transforming nature of spirit itself.

From this perspective, the functioning of the body influences the functioning of the mind and the emotions. In a like manner, thoughts and feelings have a profound and direct effect on the body. On a deeper level, many body-mind models believe that the physical, emotional, and mental aspects of human experience are a reflection of and inextricably linked to an all-pervasive spiritual essence. In different cultures and in different times, this spiritual essence has had many names: Atman, the Tao, God, energy, the force.

A body-mind discipline is an organized program of activity that seeks to awaken and activate the links between body, mind, and spirit. The practice of a body-mind discipline may involve a variety of activities, all of which aim to incorporate the physical body with the sensing, feeling, thinking, and/or intuiting faculties of the mind. Through the practice of a body-mind discipline, one develops awareness of physical sensations and mental and emotional processes. This awareness can be the basis of healing and improved health, greater efficiency and expressiveness in one's activities, more rewarding relationships and interactions, and a deeper, clearer sense of purpose in one's life.

The practice of body-mind disciplines is ancient. We have evidence that some, such as yoga and various forms of touch therapy, were widespread even well before written treatises were available. The ancient disciplines were based on one of the earliest and most perseverant of human desires—to live a long, meaningful, and healthy life. For most of human history this meant living in a state of balance and harmony, both within oneself and within one's environment. The body-mind disciplines that evolved in all cultures addressed, each in their own particular way, the many elements that create and maintain this balance and harmony.

Western culture, with its roots in the civilizations of the Fertile Crescent and Ancient Greece, once shared this same value for balance and harmony. For example, the Greek physician Hippocrates understood the importance of balance and believed his patients' health could be affected by many factors. He believed it was more important to know the kind of person he was treating than to know what kind of disease the person had. He was known to prescribe herbs, dietary changes, forms of hydrotherapy, skeletal manipulation, movement therapy, and creative arts therapies to help his patients regain a state of balance and harmony.

Over many centuries, however, there has been a gradual erosion of this holistic viewpoint as Western culture developed a highly technical and specialized perspective. By comparison, today most of us no longer have a single physician who knows us as a total human being and draws on any number of healing methods. Instead we go to one specialist for a problem in our ears, nose, and throat, another for our gastrointestinal tract, and still another for troubling emotional situations. Although each specialist may have a wealth of information regarding his or her area of expertise, no one seems to be looking at the whole picture. Often, the pharmaceutical or surgical solutions each specialist recommends address only one aspect of our problem and sometimes create new problems.

This segmented, specialized perspective is evident not only in our approach to health care, but our approach to education and the arts as well. Instead of encouraging each person to feel alive, whole, and connected to the rest of the world, this perspective seems to foster a lack of confidence in one's experience and judgment, a weakened sense of personal agency, and a feeling of spiritual isolation. For this reason, more and more people today are seeking the holistic, centering experience of body-mind disciplines.

In this volume we have tried to include all of the major disciplines with which a reader may come into contact. With a subject of such scope it was necessary to create certain limits in order to complete the task at all. We deliberately excluded any art or skill that is used primarily for performance or competition, although we recognize that any such art or skill may be practiced from a body-mind perspective. We also excluded any practice that is exclusively associated with a specific religious practice, although here again we do not diminish the value of any religious practice and its ability to incorporate body and mind. What we have included is a cross-cultural sampling of techniques and methods developing the body-mind connection that have evolved in the worlds of health care, education, physical conditioning, self-defense, spirituality, psychology, and the arts.

We have arranged the entries in sixteen sections that generally reflect the world in which the disciplines developed, highlight the multicultural approaches to a particular practice, or sometimes draw attention to historical connections. Each section is introduced by an essay that provides an overview of the histories, theoretical foundations, and methodologies of the disciplines that are included in the section. The introductory essays also help relate each individual section to other sections of the encyclopedia. It is possible to get a broad perspective of the entire world of body-mind by simply reading the sixteen introductory essays.

Most of the entries are written by certified practitioners of these disciplines. The entries describe in detail the history, philosophy, and techniques of the specific disciplines. The entries also describe what it feels like to practice or experience the discipline. It is our hope that the reader will not only gain intellectual knowledge from reading an entry, but will be stimulated on a sensory level as well.

Within each of the sections the reader will find disciplines that work along several different continuums. The broad spectrum of approaches reflects the belief of body-mind disciplines that each individual is unique and has specific strengths, weaknesses, and predilections. The first of these continuums may best be described as the percentage of physical work as compared to the percentage of mental or emotional work required of the practitioner. For example, somato respiratory integration requires the practitioner to remain relatively still, focusing the mind on physical sensations and emotional memories, whereas the Feldenkrais Method® develops awareness of mental and emotional patterns by moving the body through prescribed spatial forms. This continuum, found within individual sections of the encyclopedia, is also apparent from section to section. For example, all of the practices in the Meditation section approach the process of building the body-mind connection somewhat more from the use of the mind, whereas all of the disciplines in the somatic practices section come at the process somewhat more from the use of the body. A person may enter the world of body-mind at any point along this continuum that suits his or her needs or temperament.

Another continuum along which the various practices can be viewed concerns the degree of spontaneous action as compared to structured action used by the discipline. For example, contact improvisation and Skinner release technique work largely through improvisational forms created by the practitioner. The quality of one's conscious control of the movement patterns is loose and free flowing. By contrast, the Pilates Method and t'ai chi ch' üan use intricately structured movement sequences that rarely vary. They require a different kind of control in order to achieve a free-flowing connection of body and mind.

Another of the continuums along which one might view these disciplines concerns the degree of involvement of the practitioner, or receiver, as a whole. In any of the forms of massage therapy the receiver is relatively passive, in contrast to the very active participation required by any of the forms of martial arts. All body-mind disciplines, however, ultimately encourage the active participation of the practitioner on some level. As the practice awakens awareness of physical sensations and mental or emotional processes, the participant naturally becomes more capable of taking an active role in the practice, whether that means learning how to relax and experience physical sensations more deeply or follow complex thought, breath, and movement patterns more effortlessly and subtly. This active awareness and participation is a basic value of all body-mind disciplines.

Some of the disciplines included in this volume have as their primary goal the relief of physical pain. It may not seem immediately clear how such practices develop the body-mind connection. In body-mind terms, the response to pain can be the first step toward awakening a deeper awareness of the body. The theoretical underpinnings of every discipline included here view pain as a message from the body to the mind that some vital link between the two is not functioning. Pain is the cry of the body when it has been ignored, when the body-mind connection has not been honored. When viewed this way, pain is transformed from a symptom to be eradicated into a call to undertake a journey of self-discovery.

We hope this volume will offer the reader useful information for his or her unique journey. We wish each of you a voyage filled with the excitement of discovery, the creativity of transformation, and the joys of fulfillment.

PART I: ALTERNATIVE HEALTH MODELS

Ayurvedic Medicine • Holistic Health • Homeopathy • Naturopathic Medicine • Shamanism • Traditional Chinese Medicine • Wellness

Alternative health models consist of a variety of ways of viewing health and sickness and depicting the relationship between body and mind. Each model has developed a system of health care with associated practices and disciplines. These health models are categorized as alternative because they are different from the allopathic paradigm, the scientific framework of contemporary Western health care.

In the allopathic model the body is viewed as a self-contained machine or collection of systems that malfunction with age, injury, or when invaded by infectious microbes or germs. Allopathic health care practices developed a battery of defensive techniques for dealing with these causes of malfunction. In contrast, alternative health models see the body as one aspect of a whole person, along with mind and spirit. They view illness as an imbalance between these three interdependent aspects of a human being, or between a human being and his or her environment. Since the 1960s, because of the high cost and sometimes ineffectiveness or damaging side effects of allopathic health care practices, more and more people are exploring the possibilities of other health models.

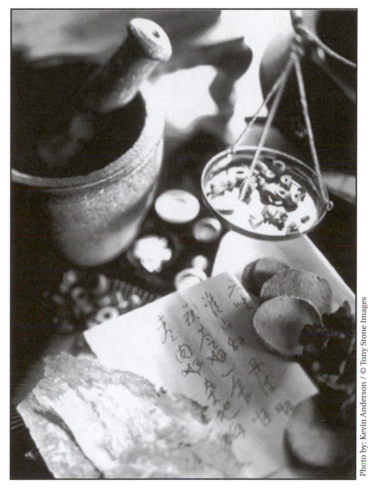

Photo by: Kevin Anderson / © Tony Stone Images

Herbal remedies play a role in many health models, including traditional Chinese medicine.

A Historical Survey of Health Models

The oldest and most widespread alternative health model is used by shamanism and contemporary shamanistic counseling. Shamanic healers believe that all things have a spirit, including rocks, rivers, the sky, and the earth. According to the shamanic model of health, spirits are responsible for the physical and psychological health or sickness of all individuals and communities. Ancient shamans developed methods of interacting with spirits to affect individual or communal health. Contemporary shamanic counselors continue to use these traditional healing techniques today.

Over time, more abstract metaphors evolved to describe the spirit world and its interactions with the material world. The concept of energy or energetic forces replaced the discussion of individualized spirits in human philosophical and medical thought. Health models such as ayurveda in India and traditional Chinese medicine in Asia developed intricate theories and practices to work with the complex patterns of energies they perceived moving through the universe and all the people in it.

The ancient Greeks also conceived of the world as a complex of energies, and many of their healing practices reflected an integrated view of spirit and matter. The philosopher Aristotle (384–322 BCE) articulated an important new tendency in Western thought. He believed that the workings of the natural world could be known through observation, experimentation, and classification. While Aristotle himself believed that spiritual truth could be known through a study of the material world, his scientific method created the possibility of a split in Western thought between spirit and matter.

During the Renaissance, many important Greek texts were rediscovered. Many of the great thinkers of the day embraced the Aristotelian scientific method of the pursuit of knowledge. This method of inquiry met with tremendous opposition from the dominant religious and political institution of that time, the Church. The Church regarded science as a threat to its most basic theological doctrines. This opposition created in Western thought a deeper schism between the material and spiritual realms.

Certain Western philosophers and scientists, however, continued to investigate health models that unify body, mind, and spirit. Health models such as Samuel Hahnemann's (1755–1843) Homeopathy, which combines the science of chemistry and biology with the belief in an invisible vital life energy, developed in Europe toward the end of the Age of Reason. Later, healers like Father Sebastian Kneipp (1821–1897) found other ways to integrate spiritual beliefs with scientific inquiry. His reexamination of ancient herbal cures and indigenous European health modalities eventually made its way to the United States in the form of naturopathy.

Spiritual and material models of health coexisted in Europe and the United States for many years. However, in the 1930s the materialistic allopathic model of health became institutionalized in organizations such as the American Medical Association, which proceeded to discredit holistic methods of healing. The successful control of infectious disease with penicillin, along with other pharmaceuticals developed throughout the 1930s to 1950s, appeared to substantiate the allopathic approach and helped it become the dominant health model.

In the 1960s dissatisfaction with social conventions and institutions, including allopathic health care, caused Westerners to investigate the ancient health models of Eastern and indigenous cultures, as well as older European-based models. Many people began to feel that allopathic strategies did not provide a complete approach to health care. Disciplines combining Western psychological insights with ancient concepts of harmony and balance, such as holistic health and wellness, became more popular.

In the 1970s and 1980s soaring health care costs and the appearance of many chronic health problems caused even greater interest in alternative health models. Today, these disciplines are practiced individually and as a complement to allopathic care. The philosophical viewpoint upon which these disciplines are based continues to exert an ever-growing and far-reaching influence on the practice of contemporary medicine.

Some Theoretical Considerations

All of the health models presented in this section believe that in addition to the physical body, human beings are comprised of nonmaterial aspects. These include thoughts, emotions, and intuitions of the mind, along with a person's spiritual essence. In these holistic models, all three aspects—body, mind, and spirit—are interdependent and determine an individual's state of health. In addition, many of the disciplines adhering to this viewpoint believe that each person's spiritual essence interacts with the spiritual essence of the universe in much the same way that his or her body interacts with the material environment. Health care modalities that developed from this philosophical viewpoint seek to maintain the balance between all aspects of human beings and their relationship with their environments.

One of the major differences between the practices based on these health models and those of allopathic health care is the emphasis they place on the maintenance of health, rather than the spectacular and dramatic treatment of illness. Maintaining health requires monitoring the subtle physical, mental, and emotional ways that the spirit manifests itself in the body.

Symptoms are viewed as physical evidence of a spiritual imbalance. They are rarely suppressed. These health models generally believe that while the suppression of symptoms may offer temporary relief from physical pain, it blocks the natural healing process and will invariably result in more serious problems. Instead of suppression, a physician follows the sequence of symptoms to find the proper way to help the body, mind, and spirit regain their state of balance.

The alternative health models included in this section believe that each individual has the potential for self-healing. While each model recognizes that there are many similarities in self-healing processes, each individual's process is respected as unique. Specialists in these modalities use various techniques to enhance a person's self-healing abilities. They help clients interpret and find patterns in their symptoms, develop greater sensitivity to their physical bodies, and create a broader awareness of the interrelationship between body, mind, and spirit. In this way, these methods encourage each person to participate in his or her own healing.

What It Might Mean to Adopt One of These Models

The health models examined in this section aim to help each individual live a happy, healthy, meaningful life. Adjusting to the methods and practices of a new health model may cause a healing crisis. Once a person no longer suppresses symptoms, old physical or emotional problems may temporarily reappear, causing a person to feel weaker or more vulnerable. Eventually these suppressed causes of illness are released, physical and emotional trauma are diminished, and the foundation has been laid for many years of continued good health and development.

—Nancy Allison, CMA

Further Reading:

Manning, Clark A., and Louis J. Vanreen. *Bioenergetic Medicines East and West: Acupuncture and Homeopathy.* Berkeley, CA: North Atlantic Books, 1988.

AYURVEDIC MEDICINE

Ayurvedic medicine, the ancient Indian science of healthy living, places great emphasis on disease prevention. It encourages the maintenance of health by paying close attention to the balance of one's body, mind, and spirit. Ayurvedic medicine teaches patients to bring about and maintain this balance through proper lifestyle, diet, exercise, herbs, and meditation. Practitioners of ayurveda learn to identify the patient's personal "constitution," understood as a unique mixture of three distinct life energies, or doshas. A healthy person employs positive thinking, diet, and lifestyle to maintain a perfect proportion of life energies.

The History of Ayurvedic Medicine

Ayurvedic medicine is considered by many scholars to be the world's oldest healing science. It dates back five thousand years to the ancient Vedic culture of the Rishis, the philosophers and religious leaders of ancient India. Ayurveda, which means "the science of life" in the ancient Indian language of Sanskrit, was passed on in the oral tradition from master to disciple for thousands of years. Some of this knowledge was published a few thousand years ago, notably in the ancient holy texts of Hinduism, one of the world's oldest existing literatures. It is believed that much of the tradition has actually been lost.

Ayurveda has been practiced in daily life in India for more than four thousand years. Western medicine has influenced (and been influenced by) ayurvedic medicine, but the traditional ayurvedic lifestyle management is, for many Indians, still the primary therapy for ailments. The principles of many natural healing methods now familiar in the West, such as homeopathy, wellness, and polarity therapy, have their roots in ayurveda.

Philosophy of Ayurveda

According to ayurvedic philosophy, the entire cosmos is made up of the five great elements—space (also known as Ether), air, fire, water, and earth. These five elements combine to form three distinct types of energy, called *doshas*, that are present in all people and things. There are no words in English to describe these energies, so we use the original Sanskrit words *vata*, *pitta*, and *kapha*. In the physical body vata, composed of air and ether, is the subtle energy associated with movement. It governs breathing, blinking, muscle and tissue movement, pulsation of the heart, and all movements in the cytoplasm and cell membranes. Pitta, made up of fire and water, is considered the body's metabolic energy. It governs digestion, absorption, assimilation, nutrition, metabolism, and body temperature. Kapha is formed from earth and water and is the energy that forms the body's structure—bones, muscles, tendons— and provides the "glue" that holds the cells together. Kapha also supplies the water for all bodily parts and systems. It lubricates joints, moisturizes the skin, and maintains immunity.

All people have *vata*, *pitta*, and *kapha*; one is usually primary, one secondary, and the third least prominent. The cause of disease in ayurveda is viewed as the lack of proper cellular function because of an excess or deficiency of one of these three energies and/or the presence of toxins.

A Balanced Life

Just as everyone has an individual face or thumbprint, according to ayurveda, each person has a particular pattern of energy—an individual combination of physical, mental, and emotional characteristics—that is his or her constitution. This constitution is determined at conception. Many factors, both internal and external, can disturb this balance, which is reflected as a change in one's constitution.

When all of the three doshas are properly proportioned, they nourish and build mental and physical health in a person. The proper amount of vata promotes creativity and flexibility; pitta engenders understanding and intelligence; kapha is expressed as love, calmness, and forgiveness.

Disease is viewed as improper body functioning that is caused by an excess or deficiency of vata, pitta, or kapha as compared to the original balance of these doshas. This imbalance can be caused by any number of factors. Genetic or congenital traits may predispose a person to develop unhealthy habits such as overeating or smoking. Accidents or other upsetting events can cause physical, mental, or emotional trauma, further disrupting the individual's balance. Furthermore, all of us have certain personal sensitivities, such as weather conditions, spicy food, and flower pollen, that can disrupt the body's function.

In all of these cases, when mind and/or body are upset, the *doshas* become imbalanced. When this happens, the process of disease begins, as fear and anxiety can raise *vata* in a person. Too much or too little *vata* can produce fear and anxiety. Similarly, *pitta* can stir anger, hate, and jealousy, and *kapha* can lead to greed, attachment, and envy.

Typical Ayurveda

In times of health, when there are no dominant outside traumas or toxins afflicting a person, practitioners of ayurveda pay strict attention to diet and lifestyle. Just as each person has a unique constitution, there exists for each person a specific "right" lifestyle, tailored to cultivate the exactly perfect levels of the three doshas. This right lifestyle engages body, mind, and spirit—three distinct but interrelated aspects of each person—in a regimen of diet, breathing exercises, meditation, and physical activity.

In times of illness, an ayurvedic physician must first determine which of the three basic constitutional types the patient is. Then the symptoms must be understood as to whether they are of vata, pitta, or kapha type. Vata heart pain is different from pitta or kapha heart pain. Accordingly, a battery of tests are applied, including taking the pulse, observing the tongue and eyes, and listening to the tone of the patient's voice. The results of these tests, coupled with a patient's physical attributes and family traits, are used to understand the cause of disease, the *dosha(s)* involved, and the stage of the disease process.

The assessment provides the doctor with a standard of the patient's normal functioning. Armed with this knowledge, the ayurvedic physician can suggest steps to help return the client's health to a balanced state. Typically this involves the implementation of a different lifestyle with a new diet, exercise, and meditation plan. In cases where disease can be attributed to toxins or other external stresses, the ayurvedic physician may prescribe additional herbal remedies, breathing exercises, and sun and massage therapies. In some cases, participation in an intensive cleansing program known as "panchakarma" is suggested to help the body rid itself of accumulated toxins.

Benefits and Risks

Ayurvedic medicine is and has been practiced throughout the world for thousands of years. Its patients claim increased longevity and better health. Proper ayurvedic practice demands adherence to a strict, carefully planned lifestyle. Furthermore, many in the ayurvedic field have integrated Western medicine into their practices, acknowledging that different systems can complement each other. For these reasons, anyone interested in pursuing ayurveda, particularly patients with preexisting conditions, should consult an established clinic or ayurvedic physician.

—*Dr. Vasant Lad*

Resources:

American Institute of Vedic Studies
1701 Sante Fe River Rd.
Sante Fe, NM 87501
Tel: (505) 983-9385
Provides information on training programs and practitioners.

American School of Ayurvedic Sciences
10025 NE 4th St.
Bellevue, WA 98004
Tel: (206) 453-8022
Offers a program in ayurvedic medicine.

Ayurvedic Foundation
P.O. Box 900413
Sandy, UT 84090-0413
Tel: (801) 943-1480
e-mail: Dean@ayur.com
Web site: www.ayur.com
Conducts workshops and custom training. Also produces cassette tapes and provides ayurvedic counseling.

Ayurvedic Institute
11311 Menaul N.E., Suite A
Albuquerque, NM 87112
Tel: (505) 291-9698
Provides a two-year program in ayurveda, as well as offering panchakarma workshops and ayurvedic herbs, supplies, and products.

Further Reading:

Chopra, Deepak, M.D. *Ageless Body, Timeless Mind.* New York: Harmony Books, 1993.

———. *Perfect Health.* New York: Harmony Books, 1991.

———. *Quantum Healing.* New York: Bantam Books, 1990.

Frawley, David, OMD. *Ayurvedic Healing.* Salt Lake City: Morson Publishing, 1990.

Lad, Vasant, M.D. *Ayurveda: The Science of Self-Healing.* Wilmot, CA: Lotus Light Press, 1984.

———. *Secrets of the Pulse: The Ancient Art of Pulse Diagnosis.* Albuquerque: The Ayurvedic Press, 1996

HOLISTIC HEALTH

Holistic health is an approach to life. Rather than focusing on illness or specific parts of the body, this ancient approach to health considers the whole person and how he or she interacts with his or her environment. It emphasizes the connection of mind, body, and spirit. The goal is to achieve maximum well-being, where everything is functioning the very best that is possible. With holistic health, people accept responsibility for their own level of well-being, and everyday choices are used to take charge of one's own health.

How Holistic Health Developed

Ancient healing traditions, as far back as 5,000 years ago in India and China, stressed living a healthy way of life in harmony with nature. Socrates (fourth century BCE) warned against treating only one part of the body "for the part can never be well unless the whole is well." Although the term *holism* was introduced by Jan Christiaan Smuts in 1926 as a way of viewing living things as "entities greater than and different from the sum of their parts," it wasn't until the 1970s that *holistic* became a common adjective in our modern vocabulary.

Holistic concepts fell temporarily out of favor in Western societies during the twentieth century. Scientific medical advances had created a dramatic shift in the concept of health. Germs were identified as outside sources causing disease. Gaining health became a process of killing microscopic invaders with synthesized drugs. People believed that they could get away with unhealthy lifestyle choices, and modern medicine would "fix" them as problems developed.

However, for some conditions medical cures have proven more harmful than the disease. In addition, many chronic conditions do not respond to scientific medical treatments. In looking for other options, people are turning back to the holistic approach to health and healing. The holistic health lifestyle is regaining popularity each year, as the holistic principles offer practical options to meet the growing desire for enjoying a high level of vitality and well-being.

The Basic Principles of Holistic Health

Holistic health is based on the law of nature that a whole is made up of interdependent parts. The earth is made up of systems, such as air, land, water, plants, and animals. If life is to be sustained, they cannot be separated, for what is happening to one system is also felt by all of the others. In the same way, an individual is a whole made up of interdependent parts, which are physical, mental, emotional, and spiritual. When one part is not working at its best, it impacts all of the other parts of that person. Furthermore, this whole person, including all of the parts, is constantly interacting with everything in the surrounding environment. For example, when an individual is anxious about a history exam or a job interview, his or her nervousness may result in a physical reaction—such as acne or a stomachache. When people suppress anger at a parent or a boss over a long period of time, they can develop a serious illness—such as migraine headaches, emphysema, or even arthritis.

The principles of holistic health state that health is more than just not being sick. A common explanation is to view wellness as a continuum along a line. The line represents all possible degrees of health. The far left end of the line represents premature death. On the far right end is the highest possible level of wellness or maximum well-being. The center point of the line represents a lack of apparent disease. This places all levels of illness on the left half of the wellness continuum. The right half shows that even when no illness seems to be present, there is still a lot of room for improvement.

Holistic health is an ongoing process. As a lifestyle, it includes a personal commitment to be moving toward the right end of the wellness continuum. No matter what their current status of health, people can improve their level of well-being. Even when there are temporary setbacks, movement is always headed toward wellness.

The U.S. Centers for Disease Control and Prevention report that the key factors influencing an individual's state of health have not changed significantly over the past twenty years. Quality of medical care is only 10 percent. Heredity accounts for 18 percent and environment is 19 percent. Everyday lifestyle choices are 53 percent. The decisions people make about their life and habits are, therefore, by far the largest factor in determining their state of wellness.

The most obvious choices people make each day are what they "consume"— both physically and mentally. The cells in a person's body are constantly being replaced. New cells are built from what is available. Harmful substances or lack of needed building blocks in the body can result in imperfect cells, unable to do what is required to keep that person healthy. Similarly, on the non-physical level, a person's mental attitudes are "built" from what he or she sees and hears.

The majority of illnesses and premature deaths can be traced back to lifestyle choices. There are the well-known dangers connected with drugs, alcohol, nicotine, and unprotected sexual activity. Less recognized is the impact of excesses in things like sugar, caffeine, and negative attitudes. Combined with deficiencies in exercise, nutritious foods, and self-esteem, these gradually accumulate harmful effects. With time they diminish the quality of the "environment" within that human being, and can set the stage for illness to take hold. Quality of life, now and in the future, is actually being determined by a multitude of seemingly unimportant choices made every day.

How Holistic Health Is Practiced

While preventing illness is important, holistic health focuses on reaching higher levels of wellness. The right half of the wellness continuum invites people to constantly explore which everyday actions work for them and discover what is appropriate to move them toward maximum well-being. People are motivated by how good it feels to have lots of energy and enthusiasm for life, knowing that what they are doing that day will allow them to continue to feel this great for years to come.

When disease and chronic conditions do occur, the holistic health principles also can be applied. The term is usually changed to holistic medicine, and additional factors are added. The health care professionals using the holistic approach work in partnership with their patients. They recommend treatments that support the body's natural healing system and consider the whole person and the whole situation.

A holistic approach to healing goes beyond just eliminating symptoms. For example, taking an aspirin for a headache would be like disconnecting the oil light on the dash of a car when it flashes. The irritation is eliminated, but the real problem still exists. In holistic medicine, a symptom is considered a message that something needs attention. So the symptom is used as a guide to look below the surface for the root cause. Then what really needs attention can be addressed.

The Benefits of Holistic Health

Holistic health supports reaching higher levels of wellness as well as preventing illness. People enjoy the vitality and well-being that results from their positive lifestyle changes, and are motivated to continue this process throughout their lives.

—Suzan Walter

Resources:

American Holistic Health Association (AHHA)
Dept. R
P.O. Box 17400
Anaheim, CA 92817-7400
Tel: (714) 779-6152
e-mail: ahha@healthy.net
Web site: www.ahha.org
This nonprofit educational organization has compiled lists of self-help resources available in the United States. These free materials and a booklet, Wellness From Within: The First Step, *which introduces the holistic approach to creating wellness, are available on the Internet or by mail.*

Graduate Certificate Program in Holistic Health Care
Director: Molly B. Vass, Ed.D.
Western Michigan University
College of Health and Human Services
Kalamazoo, MI 49008-5174
Tel: (616) 387-3800
Fax: (616) 387-3348
e-mail: Brenda.Bell@wmich.edu
Unique opportunity to study holistic health care in an accredited academic program. Consists of 18 semester hours of study in holistic health care and related topics. Can be taken as an independent certificate or can be used to supplement graduate training in related fields. Three main areas of holistic health care (promotion, prevention, and treatment) are addressed through a combination of education, research, promotion, training, administration, program planning, and program development efforts. Graduates are able to work

Training in Holistic Health

The conventional (or allopathic) medical model taught in most Western medical schools does not include the holistic principles. Complementary (or alternative) medical traditions, such as acupuncture, chiropractic, homeopathy, massage therapy, and naturopathy, include many of the principles of holistic medicine. Yet some medical doctors are holistic in how they deal with their patients, and some practitioners using complementary therapies are not holistic. Patients are learning to check for both technical expertise and whether a practitioner uses the holistic principles.

People interested in a career as a holistic practitioner must first become qualified in one or more methods of delivering health care, such as chiropractic, massage therapy, medicine, naturopathy, or psychology. Then they add on the holistic qualities and philosophy.

within their chosen professional areas from a holistic perspective.

Further Reading:

Collinge, William, Ph.D. *The American Holistic Health Association Complete Guide to Alternative Medicine.* New York: Warner Books, 1996.

Gordon, James S., M.D. *Holistic Medicine.* New York: Chelsea House Publishers, 1988.

Travis, John W., M.D., and Regina Sara Ryan. *The Wellness Workbook.* Berkeley: Ten Speed Press, 1988.

HOMEOPATHY

Homeopathy is a holistic system that is used to treat chronic and acute illness and disease. Founded by Samuel Hahnemann in the late 1700s, homeopathy is based on the concept of "like cures like," which means that remedies are matched to symptom patterns in the patient. To "match" symptoms means that the physician analyzes a patient's symptoms to find a substance, usually from plants, minerals, and animals, that induces the same symptoms in a healthy person. By ingesting small, diluted doses of these substances, the body is stimulated to fight illness. In recent times, homeopathic practices have grown dramatically in popularity as people all over the world rediscover the inexpensive, natural remedies used to cure illnesses that do not respond to conventional treatment.

History of Homeopathy

The founder of homeopathy, Samuel Hahnemann, was born in Meissen, Germany in 1755. He was thin, delicate, and highly intelligent, with an interest in the natural sciences and languages. He established his first medical practice in 1780. Hahnemann was appalled by the prevalent practices of bloodletting, purging, vomiting, and the administration of large doses of harsh drugs.

It was not until 1789, when translating *A Treatise of Materia Medica* by Dr. William Cullen, that Hahnemann first conceived of his homeopathic method. He decided to experiment on himself with *cinchona* (Peruvian bark), one of the drugs mentioned in that work. He noticed that when a healthy person took doses of cinchona, the substance from which quinine is derived, it produced many of the symptoms that it was intended to alleviate.

The official birth date of homeopathy is 1796, when Hahnemann published an article in the *Journal of Practical Medicine,* in which he delineates three methods of healing: preventative treatment, which is the removal of the causes of illness; palliative treatment by the principle of *contraria contraris*, which means the healing by opposites; and the treatment of likes with likes, namely the prescribing of medicines that cause similar symptoms in healthy individuals. Hahnemann coined the term *Homeopathy*, from the Greek words *homois*, similar, and *pathos*, meaning disease. The word *homeopathic* first appeared in print in an article he published in 1807.

Published in 1810, the *Organon of Rational Medicine* is Hahnemann's quintessential work, a complete exposition of his healing method. To this day it forms the foundation of homeopathy. The principle of *similia similibus*, first set forth in his essay of 1796, was now expanded to *similia similibus curentor*—let likes be treated by likes—the core principle of homeopathy. The reception of this work was lukewarm.

Despite the apathetic reception *Organon* had received, he attempted to teach homeopathy through his newly formed Institute for the Postgraduate Study of Homeopathy. Not one person responded to his advertisement. In 1812 Napoleon was driven from Germany, and the war flooded the area with refugees, starvation, and no less than 80,000 dead and another 80,000 wounded.

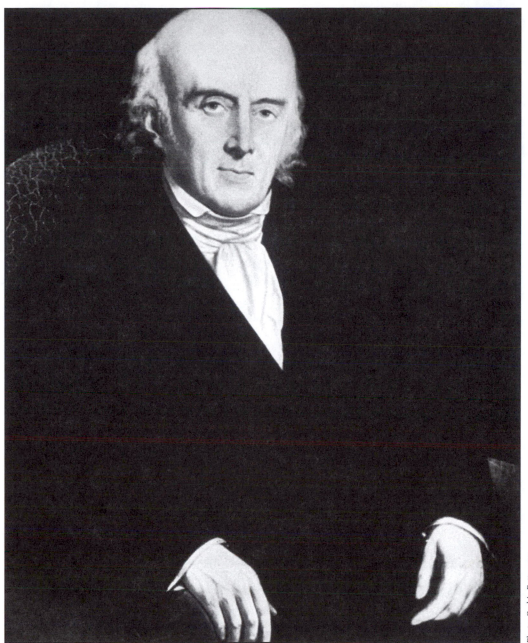

Dr. Samuel Hahnemann (1755–1843), founder of homeopathy

Hahnemann and other physicians were pressed into service trying to help the many who suffered not only from the battle but from an outbreak of typhus. Armed with twenty-six homeopathic remedies, Hahnemann achieved remarkable results in treating typhus. He would later report that only two of the 180 typhus patients he treated had died.

In 1819 a group of envious physicians and angry pharmacists filed a court action against Hahnemann to prevent him from dispensing his own medicines in Leipzig, where he was living at the time. Despite Hahnemann's growing reputation and successful treatment of royalty and famous people such as Johann Goethe, Hahnemann lost the case. Although he subsequently won in the Appeals Court of Dresden, Hahnemann closed his practice and left Leipzig for the city of Kothen in 1821.

Shortly after his arrival in Kothen, Hahnemann, through his political and social connections, procured permission from the authorities to practice homeopathy with total immunity. During these years he wrote his last great work, *Chronic Diseases: Their Peculiar Nature and Their Homeopathic Treatment.* First published in Dresden, in 1828, it ultimately ran to five volumes by 1839 and totaled in excess of 1,600 pages. This work set forth another deep insight, that not only could patients be cured of acute conditions but that their patterns of acute conditions over the years allow for a classification of chronic tendencies toward types of disease. These chronic tendencies Hahnemann called *miasms*, the patient's inherited predisposition toward certain types of illness. By knowing the miasmatic type, a homeopathic physician could now treat preventively, and this tendency could be mitigated so that the next generation's health could be improved. Hahnemann had intuited the basis for treating genetic disorders.

In 1831, a cholera epidemic swept Europe. The Hahnemannian protocol for treating cholera, which also included cleanliness, ventilation, and disinfection, resulted in a drastic reduction in mortality. Records at that time indicate that under homeopathic treatment mortality was between 2 and 20 percent while conventional treatment carried a mortality of over 50 percent.

Homeopathy began to spread to England and the United States. By 1844 the American Institute of Homeopathy was founded by homeopathic physicians from New York, Philadelphia, and Boston. The first national medical organization in the United States, it was established to promote standardization of the practice and teaching of homeopathy.

This period in American homeopathy was its golden age. There were literally thousands of homeopathic books and journals published. There were no less than twenty-two homeopathic medical schools and countless homeopathic hospitals and clinics throughout the United States. Estimates are that by the turn of the century there were about 15,000 homeopathic physicians in the United States.

Around the same time, the sciences of cellular and molecular biology, as well as physiology, began to replace the rudimentary medical knowledge of Hahnemann's time. Together these sciences produced medicines used by conventional physicians to quickly and effectively remove or modulate their patients' symptoms at relatively low costs. By the 1960s homeopathy in the United States was virtually dead and medical historians predicted the complete death of this "medical heresy" by 1980.

But instead, by the late 1970s American homeopathy was well into a revival. By 1996, the bicentennial anniversary of Hahnemann's discovery of homeopathy, more books and articles were being written about homeopathy than at any time since the turn of the century. Sales of homeopathic medicines have increased by 30 percent per year in the United States since 1990.

Eight Fundamentals

The fundamentals of homeopathy, as laid down by Hahnemann, are as follows:

1. There is a natural and universal scientific law of cure, namely, that likes can be cured by likes. This means that small amounts of any substance that causes disease in a healthy person can be used to treat that same disease in a patient.

2. The knowledge of the action of remedies is harvested from single- or double-blind experiments in which small doses are given to healthy subjects who later record their detailed reactions to the test substance. This is called a homeopathic proving. The knowledge base for a particular substance or remedy is also determined from case histories of treatment with

the substance, which has not undergone a proving but which has yielded a cure in clinical practice. Added to this is the information of symptoms produced by accidental poisonings with toxic substances. The proving, clinical, and toxicological data form the *materia medica* of the remedy.

3. The ability of an organism to feel, sense, act, or achieve homeostasis (or equilibrium) is maintained by a non-material principle called the dynamis. This dynamis, or "spirit-like" vital force is, according to Hahnemann, similar in nature to gravity or magnetism. It is a force that to date has eluded explanation or classification by the natural sciences. Diseases, therefore, are not actual material things; rather they are descriptions or classifications of symptom patterns. Symptoms are not things to be removed or suppressed by drugs; rather they are an expression of the vital force's attempt to heal. The properly prepared, selected, and administered homeopathic remedy somehow "resonates" with the vital force and stimulates the healing process.

4. A single remedy at a time is given. Single-remedy administration also allows a clear evaluation of its efficacy.

5. A minimum dose must be used. Small doses of a substance stimulate healing, medium doses paralyze the patient, and large doses kill.

6. Individualization of the treatment is essential. No two people are exactly alike in either sickness or health, and although homeopaths use classifications of disease types, finer, individual distinctions must always be made since, although the action of two remedies may often be similar, they are never exactly the same.

7. The mere removal of symptoms by suppressive means is a grave danger because it defeats the vital force's attempt at homeostasis and puts the patient at risk for a more serious disease.

8. There is a distinction between acute or epidemic diseases and chronic disease patterns of patients. Preventative homeopathic care requires an understanding of these chronic patterns.

Despite more than 200 years of clinical efficacy, the way that these remedies work is still a mystery. We do not yet possess the technology or the methodology necessary to unlock homeopathy's secrets.

Philosophically, homeopathy is holistic (not merely alternative) because the essential task is to understand the patient as a whole person. As a method, homeopathy is a synthesis of the natural science approach and the phenomenological or descriptive approach. The physician must blend his or her natural science training in anatomy, physiology, pathology, biochemistry, physical diagnosis, etc., with observation of the patient and understanding of the patient's self-description. The challenge of homeopathy, even in the treatment of apparently purely physical conditions, is to select a few probable remedies from the thousand or more possible remedies.

Just like a novel with many chapters and plot twists, so a patient's cure unfolds. The process is highly individual. The homeopathic physician will be guided by certain principles of cure: healing occurs from above downward, from the center to the periphery, from more vital organs to less vital organs and in reverse order of the appearance of the original symptoms.

Practicing Homeopathy

A typical session with a homeopathic physician begins with the patient's history. The patient is allowed to tell his or her story without interruption. Only after the patient is finished will the physician ask specific questions to understand the symptoms, namely how they vary according to time of day or season, rest or activity, temperature, bathing, position, eating, thirst, sleep, social intercourse, perspiration, external stimuli, emotions, etc.

Most important, the physician attempts to understand the patient's personality. Inquiries are made into how the patient copes with stress, and about the patient's fears and worries. The patient describes him- or herself. This process is often the most revealing.

The physician uses these descriptions to generate an understanding of the patient. He or she also obtains a conventional medical and surgical history, and finally performs a physical examination.

The physician then attempts to rank various symptoms, modalities, and generalities by degree of intensity. A list of symptoms is generated and the symptoms are then repertorized, that is, they are cross-indexed with the remedies known to have caused or cured these same symptoms. This labor-intensive process was for centuries performed by hand, but is now done by computer.

Having narrowed the field to several probable remedies, the homeopathic physician must then determine whether the patient's problem is an acute, chronic, or inherited illness, or perhaps an illness due to the suppressive effects of previous treatment.

The art of homeopathy is in the ability of the homeopathic physician to process all of this information into a synthesis, a "remedy portrait" or *gestalt*, which corresponds to the remedy likely to stimulate a healing response. Having given a dose of the indicated remedy, the patient and physician must now wait. Depending on the patient, the nature of the problem and the potency of the remedy, a return visit is scheduled weeks or months after the initial dose. While there have been miraculous homeopathic cures after just one dose, most chronic cases take months or years to cure. The process is highly individual.

Benefits of Homeopathy

Homeopathic treatment is appropriate and safe for all ages and is especially useful in childhood and during pregnancy, labor, and the postpartum period. Homeopathy has successfully treated patients with conditions such as otitis, bronchitis, pneumonia, migraines, hepatitis, pancreatitis, appendicitis, and cholecystitis. Historically, homeopathy has been used to treat potentially dangerous infections such as cholera, influenza, syphilis, gonorrhea, scarlet fever, polio, measles, and tuberculosis. Chronic conditions such as arthritis, asthma, eczema, psoriasis, and chronic fatigue syndrome have all been alleviated by homeopathic treatments. It is reported that devastating diseases such as multiple sclerosis can be brought to remission if treated early enough. Historical homeopathic literature contains many references to cures of various types of cancer, though admittedly these are some of the most difficult for any system

---

The Importance of Women in Homeopathic Medicine

Women figured prominently in the history of American homeopathy. By 1900 it is estimated that 12 percent of homeopathic physicians were women. The Cleveland Homeopathic College was one of the first coeducational medical institutions in the country. Women auxiliaries raised large amounts of money to open many of the homeopathic hospitals, and it was women, in their role of family caretaker, who were the lay prescribers introducing homeopathy to many communities. Some members of the early women's suffrage movement were either homeopathic physicians or their patients. Dr. Susan Edson, a graduate of the Cleveland Homeopathic College, was personal physician to President Garfield.

of medicine to cure and are best dealt with on a preventive basis.

—*Dr. Domenick Masiello*

Resources:

The American Institute of Homeopathy
1585 Glencoc Street, Suite 44
Denver, CO 80220-1338
Tel: (303) 321-4105
Facilitates conferences, publishes a journal, and provides referrals.

The National Center for Homeopathy
801 North Fairfax, Suite 306
Alexandria, VA 22314
Tel: (703) 548-7790
e-mail: nchinfo@igc.apc.org
Nonprofit organization that promotes homeopathy in the United States. Publishes monthly magazine entitled Homeopathy Today.

Videotape:

Winston, Julian. *The Faces of Homeopathy: A Pictorial History*. Alexandria, VA: The National Center of Homeopathy, 1995.

Further Reading:

Cook, Trevor M. *Samuel Hahnemann: His Life and Times*. Middlesex, Eng.: Homeopathic Studies Ltd., 1981.

Coulter, Harris. *Homeopathic Medicine*. St. Louis: Formur, 1972.

Hahnemann, Samuel. *Organon of Medicine*. Translated by Jost Kunzli, Alain Nuadé, and Peter Pendleton. Los Angeles: J. P. Tarcher, 1982.

———. *The Chronic Diseases: Their Peculiar Nature and Their Homeopathic Cure*. New Delhi: B. Jain Publishers, 1985.

———. Materia Medica Pura. New Delhi: B. Jain Publishers, 1984.

Kent, James Tyler. *Lectures on Homeopathic Philosophy*. Richmond, VA: North Atlantic Books, 1979.

Roberts, Herbert. *The Principles and Art of Cure by Homeopathy*. Santa Barbara, CA: Health Science Press, 1942.

Weiner, Michael, and Kathleen Gross. *The Complete Book of Homeopathy*. Garden City, NY: Avery Publishing Group, 1989.

Wright-Hubbard, Elizabeth. *A Brief Study Course in Homeopathy*. St. Louis, MO: Formur, 1977.

NATUROPATHIC MEDICINE

Naturopathic medicine is a form of health care that utilizes and integrates different natural therapies such as clinical nutrition, homeopathy, hydrotherapy, botanical medicines, minor surgery, Oriental medicine, physical medicine, lifestyle counseling, and other treatments with a knowledge of traditional diagnostic and medical therapies in order to treat a range of afflictions. A licensed doctor of naturopathy (ND) must graduate from a four-year program that specializes not only in naturopathic studies, but also basic medical science. Practitioners are then qualified to provide primary care, perform diagnostic testing, and prescribe a course of treatment that draws from a long list of natural remedies and techniques.

The Origins of Naturopathic Medicine

The development of naturopathic medicine began with Benedict Lust, a German who immigrated to the United States in 1892. A few years after arriving, Lust was struck down with tuberculosis. When American doctors couldn't help him, Lust returned to Europe and sought out Father Sebastian Kneipp, a priest living in Bavaria who was known for his "nature cure" treatments.

Kneipp did what Lust's doctor could not—he successfully treated Lust. This was a turning point in Lust's life. In 1896, Kneipp gave Lust permission to bring his treatments to America. Once back in the United States, Lust researched other natural health philosophies and used them to reshape and mold Kneipp's ideas to appeal to the American people. By broadening the scope of his work, Lust and other Kneipp disciples developed what is now known as naturopathic medicine.

In 1902, Lust bought the word "naturopathy" from a New York physician who had coined the term seven years earlier. In 1909, California became the first state to recognize the new discipline by enacting regulatory laws regarding the practice of naturopathic medicine. Popularity of naturopathy rose significantly early in the century, but began to decline with the improvement and accessibility of pharmaceutical drugs. Alternative methods of health care, including naturopathic medicine, have enjoyed a resurgence of interest as people rediscover that natural remedies are also valuable.

The Five Principles of Naturopathic Medicine

Today's brand of naturopathic medicine embodies five main principles. The first, *Vis medicatrix naturae*, means "the healing power of nature." Naturopathic physicians use therapies that help the body to heal itself.

Primum non nocere, the second principle, means "first do no harm." This translates into safe, naturopathic treatments that have no or minimal side effects. Naturopathic physicians refer patients to other health-care practitioners, such as medical doctors (M.D.s), when it is appropriate for the patient.

True health can be achieved only when your doctor practices *Tolle causam*, or "finds the cause." Diagnosing the true cause of disease and illness is fundamental to naturopathic care. Sometimes it is as simple as poor diet or sleeping habits. These basic issues can significantly affect one's health. Other times, more complex factors are responsible.

A commitment to treating the whole person is an important principle of naturopathic healing. Illness is generally the result of many factors. Part of "whole person," or holistic, care is investigating not only physical symptoms, but emotional and mental ones too. How and what you eat, lifestyle habits, genetic tendencies, as well as social interactions are all important in assessing and treating health problems.

The final principle of naturopathic medicine is the emphasis on preventative medicine. Practitioners aim to lessen and even eliminate the chance of disease by encouraging patients to take a proactive role in their health care by implementing and maintaining a healthy lifestyle.

A Visit to a Naturopathic Practitioner

Naturopathic physicians are often primary caregivers. This means they can be your family or general practitioner, except they use natural treatments. When you call an ND's office, a receptionist will greet you and ask when you'd like to make an appointment, much as in a medical doctor's office.

On the day of your visit, you'll find that a naturopathic medical office is just that—a medical office. You might fill out some forms and then be invited to see the doctor. Your naturopathic physician will ask what's wrong, and will then spend about an hour to discover the cause of your ailment.

Your ND will take a lengthy medical history and perform a thorough physical examination. Laboratory tests will be ordered as needed. An ND relies on both standard medical lab tests and specialized tests more fitting to a natural medical practice.

Your ND then recommends treatment based on his or her investigation. Diet is discussed, and perhaps vitamins or other nutrient supplements suggested. Herbs are common medicines used by NDs as well as homeopathic remedies, which are specially prepared substances used to boost healing. Various techniques like hydrotherapy, exercise, or ultrasound, just as physical therapists use, might be employed. And where appropriate, stress management or counseling is suggested.

NDs are trained to perform minor surgery such as repairing superficial wounds, but will refer you to surgeons and other doctors for major operations. Some states allow qualified NDs to prescribe some drugs like antibiotics.

It's perfectly appropriate, and sometimes desirable, to mix and match naturopathic therapies with allopathic treatment. This should be done only under professional guidance to prevent potential problems. While all naturopathic doctors are trained in the basics of Oriental medicine, there are some who specialize in acupuncture, herbal medicine, and related therapies. Some NDs offer natural childbirth, including pre- and postnatal care, for pregnant women.

Benefits of Naturopathic Medicine

Naturopathic medical care is suitable for all age groups and most acute and chronic conditions. Its whole-person, natural-care approach allows you to attain the best health possible in an effective and safe manner. Because naturopathic physicians are concerned with solving, not masking, symptoms, healing can take longer than with conventional treatment. Naturopathic medicine also requires that patients take an active role in their health care.

NDs take their role as teacher very seriously as they instruct their patients in how to stay healthy.

As primary caregivers, NDs cooperate with other medical and health professionals. An ND, like any general practitioner, is the gatekeeper for your health care. When you're sick, you see your ND first. He or she will consult with or refer you to other physicians and specialists when appropriate.

—Lauri M. Aesoph, ND

Resources:

American Association of Naturopathic Physicians (AANP)
601 Valley Street, Ste. 105
Seattle, WA 98109
Tel: (206) 298-0125
Web site: www.infinite.org/naturopathic.physician
e-mail: 74602.3715@compuserve.com
This professional organization provides referrals to naturopathic physicians in the United States. A myriad of information on naturopathic medicine is also available.

Bastyr University
14500 Juanita Dr. NE
Bothell, WA 98011
Tel: (206) 823-1300
Web site: www.bastyr.edu
Four-year postgraduate university that offers

A Naturopathic Medical Career

Before applying for naturopathic medical school, one must complete a minimum of three years of college, including specific prerequisite courses. It takes four years of graduate-level study to earn the degree of Doctor of Naturopathic Medicine. Anatomy, pharmacology, gynecology, and radiology are just some of the medical sciences taught. Training in natural therapeutics is also included, as is time spent working in a clinical setting seeing patients.

While an ND degree specifically prepares you for naturopathic medical practice, there are other career opportunities. NDs also teach, do research, work for the natural health industry, write, lecture, and work as consultants. As natural medicine expands and grows, so does the potential for naturopathic medicine.

degrees in naturopathic medicine and related health care disciplines.

Canadian Naturopathic Association
4174 Dundas Street W, Suite 304
Etobicoke, ON M8X 1X3
Canada
Tel: (416) 233-1043
Fax: (416) 233-2924
This professional group offers referrals to naturopathic doctors throughout Canada.

National College of Naturopathic Medicine
049 SW Porter
Portland, OR 97201
Tel: (503) 499-4343
Web site: www.ncnm.edu
A postgraduate, four-year institution that provides classes in naturopathic medicine.

Southwest College of Naturopathic Medicine & Health Sciences
2140 East Broadway
Tempe, AZ 85282
Tel: (602) 858-9100
Fax: (602) 858-0222
Web site: www.healthworld.com/pan/pa/naturopathic/aanp/SW/SW.college.home.html
Four-year postgraduate college that offers degrees in naturopathic medicine and related health care disciplines.

Further Reading:

Aesoph, Lauri. *How to Eat Away Arthritis.* Paramus, NJ: Prentice-Hall, 1996.

Brown, Donald. *Herbal Prescriptions for Better Health.* Rocklin, CA: Prima Publishing, 1996.

Kirchfeld, Friedhelm, and Wade Boyle. *Nature Doctors: Pioneers in Naturopathic Medicine.* East Palestine, OH: Buckeye Naturopathic Press, 1994 (distributed by Medicina Biologica, Portland, OR).

Murray, Michael, and Joseph Pizzorno. *Encyclopedia of Natural Medicine.* Rocklin, CA: Prima Publishing, 1991.

Murray, Michael. *The Healing Powers of Foods,* New York: Ballantine Fawcett, 1993.

Ullman, Robert, and Judith Reichenberg-Ullman. *The Patient's Guide to Homeopathic Medicine.* Kent, WA: Pacific Pipeline, 1995.

SHAMANISM

Shamanism is an ancient healing method that allows a person to enter and interact with an unseen world of spirits. Contemporary shamanism encompasses a wide range of spiritual practices originating in civilizations in North and South America, Siberia, Indonesia, Australia, Southeast Asia, Japan, and Tibet. Throughout history, shamanic healers have been known by many names, including medicine man or medicine woman, witch, warlock, or in African-based vodoun religions—priest or priestess. The word *shaman* was derived from the Asian word *saman* by nineteenth-century European scholars intrigued by the cultures and practices of ancient shamanism. Currently many Western medical researchers and psychologists are exploring shamanism, not as a curiosity, but as a creative and constructive way of viewing the world.

The Early Shamans

In ancient times, shamans served many roles in their societies. They performed rituals to mark the migrations of the animals that their societies hunted. Hunters consulted shamans to learn where animals could be found. The shamans also designed and performed rituals to mark the changing of seasons, the migration of their people to different locations, and individual rites of passage such as birth, the transition from adolescence to adulthood, marriage, and death.

Early shamans were also teachers. In many early societies, storytelling was an important part of the shaman's skills. Often, the stories he or she told taught lessons about the society's beliefs, fears, and traditions.

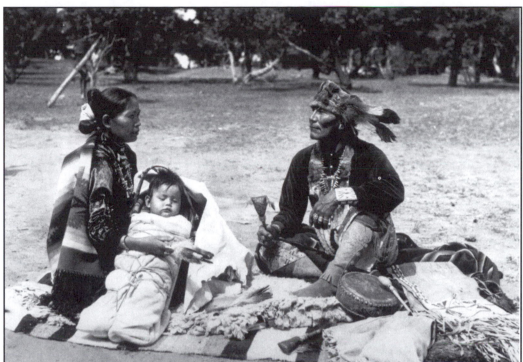

Photo: Corbis-Bettmann

A Navajo shaman ministers to a mother and baby for better health.

Shamans were also healers. Since many societies believed that all illnesses had a spiritual source, the shamans were often chosen for their ability to communicate with the spirit world. Healing rituals designed to remove harmful spirits from individuals or communities often took place in sacred spaces such as caves or mountains and included wearing ceremonial clothing, using herbs, playing drums, rattles, and flutes, and dancing.

The Unseen World
Shamans believe that there are two realities: the "seen" world, which is the world we perceive through our five senses, and the "unseen" or "invisible" world, which our five senses cannot detect. The unseen world can be compared to the world of dreams, emotions, instincts, and intuition. Emotions, such as fear, joy, love, and grief, or human sexual drives, cannot be seen but are very real forces in human life. Ancient shamanic cultures honored the forces of the unseen world in the form

of gods, goddesses, and monsters in the narratives of their mythologies.

Shamanism is founded on a belief that most diseases and grievances between individuals or nations are caused by an imbalance in the natural order of the seen and unseen worlds. A shaman interacts with the invisible world of forces and energies and restores the balance. His or her stories, rituals, and dances are used to subdue or stimulate feelings that may bring new hope, motivate a person to act, or simply increase energy for healing and change.

Shamanism in Today's World
It is unlikely that you will find the services of a shaman advertised at your family health clinic, but many clinics do refer patients to therapists who use techniques borrowed from the shamanic tradition. For example, psychologists and hypnotherapists use hypnosis and mental visualization (a traditional shamanic technique) to help people stop smoking, control their appetite,

19

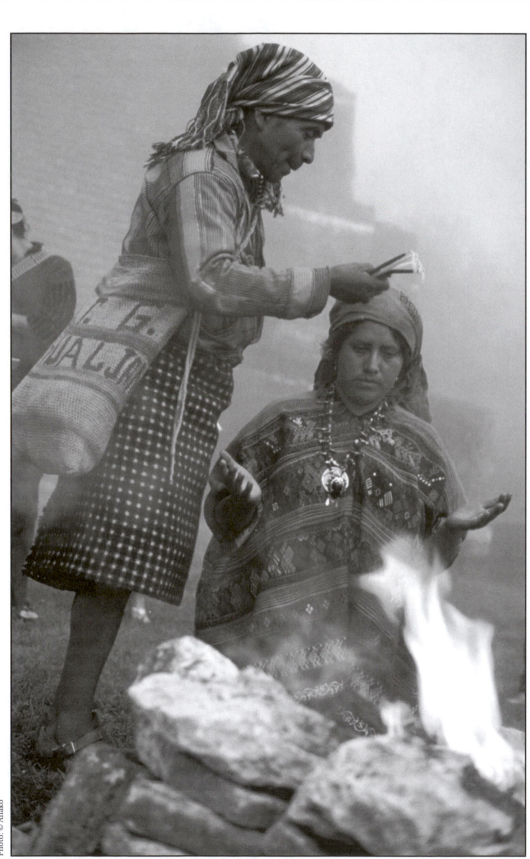

Traditional shamanic practices in Comalapa, Guatemala.

reduce anxiety, manage chronic pain, and recover from an addiction. Mental visualization is a process in which a person sets a goal by imagining himself or herself accomplishing it. For example, a person who wants to calm his or her anxiety before delivering a speech may imagine getting up on the podium, confidently delivering a successful talk, and receiving a standing ovation. For many people these images can replace the old memories that caused the fear. While shamans helped their communities by telling stories or performing rituals, today's practitioners sometimes use "guided imagery" to achieve a similar goal.

There is also an increasing number of organizations teaching traditional shamanic practices throughout the world. Courses are taught by anthropologists, psychologists, and shamans from Native American, African, Hawaiian, South American, Australian, or other traditions. Typical workshops might include lectures about basic principles of shamanism, drumming workshops, and experiences in the basic shamanistic technique of "journeying" into the unseen world.

Shamanic counseling is available today in many parts of the United States. It is used to aid a person's physical, emotional, or spiritual health. A typical session may begin with a "smudging" ceremony. This consists of burning a small amount of dried sage, often mixed with other herbs such as sweet grass and cedar. Smoke from the smudge pot might be wafted with a feathered fan over the person's body, sometimes from head to toe. Shamans believe that the person is "cleansed" as the smoke lifts away dark or negative influences and energies.

The smudging ceremony may be followed by a "journey" in which the shaman enters the unseen world in order to consult guiding spiritual forces. A person may also journey to the unseen world for him- or herself. In this practice, the shamanic counselor may begin by discussing the person's problem. The person may then be told to close his or her eyes, relax, and imagine the journey that he or she is about to make. With the image clearly in the person's mind, the shaman or shamanic counselor begins a steady rhythm with a hand drum, a rattle, or recorded music. He or she may use a rhythm similar to the human heart beat—between fifty-five and seventy beats per minute. This rhythm puts the person into a light trance, allowing him or her to relax and enter a dreamlike state.

Upon entering the trance state, the person might meet and work with an inner guide or adviser. During the journey, the person might ask his or her guide questions, listen for answers, and possibly carry on a dialogue for several minutes or more. Eventually, the shamanic counselor will change the rhythm of the drum to indicate that the person should return to the "seen" world. After returning, there might be further discussion with the shamanic counselor to help the person interpret the meaning of the journey.

Benefits of Shamanism

Although many people still view the practices of shamanism as more fiction than fact, a growing number of people value the emphasis these practices place on the unseen world of emotions, dreams, and spiritual forces to help heal illnesses and guide them in living a healthy and fulfilling life. While shamanism rarely offers a quick fix for acute illnesses, many people have reported profound physical and emotional relief through contemporary shamanic practices. With a history as long and enduring as humankind itself, it is hard to find a more time-tested method for bringing harmony and comfort to body and mind.

—*Hal Zina Bennett*

Resources:

Conference on the Study of Shamanism and Alternative Modes of Healing
Ruth-Inge Heinze, Ph.D.
2321 Russell Street, Suite 3A
Berkeley, CA 94705
Promotes shamanism as a healing practice.

Other Shamanic Techniques

Vision Quests: In this practice, a person spends a day or more alone in the wilderness. There he or she is able to fast and meditate without distractions. This can be used to help people contemplate their own inner worlds, their fears, dreams, strengths, and gifts. It can also be used to experience a oneness with nature.

Sun Dances: The sun dance was originally used to help warriors get in touch with their inner strengths and to draw strength from the spirits of nature such as those found in trees, rocks, clouds and sky. Usually over a period of several days, the young warrior was prepared through fasting, meditation, and counsel with an elder. Then small hooks or barbs were placed in the fleshy portions of his chest. Cords fastened these hooks to a tree or post and the dancer leaned back against them, naturally causing some pain. The dancers stood in this way from dawn to dusk, usually in the hot sun. It was a test of one's endurance and one's ability to deal with his or her own fears and discomforts. People who experienced the sun dance claimed to have gained dramatic self-knowledge. Even today there are those who repeat the sun dance every year.

Drumming Circles: This practice uses drums for therapeutic purposes. Usually there is a lead, or "mother," drum with a deep voice that sets a simple rhythm based on the heartbeat. People participate in these circles to help focus their energies, rather than to perform or make music. During a drumming circle, there are many conversations with the drums, which are used to teach participants how to listen and communicate with one another. Some people look upon drumming circles as times of communion, where people are brought together at a deep spiritual level.

Medicine Wheel: The medicine wheel is an important practice in most shamanic traditions; evidence of its use can be found in every part of the world. People form a wheel by gathering in a circle to discuss a problem or to bring about a change that affects them all. At the wheel, all people have equal status and an equal chance to speak. The wheel is used to allow a joining of their "spirits," that is, the inner worlds of each participant. It is understood that no single person at the wheel ever has the ultimate answer; rather, the solution is to be found as a community.

Sweat Lodge: A dome-shaped structure is constructed with willow branch poles, covered with hides or blankets. Prayers are offered and each participant is blessed upon entering the lodge. Then rocks, which have been heated at a fire outside the lodge, are brought inside and placed in the center. Water is poured over the rocks and the heat inside the lodge rises. In this steamy, hot environment, the participants meditate and contemplate their own lives or the lives of their community. The ceremonies and rituals that are performed vary with each lodge. Some create a medicine wheel. Others may sing. Still others may eat ritual herbs or peyote, a drug that produces hallucinations. The purpose of the sweat lodge, as with most shamanic practices, is to get in touch with the forces and energies of the invisible world in order to improve the quality of life.

The Foundation for Shamanic Studies
P.O. Box 1939
Mill Valley, CA 94942
Tel: (415) 380-8282
Sponsors workshops on shamanic training. Call or write for a catalog of their workshops.

Further Reading:

Books:

Andrews, Lynn. *Medicine Woman.* San Francisco: HarperCollins, 1981.

Beck, P. V., Anna Lee Walters, and Nia Francisco, eds. *The Sacred Ways of Knowledge, Sources of Life.* Flagstaff, AZ: Northland Publishing Co., 1990.

Bennett, Hal Zina. *Spirit Guides.* Ukiah, CA: Tenacity Press, 1997.

———. *Zuni Fetishes: Using Native American Objects for Meditation, Reflection, and Personal Insight.* San Francisco: HarperCollins, 1995

Campbell, Joseph. *Primitive Mythology.* New York: McGraw-Hill, 1978.

Castaneda, Carlos. *The Teachings of Don Juan: A Yaqui Way of Knowledge.* New York: Ballantine, 1968.

Harner, Michael J. *The Way of the Shaman: A Guide to Power and Healing.* San Francisco: HarperCollins, 1980.

Morgan, M. *Mutant Message.* New York: Harper-Collins, 1994.

Journals:

Shaman's Drum: A Journal of Contemporary Shamanism.

TRADITIONAL CHINESE MEDICINE

Traditional Chinese medicine (TCM) is an ancient approach to health care. Still practiced today in one form or another by almost one quarter of the world's population, TCM traces its mixture of herbal medicine, acupuncture, and massage therapy back to the origins of Taoism and Confucianism. With a heavy emphasis on understanding the patient and his or her needs, as opposed to focusing on the illness and its symptoms, TCM offers a counterpoint and complement to the bio-science of Western medicine.

TCM has been studied and practiced in many Asian countries such as Japan as long ago as 600 CE. Some Asian countries such as Korea and Japan have developed their own modifications to TCM. For this reason, the term Oriental medicine is sometimes used instead of Chinese medicine. However, all forms of traditional Oriental medicine are considered to have originated from the work done in China during the Han dynasty.

Because of the sociopolitical climate in modern China, a wide gap exists between current TCM theory and traditional TCM. Unfortunately, English translations of TCM have been available for only the past fifteen years, even then usually for a modern, officially sanctioned version of TCM. Different translations often contain confusing variations. For example, an important word we will discuss later like *qi* may be spelled *chi* (using an older translation system) or *ki* (Japanese). All three versions have the same meaning. In this essay, the modern Pinyin form of Chinese will be provided when possible. Understanding these translation principles can help you to read and understand other books and articles on the subject of TCM.

The History of TCM

In China an extremely organized system of healing developed during the period known as the Han dynasty (approximately 213 BCE–240 CE). At this time in Chinese history the country was finally reunited into one empire after hundreds of years of fighting in the Warring States period (476–221 BCE). Both Confucian and Taoist philosophies emerged from the Warring States period, and both of these philosophies had an important

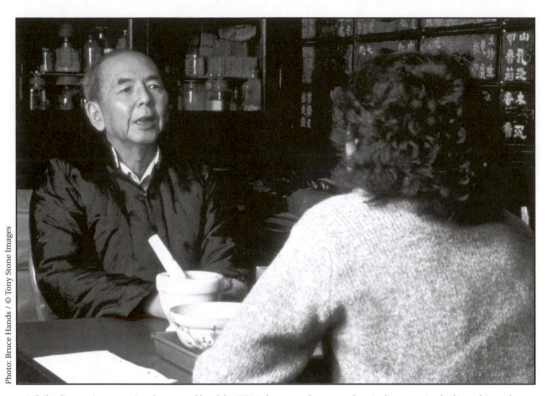

Photo: Bruce Hands / © Tony Stone Images

While discussing a patient's state of health, TCM doctors observe other indicators, including skin coloring, body structure, tone of voice, and scent.

impact on TCM. At the time of the Han dynasty there were many different kinds of healers and teachers in China. Confucianism was the main political power in court. During this time Ssu-ma Chien became the Grand Historian of the Court, and great importance was placed on organizing and recording written records.

During this time three books were written that are still considered the cornerstones of TCM. The first was called the *Yellow Emperor's Internal Classic* (*Huang di-nei Jing* or simply *Nei Jing*). The *Nei Jing* refers to both Taoist and Confucian concepts. The Taoist perspective of health emphasizes living in harmony with nature and achieving longevity. The Confucian ideals describe an integrated system within the human body that reflected the orderly social structure finally made possible in one unified state.

This organized structure was eventually mapped into the specific lines and pathways we see on acupuncture charts.

The lines or pathways are usually called meridians. Places where the *qi* comes right up to the surface are called acupoints. The *qi* is believed to circulate through this system connecting the deepest internal organs to places on the skin where the energy can be influenced and treated. The points can be treated with needles (acupuncture), heat (moxibustion), or manipulation (acupressure).

The *qi* system was described in more detail in the second book, called the *Classic of Difficult Issues* (*Nan Jing*). The *Nan Jing* is believed to have been written at least one hundred years after the *Nei Jing*. The *Nan Jing* refers to information in the *Nei Jing* and expands on those ideas. The *Nan Jing* goes so far as to say that a person's health can be directly analyzed just from carefully feeling the *qi* and blood as it moves through the radial artery in the wrist. This is called the radial pulse. Modern practices of TCM still use this map of the *qi* system to diagnose and treat their clients.

The third book is believed to have been written around 220 CE. Written by a very famous physician and scholar named Zhang Zhong-Jing, it is called the *Treatise on Harm Caused by Cold* (*Shang Han Lun*). This book deals with how outside influences such as colds, flu viruses, and plagues can attack and make people sick, and describes how to treat these problems with Chinese herbal medicine.

Zhang Zhong-Jing described six specific layers of the body's defense system and matched these with already recognized meridian pathways. He described the qualities of illness as they invaded each layer and gave specific herbal formulas that could be used for treatment. Using a wide variety of herbs given in specific dosages, he created formulas that could match detailed patterns of diagnosis. Zhang's use of herbal medicine introduced a whole new level of sophistication within the possibilities of TCM. While he cannot be credited with inventing Chinese herbal formulas, his ability to understand and match patterns of illness with the herbs that will cure them place him as one of the founding fathers of Chinese herbal medicine.

Over the next 1,500 years, China continued to develop and perfect the ideas that originated in the Han dynasty. Many physicians and scholars continued to practice and write about their ideas and results. Ideas that were originally used by particular authors and schools of thought were eventually homogenized into guiding principles for one predominant system of medicine.

By the end of the Ming dynasty (1643 CE) another idea, now described as the eight principles, began to emerge. This model included all of the dynamics that impact health. These are internal and external factors, hot and cold, yin and yang, and excess vs. deficiency. This model was used to integrate many of the previous models in TCM. The Ming was the last dynasty in which traditional Chinese medicine continued to evolve and flourish without being influenced by Western thought and medicine.

The introduction of Western culture in China began a period of slow decline for TCM. The obvious realities revealed through anatomical study made many Chinese physicians and scholars feel less confident in some of TCM's less tangible theories. The Chinese government also applied political pressures that affected the publication of certain literature. Eventually there began a trend to weed out the more "esoteric" ideas from Chinese medical literature. While ideas as fundamental as the *qi* and blood remained intact, references to the spiritual components became more and more simplified. Under the Communist regime, many ideas came to be viewed as superstitious and unscientific. These ideas were disregarded and systematically eliminated from revised texts.

To this day very little of original TCM literature has been translated into Western languages. Subsequently, TCM is often described in terms of the clinical approach presently being used in hospitals in mainland China. While this system offers very effective clinical applications for the treatment of disease, much of the broader perspective and theories remain buried in literary Chinese characters.

Guiding Principles

Influenced by its Taoist origins, TCM views the human body as an image of the natural world. This is reflected in the terminology of TCM. Energy is said to flow through the body in "rivers," often to a bodily "reservoir" or "sea." A diagnosis might describe an ailment as "liver fire," or an entire organ system as part of the water element. These terms do not reflect a lack of sophistication on the part of TCM, but rather a conscious decision to accept that the human body is a participating, not an isolated, part of the surrounding world. The language of TCM reflects how the ancients tried to reconcile their observations of the human body with what they observed in nature.

Continuous, dynamic movement is something the ancient Chinese observed in both the human body and in all nature. They viewed this movement as an interaction between two opposite but complementary energies that they called yin and yang. In Chinese philosophy these forces are understood to complement and help nourish each other. Neither can exist without the other. Examples of dynamic interaction between pairs of opposites can be seen in the constant interplay of day and night, male and female, or hot and cold. All the organs and actions of the body may be categorized as either yin or yang.

TCM identifies five "essential substances" at work in the human body:

1. Spirit (shen), which determines how people direct and conduct themselves in life.
2. Energy or electromagnetic force (*qi*), a Chinese concept that cannot be translated into just one English word. *Qi* is how the spirit moves and becomes materialized in the body. It describes both activity and a material substance. The concept of *qi* bridges the line of distinction that the English language makes between energy and matter.
3. Blood is the same blood we refer to from a Western anatomical view, but from the TCM perspective, it is imbued with the nutritional and energetic qualities TCM attributes to *qi*. This aspect of blood is called the *ying qi* and it circulates with and in the blood, as it moves through the vessels and performs its various functions.
4. Body fluids (jin ye), which include sweat, tears, cerebral spinal fluid, and other fluids of the body.
5. Essence (jing), which in English may be understood as potential. This includes our genetic potential as well as the potential of any person or thing to take an action.

These essential substances are understood to exist as a continuum of each other. None can be considered as entirely separate, just as no one part of the body can be treated as entirely separate from the whole.

TCM uses the term *resonance* to describe the relationship between the five essential substances and their role in our health. Resonance describes the idea that certain qualities may be identified as similar within different spheres of existence. For example, the morning time of day has a quality of energy that is similar to or resonates with the spring time of the year. This quality of rising energy identifies them as a particular stage in a cycle of change.

Such stages of change are referred to as elements or transformations. The spring and morning are categorized as belonging to the wood element stage of what is known as the five-element cycle. This cycle is used to explain how energy is constantly changing. It can be applied to the day, the year, the human body, or anything else we want to understand.

In TCM the five-element cycle has proved to be an exceptionally versatile frame of reference for explaining the patterns of dynamic change in our physical bodies. Each of our ten primary organs is correlated with one of the five elements of nature: fire, soil, metal, water, and wood. Doctors of Chinese medicine then correlate the ways in which these elements interact in nature at large with the way these organs and the dynamic qualities of yin and yang work together in the physical body. For example, an inflamed liver might be seen as having too much fire. The solution to the problem is best deduced from the way nature cools fire with water. In the case of "liver fire," a yang excess condition, the patient will naturally be very thirsty and want to drink large quantities of cold water. The practitioner treating such a condition knows that the excess "fire" needs to be dispersed or drained and more "water" quality added to the meridian in order to keep the fire in check. Using either needles, acupressure, magnets, or other techniques, a skilled practitioner will choose to use a dispersing technique on the fire point of the liver meridian and will tonify the water point. Understanding that the entire kidney organ system reflects the water element, a practitioner may also choose to bring in more water or yin quality using specific kidney meridian points.

Just as the five essential substances are all seen as part of one living whole, the dynamic interplay of yin and yang energies and the five elements are understood as having a complex interactive relationship with one another. Extensive study of Chinese medicine is needed to truly understand and effectively direct these complex interactions.

Traditional Chinese Herbal Medicine

Over the last two decades, the ancient arts of acupuncture, Chinese herbology, and Oriental bodywork therapy have emerged from the privacy of Asian-American communities and into the greater American consciousness.

Unlike acupuncture and Oriental bodywork therapy, which use physical pressure and manipulation to effect changes in the way a patient's body functions, Chinese herbal medicine counts on the properties of different plants and foods to stimulate or calm different parts of the body. In many ways, this is similar to the drugs of Western medicine, but because Chinese herbal medicine employs "whole" naturally occurring food substances, the risk of causing harmful side effects is greatly reduced.

Chinese herbal medicine must be studied as a distinct skill. Its practitioners must learn the *pharmacopiae*, a name for the knowledge of the names, characteristics, and actions in the body of all the individual herbs. Dosage formulas must be memorized along with various modifications for each. Knowledge of contraindications and hidden effects for specific herbs is an important part of what must be studied. This information can take years to assimilate. Nevertheless, all this information is necessary for the experienced clini-

cian to create formulas that skillfully match the patient's condition.

Chinese herbal medicine stores can usually be found in any major city of the United States where there is a significant Asian population. Often these herb shops are owned or run by practitioners or "doctors" of Chinese herbal medicine. When this is the case "customers" have the option of becoming "patients" when they go into the store. Often a number of practitioners in one area will refer all their patients to one local herb store in order to have their herbal prescriptions filled. In this way Chinese herbal medicine stores act as pharmacies.

Four Examinations

TCM practitioners use a system called the "four examinations" to diagnose a patient and determine a proper course of treatment. The examinations include the following steps:

1. *Questioning*: Starting with information about a specific complaint or condition, the experienced practitioner asks about other symptoms and signs that can help point toward a specific pattern. In the Ming dynasty Zhang Jie-Bin developed a set of ten specific questions, and modified versions of this are still useful today.

2. *Looking*: The practitioner carefully observes the patient's appearance. This usually includes looking at the person's tongue, face, and body structure.

3. *Touching*: The practitioner carefully feels the radial pulse in the patient's wrist for a very specific assessment of the patient's *qi*, blood, and other essences. Some practitioners can get most of their information from this one source. If the person's complaint is a pain or injury, then the practitioner must examine the injured or painful area. A number of other sets of points and microsystems (the hand, foot, ear) may also be used for palpation.

4. *Listening and smelling*: This aspect of the four examinations involves listening to the patient's voice, noticing any strange odors (which could, for example, indicate infection), and otherwise gleaning information that a patient does not actually report to the practitioner.

Once the assessment is clear, the doctor of herbal medicine writes out a prescription to be filled with exact dosages of each herb. Some prescriptions call for bags or batches of herbs, which are often packed in wrapped paper. For such prescriptions, dosage is determined by the number of bags to be cooked and used within a specified time frame. Patients who are unfamiliar with their formulas need to be instructed on how to cook their prescription into a tea or soup. Sometimes one or two herbs need to be added separately to make their cooking time longer or shorter than other ingredients. For less serious problems, experienced customers are able to use the herbal store as a pharmacy, buying familiar, simple remedies without a prescription.

Benefits and Risks

The three disciplines of traditional Chinese medicine have evolved over thousands of years and are considered to be safe for almost anyone who wishes to try them. Many schools for TCM have adjusted their programs to incorporate more training in modern Western science. More medical schools, such as Harvard Medical School, are including courses to help Western physicians to refer to and work with alternative medicine. For this reason, anyone thinking about choosing a full program of TCM should consult with both TCM and Western doctors to understand the strengths and shortcomings of each.

As with all health programs, choosing a therapist is a crucial decision. To decide whether your herbalist or therapist is properly qualified, a prospective patient should carefully ask the doctor where and how he or she learned this discipline. For Chinese herbal medicine, national

certification through the National Commission for Certification of Acupuncture and Oriental Medicine (NCCAOM) is one clear way to be sure that a practitioner is at least competent. It is quite possible, however, to find master-level practitioners who have not chosen to get such a credential.

—*Cindy Banker*

Resources:

American Association of Acupuncture and Oriental Medicine
4101 Lake Boone Trail, Suite 201
Raleigh, NC 27607
Tel: (919) 787-5181
Offers information on TCM.

National Commission for Certification of Acupuncture and Oriental Medicine (NCCAOM)
1424 16th St. NW, Suite 501
Washington, DC 20026
Provides certification for practitioners of acupuncture, Chinese herbal medicine, and Oriental bodywork therapy.

The New Center for Wholistic Health, Education and Research
6801 Jericho Turnpike
Syosset, NY 11791
Promotes the study and practice of TCM.

Further Reading:

Cheng, Xinnong, editor. *Chinese Acupuncture and Moxibustion*. Beijing: Foreign Language Press, 1987.

Enqing, Dr. Zhang, editor. *Practical English-Chinese Library of traditional Chinese medicine*. Shanghai: Publishing House of Shanghai College, 1990.

Kaptchuk, Ted J. *The Web That Has No Weaver*. New York: Congdon & Weed, 1983.

Unschuld, Paul, editor. *Introductory Readings in Classical Chinese Medicine*. Dordrecht, Netherlands: Kluwar Academic Publishers, 1988.

Yubin, L. & L. Chengcai. *Advanced Traditional Chinese Medicine Series*. Amsterdam: IOS Press, 1996.

WELLNESS

Wellness programs are based on holism, sometimes called holistic wellness, a philosophy of health that believes well-being is not just a condition of physical health or the absence of disease and illness. Rather, health is a balance of elements that include the mental, emotional, spiritual, and physical aspects of the human condition. In other words, wellness is the integration, balance, and harmony of mind, body, spirit, and emotions, where the whole is thought to be greater than the sum of the parts. Wellness professionals believe that the lines separating the mental, physical, emotional, and spiritual aspects exist in theory, but not in actuality. Research in the field of psychoneuroimmunology (the relationship between emotions and the body) reveals that there is no division between these aspects, and they should be regarded as one.

History of the Wellness Approach

Although the concept of wellness is thousands of years old, the word *wellness* was introduced into the American vernacular in the 1960s. Thought by many to be an expansion of the fitness movement of the late 1970s and early 1980s, wellness is considered to be a more comprehensive approach to optimal health than standard health education programs that treated specific symptoms or were used to prevent disease. Addressing more than physical ailments, wellness programs integrate, balance, and harmonize the physical, mental, emotional, and spiritual aspects of the wellness paradigm. Today programs are offered in corporate, community, hospital, and fitness club settings.

The Basic Principles of Wellness

It may seem as if mind, body, spirit, and emotions are separate aspects—a premise proposed by the French philosopher René Descartes (1596–1650) stated that the mind and body are separate entities. Descartes' premise, known as the Cartesian Principle, led to the mechanistic paradigm, which eventually led to the belief that the human body acts like a machine and the way to treat disease and illness (the opposite of health) was through medications and surgery.

The wellness paradigm holds that there is no separation between mind, body, spirit, and emotions. All aspects of the human condition are so tightly connected that it is impossible to distinguish one from the other. An ancient theory that is supported by many experts in several disciplines suggests that each aspect of the human condition is comprised of energy, with the most dense energy being the most obvious and tangible: the physical body. Here then are definitions for each aspect of the wellness paradigm:

- Emotional well-being is best defined as the ability to feel and express the entire range of human emotions from anger to love, and to control them, not be controlled by them.
- Physical well-being is defined as the optimal condition of each of the body's physiological systems. These include pulmonary, cardiovascular, nervous, immune, reproductive, urinary, endocrine, musculoskeletal and digestive.
- Mental well-being is understood as the ability to gather, process, recall, and communicate information. Like a computer, the mind can gather and store mass quantities of information.
- Spiritual well-being is defined as the maturation of higher consciousness as developed through the dynamic integration of three facets: relationships (internal, how you relate to yourself and a higher power, however you conceive this to be; and external, how you relate and interact with all people in your life), a personal value system, and a meaningful purpose in life.

An important figure in the wellness area, Dr. Elizabeth Kübler-Ross, outlines a theory that suggests that although all

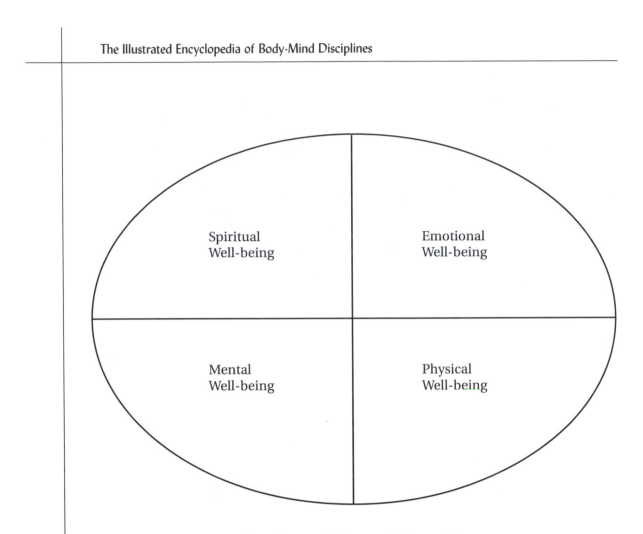

The wellness model of a complete human being.

four components are always present in the human condition, each component dominates in our lives as we journey through the life cycle. The first component is the emotional, in which we experience the array of human emotions. During this time, we may be conditioned by parents, guardians, or even society to suppress our feelings, which could likely result in emotional dysfunction later in life. The influence of physical development begins to dominate at puberty and continues well throughout the teen years. The mental or intellectual aspect kicks in during the college years and endures well into mid-life, as we exercise our mental capabilities through the thinking processes of the right and left brain and the conscious and unconscious minds. The last section of the wellness paradigm, the spiritual, emerges during the mid-life

years. As Kübler-Ross and others note, there are many people who never move into this phase of development because of laziness, mistrust, or fear.

How Wellness Works

With the help of a thorough personal history and open discussions between the patient and practitioner, the practitioner will be able to recognize an imbalance or problem in one of the four areas. He or she will then be able to guide the patient to a program or services that address the patient's needs. The wellness professional has a whole range of programs to choose from and is aware of how these services and programs interact and affect the patient. Wellness professionals work in partnership with their patients and recommend treatments that support the body's natural healing system.

Wellness Programming

When evaluating the dynamics of wellness applications, there are many programs and services that need to be considered. Below is a partial list of wellness program services, by their respective holistic components. Keep in mind that a service listed in one area has a crossover effect in all the other areas.

Physical Well-being:
Aerobic Fitness
Cholesterol Screenings
Blood Pressure Screenings
Blood Sugar Screenings
Weight Training
Nutritional Assessments
Biofeedback
Massage Therapy
Hatha Yoga
T'ai Chi

Spiritual Well-being:
Values Clarification and Assessment
Journal Writing
Dance Therapy
Meditation
Communing with Nature
Inner Resource Development
Human Potential Development
Community Service Projects
Social Support Group

Mental Well-being:
Meditation
Mental Imagery
Stress Management
Time Management
Creativity & Creative Problem Solving
Communication Skills
Dream Analysis

Emotional Well-being:
Humor Therapy
Music and Art Therapy
Aromatherapy
Codependency Therapy
Grieving Therapy
Communication Skills
Creative Anger Management
Stress Management

The Benefits of a Wellness Approach to Health

Wellness programs focus on reaching higher levels of wellness as well as preventing illness. Many patients are motivated by the energy and vitality that result from a holistic approach to life, especially when they realize that the benefits could continue and allow them to feel good for many years.

—*Brian Luke Seaward, Ph.D.*

Resources:

National Wellness Association (NWA)
1045 Clark St., Suite 210
Stevens Point, WI 54481-0827
Tel: (715) 342-2969
Fax: (715) 342-2979
e-mail: nwa@wellnesswi.org
Web site: www.wellnesswi.org/nwa.html
A nonprofit professional membership organization that disseminates information and provides services to professionals working in wellness areas.

National Wellness Institute
1045 Clark St., Suite 210
Stevens Point, WI 54481-0827
Tel: (800) 243-8694
Fax: (715) 342-2979
Founded in 1977, this is a full resource center for wellness practitioners and those interested in wellness programs.

Further Reading:

Edlin, Gordon, Eric Golanty, and Kelli McCormack Brown. *Health and Wellness.* Sudbury, MA: Jones and Bartlett, 1996.

Travis, John, and Regina S. Ryan. *The Wellness Workbook*, Second Edition. Berkeley, CA: Ten Speed Press, 1988.

PART II: SKELETAL MANIPULATION METHODS

Chiropractic • CranioSacral Therapy • Network Chiropractic • Osteopathy • Zero Balancing®

Skeletal manipulation methods are a group of healing practices that focus on the form of the skeleton to improve the functioning of the whole person. They are part of a larger group of practices that have come to be known collectively as bodywork. Bodywork is a general term describing a wide variety of methods that use touch to improve awareness of feelings and sensations in the body and improve physical functioning. Bodywork methods are also used to relieve pain and encourage relaxation. There are many disciplines in this book included in the bodywork category. They can be found in the sections entitled Acupuncture and Asian Bodywork, Body-Oriented Psychotherapies, Massage, Movement Therapy Methods, Somatic Practices, and Subtle Energy Practices.

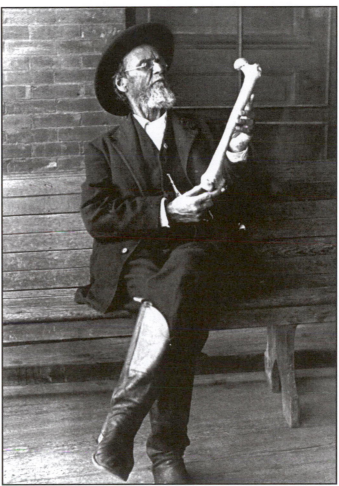

Photo: Still National Osteopathic Museum, Kirksville, MO

Dr. Andrew Taylor Still, founder of osteopathy, championed the idea that a thorough knowledge of the human skeleton could be the basis for a complete health care method.

The oldest methods in this section, chiropractic and osteopathy, developed in response to the conventional medical practices prevalent in America in the mid- to late nineteenth century. The other skeletal manipulation methods evolved from these seminal practices. In addition to their historical roots, these methods also share a theoretical framework. They view the human being as an integrated whole of body, mind, and spirit, possessing its own innate healing and balancing mechanisms that guide communication between the interrelated systems of the body. The goal of all of these drugless methods is to remove any structural alterations to the natural skeletal alignment that may impede the operation of these innate healing and balancing mechanisms. The older methods, osteopathy and chiropractic, are used by millions as primary health care modalities for treating a wide variety of health problems. The younger methods derived from them are generally used to treat specific problems or to enhance general physical health and emotional well-being.

The Development of Skeletal Manipulation for Health

The practice of manipulating the skeleton for optimal health is ancient and widespread. Some medical historians report that the Egyptians used such techniques. The earliest written record of skeletal manipulation comes to us from China, where methods of bodywork were developed several thousand years ago as part of a complete health care system. The Asian bodywork methods practiced today that are derived from these ancient practices are similar to the skeletal manipulation methods described in this section in that both of them manipulate the physical body with the goal of influencing a vital life force. There is no evidence that these Eastern practices directly influenced the development of the earliest skeletal manipulation methods. But it is very likely that the philosophy upon which these Eastern practices are based, which was introduced into American cultural discourse in the late nineteenth century, indirectly influenced the founders of chiropractic and osteopathy.

Hippocrates (c. 430–377 BCE), the father of modern Western medicine, is reputed to have said that dislocations of the spine are the origin of many ailments, but it is unclear how this belief affected his medical practice. The recorded history of manipulating the skeleton as a means of treating disease and creating optimum health begins in the West with the work of Andrew Taylor Still (1838–1917). A controversial figure in American medical history, Still rebelled against the medical practices of his day, which included heavy use of drugs, purging, and bloodletting. He formulated the gentle, drugless, noninvasive principles and techniques of osteopathy and established its first school in Kirksville, Missouri, in 1892.

Unlike Still, Daniel David Palmer (1845–1913), the founder of chiropractic, had no formal medical training, but practiced various forms of energy healing popular at the end of the nineteenth century. Chiropractic was formally introduced as a healing modality in 1895. Some medical historians report that Palmer was treated by Still in Kirksville in 1893. Whether or not this particular treatment occurred, given Palmer's lifelong interest in unconventional healing techniques, it is certainly probable that he was familiar with Still's groundbreaking work.

Both osteopathy and chiropractic have had long, arduous struggles for acceptance within the conventional medical establishment. Today doctors of osteopathy (D.O.s) and doctors of chiropractic (DCs) are licensed to practice throughout the United States and Canada. In recent years a number of D.O.s and DCs have added their own insights to these century-old healing modalities to create more personalized approaches to healing the whole person through manipulation of the skeleton. These new methods include CranioSacral therapy, which focuses primarily on manipulating the bones of the skull; network chiropractic, which blends Western psychotherapeutic theory with gentle chiropractic techniques; and Zero Balancing®, which integrates Eastern concepts of energy with skeletal manipulation.

Using the Body's Inborn Healing Potential

All the methods described in this section believe that the body has an inborn healing potential. This potential is called by many names, such as "energy," "spirit," or "innate intelligence," by the practitioners of these methods. Andrew Taylor Still believed this energy was transmitted primarily through the blood, whereas Daniel David Palmer postulated that it moved primarily through the nervous system. In either event, both methods, and all the methods derived from them, when practiced in their most pure form, are drugless, concentrating on releasing structural misalignments in the skeleton and thereby allowing the body's own internal healing and balancing systems to work freely.

Practitioners of skeletal manipulation methods see the relationship between structure and function in the body to be interdependent. Just as the wooden or steel frame of a building supports its heating, plumbing, and electrical systems, practitioners of skeletal manipulation methods see our bones as the supporting framework of all other systems of our body. If the framework is faulty or collapsing at any point, it is likely to cause damage to the interior systems. Likewise, if there is a problem in an interior system such as a leaky pipe, which on a body level might correspond to a diseased organ such as kidney, liver, or heart, that malfunction will eventually cause a structural defect in the building such as a bulge in a wall with peeling paint, or buckling wallpaper. On a body level these changes in structure will appear as misalignments in the skeleton and as pain caused by muscles responding to the skeletal changes.

Furthermore, skeletal manipulation methods view the systems of the body as interrelated. A common everyday activity such as reaching high for something tucked away on a closet shelf or vigorously swinging a baseball bat could initiate a series of systemic changes that begin as a small change in the alignment of the upper spine. If left unchecked this dislocation could cause localized muscular pain in the shoulder or upper back area, and then shortness of breath as muscles between the ribs in the upper torso contract in response to the structural change. Restricted breath may in turn lead to any number of complicated health problems, including bronchitis, asthma, heart conditions, and even depression.

In a like manner, emotional problems such as a traumatic experience, phobias, and even addictions, which can cause chemical toxicity, are seen as possible causes of structural changes in the body. These structural changes then initiate a chain reaction in the interdependent systems of the body, which stimulates further emotional or physical cravings. Many practitioners of skeletal manipulation methods extend this holistic view of the causes and effects of alterations to skeletal alignment to every aspect of a person's life including genetic inheritance, diet, exercise, daily activities, and stress from work and personal relationships.

Experiencing Skeletal Manipulation

Practitioners of skeletal manipulation methods rely predominantly on the use of the hands, physical contact, and knowledge of anatomy to diagnose patients. Touching and physically moving the patient in various ways allows the practitioner to feel the alignment of the skeleton and the state of the muscular system. In this way they are able to treat a spectrum of chronic and acute health problems.

Each of these disciplines has its standard techniques for manipulating the skeleton. Chiropractors focus on the manipulation of the spine itself. They see the flow of information from the central nervous system housed inside the spine as the primary self-regulating system of the body. CranioSacral therapists focus on the relationship of the bones of the skull to each other to monitor the wavelike flow of cerebrospinal fluid, which they believe to be a barometer of healthy functioning throughout all the systems of the body. Zero Balancers focus on special joints, called foundation joints, which they believe are the primary regulators of energy throughout the body. Osteopaths may manipulate the spine, including the skull, or any other joint of the skeleton where they feel skeletal misalignment is negatively affecting the whole person. Although in their original and most pure forms osteopathy and chiropractic used only manipulation techniques, today many D.O.s and DCs add other techniques to treatment plans, including recommendations of specific exercises, dietary or lifestyle changes, and in some cases herbal or pharmaceutical remedies.

Providing Relief for Millions of People Each Year

Skeletal manipulation methods are reported to help more than 15 million people each year who are suffering from a variety of physical and emotional problems. They have been found to help with problems that have not responded to conventional Western medical practices. Whether you are looking for a comprehensive health modality or relief from a specific pain or condition, these methods may offer unique, drug-free, holistic approaches to healing and maintaining optimum health of body and mind.

—*Nancy Allison, CMA*

Resources:

American Chiropractic Association
1701 Clarendon Boulevard
Arlington, VA 22209
Tel: (703) 276-8800
Provides information about chiropractic, including monthly publications, newsletters, and clinical councils.

American Association of College of Osteopathic Medicine (AACOM)
5550 Friendship Blvd. Suite 310
Chevy Chase, MD 20815-7231
Tel: (800) 621-1773, ext. 7401

Fax: (312) 280-3860
Web site: www.aacom.org
Offers educational and professional support to osteopathic physicians.

Further Reading:

Montague, Ashley. *Touching: The Human Significance of Skin.* New York: Columbia University Press, 1986.

CHIROPRACTIC

Chiropractic is a mode of bodywork that promotes self-healing by manipulating the spine so as to remove blocks in the transmission of nerve impulses from the brain through the spinal nerves and out to all parts of the body. It postulates that malfunction in any aspect of the individual can be attributed to subluxations, misalignments of the vertebrae that disturb the spinal nerves in their mediation of mind and body. Further, chiropractic subscribes to the basic principle that the immune system will function perfectly and maintain the person in robust, good health as long as misalignments of the spine do not constrict the nervous system. Other therapeutic methods such as nutritional counseling may be included in chiropractic, but treatment always focuses upon detection and adjustment of vertebral misalignments. Chiropractic is the second-largest primary health care field in the world. Proponents credit it with a wide range of benefits, from relief of chronic back pain to successful treatment of asthma and depression.

A Long History

There is strong evidence that adjustment of the spine has been used as a form of medical treatment since civilization first began. A Chinese manuscript of 2700 BCE records details of soft tissue manipulation, and the Greeks are known to have developed similar practices around 1500 BCE. In a treatise of the fifth century BCE, Hippocrates encouraged his patients to "get knowledge of the spine, for many diseases have their origin in dislocations of the vertebral column."

David Daniel Palmer is responsible for developing the form of spinal adjustment used today. Born in 1845, Palmer was an American who worked as a healer through most of his life but had no formal medical training. While its Greek name, chiropractic, meaning

"done by hand," evokes ancient Hippocratic teachings, virtually all its principles and techniques are late nineteenth century in derivation. Manual "bone-setting" was accepted practice, and irregularities in the nervous system were commonly viewed as the cause of illness. The third major component in chiropractic, the use of the hands to harmonize the circulation of nervous energy, came from Palmer's experience as a magnetic healer, or Mesmerist. In Mesmerism the hands are passed over the person's field of electromagnetic energy with the aim of correcting imbalances regarded as the cause of illness.

Palmer advanced beyond Mesmerist concepts as his work progressed, but he never relinquished its vision of a treatment that bypasses drugs and surgery in favor of direct contact between the hands of the healer and the life force of the person. By 1895 he had put together the basic principles of chiropractic and was winning renown throughout the Midwest for "miracle cures" of apparently irreversible problems.

Palmer's son, Bartlett Joshua Palmer (1881–1961), transformed chiropractic into a profession with a following that was devoted but rocked by persistent controversy. Doctors of medicine were generally opposed to the growth of a competing system of health care and led efforts to make chiropractic illegal. Attacks on its lack of scientific rigor intensified debate about the interpretation of Palmer's legacy within the chiropractic community. "Straights" argued that chiropractic should consist solely of hands-on vertebral adjustment and condemned as traitors those who "mixed" spinal adjustment with other forms of therapy or used mechanical devices in lieu of their hands.

Present-day chiropractors continue to identify themselves as either "straights" or "mixers," but the struggle to win public respect and authority for chiropractic is largely over. During the 1930s John J. Nugent started a movement that gradually raised the standards at chiropractic schools and set up chiropractic licensing

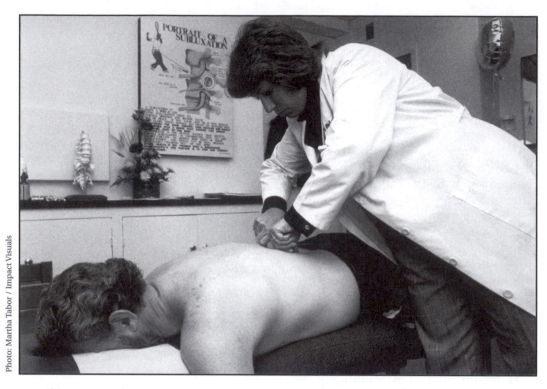

Chiropractic techniques manipulate the spine to aid the healing process in any part of the body.

Photo: Martha Tabor / Impact Visuals

laws in all the states. More recently chiropractic has benefited from a swing toward natural medicine that stimulated broad interest in its history and potential as an alternative mode of health care. Because of the experiments of "mixers," chiropractic is rapidly becoming more diversified and offers nutritional counseling, massage, and an increasing use of mechanical devices.

Finding the True Cause

Palmer believed the human being is born with an ever vigilant "innate intelligence" or "innate mind" that superintends all the body's functions and seeks to achieve homeostasis, a state of balance that extends "to every individual cell in the living organism." Thus in chiropractic, much as in therapeutic touch or osteopathy, virtually unlimited powers of self-healing are imputed to the person, and drugs are seen as detrimental to the workings of the body's own defense mechanisms. Palmer also taught that diagnosis of disease through

study of symptoms generally overlooks the true cause of the crisis. Ninety-five percent of all disease, he contended, is attributable to vertebral misalignment that interferes with the transmission of information from the "innate intelligence" to the spinal nerves.

Contemporary chiropractors are more apt to speak of an inborn switchboard than of "innate intelligence," but they adhere to Palmer's belief that illnesses are often caused by subluxated vertebrae and in numerous instances are misdiagnosed because the symptoms do not point directly to back trouble. For example, chronic bladder infection may be the result of a misalignment of the lower vertebrae that irritates the nerves leading to the bladder. Palmer performed his most famous cure, restoring the hearing of a man deaf for seventeen years, by correcting a subluxation of the upper spine.

Diagnosis and treatment in chiropractic are therefore organized, not around disease, but around signs of systemic malfunction likely to start in vertebral misalignment: aberration of musculoskeletal development, or kinesiopathology; abnormality in the muscles proper, or myopathology; irritation of the nerves, or neuropathology; inflammation indicative of abnormality in the blood cells, or histiopathology; and deterioration of the sense of mental and physical well-being, or pathophysiology. The misalignments themselves are attributed to any of several causes, such as injury, mental or physical stress, and genetic defect or predisposition.

Experiencing Chiropractic

Chiropractic treatment begins with the taking of a thorough case history and a physical examination that includes analysis and touching of the spine to determine imbalances and subluxations. X rays of the spine are sometimes made to get additional information. Recommendations for rest, physical therapy, or diet may be made as part of a therapy plan that generally entails spinal adjustments carried out over a series of sessions. The adjustments are done through hands-on contact that varies from gentle touch to firm pressure depending on the needs of the patient and the orientation of the chiropractor. Some advocate a maneuver in which the joint is stretched to just beyond its normal range of motion and makes an audible click. Others rely upon a repertory of "non-force" techniques to manipulate the vertebrae. The adjustments are not painful and are often described as relaxing, relieving, liberating, or energizing. Length and frequency of the sessions are established by the chiropractor and patient and depend on the nature of the problem.

The Benefits of Chiropractic

A wide variety of health problems respond favorably to chiropractic treatment. It is beneficial for musculoskeletal disorders, particularly whiplash injuries, neck and back pain, scoliosis, sciatica, arthritis, and bursitis. It can be effective in alleviating migraine headaches and other organic conditions, sinusitis, gastrointestinal disorder, bronchial asthma, high blood pressure, and heart trouble. Spinal adjustment is also regarded as a drug-free means of releasing nervous tension that contributes to the formation of mental and physical disability. Extensive research today is also testing the efficiency of chiropractic in the treatment of addictions.

—Dr. Trina Marx

Resources:

American Chiropractic Association
1701 Clarendon Boulevard
Arlington, VA 22209
Tel: (703) 276-8800
Provides a myriad of information about chiropractic, including monthly publications, newsletters, and clinical councils.

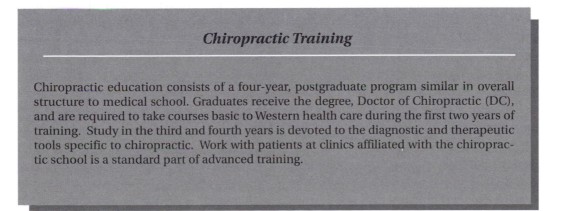

Chiropractic Training

Chiropractic education consists of a four-year, postgraduate program similar in overall structure to medical school. Graduates receive the degree, Doctor of Chiropractic (DC), and are required to take courses basic to Western health care during the first two years of training. Study in the third and fourth years is devoted to the diagnostic and therapeutic tools specific to chiropractic. Work with patients at clinics affiliated with the chiropractic school is a standard part of advanced training.

International Chiropractors Association
1110 North Glebe Road
Suite 1000
Arlington, VA 22201
Tel: (703) 528-5000
A professional organization dedicated to chiro-practic.

World Chiropractic Alliance
2950 N. Dobson Road, Suite 1
Chandler, AZ 85224
Tel: (800) 347-1011
Fax: (602) 732-9313
Web site: worldall@ix.netcom.com
A professional support group that provides refer-rals for chiropractors nationwide.

Further Reading:

Coplan-Griffiths, Michael. *Dynamic Chiropractic Today: The Complete and Major Guide to This Major Therapy.* San Francisco: Harper-Collins, 1991.

Gevitz, Norman. *Other Healers: Unorthodox Medi-cine in America.* Baltimore: The Johns Hopkins University Press, 1988.

Martin, Raquel. *Today's Health Alternative.* Tehachapi, CA: American West Publishers, 1992.

Moore, J. Stuart. *Chiropractic in America: The His-tory of a Medical Alternative.* Baltimore: The Johns Hopkins University Press, 1993.

Palmer, Daniel D. *The Chiropractor's Adjuster.* Davenport, IA: Palmer College Press, 1992 (first published 1910).

CRANIOSACRAL THERAPY

CranioSacral therapy is a gentle form of bodywork based on releas-ing restrictions in the craniosacral system to help people achieve their high-est levels of physical, mental, and emo-tional well-being. It was developed over a twenty-year period by Dr. William Sutherland, an osteopathic physician intrigued by the movement of different bones in the skull. He discovered that by exerting gentle pressure on selected areas of the skull or the rest of the body, a craniosacral therapist can effectively treat chronic pain, lowered vitality, recurring infections, and dysfunctions affecting the head, spine, and whole body.

Origins of CranioSacral Therapy

CranioSacral therapy developed from cranial osteopathy, the origin of which dates back to the 1890s, when Dr. Andrew Still founded the osteopathic profession. Distraught by the death of his wife and two children from meningi-tis and not knowing whether the disease or the mercury used to treat them was responsible, Dr. Still began an intensive study of anatomy and non-drug-based healing ways. He realized everything in nature was ordered: that the body func-tions as a unified whole; structure and function are interrelated; the body has an inherent self-corrective mechanism; and that drugs can be harmful. Based upon these principles, Dr. Still founded the first osteopathic college.

Dr. Still's star student was William Sutherland. Dr. Sutherland was intrigued by the idea that the bones of the skull were structured to allow for movement. For more than twenty years he explored this concept, eventually developing a system of treatment known as cranial osteopathy.

In 1970 osteopathic physician John E. Upledger observed the rhythmic movement of the craniosacral system during surgery. Dr. Upledger and his colleagues could not find an explana-tion for this mysterious movement.

After studying the work of Dr. Suther-land, Dr. Upledger worked to scientifically confirm the mobility of the cranial bones and the subsequent existence of the cran-iosacral system. From 1975 to 1983, he served as clinical researcher and a profes-sor of biomechanics at Michigan State

University. There he supervised a high-level team of anatomists, physiologists, biophysicists, and bioengineers to test and document the influence of therapy on the craniosacral system.

This team developed the theoretical PressureStat Model to describe how the craniosacral system functions. Dr. Upledger's continued work in the field resulted in the further development of CranioSacral therapy, including a ten-step protocol used to alleviate a range of conditions.

Insights Through Touch

The craniosacral system consists of the central nervous system, brain, and spinal cord, as well as the membranes and cerebrospinal fluid that surrounds and protects the cord. The central nervous system interconnects with the connective tissue that surrounds it, which in turn interconnects with all other bodily structures. Functionally there is one uninterrupted tissue sheath from the top of your head to the tips of your toes. Therefore, CranioSacral therapists are highly trained in sensing through touch a restriction in your system and determining how it affects other areas in your body. For instance, practitioners believe a restriction in your leg might have a profound effect on your lower back, shoulder, neck, or even head. CranioSacral therapists are highly trained in sensing through touch to track, identify, and release root restrictions affecting the person.

How does CranioSacral therapy work? First, as cerebrospinal fluid filters into the craniosacral system, pressure builds. As the amount of fluid increases, the increased pressure forces the fluid to travel down the spinal cord. As the fluid moves, the membranes surrounding the fluid and the interconnected fascial tissue of the entire body pulse in a rhythmic fashion, normally at a rate of six to twelve cycles per minute. It is this rhythm that the therapist monitors when evaluating and performing a CranioSacral therapy session.

One unique feature of CranioSacral therapy is its emphasis on very delicate palpation. Therapists are taught to use, appreciate, and develop profound insights through applying a very light, gentle touch—generally the pressure is equal to the weight of a nickel. It is believed that this light touch allows the therapist to receive as much information as possible from the patient's body, and to interact in a respectful, highly therapeutic manner.

Another distinction of CranioSacral therapy relates to its facilitation of the body's self-corrective ability. CranioSacral therapists believe engaging body restrictions with a gentle touch can break down tissue, emotional, and energetic blocks to self-release. CranioSacral therapy is not a manipulative therapeutic modality in which therapists impose what they think should happen on their patients. Rather, therapists are trained to follow their patients' bodies to facilitate their own healing process.

CranioSacral therapy aims to be very direct yet highly respectful of the patient. A gentle touch directed toward a patient's primary restrictions is believed to provide profound access to the very fabric of an individual's being. This respect for the patient's own healing abilities reflected through touch creates a safe environment for people to frequently access deep, non-conscious parts of themselves they may have blocked or simply couldn't access by themselves.

The training of a therapist's touch by the CranioSacral therapy technique is recognized as a profound foundation for advancement in manual therapies, massage, and therapeutic bodywork.

Practicing CranioSacral Therapy

A typical session of CranioSacral therapy lasts forty-five minutes to an hour. The client is fully clothed and lies on a comfortable, padded table. In a very gentle manner, the therapist evaluates the patient by testing for craniosacral motion in various parts of the patient's body. Experienced practitioners are able to feel the craniosacral rhythm anywhere on a patient's body. They can quickly gain valuable information by palpating the craniosacral motion for rate, amplitude, symmetry, and quality.

Lack of craniosacral rhythm or an asymmetrical craniosacral rhythm is used to locate problems throughout the body. The problem may be any type that causes loss of natural physiological responses, pain, trauma, adhesions, neurological and orthopedic disorders, systemic disease processes, and others. The therapist's job is to restore the symmetrical craniosacral motion to problem areas. As the asymmetry is eliminated and normal physiological motion is restored, the problem is being or has been alleviated.

Benefits of CranioSacral Therapy

CranioSacral therapy has been used to improve the functioning of the brain and spinal cord, to alleviate pain and the effects of stress, and to enhance general health as well as resistance to illness and disease. It has been especially effective for conditions such as migraines, hyperactivity, chronic neck and back pain, TMJ pain and dysfunction, chronic fatigue, eye difficulties, stress and tension-related problems, scoliosis, emotional difficulties, motor-coordination impairments, central nervous system disorders, learning disabilities, childhood developmental disabilities, and many others.

—*Kenneth I. Frey, PT, Diplomate CST*

Resources:

Kenneth I. Frey, PT, Diplomate CST
Director, Institute of Physical Therapy
30 W. 60th St., Suite 1BC
New York, NY 10023
Tel: (212) 245-1700
World recognized for its clinical services and as a educational resource center in New York City dedicated to the application and development of advanced holistic physical therapies. Treatment integrates whole body evaluation and advanced manual therapies, clinical sciences, and therapeutic exercise.

The Upledger Institute, Inc.
11211 Prosperity Farms Rd., D-325
Palm Beach Gardens, FL 33410-3487
Tel: (800) 233-5880 ext. 9283
An educational and clinical resource center that integrates the best of conventional health care with advanced complementary techniques. Dedicated to the natural enhancement of health, it is recognized worldwide for its continuing education programs, clinical research, and therapeutic services.

Further Reading:

Claire, Thomas. *Bodywork*. New York: William Morrow, 1995.

Sutherland, William. *Teachings in the Science of Osteopathy*. Portland, OR: Rudra Press, 1990.

Upledger, John E., and Jon D. Vredevoogd. *CranioSacral Therapy*. Chicago: Eastland Press, 1983.

Upledger, John. *Your Inner Physician and You*. Berkeley, CA: North Atlantic Books, 1991.

The Growth of CranioSacral Therapy

Dr. Upledger is credited with introducing CranioSacral Therapy to a broad spectrum of the world's health care professionals representing diverse specialties. In 1985 he founded The Upledger Institute to educate the public and health care practitioners about the benefits of CranioSacral Therapy. To date, this health care resource center and clinic based in Palm Beach Gardens, Florida, has trained more than 25,000 health care practitioners worldwide in the use of CranioSacral Therapy. Alumni include osteopaths, medical doctors, psychiatrists, psychologists, dentists, physical therapists, occupational therapists, acupuncturists, doctors of chiropractic, nurse practitioners, massage therapists, and bodyworkers.

Network Chiropractic

Network chiropractic is a branch of chiropractic, a health care method that views all health as a result of the body's inability to express, relay, and distribute energy and information through the nervous system. Chiropractors aim to enable the brain and the body to better communicate through the elimination of disruptions in the central nervous system, which is housed in the protective bones of the spinal column. To do this, they use gentle manual pressure and adjustment to reduce muscular tension, skeletal torsion or twisting, and compression of the spinal cord or the nerves branching from it which may result in a disruption of the body's essential energy and information highway.

Network chiropractic is a form of chiropractic that seeks to develop the body's self-corrective mechanism. It is believed that this improvement will enhance a person's health, wellness, and quality of life.

Establishing a Network
Donald Epstein, D.CA., a 1977 graduate of New York Chiropractic College, developed this method of chiropractic, which has been researched through the Department of Anatomy and Neurobiology and Sociology at the College of Medicine at the University of California–Irvine, and at the University of Southern California, Department of Engineering. Epstein's method resulted from his efforts to incorporate many different approaches and theories into a single "network" of established chiropractic techniques. Also known as network spinal analysis, the system has been evolving since 1982 and is currently practiced by chiropractors under the trade name network chiropractic.

Enhancing Communication
Adjustment is a central technique of chiropractic doctors. Adjustment means using the hands to apply leverage and thrust to a joint to restore function to the joint or muscles, nerves, and tissue around the joint. This therapy relies on the body's ability to recover without surgery or drugs.

Network shares the historical philosophy of chiropractic, which is based on the concept that the information the body needs to function is conveyed through oscillation, or vibration. The nervous system coordinates all vibration through the body, relaying energy and information to all body parts, and influencing all body functions. Tension on the spinal cord or the nerves exiting from the spinal cord causes an energy disturbance. Network chiropractic seeks to enhance communication between the brain and the body through the correction (adjustment) of vertebral subluxations.

Network practitioners believe that subluxations are caused by physical, emotional, mental, or chemical stresses. In network care it is common for the body to express the energy unavailable to the body as spontaneous muscular movement, stretching, or the outward expression of emotion such as laughter or crying. This liberates the spine from the interference caused by the inability to effectively "move the energy" and circulates the body's information.

The Practice of Network Chiropractic
Before beginning sessions, the chiropractor will request that individuals complete a questionnaire that discusses the individual's physical, emotional, mental, and chemical stresses and history. The spine will be evaluated for posture, muscle tension patterns, tension in the extremities that may be related to spinal cord tension, range of motion, or the involvement of spinal motion with respiration. Some practitioners may utilize various noninvasive instrumentation to further assess the functioning of the nervous system. Spinal X rays are not routine, however, and are taken as indicated on an individual basis.

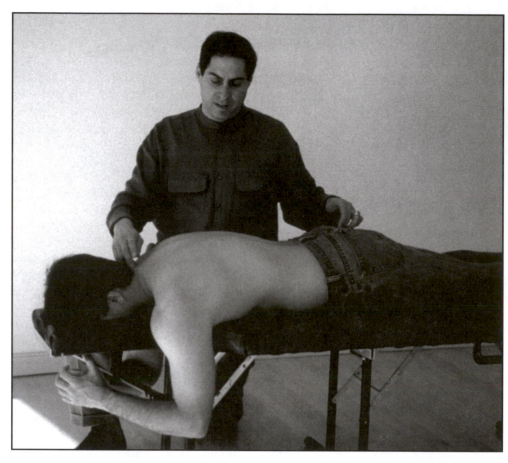

Photo: courtesy of Dr. Donald Epstein

Dr. Donald Epstein, founder of network chiropractic, demonstrates the light pressure techniques he developed to release tension.

A chiropractor's office usually contains a special device called an adjusting table, which allows patients to sit or lie in the optimal position for receiving care, whether that be faceup, facedown, seated, or on the side. Time spent on the adjusting table is often ten minutes or so—not an extended period.

Rather than addressing the structural misalignment as a primary distortion, the network practitioner views it as a protection for a spinal cord under tension. The doctor begins with light pressure applied to the tissue around the spine. Precise touch adjustments and touches are used to release tension in the spinal cord and to assist the body in recognizing the distortion and generate self-correction.

It is common that as tension is relieved from the spine a spontaneous release of emotional tension occurs. The practitioner will reassess the patient regularly, perhaps every two months, until the desired improvement has been made.

Benefits and Risks

Network chiropractic is one of the most nonaggressive types of adjustment available. Adjustments are not given in the areas of maximum tension, fixation, swelling, or pain. Most adjustments are very gentle. The practitioner is not seeking to inhibit the body or alter pain; instead, the objective is to enhance the body's own self-corrective, self-healing mechanism. For these reasons, network is considered a very safe application of chiropractic.

—Donald Epstein, D.CA.

Resources:

Association for Network Chiropractors
444 North Maine Street
Longmont, CO 80501
Tel: (303) 678-8101
Professional organization of network chiropractors.

International Chiropractors Association
1110 North Glebe Rd.
Suite 1000
Arlington, VA 22201
Tel: (703) 528-5000
Provides information on practitioners.

World Chiropractic Alliance
2950 N. Dobson Rd., Suite 1
Chandler, AZ 85224
Tel: (800) 347-1011
Promotes the practice of network chiropractic.

Further Reading:

Books:

Epstein, Donald, and Nathaniel Altman. *The Twelve Stages of Healing: A Network Approach to Wholeness.* San Rafael, CA: Amber-Allen Publishing, 1994.

Maynard, Joseph E. *Healing Hands: The Story of the Palmer Family, Discoverers and Developers of Chiropractic.* Fourth edition. Woodstock, GA: Jonorm Publishers, 1992.

Woodham and Peters. *Encyclopedia of Healing Therapies.* New York: DK Publishers, 1997.

Journals:
Journal of Vertebral Subluxation Research, Vol. 1, No. 1 (1996).

OSTEOPATHY

Osteopathy is a holistic and drugless approach to health and disease. It is based on the idea that a human being is not merely a collection of parts but a totality imbued with spirit. The human body functions as a unit and possesses self-healing and self-regulating mechanisms. Osteopathy maintains that there is a reciprocal relationship between structure and function, that is, an alteration in structure (the musculoskeletal system) through injury, will result in a change in function (in internal organs), namely, disease. Likewise, a diseased internal organ will result in an alteration in the musculoskeletal system. The osteopathic physician, by his or her intimate knowledge of human anatomy, can recognize even subtle deviations from normal bodily functioning and by the application of various techniques can restore the proper structure and function and assist the inherent self-healing powers of the body.

A Rejection of Conventional Medicine

The practice of osteopathy was developed by Andrew Taylor Still, M.D.

Health and Well-Being

The largest study of health and wellness benefits of a chiropractic method was performed at the University of California–Irvine. Patients evaluated their own improvements through a wide range of health and wellness indicators. The study showed evidence of significant improvement in the areas of physical symptoms, emotional and mental state, stress evaluation, life enjoyment and overall quality of life.

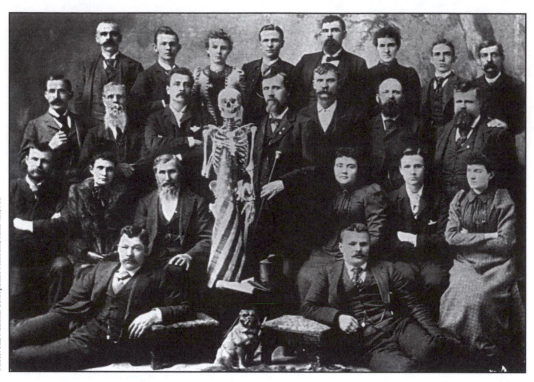

Photo: Still National Osteopathic Museum, Kirksville, MO

The first class of the American School of Osteopathy in Kirksville, Missouri, winter term (1892-1893).

(1828–1917), the son of an itinerant Methodist preacher who supported his family by farming and practicing medicine. It was during the time spent with his father tending to the medical needs of Native Americans that Still decided to take up medicine himself, under the guidance of his father. He studied the standard medical texts of the time, including ones on anatomy, physiology, pathology, surgery, and other topics.

Early on, Still became aware of the limitations of the medical practice of his day, particularly the almost total preoccupation of conventional, or "allopathic," medicine that focused on identifying symptoms and suppressing them. Still thought that this understanding of disease was crude at best and was based on vague notions of "physiological tension" that needed to be relieved by such devices as purging, bloodletting, and the administering of large doses of morphine, opium, alcohol, and mercury. Still believed that rather than treating only the symptoms

of a disease with such agents, a doctor should attempt to discover the cause of the disease itself. He originated the concept of wellness and developed principles of proper exercise and diet to prevent disease. He also created a system of manipulating various joints and tissues to realign the bones and muscles and thereby increase blood circulation and nerve functioning.

In the 1870s, in America, this holistic perspective was heresy. Still's early life provided many unfortunate opportunities to witness the shortcomings of conventional medicine. He lost his first wife and six children to infectious diseases of one kind or another. He saw the impotency of medical care during his service as an Army field surgeon and when he cared for Native Americans during epidemics. He had pneumonia for three months and took three years to recover from typhoid. In many ways osteopathy was Still's unique synthesis of his personal experience and several major intellectual and philosophical movements making their way across America during his lifetime.

Over the years Still continued to practice conventional medicine—including service as a surgeon in the Union army during the Civil War—and to develop his unique healing methods. He devised a system of manipulation and spinal reflexes with which he treated all types of conditions.

Despite his therapeutic successes he was viewed as a medical heretic, a grave robber, and a "crazy crank" because of his unorthodox views, study of corpses, long hours of solitary study, and casual dress. His methods obtained results that were seemingly inexplicable, so some viewed his practice as the work of the devil. In 1873, while living in Kirksville, Missouri, Still saved many lives during an epidemic of infectious diarrhea, without the use of any drugs. Despite this success, his reputation as an eccentric followed him and he was shunned by most until he cured a prominent Presbyterian minister's crippled daughter.

In 1874 Still severed his ties to conventional medicine and announced the founding of his new medical science, which he called osteopathy. This new school of medical thought was conceived as a reformation or improvement of conventional medicine, not an alternative system. During the 1880s he continued to refine his science and made several attempts to train others. Although he initially had trouble training others in the practice of osteopathy, Still hoped to establish an osteopathic school. During this time patients flocked to Kirksville from all over America for his treatment. Hotels were built in the town to house the many patients arriving daily, and several railroad companies advertised train service to Kirksville.

On November 1, 1892, the American School of Osteopathy was opened. The first class of eleven students consisted of former patients, family friends, and five of Still's children. Five women were among the members of this first class,

and Still was later reported to have said that he thought women made better osteopaths than men.

Still was assisted in his teaching by William Smith, M.D., an 1889 graduate of the University of Edinburgh. After one year Still determined that for the most part his attempt to teach osteopathy was a failure. He issued certificates but beseeched the graduates to return for another year of instruction. Some did not return.

However, in 1893, Still did receive some confirmation that his method could be successfully learned when two of his sons saved many lives during a black diphtheria epidemic in Minnesota. Graduation for those members of the first class who had returned was held on March 4, 1894. Slowly, the curriculum improved, more and better students graduated, and an infirmary was built in 1895. In that year Still and his students performed thirty thousand osteopathic treatments. By the late 1890s his school, infirmary, and new surgical hospital were increasingly successful, both academically and financially.

In its struggle for acceptance, organized osteopathy had to battle the powerful American Medical Association, which sought to maintain its control of the practice of medicine in America. Denied the right to serve as physicians in the military and other government jobs, the osteopathic profession lobbied hard for inclusion.

It wasn't until the Vietnam War that osteopaths were allowed to serve their country as physicians. Today there are seventeen osteopathic colleges. Some are state-supported schools where faculty and facilities are shared with students of allopathic medicine. Osteopathic physicians can now practice in all medical and surgical specialties and serve in all branches of the military and government health service organizations.

The curriculum at osteopathic schools is identical to its allopathic counterpart with the exception that D.O.s learn osteopathic philosophy and manipulation. However, with equality comes paradox.

As the osteopathic curriculum improved over the years, it became more like conventional medicine. Today there are approximately 35,000 osteopathic physicians in practice in the United States. Only about 3 to 5 percent of osteopaths practice the original healing art as envisioned by Still. Yet the original osteopathic concept is powerful and has made a lasting impression on medicine throughout the world. Chiropractic, Rolfing, and CranioSacral therapy borrow heavily from much of Still's pioneering work.

The osteopathic concept has also spread worldwide. There are colleges in England, Canada, and Europe. To date, thirty-two countries have granted osteopathic physicians unlimited practice privileges, with an additional nine countries granting privileges limited to manipulation.

Holistic Approach to the Body

In many ways osteopathy was Still's unique synthesis of his personal experience and several major intellectual and philosophical movements that were making their way across America during his lifetime. He viewed disease as an effect of derangement from the anatomical perfection intended by God, the divine architect.

Still was most influenced by Herbert Spencer, a nineteenth-century British philosopher who coined the term "evolution" and influenced the thinking of Charles Darwin. In Still's philosophy of osteopathy one can find many of Spencer's ideas—the concepts of cause and effect, the relationship between structure and function, the holistic nature of humans, and the interrelatedness of parts. The fascinations with phrenology, spiritualism, and Mesmerism, prevalent in the nineteenth century, also had an influence on Still.

These systems theorized the existence of the flow of certain healing and self-regulating electromagnetic and spiritlike fluids in the body, and Still incorporated these concepts into his notion of the healing effects of an unimpeded flow of blood. According to Still, osteopathic manipulation could relieve the restrictions to the free flow of blood and nerve power by removing the bony dislocations and easing muscle contractions. Moreover, Still revealed to one of his students toward the end of his life that he was able to see the human aura, the human energy field.

Modern doctors of osteopathy take a holistic approach to the human body and mind and, accordingly, take a patient's emotional and mental states into consideration, as well as his or her physical condition. Osteopaths emphasize the interaction between the brain and nervous system and the musculoskeletal system, paying particular attention to the musculoskeletal system, which they believe influences all other organs and systems. They contend that physical and emotional disease is brought about by interrupted nerve flow caused by muscle spasms, injury, or improper alignment of the spine and other bones. By applying hands-on manipulation, palpation, and other physical therapies to the spine, bones, muscles, and connective tissues, D.O.s (doctors of osteopathy) treat a variety of disorders.

Experiencing Osteopathy

A typical office session with an osteopath begins by taking a history of the current problem, including all medications or other therapies being used. This is augmented to include all past medical and surgical treatments and, especially, any physical or emotional traumas. Family and occupational histories are also obtained. In the case of an infant or child, the medical history includes the details of the pregnancy, labor, delivery, and perinatal period for that individual, and questions about developmental milestones are asked. Next comes a physical exam based on the patient's history, and laboratory and imaging studies (X rays, CT scans) may be ordered if appropriate.

In addition, the osteopathic physician performs either a regional (focusing just on the problem area) or a complete body examination, searching for areas of somatic (body) dysfunction, that is, impaired or altered functioning of parts of the musculoskeletal system. The dysfunction may lie in bone, joint, fascia, and muscle, or in related vascular, lymphatic, cerebrospinal, and neural elements. Once a diagnosis is made, treatment can begin. The entire body may be treated with a wide variety of natural techniques, using varying degrees of force according to the nature of the problem and the patient. Any point on or within the body that can be reached with the hands can be treated osteopathically.

The treatments are given on a padded table to a patient wearing comfortable, loose-fitting clothing (although the patient may have to undress partially for the initial screening examination). If it is performed properly, there is no contraindication for osteopathic manipulative treatment.

In osteopathic hospitals treatments are given to patients in intensive care units, emergency rooms, labor and delivery rooms, and newborn nurseries, as well as in general medical and surgical units. After the first session the patient's condition and treatment plan are discussed. Return visits are scheduled based on the individual's response to the first treatment and not on a fixed or routine schedule.

—*Dr. Domenick Masiello*

Resources:

American Association of College of Osteopathic Medicine (AACOM)
5550 Friendship Blvd. Suite 310
Chevy Chase, MD 20815-7231
Web site: http://www.aacom.org
Promotes the study of osteopathic medicine. Provides information on the seventeen osteopathic schools in the United States.

American Osteopathic Association (AOA)
142 E. Ontario St.
Chicago, IL 60611
Tel: (800) 621-1773, ext. 7401
Fax: (312) 280–3860
Web site: www.am-osteo-assn.org
Offers educational and professional support to osteopathic physicians.

Further Reading:

Gevitz, Norman. *The D.O.'s: Osteopathic Medicine in America.* Baltimore: Johns Hopkins Press, 1982.

Hildreth, Arthur Grant. *The Lengthening Shadow of Dr. A.T. Still.* 3rd ed. Kirksville, MO: Osteopathic Enterprise, 1988.

Magoun, Harold Ives, Sr. *Osteopathy in the Cranial Field.* 3rd ed. Kirksville, MO: Journal Printing Company, 1976.

Still, A. T. *Autobiography.* Kirksville, MO: privately printed, 1897.

Popularity of Osteopathy

There are currently around 35,000 osteopathic physicians in the United States, yet only about 500 osteopaths practice the original healing art, as many use manipulation techniques merely as an adjunct to their conventional practices. Nevertheless, the original osteopathic concept has made a lasting impression on medicine throughout the world. Osteopathic and conventional forms of research have validated and confirmed many of Still's original ideas. Today even the conventional medical world has many manual medicine societies, and the specialties of psychiatry and rehabilitation medicine benefit from Still's pioneering work. The osteopathic concept has also spread worldwide. There are colleges in England, Canada, and continental Europe. To date, thirty-two countries have granted osteopathic physicians unlimited practice privileges, with an additional nine countries granting privileges limited to manipulation techniques.

———. *Philosophy of Osteopathy.* Kirksville, MO: privately printed, 1899.

———. *Philosophy and Mechanical Principles of Osteopathy.* Kirksville, MO: privately printed, 1902.

———. *Osteopathy: Research and Practice.* Kirksville, MO: privately printed, 1910.

Still, Charles F., Jr. *Frontier Doctor, Medical Pioneer: The Life and Times of A.T. Still and His Family.* Kirksville, MO: The Thomas Jefferson University Press, 1991.

Sutherland, William Garner, and Ann L. Wales, eds. *Teachings in the Science of Osteopathy.* Fort Worth, TX: Sutherland Cranial Teaching Foundation, Inc., 1990.

Trowbridge, Carol. *Andrew Taylor Still: 1828–1917.* Kirksville, MO: The Thomas Jefferson University Press, 1991.

Ward, Robert C., ed. *Foundations for Osteopathic Medicine.* Baltimore: Williams & Wilkins, 1997.

ZERO BALANCING®

Zero Balancing® (ZB) is a hands-on body-balancing and integrating approach that aligns body energy fields with body structure. ZB is based on the Western understanding of anatomy and physiology but is distinct in that it uses Eastern concepts of energy as working tools as well as guiding principles for the integration of the whole person. Alignment through ZB balances body energy and structure, creates clearer fields of vibration throughout the body, releases tension patterns from the body tissue, the mind, and the emotions, and allows the vibration of stress to pass more freely through the person.

The History of Zero Balancing®
Fritz Frederick Smith, M.D., developed the system of Zero Balancing over several years. The son of a prominent chiropractor, Smith trained as an osteopath and medical doctor in the 1950s, and later as a five element acupuncturist with Professor J. R. Worsley. He was also a student of shakti yoga as taught by Swami Muktananda, a massage therapist and certified Rolfer (while he was studying with Ida Rolf he was her model for seven of the ten-hour sessions). Out of these various experiences he formulated his own distinct set of ideas and techniques that later became known as Zero Balancing.

The Basic Principles of ZB
According to Dr. Smith, Zero Balancing draws from Eastern concepts of energy and yet is fully consistent with contemporary quantum physics and the viewpoint that matter is composed of both particle and wave. In ZB the practitioner considers both of these components as they are found in the body—particle is represented by structure or matter, and wave by energy or vibration. If we compared the body to a sailboat, the sail would represent the structure and the wind the energy. ZB focuses on the interface and relationship of where the wind meets the sail—where the energy meets structure within the body and mind—knowing on another level that all these aspects are forms of energy.

Smith postulates that the strongest fields of energy are in the bones of the skeletal system. This is the densest tissue in the body and therefore entraps the densest energy of the body. Whereas ZB also addresses soft tissue, its main focus is on the skeletal system. Within the skeletal system its main focus is on the foundation and semi-foundation joints of the body—those joints that have more to do with the transmission, absorption, and equalization of energy in the body than with locomotion or movement. Examples of these joints are the sacroiliac joints, the tarsal and carpal joints of the feet and hands, and the inter- and costo-vertebral articulations of the spine.

In addition to being intimately involved with energy forces in the body, these joints have several other characteristics that make them especially important in energy medicine. They have small ranges of motion, and when they become compromised in function the body tends to compensate around the dysfunction rather than resolve it directly. The compensatory patterns that result impact not only the physical body but the mind, emotions, and spirit as well. This means that these joints (and other tissues that hold vibration) can lock imbalances within the whole person. Many of these imbalances are at first subtle and do not come to the level of a person's awareness until symptoms (such as muscle pulls, increasing irritability, stress burnout) have ensued and magnified the problem. The structural/energetic work of ZB can release these patterns while they are still hidden from awareness and before they create symptoms. ZB can also improve the fundamental imbalance after a person develops symptoms and create a climate in which nature can improve or heal the person's complaint.

ZB is taught as a postgraduate studies program for the health care practitioner. It is not designed as a start-up program for the beginning student of health care. A program of training has been established; the graduate of the program receives in-house recognition as a certified Zero Balancer and is given permission to use the registered trademark of ZB. It is not designed or intended to give the student any specific legal recognition or permission to work in the health care field. ZB is practiced under the umbrella of other health care studies.

ZB in Practice

The Zone Balancer assesses the body by testing and evaluating the currents and/or stagnation of energy within bone, within the foundation joints of the skeleton, and within certain soft tissues of the body. In places where the energy and structure are not well balanced, the ZBer uses touch to create a fulcrum or balance point in the tissue. When this balancing field of tension is held stationary for a few seconds it allows the two variables—energy and structure—to reorganize in terms of each other. Improved function, movement of energy, and feelings of well-being ensue. By repeated use of fulcra, placed properly and where necessary, the skilled Zero Balancing practitioner can balance a person in terms of the person's own energy and structure.

A typical ZB session requires about thirty to forty minutes and is done with a person fully clothed. It is done in two positions, with a person first sitting and then lying on his back, comfortably, on a massage table. Everything in ZB should either feel good to the client or "hurt good." If any of the Zero Balancing is

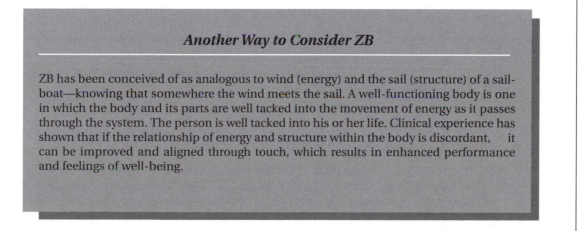

Another Way to Consider ZB

ZB has been conceived of as analogous to wind (energy) and the sail (structure) of a sailboat—knowing that somewhere the wind meets the sail. A well-functioning body is one in which the body and its parts are well tacked into the movement of energy as it passes through the system. The person is well tacked into his or her life. Clinical experience has shown that if the relationship of energy and structure within the body is discordant, it can be improved and aligned through touch, which results in enhanced performance and feelings of well-being.

ever uncomfortable or "hurts bad," the client should notify the ZBer.

Why Practice ZB?

Zone Balancing's major strength arises from the ability to balance and integrate a person in terms of his or her own body energy and body structure. This ability comes from integrating Eastern concepts of energy as working principles and tools into the practice of body handling. ZB is extremely effective in relieving stress and assisting a person as he or she is going through stressful periods in life. When a person is well balanced between energy and structure, the vibration of stress passes through the body more easily and has less tendency to become stuck, to cause tension patterns, and to progress to physical or emotional dysfunction. ZB also has a particularly important place in relieving pain and suffering if they are the result of blocked energy.

Of course, like any system of balancing or healing, it is not always the appropriate therapy for a given situation. The ZBer is schooled as to where ZB is of particular value, as to specific risks for the use of ZB, and to situations where a medical opinion is mandatory. ZBing is not meant to delay or replace standard medical care, but rather is an adjunct to high-level function and feelings of well-being.

—*Fritz Smith, M.D.*

Resources:

Zero Balancing® Association
P.O. Box 1727
Capitola, CA 95010
Tel/fax: (408) 476-0665
e-mail: zbaoffice@aol.com
Web site: www.zba.com
Conducts training programs throughout North America. Continuing education credit is granted for most programs by the Board of Nurses (California), Acupuncture Committee (California), and the National Certification Board for Therapeutic Massage and Bodywork [NCBTMB].

Further Reading:

Smith, Fritz Frederick, M.D. *Inner Bridges: A Guide to Energy Movement and Body.* Atlanta: Humanics New Age, 1990.

PART III: NUTRITIONAL AND DIETARY PRACTICES

Herbal Medicine • Orthomolecular Medicine

Nutritional and dietary practices are body-mind disciplines that adhere to the popular adage, "You are what you eat." Advocates of these practices believe that everything you ingest becomes a part of you, affecting your physical health, mental abilities, and emotional outlook. Nutritional and dietary practices are some of the oldest body-mind disciplines known to humankind. Although there are many specific practices popular today, this section examines one ancient and one modern practice currently used to maintain wellness, prevent disease, and treat specific conditions, both chronic and acute.

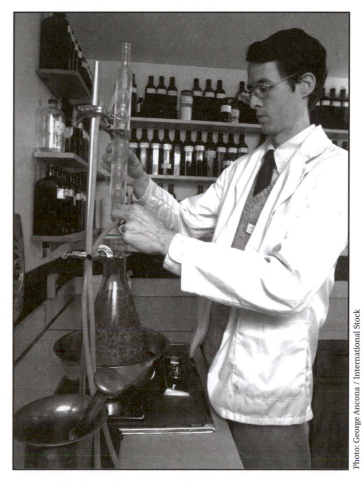

Herbs are the primary ingredient in many commercial pharmaceuticals.

Photo: George Ancona / International Stock

The Development of Nutritional and Dietary Practices

The roots of nutritional and dietary practices are firmly planted in the deepest biological and psychological instincts of the human race. When ill, humans and many other animals instinctively fast, which cleanses and rests the digestive system. In addition, animals have been observed in their natural environments searching out and eating specific plants for medicinal purposes.

Indigenous peoples also use plants from their surrounding environment for medicinal purposes. Much of our knowledge of herbal medicine comes from anthropologists who have lived with these peoples and learned their age-old wisdom. The diets of these peoples invariably include a variety of fruits, vegetables, grains, and sometimes animal products native to their area. These locally produced diets create a chemical balance within each person's body and between the people and their environment.

Nutritional practices and herbal medicine form an integral part of all classical healing systems. Both ayurvedic and traditional Chinese medicine doctors diagnose patients, in part, by knowledge of their dietary preferences and cravings. Both systems prescribe dietary changes and herbal medicines to balance the body-mind disharmonies they perceive through their diagnostic methods. Like those of indigenous peoples, both of these highly developed healing systems are based on a belief that disharmony of body and mind, or of the body-mind complex and the surrounding environment, is the root cause of disease.

In classical Greece, where the modern Western healing system originated, the physician Hippocrates (c. 460–c. 377 BCE) also believed in health as a balance between the individual and his or her environment. Discussing the prescription of food as medicine, Hippocrates is believed to have said, "Food or drink which is in itself slightly inferior, but more pleasant should be preferred to that which is better in itself, but less pleasant." In this recommendation Hippocrates seems to affirm not only a belief that food could be used as medicine, but that the human organism has the innate ability to direct its own healing, in part at least, through the sense of taste.

Throughout European history people continued to rely on their sense of taste to develop a varied, balanced, moderate diet that made use of local fruits, grains, and animal products. They also used various herbs and foods to heal specific conditions. For example, garlic has been used by people in many European countries for centuries to heal infections. Chamomile tea has long been recommended to calm the nerves.

The French chemist Louis Pasteur (1822–1895) was the first person to see bacteria under a microscope. This momentous discovery led to many innovations in Western health care including sterilization of surgical instruments, hygienic standards of cleanliness in hospitals, and the process known as pasteurization of milk and other liquids. It also led to the development of the germ theory of disease in which all disease was believed to be caused by outside organisms invading the human body.

In order to fight the outside invaders, biochemists developed an arsenal of antibiotics and other pharmaceutical germ-killers. These medicines appeared to work more quickly and to be more effective than the traditional dietary and herbal cures. Doctors began to pay less and less attention to the diet of their patients. Instead they began to rely more and more on a growing stockpile of synthesized drugs to relieve painful and uncomfortable symptoms.

Throughout the nineteenth and early twentieth centuries there were many voices of dissent against this shift away from natural whole-food diets and toward dependence on pharmaceutical drugs for healing. Some of those voices, such as that of American doctor Sylvester Graham (1794–1851), were dismissed as alarmists by allopathic, or conventional Western, doctors. Other individuals such as Japanese doctor Michio Kushi, a leading proponent of macrobiotics, were dismissed as exotic and extremist.

In the mid-twentieth century scientists such as two-time Nobel Prize winner Linus Pauling (1901–1994) began using Western biochemical methods to study the effects of the individual vitamins found in foods on various physical, mental, and emotional conditions. The discoveries made by Pauling and other scientists form the basis of orthomolecular medicine, a contemporary scientific nutritional practice that recommends individualized whole food diets and high doses of vitamins instead of drugs to heal disease and create optimum health.

In the 1960s a growing number of people became increasingly disillusioned with the use of pharmaceutical drugs. Some people felt, as many feel today, that the drugs are costly, increasingly ineffective, and that they often produce as many side effects and complications as they appear to cure. For these reasons many individuals, and eventually the U.S. government through the National Institutes of Health, began to reconsider nutritional and dietary practices as a safe and effective means of disease prevention and health care.

Eating to Maintain the Body's Natural Chemical Balance

The basic theoretical foundation of all dietary and nutritional practices is the belief that whatever we take into our bodies will affect our bodies. If we eat a diet that maintains the natural chemical balance of our cells and provides for extra vitamins and minerals in times of stress or high demand, we will remain healthy. However, if we don't eat a balanced diet we may create an imbalance in our cellular chemistry. This may lead our organs and systems to malfunction and eventually may lead to disease and illness.

Many scientific studies conducted by the National Institutes of Health and private foundations such as the National Cancer Institute have pointed to a strong connection linking diets high in fats, especially saturated fats, and low in fiber to diseases and conditions such as coronary artery disease, strokes, diabetes, high blood pressure, and breast and colon cancer. Conversely, changes in diet or eating specific herbs and nutrients seem to activate the body's natural defenses, enabling it to heal itself. Today scientists are looking at whole foods, specific vitamins, and herbs to discover, in scientific terms, how diet can prevent and cure illnesses. Among the things they have discovered are that orange and dark green vegetables like carrots, sweet potatoes, pumpkins, spinach, broccoli, and kale, which all contain high levels of beta carotene, seem to help prevent certain kinds of cancer. High doses of vitamin B_3 (niacin) have been used with positive results to help people suffering from a variety of mental and emotional symptoms often diagnosed as schizophrenia. And *Hypericum perforatum*, more commonly known as St. John's wort, seems to be a safe and effective remedy against mild to moderate depressions.

Nutritional and Dietary Methods in Practice

Many different nutritional and dietary practices are in use today. Naturopaths, traditional Chinese medicine doctors, ayurvedic physicians, osteopaths, chiropractors, and bodyworkers may prescribe or suggest nutritional or dietary practices during a course of treatment. Herbalists and orthomolecular physicians are two types of practitioners who focus specifically on dietary or herbal practices as a means of maintaining health and curing disease.

A visit to one of these practitioners can be like a visit to a general practitioner. Both will want to know about the nature of your problems and information about your diet. The orthomolecular physician may make use of tests, whereas the herbalist may rely more on his or her physical observations and questioning of you to arrive at a diagnosis.

Once diagnosed, both will probably recommend changes in your diet and prescribe specific supplements. An herbalist may recommend that you buy a specific herb or combination of herbs that can be prepared and eaten in various ways, whereas the orthomolecular physician may recommend various doses of vitamins. Whichever practice you follow, these practitioners work with you and your other health care professionals to help you attain your maximum state of health.

Learning About Your Body

Like other body-mind disciplines, nutritional and dietary practices require that you take responsibility for your own health and healing. After all, an herbalist or orthomolecular physician can prescribe a course of treatment, but no one can make you prepare the prescription or take it!

Some people enjoy the heightened awareness of the body-mind connection that develops over time as they participate in a particular dietary or nutritional practice. Others find the process cumbersome, time consuming, or too restrictive. In addition, some people find the scents and tastes of various herbal cures unpleasant, whereas others enjoy the experience of preparing their own remedies and tonics.

Nutritional and dietary practices are designed to balance your body chemistry in order to develop its natural resilience and resistance to disease. After working with a dietary or nutrition professional, balancing your body chemistry, and becoming more knowledgeable about your nutritional needs, you may formulate a delicious and enjoyable diet that will help you heal minor ailments, prevent disease, and create optimum health of both body and mind.

—Nancy Allison, CMA

Resources:

American Botanical Council (ABC)
P.O. Box 201660
Austin, TX 78720-1660
Tel:(800) 373-7105
Fax:(512) 331-1924
e-mail: custserv@herbalgram.org
Web site: www.herbalgram.org
Nonprofit research and educational organization. Offers a quarterly magazine called HerbalGram, *which publishes the latest herbal research, legal and regulatory issues regarding herbal medicine, detailed profiles of herbs, conference reports, and book reviews.*

The International Society for Orthomolecular Medicine
16 Florence Avenue
Toronto, ON M2N 1E9
Canada
e-mail: centre@orthomed.org

Web site: www.orthomed.org
Founded in 1994, this organization lists and recommends orthomolecular practitioners in Canada. Also publishes the periodical Journal of Orthomolecular Medicine.

Further Reading:

Books:
Gladstar, Rosemary. *Herbal Healing for Women.* New York: Simon & Schuster, 1993.

Kowalchik, Claire, and Hylton Williams, eds. *Rodale's Illustrated Encyclopedia of Herbs.* Emmaus, PA: Rodale Press,1987.

Santillo, Humbert B.S., MH. *Natural Healing with Herbs.* Prescott Valley, AZ: Hohm Press, 1984.

Journals:
Willoughby, John, "Primal Prescription." *Eating Well ™ Inc.* (May-June 1991).

HERBAL MEDICINE

Herbal medicine has become one of the most popular forms of alternative medicine in the United States today. People use herbal remedies for a variety of reasons: to aid digestion; to relax; to alleviate minor aches, pains, and headaches; to stave off disease; and to diminish the symptoms of the common cold or flu. Besides addressing specific symptoms or needs, some herbalists believe that these remedies bring the body and mind into balance and can therefore cure chronic or long-term illnesses.

Herbal Medicine Throughout the Ages

Herbal remedies have been utilized in many cultures throughout time to alleviate pain and cure disease. The ways that herbs are used in diverse geographical areas reflect the philosophy and values of each particular culture as well as what herbs are available in each region. For instance, in traditional Chinese medicine, herbs are used to restore balance in the body and are part of a long-term treatment that seeks to maintain the health of both mind and body. In Western medicine, herbal medications have been developed to treat particular physical symptoms immediately. This pharmacologically based system has been especially successful in the treatment of acute illness.

Herbs form the basis of many modern pharmaceutical drugs. Today, about 25 percent of all prescription medicines are derived from medicinal plants. Pharmaceutical companies are doing research on herbs from the Brazilian rain forests. In fact, the word *drug* derives from the old Dutch word *droge,* which means "to dry." During the Middle Ages, Dutch pharmacists dried plants for use as medicines.

In 1994 an estimated 17 percent of all Americans used herbs for some medicinal or health reason. The herbal industry is estimated to have earned $2 billion in sales in the United States in 1996, and sales are increasing at the rate of about 25 percent per year. A poll conducted in early 1997 indicated that one-third of adult Americans are using herbal medicines, spending an average of $54 per person annually, thus creating a total estimated retail market of $3.24 billion. Once found only in health food stores, mail-order catalogs, and marketing organizations, herbal medicines are now sold in drugstores, supermarkets, and mass-market retailers, where herbal preparations constitute one of the fastest growing areas.

Increased popular interest in herbs has been fueled in part by the passage of the Dietary Supplement Health and Education Act of 1994 (DSHEA). In 1993 and 1994, when the act was being considered, Congress received more mail from American voters concerning this new law than they had concerning any other single issue since the Vietnam War. This overwhelming response suggests that consumers are interested in using herbs and other dietary supplements for their health.

In addition, the heightened interest in herbal medicine reflects consumer concern about the high cost of Western medicine in general and pharmaceutical drugs in particular. Further, there is a growing perception among consumers that many conventional medicines are toxic and produce adverse side effects, despite the fact that they have been approved by the Food and Drug Administration (FDA). These concerns have revived interest in many traditional herbs and medicinal plants, as well as other forms of alternative medicine. Many Americans have also become interested in this area because of the increased media coverage in alternative medicine and the creation of the Office of Alternative Medicine (OAM) at the National Institutes of Health (NIH) to study herbs and other alternative modalities.

A Description of Herbal Medicines

Herbs are popular all over the world. The World Health Organization (WHO)

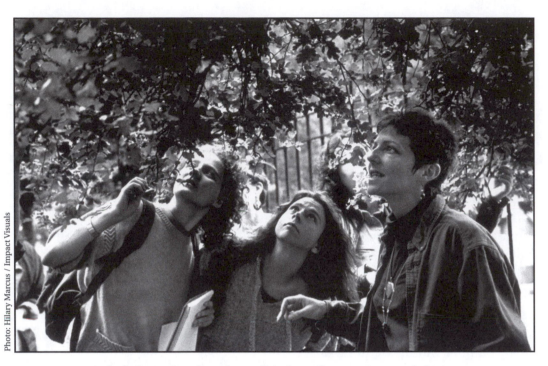

Photo: Hilary Marcus / Impact Visuals

An herbalist teaches about the medicinal use of common trees and plants.

estimates that about 80 percent of people in developing countries still rely on some form of traditional medicine for primary health care. In every type of traditional medicine, that is, medicine based on historical uses and used by indigenous cultures, herbs and medicinal plants constitute the major basis for the remedies used.

In a very real sense, herbs are not alternative medicine; they are integral to the development of all medicinal systems, both modern and traditional. Despite the fact that many modern drugs are derived from plants, there is a major distinction between a plant-derived drug (e.g., quinine) and an herbal medicine. Plant-derived drugs are single chemical compounds that are extracted and purified from plants. Herbal medicines, on the other hand, can be defined as a whole plant or plant part that is used for its medicinal properties. Thus, an herbal remedy contains small amounts of many naturally occurring chemicals from the plant.

Most herbal medicines are used for minor, self-limiting conditions or illnesses.

Herbal medicines can be as simple as a cup of chamomile tea (*Matricaria recutita*) to help digestion after a big meal, to ease an upset stomach, or to help as a relaxing beverage before bedtime. Other simple herbal medicines include an extract of the roots or leaves of echinacea (*Echinacea* spp.) to help reduce the severity or duration of a cold or flu, especially when taken at the onset of symptoms; the use of feverfew leaf (*Tanacetum parthenium*) to allay migraine headaches; and valerian root (*Valeriana officinalis*) to help assure a good night's sleep, especially for persons with insomnia or other sleep disorders.

Today many people are also using herbs to help prevent long-term illness. Cardiovascular disease is the the biggest killer of all Americans. Millions of Americans are turning to such simple remedies as garlic (*Allium sativum*) to help reduce cardiovascular risk factors. In fact, the German government approves garlic for such use, including lowering of the LDL cholesterol, known as the "bad" cholesterol—a property of garlic that has been documented in more than two dozen clinical studies. Because the German government allows such claims on garlic tablets, garlic is the biggest-selling over-the-counter medicine sold in German pharmacies.

Another increasingly popular use for herbs is as alternatives to modern synthetic prescription drugs. Millions of American men have begun to use the extract of the fruits of the native American saw palmetto plant (*Serenoa repens*) as a safe and clinically documented remedy for benign prostatic hyperplasia (BPH), nonmalignant enlargement of the prostate that affects about half of men over fifty years of age. Gaining popularity is the standardized extract of St. John's wort (*Hypericum perforatum*), which is considered a safe and effective remedy for mild to moderate depression. The efficacy of this herb, called a phytomedicine in Europe, has been established in numerous clinical studies.

There are many more examples. Standardized extract of ginkgo leaf (*Ginkgo biloba*) has been shown in many clinical studies to be safe and effective in stimulating peripheral circulation, especially in the brain. This herb is especially useful in geriatric care to help treat senile dementia and short-term memory loss in elderly patients. Another useful phytomedicine is the standardized extract of milk thistle fruits (*Silybum marianum*). This preparation is a safe and effective tonic to the liver, especially for persons who suffer from alcohol-induced cirrhosis of the liver, who have been exposed to toxic industrial chemicals, or who suffer from certain types of hepatitis.

How Herbal Remedies Are Used

Herbal medicines can be taken as teas that have been either steeped or boiled in water, known as an infusion and decoction, respectively. They can be ingested as powdered herbs in capsules and tablets, or as liquid extracts made with water and alcohol or just alcohol. They can also be taken as standardized extracts, which have recently been developed. In these extracts, the level of one naturally occurring chemical compound or group of compounds is chemically guaranteed from one batch to another in order to ensure reliable content.

Herbs can also be used topically. Fresh aloe gel (*Aloe vera*) can be directly applied to the skin to help reduce the

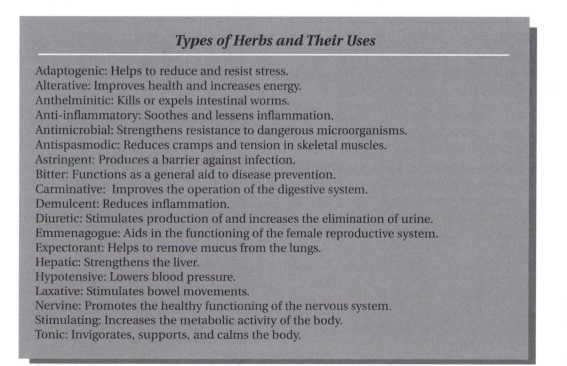

Types of Herbs and Their Uses

Adaptogenic: Helps to reduce and resist stress.
Alterative: Improves health and increases energy.
Anthelminitic: Kills or expels intestinal worms.
Anti-inflammatory: Soothes and lessens inflammation.
Antimicrobial: Strengthens resistance to dangerous microorganisms.
Antispasmodic: Reduces cramps and tension in skeletal muscles.
Astringent: Produces a barrier against infection.
Bitter: Functions as a general aid to disease prevention.
Carminative: Improves the operation of the digestive system.
Demulcent: Reduces inflammation.
Diuretic: Stimulates production of and increases the elimination of urine.
Emmenagogue: Aids in the functioning of the female reproductive system.
Expectorant: Helps to remove mucus from the lungs.
Hepatic: Strengthens the liver.
Hypotensive: Lowers blood pressure.
Laxative: Stimulates bowel movements.
Nervine: Promotes the healthy functioning of the nervous system.
Stimulating: Increases the metabolic activity of the body.
Tonic: Invigorates, supports, and calms the body.

pain of a minor burn or sunburn. Aloe is used as an ingredient in sunburn creams, skin lotions, and even shaving creams—all of which attests to the popularity and widespread acceptance of the healing dermatological properties of this plant recognized since ancient times. In addition, in Germany many skin-care products rely on extracts of chamomile for their scientifically proven skin-healing properties. Also in Germany, manufacturers sell echinacea products intended for external use for slow-healing wounds.

Enduring Popularity of Herbal Medicine

A qualified herbalist or a well-respected herbal guide or specialist should be consulted for the most effective herbal treatment. Herbs have certain qualities and must be used with care. Like conventional drugs, they are not recommended in every instance. For example, the herb ephedra (*Ephedra sinia,* commonly called by its Chinese name, ma huang), functions as a stimulant and is not recommended for those with high blood pressure, diabetes, glaucoma, and related conditions where hypertensives are contraindicated.

The world of plants is rich and diversified and produces numerous herbal remedies that have been used for thousands of years. Modern scientific research continues to document and validate the historical traditional uses of many herbs as well as new uses of some traditional medicines. The safe and responsible use of herbal medicines offers an important way to lower health care costs and increase the wellness of the American public. It is most likely that more scientific research will continue to place herbs in a position to offer many benefits in the new medicine of the twenty-first century.

—*Mark Blumenthal*

Resources:

American Botanical Council (ABC)
P.O. Box 201660

Austin, TX 78720-1660
Tel: 1-800-373-7105
Fax: (512) 331-1924
e-mail: custserv@herbalgram.org
Web site: www.herbalgram.org
Leading nonprofit research and educational organization. Offers a quarterly magazine called HerbalGram, *which publishes the latest herbal research, legal and regulatory issues regarding herbal medicine, detailed profiles of herbs, conference reports, and book reviews.*

American Herbalists Guild
P.O. Box 1683
Sequel, CA 95073
Provides a directory of schools and teachers of herbal medicine.

Further Reading:

Castleman, Michael. *The Healing Herbs.* Emmaus, PA: Rodale Press, 1991.

Foster, Steven. *50 Herbs for Your Health.* Loveland, CO: Interweave Press, 1996.

Hoffmann, David. *The New Holistic Herbal.* Rockport, MA: Element Books, 1992.

Tierra, Leslie. *The Herbs of Life.* Freedom, CA: Crossing Press, 1992.

ORTHOMOLECULAR MEDICINE

Orthomolecular medicine strives to achieve optimum health of its patients, as well as treat and prevent disease, by creating the uniquely individual levels of nutrients needed in each body through diet, vitamin supplementation, and lifestyle changes. Practitioners employ what is more commonly known as megavitamin therapy, which is the use of large doses of certain vitamins based on thorough biochemical analysis to correct ineffective or destructive chemical balances in the body. Ortho-molecular medicine also addresses a variety of psychiatric disorders, such as schizophrenia and severe depression.

History of Orthomolecular Medicine

It was Linus Pauling, the two-time Nobel Prize winner (one for chemistry, the other for peace), who, in 1968, first coined the term *orthomolecular medicine* to describe more accurately what had been popularly known as megavitamin therapy.

Pauling's concept was to create an optimum nutritional micro-environment for every cell in the body by giving it the "right amounts of the right molecules"—vitamins, minerals, amino acids, enzymes, and other substances used by the body. This would not just correct the deficiencies or imbalances that make us more susceptible to disease and degeneration. It would also promote the highest level of health, enabling us to reach our physical, mental, and spiritual potential and enjoy a maximum life span. The path to this goal, according to Pauling, is accomplished through dietary changes and supplementation.

For many years before his death in 1994 at the age of ninety-three, Pauling was an outspoken champion of non-toxic therapies and nutritional supplementation. He attracted considerable attention—and controversy—with his books on the beneficial effects of vitamin C supplementation against the common cold and cancer.

Pauling formulated a modern nutritional paradigm—an approach emphasizing optimum intake of nutrients for achieving powerful prevention and healing benefits. Orthomolecular physicians have used this approach to successfully treat schizophrenia, depression, alcoholism, drug abuse, and individuals with gastrointestinal disorders, arthritis, cardiovascular disease, and even cancer.

During the first half of the twentieth century, there was much excitement and interest in vitamins because people believed that they were a quick way to good health. From 1925 to 1940, many were isolated from food, then identified and synthesized. Nutritional pioneers began exploring the clinical uses of these newly available substances and using amounts that were above the levels considered necessary to prevent deficiency-state diseases such as scurvy, beri-beri, and pellagra.

In North Carolina, a country doctor named Fred Klenner used large doses of vitamin C effectively against viral illness. The infants delivered by mothers on his supplement program were so robust and healthy that the local hospital staff nicknamed them the "vitamin C babies." In Canada, two physician brothers, Evan and Wilfrid Shute, found that vitamin E offered a valuable treatment against heart disease.

In the early 1950s, two other Canadian physicians, Abram Hoffer and Humphrey Osmond, began to use high doses of niacin (vitamin B_3) and other nutrients to help schizophrenic patients. The nutritional treatments they pioneered for a variety of mental conditions were later formalized into orthomolecular psychiatry.

Over the years, the orthomolecular arsenal has expanded dynamically from just a few vitamins. Today, it includes a broad spectrum of vitamins, minerals, amino acids, enzymes, hormones, and plant-derived supplements.

Many commentators believe that allopathic, or more conventional, medicine has given little respect to nutritional therapy in an age of pharmaceutical, surgical, and high-tech techniques. In the past, vitamins and minerals were considered necessary only in tiny amounts in order to prevent certain diseases; furthermore, conventional Western medical practitioners maintained that if people ate right, it would result in obtaining enough nutrients from food. As a result, conventional medical schools have not thoroughly educated their students about the role of nutrition in causing and healing disease.

Times may finally be changing. There is a growing interest in alternative treatments because of the cost and side effects of pharmaceuticals and the failings of modern conventional medicine to impact the crisis of chronic disease and runaway medical costs. A growing number of medical schools are offering programs in nontoxic treatments and clinical nutrition. In addition, there has been quite a bit of research proving that vitamin supplementation, at doses higher than those usually present in the diet, has a significant preventive and therapeutic effect and represents a potent, safe, and inexpensive medical option.

In 1992, the New York Academy of Science convened a landmark conference called "Beyond Deficiency: New Views on the Function and Health Effects of Vitamins." At this meeting, researchers presented new findings on the positive effects of vitamins and minerals against cancer, heart disease, and other illnesses. A joint United Nations and World Health Organization conference in 1996 on healthy aging reflected a growing recognition of nutrition in the fight against disease.

The Basic Principles of
Orthomolecular Medicine

"Let food be thy medicine and thy medicine be thy food," said Hippocrates to his students. More than 2,500 years later, this advice from the "father of medicine" has been overlooked, but not altogether ignored, by modern doctors using pharmaceutical drugs and sophisticated technology. Practitioners of alternative medicine, among them orthomolecular physicians, regard food and nutrition as the bedrock of their professions.

Orthos is a Greek word meaning "straight." Just as orthopedic medicine refers to the straightening of deformed or broken bones, and orthodontics to the straightening of crooked teeth, orthomolecular medicine literally means to straighten or correct the body's molecules.

Orthomolecular practitioners base their recommendations to patients on the concept of biochemical individuality, an idea put forward by Roger Williams, Ph.D., the University of Texas scientist who discovered vitamin B_5. This concept holds that each of us is uniquely different. We look different, react to stress and chemicals differently, live and work in different environments, have different genetic makeup, drink different water and eat different food, and have different requirements for various nutrients. Although the number of necessary nutrients is the same for each of us, the optimum amounts we need individually are very different.

For this fundamental reason, orthomolecular physicians regard the government-promoted RDAs (recommended daily allowances) and MDRs (minimum daily requirements) as irrelevant. "Even if 90 percent of any population required only the minimal daily requirement of

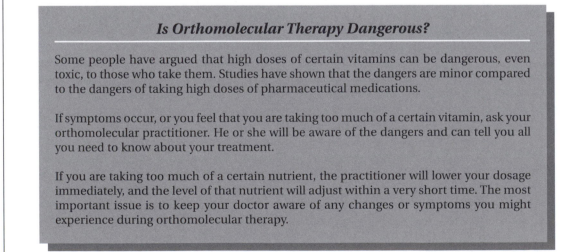

Is Orthomolecular Therapy Dangerous?

Some people have argued that high doses of certain vitamins can be dangerous, even toxic, to those who take them. Studies have shown that the dangers are minor compared to the dangers of taking high doses of pharmaceutical medications.

If symptoms occur, or you feel that you are taking too much of a certain vitamin, ask your orthomolecular practitioner. He or she will be aware of the dangers and can tell you all you need to know about your treatment.

If you are taking too much of a certain nutrient, the practitioner will lower your dosage immediately, and the level of that nutrient will adjust within a very short time. The most important issue is to keep your doctor aware of any changes or symptoms you might experience during orthomolecular therapy.

vitamins, it would leave huge numbers of people needing 10, 100, or 1,000 times as much," contends orthomolecular physician Abram Hoffer. "With sick people the range of need is many times greater."

The perspective of pioneers like Hoffer and other orthomolecular specialists is that their form of medicine is not a cure-all or a replacement for conventional treatment. Rather, explains Hoffer, "a proportion of patients will require orthodox treatment, a proportion will do better on orthomolecular treatment, and the rest will need a skillful blend of both."

How Orthomolecular Physicians Can Help

Orthomolecular physicians practice throughout the world. They are primarily medical doctors (M.D.s), but also osteopaths (D.O.s), naturopaths (NDs), and chiropractors (DCs).

Orthomolecular practitioners zero in on the individuality of patients through laboratory tests and comprehensive medical reviews that consider diet, stress, exercise, levels of sensitivity to foods or chemicals, and the use of alcohol, drugs, or pharmaceuticals. These tests are performed in a physician's office.

Recommendations typically involve not just nutritional supplements but also the elimination or reduction of drugs, contaminants, and allergens, and the replacement of junk food and nutrient-poor diets with complete, fresh, and nourishing diets.

Benefits and Risks

Orthomolecular medicine is beneficial for a wide range of physical and mental conditions, and its concepts are widely practiced by health-conscious individuals concerned about preventative care.

To get comprehensive and effective treatment, one should see an orthomolecular specialist first rather than trying to attempt self-treatment.

—*Martin Zucker*

Resources:

International Academy of Nutrition & Preventive Medicine
P.O. Box 18433
Asheville, NC 28814
Tel: (704) 258-3243
Offers a list of practitioners by state. Publishes the Journal of Applied Nutrition, *a quarterly journal that covers nutritional issues.*

The International Society for Orthomolecular Medicine
16 Florence Avenue
Toronto, ON M2N 1E9
Canada
e-mail: centre@orthomed.org
Web site: www.orthomed.org
Founded in 1994, this organization lists and recommends orthomolecular practitioners in Canada. Also publishes the periodical Journal of Orthomolecular Medicine.

The Society for Orthomolecular Medicine of America
2698 Pacific Avenue
San Francisco, CA 94115
Tel: (415) 922-6462
Provides information on orthomolecular practitioners in the United States.

Further Reading:

Hoffer, Abram, and Morton Walker. *Putting It All Together: The New Orthomolecular Nutrition.* New Canaan, CT: Keats Publishing, 1996.

Hoffer, Abram. *Orthomolecular Medicine for Physicians—A Survey/Introduction Textbook.* New Canaan, CT: Keats Publishing, 1989.

Janson, Michael. *The Vitamin Revolution in Health Care.* Greenville, NH: Arcadia Press, 1996.

Pauling, Linus. *Vitamin C and the Common Cold.* San Francisco: W. H. Freeman, 1970.

Pauling, Linus, with Ewan Cameron. *Cancer and Vitamin C.* New York: Linus Pauling Institute of Science and Medicine, 1979.

Part IV: Mind/Body Medicine

Biofeedback Training • Guided Imagery • Hypnotherapy • Interactive Guided Imagery[SM] • Psychoneuroimmunology

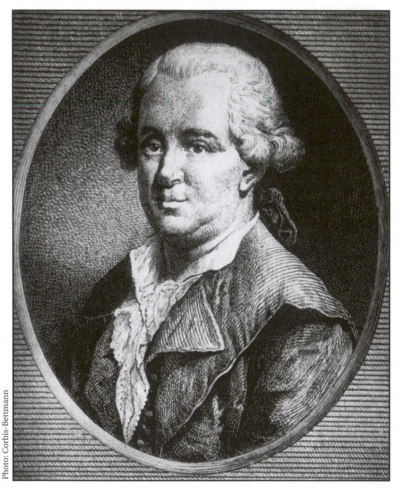

Photo: Corbis-Bettmann

Franz Anton Mesmer (1734–1815), now called the "Father of Hypnosis," was one of the earliest Western scientists to investigate the connection between body and mind.

Mind/body medicine is a contemporary term used to describe a number of disciplines that study or approach healing the physical body, or transforming human behavior, by engaging the conscious or unconscious powers of the mind. While "mind/body medicine" is a term used in this section of the encyclopedia to describe a growing field of study and practice in contemporary Western medicine, it is also used by others to describe ancient Eastern disciplines such as yoga, meditation, traditional Chinese medicine, and subtle energy therapies. The variety of disciplines that comprise mind/body medicine in this encyclopedia combine a theory of the relationship between body and mind that has much in common with these ancient Eastern disciplines with Western scientific models of biology and chemistry. These disciplines are also characterized by an emphasis on individual motivation in the healing process and a more personal relationship between caregiver and receiver. These practices have been used to treat stress-related conditions, such as chronic pain, allergies, chemical and emotional dependencies, and performance anxiety.

Mind/Body Medicine—Ancient and Modern

While the disciplines discussed in this section emerged from a context of contemporary Western science, the theories and techniques they use have much in common with approaches to healing developed by ancient cultures and still in use worldwide. Both ancient and modern approaches to mind/body medicine believe that the cause of disease is not restricted to the physical body. For ancient disciplines, the non-physical causes of disease may include spirits, emotions, or the mind, which bridges spirit and body. Contemporary Western methods of mind/body medicine attempt to understand the cause of disease by investigating the effect of thoughts or emotions on behavior and the physical workings of the body.

Shamanism, an ancient method of healing, is based on the belief that all illness is a result of disharmony between the spirit world and the material world. Traditional shamanic practices include trance states and mental focusing techniques similar to those used by hypnotherapy and guided imagery today.

The highly disciplined Indian practice of hatha yoga is driven by the belief that all matter is a materialized form of the one great spirit motivating the universe. It includes numerous health-enhancing physical exercises, internal cleansing techniques, and breathing practices to help people refine the physical body and experience its spiritual nature. Hatha yoga practitioners develop a control of the body similar to that developed through biofeedback today.

In China, healers practiced within the framework of the ancient Chinese religion of Taoism, which seeks a balanced, harmonious existence between humankind and nature. Over thousands of years, Chinese herbal treatments evolved by correlating observations of the interaction of elements in nature with the physical, emotional, and mental characteristics associated with human illnesses. The relationships Chinese healers noted between elemental balances, emotional states, and physical health are similar to those recognized by psychoneuroimmunology today.

The Development of Mind/Body Medicine in the West

While ancient Greek medical practices were originally holistic, ways of viewing the body began to change with the influence of the philosophical pragmatism of Aristotle (c.384–c.332 BCE) and his desire to know and categorize all aspects of the material world. Ancient Greeks began to separate the observation and treatment of matter, or body, from the observation and treatment of spirit, or mind. This trend in Western thinking and healing was later reinforced by the medieval Christian church, which glorified the devoted mind of humankind as the true channel to the spirit of God while denigrating the physical body as an instrument of the devil. In the seventeenth century, the French philosopher René Descartes helped establish the philosophical foundation of the Enlightenment by proclaiming the mind a non-material, transcendent aspect of human beings, to be separate and infinitely more valuable than the physical body.

Split off from philosophical or spiritual inquiry, Western medical science developed by studying the physical body and treating it as a purely mechanical instrument that could be broken down into smaller and more knowable components. While this approach yielded many amazing, lifesaving achievements over the last 300 years, it investigated only the physical treatment of ailments. The relationship of the mind and body was not fully investigated by Western medicine until the beginning of this century, gaining ever more momentum in the last thirty-five years. The neurologist Sigmund Freud's (1856–1939) theory of the unconscious mind opened new ways of considering the mind's effect on behavior and physical health. The research that inspired Freud's theories employed many of the techniques that are a part of hypnotherapy and guided imagery practices.

Throughout the twentieth century, data pointing to a relationship between our thoughts, emotions, and health began to appear from many branches of science, including sociology, anthropology, and psychology. For example, in 1956 Hans Selye, a Canadian physiologist, revealed the devastating effects of traumatic experiences, which he termed stress, on an organism's health. Then in the 1960s a more specific clue to the connections between mind and body appeared. Drs. Elmer and Alyce Green, pioneering researchers in biofeedback, documented the profound abilities of advanced yoga practitioners to control consciously their heart rate, temperature, and brain wave patterns. As the century continued, scientists in the newly developing field of psychoneuroimmunology presented evidence linking particular chemical substances, such as endorphins, to specific human emotions, such as pleasure. They showed how certain levels of endorphins in the body may act as a chemical shield against invading viruses or germs.

Today mind/body medicine practices are a respected part of treatment in many major hospitals and clinics throughout the United States. They may be used for relief of pain before or during surgery and to aid in the postoperative process. In addition, individuals seeking help for a variety of chronic physical conditions, including cancer and AIDS, as well as those seeking to change painful and destructive behavior patterns, such as chemical addictions or eating disorders, are enhancing traditional Western methods of treatment with mind/body medicine practices.

Some Basic Mind/Body Medicine Beliefs

The disciplines discussed in this section represent an expansion of traditional Western approaches to medicine. While research in each discipline has yielded different theories and techniques, together these fields share certain basic principles. First, approaches to mind/body medicine are unified by their belief that real and useful connections exist between our bodies and our minds. Whether the discipline uses the powers of the conscious mind to interact with and affect the systems of the body, as in biofeedback, or employs the powers of the unconscious mind to effect changes in behavior, as in hypnotherapy, the pathways between body and mind are at the heart of these healing modalities.

The disciplines discussed in this section share the belief that a person's emotions and attitudes will influence his or her body's innate ability to heal. In clinical studies in the 1940s and 1950s patients were given a placebo, or neutral substance such as sugared water, and told that it would relieve their chronic pain. The patients' emotional attitudes about their pain, as well as their physical progress, were closely monitored. The results showed that patients who believe they will recover are much more likely to do so than those who think they won't, or those who think they will get worse. Mind/body medicine practitioners believe that these results strongly suggest that emotions and mental attitudes play an important role in the body's ability to heal.

Finally, all mind/body medicine practices believe in the importance of personal motivation in the healing process. This belief is supported by clinical research, which shows that cancer patients who become actively involved in their treatment are more likely to recover than those who passively accept their diagnosis and fail to examine their treatment options. Taking charge of one's life fends off feelings of hopelessness and lack of control, both of which have been shown through psychoneuroimmunology studies to reduce the number of disease-fighting cells in the body. By emphasizing personal responsibility, mind/body medicine practitioners aim to empower patients to make a successful healing journey.

Because mind/body medicine practitioners emphasize the individual's participation in the healing process, special attention is given to the relationship between caregiver and receiver. For instance, in guided imagery the caregiver is often referred to as a guide or knowledgeable aide. The guide's role is viewed as helping the receiver access his or her own inner sources of physical, mental, and emotional health and offering positive reinforcement as he or she learns to navigate the channels between body and mind.

The Future of Mind/Body Medicine

Mind/body medicine practices have helped millions of people find relief from a multitude of physical and emotional problems. People suffering from migraine headaches, insomnia, hypertension, asthma and other respiratory conditions, ulcers and other gastrointestinal disorders, incontinence, cardiac and vascular irregularities, muscular problems caused by strokes or accidents, arthritis, anxiety, attention and learning disorders, depression, chemical and emotional addictions, and phobias and other stress-related disorders have all been helped by mind/body medicine practices. Although the field is still young, with continued research, creative and caring practitioners, and courageous health care consumers willing to view illness as a message from the body to begin an active healing journey, mind/body medicine may provide new solutions for health care in the twenty-first century.

—*Nancy Allison, CMA*

Further Reading:

Borysenko, Joan. *Minding the Body, Mending the Mind.* New York: Bantam Books, 1988.

Chopra, Deepak. *Quantum Healing.* New York: Bantam Books, 1989.

BIOFEEDBACK TRAINING

Biofeedback training is a means of enhancing mental awareness of body changes. It is a process that offers techniques for regulating the body's vital functions and fostering overall health. Electronic biofeedback instruments supply information about the body not usually available to the consciousness. Heart rate, muscle tension, blood circulation, brain wave activity, and other body functions are made perceptible as visual and auditory signals that enable an individual to monitor his or her physiological reaction to various stimuli or situations. With the help of the biofeedback instrument it is possible to develop new, healthier patterns of response throughout the body's systems, even those previously regarded as involuntary and outside the reach of the conscious mind. Biofeedback training has a vast range of diagnostic, therapeutic, and preventive applications, particularly in cases where stress and related psychological factors play a role.

The History of Biofeedback Training

The use of biofeedback devices to modify behavior started in 1938, when Hobart G. Mowrer introduced an alarm triggered by urine to stop children from wetting their beds. Beginning in the 1940s muscle-tension biofeedback was successfully used in the field of neuromuscular rehabilitation. Biofeedback developed rapidly in America during the 1950s and 1960s because of a coincidence of two factors. There was growing awareness that stress was a principal cause of disease and an accompanying interest in expanding the mind's ability to respond to stress more positively and nurture all parts of one's self. At the same time the invention of the electroencephalograph machine (EEG) and similar electronic equipment gave scientists new tools for monitoring the internal workings of the body-mind connection. Alyce and Elmer Green used the EEG to study the techniques that enable masters of yoga meditation to alter the rhythms and responses of the body so extensively that they can become impervious to extremes of temperature and pain. Under the direction of Joe Kamiya, volunteers in another study learned to use feedback from the EEG to recognize and achieve the alpha state, an alert sense of effortless well-being normally associated with advanced stages of meditation.

During the late 1960s the excitement generated by the initial findings of biofeedback research led to overly optimistic claims about "miracle cures" of the future. Nonetheless, it was clear that a fundamental concept in the human sciences, the distinction between voluntary and involuntary nervous activity, had been discredited. Vital functions like blood pressure were now seen as subject to the control of the individual. Behavioral modification accordingly became an ever more accepted mode of health care. The first professional meeting of feedback researchers was held in 1968, chaired by Les Fehmi. In 1969 biofeedback researchers founded a professional support group, the Biofeedback Research Society, later renamed the Association for Applied Psychophysiology and Biofeedback (AAPB). The voluminous scholarly literature on various aspects of biofeedback attests to the interest it has attracted in the scientific community.

The Theory of Biofeedback Training

Biofeedback training approaches the brain as a control center that sends impulses through the nervous system to program the body's vital functions: heart rate, blood pressure, circulation, digestion, breath, perspiration, and so forth. By automatically signaling the different systems when to turn on or off, people live safely and comfortably in their surroundings without deliberating over the body's basic activities. But stress, illness, or an accident can disrupt the natural process and cause it to

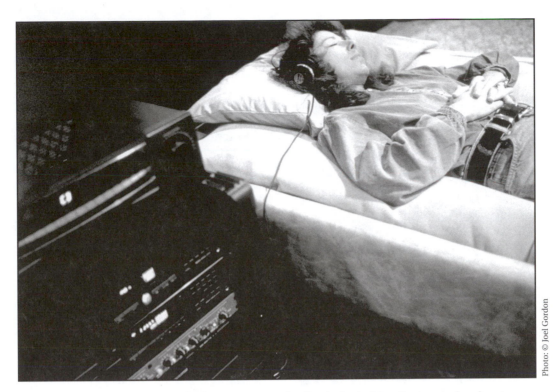

Photo: © Joel Gordon

A biofeedback machine translates some aspects of a client's physical functioning, such as heart rate or blood pressure, into a sound or visual signal.

send signals that produce common health problems like insomnia, muscular or vascular pain, and irritable bowel syndrome, to name just a few. While these stress-aggravated processes make the body seem unpredictable and beyond control, biofeedback training can help reverse overreactions.

The use of electronic instruments to measure and reflect the status of body functions is only one element of biofeedback training. It also uses relaxation techniques derived from ancient meditation practice and requires participants to be open to the idea of attentional flexibility. Contrary to popular belief, the machines do not intervene in the information traveling between the body and mind. Instead, the instruments act as a mirror of one's internal reactions, allowing an individual to observe this behavior and to be aware of harmful reactions. This information helps uncover hidden patterns of physiological reactions to stress, for example, tensing of

muscles and a fall in body temperature, that the person may never have noticed. Furthermore, the machines serve as a precise, objective gauge of the physiological effects accomplished by using a relaxation technique such as visualizing a pleasant scene or soothing color. The true source of the self-healing promoted and reflected by biofeedback training are techniques that normalize physiological functioning. These techniques enable the person to stabilize erratic or unhealthy physical responses and to take responsibility for his or her own well-being.

Biofeedback Training in Practice

In its most frequent application, biofeedback training is used to teach people techniques for coping with health problems that have already been diagnosed by a medical doctor or psychologist. The role of the certified practitioners who administer biofeedback training is to show the client how to interpret control and the electronic biofeedback. The client sits during training and remains fully clothed, though sensors are placed on the skin over the region to be monitored. The sensors do not cause pain or discomfort. Body information from the biofeedback instrument is presented in any of several forms: flashing lights, beeping sounds, patterns on a computer screen, or tactile sensations. Currently available instruments have the capacity to monitor skin temperature, electrical conductivity in the skin, muscle tension, heart rate, brain wave activity, and other body processes.

The nature of the work in a training session varies according to the needs of the client. In the case of compulsive teeth grinding and temporomandibular joint (TMJ) disorder, for example, training focuses on regulation of muscular tension in the jaw. Attention deficit disorder can be addressed by means of a computer game controlled by brain wave activity. The client watches the game but cannot play unless he or she produces brain waves of an appropriate pattern. In this way the client becomes minutely attuned to different levels of concentration and learns how to heighten, expand, and focus his or her attention.

As a biofeedback training session unfolds, the practitioner recommends techniques for attaining the desired result and provides positive reinforcement. Learning and achieving the body-mind benefits of a training program generally requires several sessions with a practitioner, who may advise additional work with home biofeedback instruments or audio tapes. Success in biofeedback training generally depends on the effort expended by the client. Over time, and with consistent practice, one progresses to the point where one can monitor and adjust body processes without the aid of electronic instruments.

Benefits of Biofeedback Training

Most practitioners still limit their practice of biofeedback to EMG and blood flow biofeedback. However, there is a growing movement toward providing other types, especially neurofeedback, for a variety of disorders. The most common applications are for headaches, pain management or pain dissolution, and general stress reduction. Stress reduction is therapeutic for a variety of symptoms such as irritable bowel syndrome, migraine headaches, hypertension, breathing difficulties, cardiac and vascular irregularities, anxiety, depression, insomnia, as well as symptoms related to addiction, attention disorders, and for the reduction of other learning disabilities. The AAPB can provide a list of clinical symptoms that have responded favorably to biofeedback treatment as well as a referral to a certified biofeedback provider in your area.

—*Les Fehmi, Ph.D.*

Resources:

Association for Applied Psychophysiology and Biofeedback
10200 West 44th Avenue, Suite 304
Wheat Ridge, CO 80033
Tel:(303)422-8436
Provides a nationwide referral service. To receive a free copy of their brochure "What Is Biofeedback?" send a self-addressed stamped envelope to the address above.

Biofeedback Certification Institute of America (BCIA)
10200 West 44th Avenue, Suite 304
Wheat Ridge, CO 80033
Tel:(303)420-2902
A professional organization that determines minimum standards for certification in biofeedback training. BCIA also certifies organizations that provide training for biofeedback practitioners.

Further Reading:

Crow, Mark, and David Danskin. *Biofeedback: An Introduction.* Palo Alto, CA: Mayfield Publishing Co., 1981.

GUIDED IMAGERY

Guided imagery is a therapeutic technique in which a person withdraws into his or her mind to focus on scenes and symbols pertaining to an illness, accident, or personal issue. Within one's imagination, problems are replaced with a "make-believe" story of recovered health and happiness. Guided imagery is based on the principle that the imagination has the capacity to relieve pain and promote healing when it is optimistic and confident and, inversely, can help trigger a breakdown when it is consumed by worry. The techniques of guided imagery are designed to teach individuals how to use their own powers of imagination to steer away from negative thoughts toward models of well-being. Guided imagery generally serves as an adjunct to medical treatment and has been incorporated in sports training programs and methods of self-care.

The Development of Guided Imagery for Healing

What is now called guided imagery can be traced back to practices found in early civilizations around the world. Symbols and spirits were summoned to promote healing, and envisioning one's health was a key element in rituals performed by shamans. When medicine was first separated from religion in classical Greek culture, imagery continued to be regarded as a valuable tool in the maintenance of physical and mental well-being. According to the Greek philosopher Hippocrates, inner pictures produce a "spirit" that arouses the heart and other parts of the body. They need to be controlled if the person is to be healthy. Renaissance doctors took a similar view of the role of the imagination. Paracelsus, for example, wrote that "the power of the imagination is a great factor in medicine. It may produce diseases . . . and it may cure them."

After the Renaissance, interest in therapeutic imagery declined because of radical changes in the interpretation of the links between mind and body. Following the precepts of René Descartes, the body was considered a mechanical structure, and the imagination's role in either the body or the operations of the intellect was severely restricted. Sigmund Freud's study of hysteria, a psychosomatic disorder, marks the beginning of a revolution in medicine that can be viewed as a revival of ancient and Renaissance teachings about the power of the imagination. By explaining hysteria as a physical manifestation of emotional trauma, Freud challenged Descartes' notion that illnesses may have only a physical cause. He believed that an effective treatment must also address the patient's inner experiences.

The current American approach to guided imagery is based on Carl Simonton's work with cancer patients during the 1970s. He instructed cancer patients to imagine white cells as warriors defeating the cancer cells and discovered that these patients lived twice as long as those relying on medical treatment alone. After Bernie Siegel conducted an equally successful pilot program at Yale University, there was a rapid expansion in medical research into the benefits and workings of systems of internal visualization from daydreaming to self-hypnosis to doodling and drawing. By 1990, guided imagery had emerged as an established mode of treatment, acclaimed by advocates of both traditional and alternative medicine.

The Theory of Guided Imagery

Recent research has suggested that mental imagery can modify the functioning of the body. The brain responds to an image much as if it were the real thing, recalling past experiences and triggering a set of responses that lead from the cerebral cortex to the hypothalamus. The hypothalamus, in turn, transmits messages to the autonomic nerves controlling the body's involuntary functions—heart rate, blood pressure, breathing, digestion, temperature, sexual arousal, and immunity. As a result, a seemingly passive activity, like guided imagery, can bring about changes beneficial to physical health.

While guided imagery resembles other relaxation techniques that intervene in the autonomic nervous system, such as biofeedback training, it is distinctive in one regard. By releasing the imagination, it allows the person to get in touch with repressed emotions that may be at the root of his or her health problems. By finding a concrete image for a persistent problem, participants often bring troublesome needs and conflicts out into the open, where they can be resolved.

Guided Imagery in Practice

It is possible to learn guided imagery from a self-help manual or tape, but most people begin by working with a therapist at a doctor's office or health care center. The exact nature of the training depends on the individual's goals and the professional background of his or her therapist. Some therapists rely on a prepared script of healing images, whereas others encourage individuals to let their imaginations roam. Another major difference in approach concerns the use of imagery. In some techniques, it is directed toward relaxation and healing. In a variant of guided imagery, known as Interactive Guided Imagery™, the emphasis is shifted away from creating ideal images to picturing symbolic scenes that may reveal hidden emotions. Given the many variants that are now available, it is advisable to ask a prospective therapist to explain the course of therapy before starting a training program.

Guided imagery training generally involves learning a procedure to follow at home or work, two or even three times a day for five to twenty-five minutes. In many instances, the first steps of the procedure parallel those followed in meditation: the person withdraws to a quiet place, assumes a comfortable position, and turns his or her thoughts inward. But, unlike meditation, in guided imagery a person fashions an alternative version of his or her circumstances. Frequently, participants are instructed to imagine themselves mounting stairs that lead to a place where they feel secure and content, then to picture themselves gradually getting well. To exit from the imagery exercise they reverse the process: they imagine themselves leaving the pleasant place, descending the stairs, and returning to normal activity.

When guided imagery was first introduced in American medicine, it employed aggressive images of combat between the forces of health and disease. Over the past decades, researchers have discovered the importance of adjusting imagery to suit the individual's personality and have broadened the range of things considered "imagery." For instance, among participants without a strong visual sense, listening to music may take the place of imagining pictures. There has also been increased stress on "sensory recruitment" in the imaging process. Rather than rely simply on one sense, individuals are urged to incorporate all the senses—sight, hearing, touch, smell, and taste—into their imagery exercises. In this way, they intensify the impact of the healing messages that the autonomic nervous system sends to the immune system and other vital functions of the body.

The Benefits of Guided Imagery

Daily practice with a routine of guided imagery has been used to relieve headaches and chronic pain. It has also helped people tolerate medical procedures, stimulate healing, and explore the emotions that may have caused an illness. Guided imagery can also give people a heightened sense of their own potential and encourage them to find creative solutions to personal and professional problems.

Resources:

Academy for Guided Imagery
P.O. Box 2070
Mill Valley, CA 94942
Tel: (800)726-2070
Offers a training program in guided imagery for health professionals; also provides information about guided imagery, including a list of practitioners, books, and videotapes.

Exceptional Cancer Patients
1302 Chapel Street
New Haven, CT 06511
Tel: (203)865-8392
Organization that maintains a referral list of imagery practitioners who work with cancer patients and offers books and tapes about guided imagery.

Health Associates, Inc.
P.O. Box 220
Big Sur, CA 93920
Fax: (408)667-0248
Provides workshops on various uses of guided imagery.

Further Reading:

Achterberg, Jeanne. *Imagery in Healing: Shamanism and Modern Medicine.* Boston: New Science Library/Shambala, 1985.

Borysenko, Joan. *Minding the Body, Mending the Mind.* Reading, MA: Bantam, 1988.

Rossman, Martin. *Healing Yourself: A Step-by-Step Program for Better Health Through Imagery.* New York: Pocket Books, 1989.

Siegel, Bernie. *Peace, Love, and Healing.* New York: Harper & Row, 1989.

Simonton, Carl, Stephanie Simonton, and Creighton Simonton. *Getting Well Again.* Los Angeles: Jeremy P. Tarcher, 1978.

HYPNOTHERAPY

Hypnotherapy is the use of hypnosis, trance states, and suggestion for therapeutic results. It is used to address a diversity of problems, including anxiety, phobias, and emotional problems and to help break habits like smoking. Doctors and dentists are increasingly using hypnosis with patients to help relieve pain and assist healing. It is also used to improve performance in sports activities, examinations or public speaking and social activities. By inducing altered states of consciousness, hypnotherapists help clients use the resources of the unconscious mind to bring about psychological and physical benefits. Hypnotherapy asserts that the unconscious mind is a vast reservoir of learnings and skills.

Founders of Hypnotherapy

Franz Anton Mesmer (1734–1815), now called the "Father of Hypnosis," is responsible for beginning the scientific investigation of trances. Mesmer used auspicious passes of the hands, dramatic gestures, and magnetic apparatuses to induce sleeplike states in willing subjects. He termed the phenomenon "animal magnetism," believing that a magnetic fluid had passed from his hands to the subject. In 1784, a commission for the Academy of Science in France (including Benjamin Franklin) was appointed to investigate Dr. Mesmer's practices and concluded, "Imagination is everything, magnetism nothing." However, future researchers would confirm the power of suggestion.

James Braid (1795–1860), a Scottish surgeon, used Mesmer's hand gestures to produce anesthesia in patients in his hospital in India, reducing his infection rate from 50 percent to 5 percent in the process. He first coined the term "hypnosis," shortened from neuro-hypnosis, meaning nervous sleep. Braid noted that a trance consisted of fixed and focused concentration that rendered a subject open to suggestion.

Auguste Ambroise Liebault (1823–1904) began the first scientific investigation of hypnotic phenomena, founding the School of Nancy in France and developing the doctrine of suggestive therapeutics. Working under him, as a professor of internal medicine, Hyppolyte Bernheim (1837–1919) gave us the foundation of our current understanding of hypnotic suggestion. He asserted that hypnosis is not a disorder of the nervous system, as many medical authorities of the day believed. It is instead a product of suggestion. He also believed that suggestion was a common occurrence in all interactions and not specific to a hypnotist's gestures.

One of the most famous suggestions in hypnotherapy comes from Émile Coué (1857–1926), another pupil of Liebault. He thought that all suggestion is really self-suggestion. His exercise involved repeating the phrase, "Every day in every way I am getting better and better." He found that slowly repeated suggestions, such as this, can become absorbed into the unconscious and affect one's life. This is the basis for all the audio tapes on the market promising reprogramming of the unconscious.

Sigmund Freud (1856–1939), although initially interested in the psychological use of hypnosis, abandoned it in treatment because he was not able to obtain successful trances in his neurology patients. He became more interested in the causes of neurosis and instead used free association for his "analytic inquiry."

Freud's influence on the medical establishment's view of mental illness and its treatment set back the acceptance of hypnosis until Clark Hull, an American professor of psychology at the University of Wisconsin, published the book *Hypnosis and Suggestibility* in 1933. It describes some of the first experimental research on hypnosis. A student of Hull's, Milton H. Erickson (1910–1980), who founded the American Society for Clinical Hypnosis, is credited with bringing the techniques of hypnotherapy into mainstream medical and psychological practice and developing its most comprehensive form.

He stressed that hypnotherapy is most effective when it is part of a unique program of therapy, developed for each patient according to his or her situation or needs. Erickson believed that hypnosis is a specialized form of communication in which both conscious and unconscious channels can learn. A patient's natural capacities and unique ways of learning and responding are utilized as part of the therapy. So, rather than being controlled by suggestions, a patient is actively finding solutions. In this model, indirect suggestions in the form of metaphors or stories are used in addition to direct and authoritative suggestions. This is intended to facilitate unconscious learning and bypass conscious imitation and resistance.

What Is a Hypnotic Trance and Hypnosis?

While the word *trance* may conjure up the idea of a zombielike state from a horror movie, in reality we all experience different trance states every day. When we become absorbed in reading or watching television we often shift into a trance state where time is suspended, cares and worries are forgotten, or surrounding stimuli are tuned out. More intense trances can occur during meditation or prayer, or under states of extreme emotion, such as falling in love. More tranquil trances often are induced during procedures like relaxation training, guided imagery, or massage. Most therapeutic trances are very relaxing, but they can also be arousing and invigorating.

A hypnotherapist induces trances to suspend the limitations of the conscious, analytical mind. This allows all the possibilities of a person's imagination and unconscious to solve, reinterpret, or reorganize an experience, issue, or problem.

Using Hypnosis for Therapy

Trances in and of themselves have little therapeutic value. But they greatly facilitate therapeutic goals. Unlike traditional psychotherapy, in which unconscious thoughts and impulses are brought to consciousness for analysis and understanding, in hypnotherapy the patient

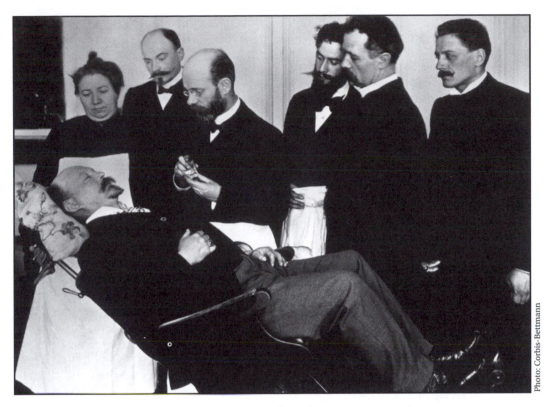

Photo: Corbis-Bettmann

A group of French doctors in the 1890s watch a colleague put a patient into a trance.

is trained in using trance to learn and practice new skills for alleviating symptoms or changing behavior. Suggestions may be incorporated unconsciously and can be brought to normal consciousness when that part of the mind is ready.

At the start of a typical hypnotherapy session, the therapist first will ask questions about the client's problem and what he or she hopes to gain from the treatment. After discussing the problem, the procedure to be used, and the goals to be realized, the therapist then will explain what is to be done and answer any questions or concerns. A series of instructions will be provided that help guide the person into a relaxed trance state. Since hypnosis is a learned skill, the induction process is practiced slowly until the person feels comfortable and is able to relax and focus. Suggestions then are offered to help with the problem or issue at hand. As a person's conscious thinking is

increasingly withdrawn from the outside environment, while suggestions engage more and more of his or her inner awareness, the trance will become deeper. The goal of the trance is to allow one to experience an expanded awareness, unhindered by ordinary limitations. In this state intuitive, instinctive, and imaginative thoughts and feelings are used to address the issue at hand. Most work is done in light or medium trances, but catalepsy, a condition where the limbs stay where they are placed, often occurs. Unconscious hand levitation is a common technique for verifying and deepening the trance experience. The session is usually ended with suggestions to feel refreshed, alert, and completely ready for the rest of the day.

The induction procedure is often taught to the client so that it can be practiced at home, or used when needed, for example, at times of stress. Appropriate suggestions are prepared ahead of time. For example, a person may rehearse by visualizing himself or herself accomplishing a goal and feeling prepared. Another method of self-hypnosis is to repeat simple affirmations until they become absorbed into behavior. For example, a person may repeat, "I will become naturally more confident as I practice these skills."

Benefits of Hypnotherapy

The uses of hypnosis in psychological therapy are well known. People may enter hypnotherapy to gain greater confidence in their own resources for dealing with problems and difficulties. Hypnosis is also used to produce relaxation and relieve anxiety. Learning the ability to control emotions, impulses, and urges is used to bring greater self-confidence, self-control, and mastery. These general results occur from most hypnotherapy interventions, even when the focus or problem is quite specific.

Common issues include smoking, overeating, insomnia, and fears such as flying, public speaking, or performing in sports or examinations. The range of problems addressed by hypnosis is expanding as scientific knowledge about unconscious communication and motivational processes increases.

Its use in medical situations is increasing as more and more hospitals employ hypnotherapists to help create optimal conditions for patient recovery and health. For decades, it has been used successfully to manage pain and stress, often in preparation for childbirth and surgery. Migraines, respiratory conditions, ulcers, and arthritis are some of the medical conditions commonly treated.

Precautions

Anyone interested in pursuing hypnotherapy should take certain precautions. While inducing trance is easy and can be learned by anyone, only trained practitioners with the appropriate licensing, experience, and knowledge in psychology and physiology should be consulted. Learn about the hypnotherapist's background, credentials, and education and experience. The American Society for Clinical Hypnosis and the Milton H. Erickson Institutes in the United States set the guidelines for proper training and certification for hypnotherapists. The International Medical and Dental Hypnotherapy Association, the Society for Clinical and Experimental Hypnosis, and the American Association of Professional Hypnotherapists are also long-standing associations with much experience in all aspects of hypnotherapy. Finally, be aware of the limitations of hypnosis. It is not a cure-all, and its effects depend completely on the abilities and limitations of the client. Skilled hypnotherapists utilize a client's internal resources but do not replace a person's own skills and capacities. It is highly individual. Avoid practitioners who make exaggerated claims and promise all-purpose cures. While hypnotherapy is a powerful tool, it is not able to solve every problem.

—*Oscar A. Gillespie, Ph.D.*

Resources:

American Association of Professional Hypnotherapists
P.O. Box 29
Boones Mill, VA 24065
Tel: (540) 334-3035

So far as I know hypnosis as a human activity has been used since the beginning of the human race.

—Milton H. Erickson.

All suggestion is self-suggestion.

—Émil Coué.

The American Society of Clinical Hypnosis
2250 E. Devon Avenue., Suite 336
Des Plaines, IL. 60018
Tel: (847) 297-3317
Has sections in major cities in the United States. Publishes the newsletter American Journal of Clinical Hypnosis *and has regional workshops for professionals throughout the year. ASCH provides the most rigorous credentialing process for professionals.*

International Medical and Dental Hypnotherapy Association
4110 Edgeland, Suite 800
Royal Oak, MI 49073
Tel: (248) 549-5594
Toll-free: (800) 257-5467

The Milton H. Erickson Foundation, Inc.
3606 N. 24th Street
Phoenix, AZ 85016
(602) 956-6196
Presents the National and International Erickson Congresses and publishes a newsletter that includes information on training programs. Separate Erickson Institutes and Societies can be found in major cities in the United States and in several other countries.

The New York Milton H. Erickson Society for Psychotherapy and Hypnosis (NYSEPH)
440 West End Avenue, #1C
New York, NY 10024
Tel: (212) 873-6459
Provides a 100-hour comprehensive training program (chartered by the Board of Regents of New York State) in Ericksonian approaches in psychotherapy and hypnotherapy and a referral service for the New York tristate area.

The Society for Clinical and Experimental Hypnosis, Inc.
111 North 49th Street
Philadelphia, PA 19139
Publishes The International Journal of Clinical and Experimental Hypnosis.

Further Reading:

Cheek, David B., and L.M. LeCaron. *Clinical Hypnotherapy.* New York: Grune and Stratton, 1968.

Hammond, D. Corydon, ed. *Hypnotic Suggestions and Metaphors.* New York: W. W. Norton, 1990.

Hunter, Marlene Elva. *Creative Scripts for Hypnotherapy.* New York: Brunner/Mazel, 1994.

Lynn, Steven Jay, and Judith W. Rhue, eds. *Theories of Hypnosis: Current Models and Perspectives.* New York: Guilford Press, 1991.

Phillips, Maggie, and Claire Frederick. *Healing the Divided Self: Clinical and Ericksonian Hypnotherapy for Post-traumatic and Dissociative Conditions.* New York: W.W. Norton & Co., 1995.

Rowley, David T. *Hypnosis and Hypnotherapy.* Philadelphia: Charles Press, 1986.

Rosen, Sydney. *My Voice Will Go with You : The Teaching Tales of Milton H. Erickson.* New York: W. W. Norton, 1982.

Yapko, Michael D. *Trancework: An Introduction to the Practice of Clinical Hypnosis.* New York: Brunner/Mazel, 1989.

INTERACTIVE GUIDED IMAGERY^{SM}

Interactive Guided Imagery^{SM} is a method of using the mind to support healing and growth. An expert will use certain techniques to help a person enhance his or her awareness of unconscious images and help him or her to learn to effectively interact with them. With the aid of a guide, people use Interactive Guided Imagery sessions to learn to relax, relieve stress, enhance body-mind communication, sharpen intuition, and become more effective at reaching goals. It is used to mobilize the latent, innate healing abilities of the client to support rehabilitation, recovery, and health.

Interactive Guided Imagery was created by Martin L. Rossman, a medical doctor, and David E. Bresler, a health psychologist. Both had been independently researching clinical applications of body-mind effects in health since the late 1960s. In 1982 Dr. Rossman co-created the Power of Imagination Conference, where leading clinicians and researchers introduced to more than 1,400 health professionals nationwide the practical applications of imagery work. Frequent requests for clinical training led to the creation of "clinical guided imagery" courses taught by Drs. Rossman and Bresler around the United States from 1982 to 1989. In 1989, Dr. Rossman and Dr. Bresler founded the Academy for Guided Imagery. In 1995, the mission of the academy was expanded to include teaching the public and organizations to work with the imagery methods the academy had refined over the years.

A session in Interactive Guided Imagery begins with a simple relaxation technique used to help a client focus his or her attention inward. The guide will then teach skills to help with problem solving, conflict resolution, goal setting, stimulating healing responses in the body, or using personal strengths and resources most effectively. Participants are fully aware of their guide's suggestions and questions, and are engaged in an active dialogue at all times. In one typical technique, a client is asked to close his or her eyes to allow the mind to present a picture representing the experience of his or her problem. The client may then be guided in an imaginary dialogue with this image to explore and reveal its meaning and relevance to the problem or issue. These images can provide information not only about the problem, but also about clients' beliefs, hopes, expectations, fears, resources, and solutions. The imagery process is used to reveal the clients' intuitions about a problem and its solution.

The guide works to make a person become more aware of his or her own thoughts, feelings, and body responses, allowing him or her to have more control of how he or she feels. Many Interactive Guided Imagery self-care techniques can be learned from books, home study programs, and tapes. A certified guide can assist a person with these approaches.

Interactive Guided Imagery seeks to help a person learn to relax, mentally and physically, relieve pain or other physical symptoms, stimulate healing responses in the body, solve difficult problems, resolve emotional issues, and envision and plan for the future. It may be used for self-care or by physicians, psychotherapists, nurses, and other professionals.

Interactive Guided Imagery can pose certain risks when used by poorly trained personnel. There is a possibility of uncovering traumatic insight or overwhelming effects. A certified Interactive Guided Imagery guide is trained and prepared to help prevent this whenever possible, and to help a person work through it, should it occur.

—*Martin Rossman, M.D.*

Resources:

Academy for Guided Imagery
P.O. Box 2070
Mill Valley, CA 94942
Tel: (800) 726-2070
Fax: (415) 389-9342
Sponsors professional training conferences, seminars, and retreats, and produces educational books and tapes to teach imagery skills to professionals, businesses, and the general public.

Further Reading:

Bresler, David. *Free Yourself from Pain.* New York: Simon & Schuster, 1979.

Rossman, Martin. *Healing Yourself: A Step-by-Step Program for Better Health Through Imagery.* New York: Pocket Books, 1989.

PSYCHONEUROIMMUNOLOGY

Psychoneuroimmunology, also commonly referred to as PNI, is the study of how thoughts and emotions may affect the body's immune system. The immune system is the body's elaborate and varied defense mechanism that fights against disease and illness. Advocates of this discipline have observed that the quality of a person's mental state, when improved through humor, positive thinking, and relaxation, can improve his or her body's ability to fight disease. Accordingly, stress, grief, and pain are seen to cause the body's defenses to weaken. Many supporters of this theory promote the use of relaxation techniques as a preventive measure for ensuring physical well-being. Some also see these techniques as a part of treatment for patients with chronic illnesses.

PNI Research

For most of this century, science has taught that the nervous system, including the brain, and the immune system function independently. The body's ability to fight disease was thought to be beyond our conscious control. In the 1960s, several researchers suggested that there is actually a complex network linking these two systems. Nerve cells, for instance, penetrate into the principal organs of the immune system, including the thyroid, spleen, and lymph glands, where lymphocytes, or disease-fighting cells, reside until they are called into action. Researchers also discovered that the chemicals nerve cells use to communicate with one another lock onto the membranes of lymphocytes; thus the information that the brain is sending and receiving is also shared with the immune system.

The idea of the connection between the nervous and immune systems gained attention after an experiment in 1975 appeared to confirm that the mind could affect physical health. Researchers fed rats saccharin-flavored water along with a drug that suppressed their immune functions. Later, when the rats were given the saccharin-flavored water without the drug, the researchers found that the rats' immune systems did not recover. As a result, the rats became ill and some died. Researchers believed that the rats had learned to associate the sweet water with the effect of the drug, thus proving that a thought or mental association could alter an animal's immune system. This experiment inspired similar studies that concluded that mental attributes, such as attitudes, sensations, memories, and emotions could change the immune system's ability to resist infections.

These early experiments developed into the field of study known today as PNI. Much of current PNI research investigates the physical effects of stress. Some researchers believe that stress, especially over long periods of time, can weaken the body's ability to recover from illnesses. To find out the physical effects of stress, researchers have tested the concentrations of lymphocytes in people's bodies while they were experiencing stressful situations. In one of these experiments, widowers were tested during the months following the death of their wives. The widowers' immune systems were found to be functioning more weakly than those of men who had not suffered the loss of their partner. In another experiment, medical students' immune systems appeared to weaken before they took exams. As a result of these studies, some researchers claim that reducing stress can help a person's immune system.

The Benefits of Positive Thinking

The case of noted journalist and commentator Norman Cousins changed the way many people thought about the relationship between body and mind. In 1976, Cousins was diagnosed with a severe, crippling disease of the spine (ankylosing spondylitis), and there was no known therapy that offered any real promise for recovery. Cousins decided to confront his gloomy future with humor—with an intense diet of movies by Laurel and Hardy, the Marx Brothers, and other famous comedians—and by prescribing for himself large doses of vitamin C. After months of laughter and good feelings,

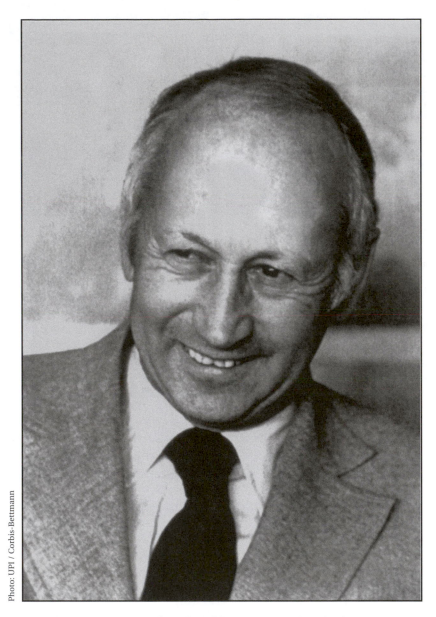

Photo: UPI / Corbis-Bettmann

Author Norman Cousins brought public attention to the role of emotions
in the healing process by his account of how he used laughter to recover
from a debilitating spinal disease.

his debilitating spinal condition disappeared. Cousins went on to live fourteen more years and wrote a book, *Anatomy of an Illness as Perceived by the Patient: Reflections on Healing and Regeneration*, detailing his personal path to recovery. His story led many people to believe that positive thinking may help the body's ability to heal.

Applications of PNI Research

Some health care workers have begun to consider findings from PNI research when designing new therapies. Biofeedback is used to relieve stress in an attempt to reduce its burdens on the immune system. Guided imagery techniques are being used to direct the immune system responses to certain areas of the body. People with chronic illnesses are often encouraged to join support groups where they can share their experiences, unburden themselves of fear, and draw strength and positive encouragement from others. All of these contribute to easing emotional strains, and possibly to bettering chances for recovery. The lessons learned from PNI research may also help explain other models of healing, such as Chinese acupuncture and Native American shamanism.

PNI is a recent and widely debated field of study. Not all PNI researchers are convinced that the physical effects of stress or trauma are significant beyond extreme or chronic cases. It is far too simple to say that thinking positive thoughts will make us healthy and negative thoughts will make us sick. Sudden and rapid recoveries like Cousins' are very uncommon. PNI is intended to enhance, not replace, the physical treatment of illnesses.

—*Leonard Wisneski, M.D.*

Resources:

Integral Health Foundation
4300 Crossway Court
Rockville, MD 20835
Tel: (301) 871-8384
Promotes a greater understanding of the integral nature of the spirit, mind, and body in the healing process through interdisciplinary cooperation in research, education, and practice.

Further Reading:

Benson, Herbert. *Timeless Healing: The Power and Biology of Belief.* New York: Simon & Schuster, 1994.

Cousins, Norman. *Anatomy of an Illness as Perceived by the Patient: Reflections on Healing and Regeneration.* New York: W.W. Norton, 1979.

Locke, S., and D. Colligan. *The Healer Within.* New York: Dutton, 1996.

Ornstein, R., and D. Sobel. *The Amazing Brain.* New York: Simon & Schuster, 1987.

Many researchers in psychoneuroimmunology have observed some startling findings that may reveal the ways that emotions and stress can change a person's immune system:

• Early in the U.S. space program, NASA found that astronauts had reduced white blood cell counts after returning from space. Many scientists believed that it was a result of the stress of reentry.

• Subjects who viewed a film of Mother Teresa ministering to the poor were found to have increased levels of immune chemicals in their saliva.

• Researchers observed that women with breast cancer who attended support groups tended to survive longer than women who faced their illness alone.

• People who experienced the stress of being responsible for the care of another person were found to have fewer infection-fighting cells, suffer more upper-respiratory infections, and take longer to heal wounds.

PART V: SENSORY THERAPIES

Aromatherapy • Bates Method • Behavioral Vision Therapy
Eye Movement Desensitization and Reprocessing • Flower Remedies
Hydrotherapy • Light Therapy • Sounding • Tomatis Method

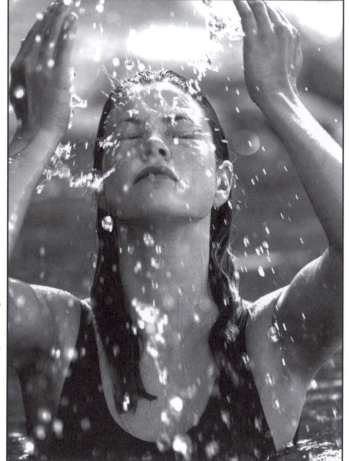

Photo: Caroline Wood / © Tony Stone Images

Through the five senses, sensory therapies awaken one's innate healing potential.

Sensory therapies use one of the five senses as the means to adjust chemical or other imbalances within the body that may be the cause of physical or psychological problems. While the name *sensory therapies* generally refers to those methods that work with the senses of sight, sound, or smell, this section also includes some disciplines that work with the sense of taste or touch. There are also many body-mind disciplines that work with the kinesthetic sense, or sense of body movement. These disciplines can be found throughout the encyclopedia in the sections entitled Subtle Energy Therapies, Mind/Body Medicine, Yoga, Martial Arts, Massage, Acupuncture and Asian Bodywork, Movement Therapy Methods, Somatic Practices, Expressive and Creative Arts Therapies, and Body-Oriented Psychotherapies.

While the idea of treating physical and psychological problems by manipulating the senses is ancient, most of the methods described in this section were developed in the twentieth century by creative Western physicians, often working outside or on the fringes of accepted allopathic medical practice. Through their pioneering work many sense-organ exercises and treatments, often involving special equipment, or combined with more traditional psychotherapeutic practices, were developed. Many of these methods are prescribed as part of naturopathic cures. They have been effective in treating a wide variety of specific physical or emotional ailments such as post-traumatic stress disorder, nearsightedness, hearing loss, chemical addictions, depression, anorexia, and bulimia while offering interesting and effective practices to strengthen the immune system and reduce the many harmful effects of stress on the body and mind.

Sensory Therapy: Practices Ancient and Modern

Many diverse cultures, including Native American, Indian, Chinese, and Egyptian, used sensory therapies such as aromatherapy and hydrotherapy for healing the body and mind. Living in concert with the world around them, these cultures recognized the healing potential of plant essences, which they used to create pungent or sweet-smelling cosmetics, medicines, and incense. Water, one of the most basic ingredients necessary for life, was used for therapeutic baths, as an elixir, and in purifying rituals.

The ancient Greeks and Romans also made use of these natural methods of life enhancement, health maintenance, and healing. Hippocrates (c. 460–377 BCE), often called the father of modern medicine, was known to have prescribed both hydrotherapy and sunlight (the most basic form of all light therapy) for many conditions. The Romans had bathhouses where people went for relaxation, hygiene, and recreation, much the way health clubs are used today.

Hydrotherapy has been used fairly constantly throughout Western history. Spas were built throughout Europe in the eighteenth century in places such as Spa, Belgium; Baden-Baden, Germany; and Vichy, France, where people went to "take the waters."

Sensory Therapies in Western Medical Practice

At the beginning of the nineteenth century sensory therapies grew more popular, and more uses for them developed. At that time Vincent Priessnitz (1799–1852), an Austrian peasant, intuitively used hydrotherapy to heal his broken ribs. Father Sebastian Kneipp (1821–1897), a German priest, used hydrotherapy for a variety of ailments. In France in the mid-1800s Dr. Emile Javal, an ophthalmologist, was designing eye exercises as an alternative to the destructive eye surgery practices of the day. These exercises became the basis of present-day behavioral vision therapy.

By the early part of the twentieth century sensory therapies had become an accepted part of Western medical practice. Father Sebastian Kneipp's methods, which came to be known as naturopathy, spread throughout Europe and America through the work of Benedict Lust, a German-American cured of tuberculosis by Kneipp in 1892. The sun cure, the therapeutic use of sunbathing, was used in many hospitals and sanatoriums, including the prestigious Charing Cross Hospital in London.

Meanwhile more doctors began to experiment with these drug-free, nonsurgical methods, developing deeper insights into the connections between the senses and the mind. For example, in the 1930s Dr. Edward Bach, a British physician, began experimenting with methods of imbibing plant essences to alleviate the psychological problems he observed as the precursors and hindrances to healing of the physical ailments presented by his patients. The thirty-eight remedies and methods he discovered are the basis of present-day flower remedies.

Pharmaceuticals Overshadow Sensory Therapies

After 1928, with the discovery of penicillin and other powerful antibiotics, the Western medical establishment began to lose interest in sensory therapies. These newly discovered drugs worked quickly and were thought to be more effective than the slower-working sensory therapies. As pharmaceutical research exploded, scientists manufactured a multitude of synthetic drugs that were applied to numerous physical and psychological illnesses.

Throughout the mid-twentieth century interest in sensory therapies was kept alive by curious and dedicated individuals such as the American physician Harry Spitler. Spitler expanded the range of light therapy by exploring the effects of various colored lights on the emotions. In the 1950s Dr. Alfred Tomatis (1920–), a French physician, discovered that the ability to speak is directly related to the ability to hear and that both abilities affect creativity, motivation, and the ability to learn. His series of exercises, known as the Tomatis method, helps people regain the abilities to listen and concentrate.

A Revival for Sensory Therapies

In the 1960s a confluence of forces in science and culture created a resurgence of interest in sensory therapies, as well as other holistic health and living practices. Many people were becoming disillusioned with conventional medicine, which relied more and more on pharmaceutical solutions, which often create dangerous side effects and debilitating conditions. The social revolution of the decade brought a greater awareness of the value of the senses in living life fully. Many people, young and old, began turning to more natural sources of healing.

With the approach of the twenty-first century, scientists and healers in many areas continue to explore the ways in which we can use the senses to affect our physical and emotional functioning and enhance our experience of life. Today a wide variety of sensory therapies are used individually or combined with other natural healing modalities such as bodywork and massage, psychotherapy, diet, and movement practices to heal specific injuries and conditions, to alleviate the detrimental effects of stress, and to improve the quality of life.

The methods in this section share many philosophical beliefs with the other body-mind disciplines presented in this book. They all see human beings as complex organisms of interconnected aspects, complete with their own self-healing/self-regulating mechanisms. Illness, whether viewed as a chemical imbalance or as a breakdown in an interconnected process involving body and mind, is believed to be continually perpetuated by a malfunction or block in the self-regulating mechanism. The goal of each of the methods described in this section is to remove blocks in the self-regulating mechanism so that it can bring the body and mind back into balance.

Because sensory therapies view human beings as an integral part of nature, they believe the means to remove these blocks, or stimulate the self-healing mechanism, can be found in natural elements and processes. What distinguishes these methods from any other holistic healing modalities is their use of the sense organ —eyes, ears, nose, taste buds, and skin—as the primary entry point to the interconnected systems of body, mind, and spirit.

Western Science's Theories on Sensory Therapies

Although human beings have reaped the benefits of sensory therapies for centuries, advances in scientific research in the latter part of the twentieth century have given the Western medical community new information about the connections between the senses and other systems of the body.

Today scientists have identified that the limbic system, which controls heart rate, blood pressure, breath rate, and hormone levels, is highly sensitive to odors and also stores emotional memories. It is believed to be the system activated through aromatherapy and the use of flower remedies. The nervous system, with its thousands of receptors on the surface of the skin and access to every organ of the body, is thought to be the primary system activated through the many external forms of hydrotherapy. Light therapy seems to achieve its effects through the endocrine system. This system is stimulated when light- and color-sensitive photo receptors in the eyes convert sunlight into electrical impulses, which are sent along the optic nerve to the brain.

While this scientific information may be reassuring to some, it is admittedly sketchy to others, and few advocates of sensory therapies would aim to convince a prospective practitioner of a method's efficacy based solely on current Western scientific knowledge. But with ever greater interest in drug-free, nonsurgical methods of health maintenance and healing and ever greater development of scientific research methods, the time may not be distant when the many healing effects of these methods will be fully understood.

—Nancy Allison, CMA

Further Reading:

Bates, William H., M.D. *The Bates Method for Better Eyesight Without Glasses.* New York: Henry Holt, 1940.

Buchman, Dian Dincin. *The Complete Book of Water Therapy.* New Canaan, CT: Keats Publishing, Inc., 1994.

Devi, Lila. *The Essential Flower Essence Handbook.* Carlsbad, CA: Hay House, Inc., 1996.

Dewhurst-Maddock, Olivea. *The Book of Sound Therapy: Heal Yourself with Music and Voice.* New York: Simon & Schuster, Inc., 1993.

Kelville, Kathi, and Mindy Green. *Aromatherapy: A Complete Guide to the Healing Art.* Freedom, CA: The Crossing Press, 1997.

Kennedy, Teresa. *Sensual Healing: An Elemental Guide to Feeling Good.* New York: M. Evans and Company, Inc., 1996.

Scheffer, Mechthild. *Bach Flower Therapy: Theory and Practice.* Rochester, VT: Healing Arts Press, 1988.

AROMATHERAPY

Aromatherapy is a branch of herbal medicine in which aromatic plant extracts are inhaled or applied to the skin as a means of treating illness and promoting beneficial changes in mood and outlook. Though aromatherapy and herbal medicine use many of the same plants, in aromatherapy the plants are distilled into oils of exceptional potency. As much as three thousand pounds of a plant may be consumed in the production of one pound of "essential oil" suitable for aromatherapy.

The therapeutic power of such oils is generally attributed to their ability to influence the workings of the limbic system, the "switchboard" in the brain that coordinates mind and body activity. When a small amount of oil is rubbed into the skin or inhaled, it sets off a chain reaction that leads to rapid, profound alteration in memory, heart rate, and other bodily processes. Most recipients choose oils that promote relaxation, but certain oils can boost energy, and others are thought to have pharmaceutical properties.

The 1990s saw an explosion of scientific interest in all aspects of aromatherapy. It is, however, an ancient mode of medicine that can be traced back to the dawn of civilization.

A Long History

In ancient Egypt, extracts of plants were mixed with animal oil to form aromatic balms thought to be of inestimable worth in proper care of the person's whole being, mind, body, and soul. The balms were rubbed into the skin and hair for medicinal as well as cosmetic purposes and burned in religious rituals at temples and tombs. The practice of mummification was itself a type of aromatherapy, since the body was preserved and purified through the systematic application of balms.

While the ancient Greeks and Romans did not practice mummification, they employed aromatic balms much as the Egyptians had. Balms were regarded as medicine, as luxurious items of personal care, and as offerings in religious rituals. Renaissance paintings that depict the Three Wise Men presenting gifts of frankincense and myrrh to the infant Christ are an example of the ancient ritual use of aromatic balms.

Modern aromatherapy is based on the research of a French chemist, René-Maurice Gattefosse, who recognized the healing powers of the substances routinely made into perfumes. In 1928, he published a paper that gave the medicinal use of plant oils a name, "aromatherapy," as well as introducing a set of principles.

These principles were developed by a handful of French and English scientists, most notably Marguerite Maury and Jean Valnet, who compiled data and published a number of books, including Valnet's classic, *The Practice of Aromatherapy*. But awareness of the benefits of aromatherapy was confined to European circles until the advent of holistic medicine swept it into prominence in the United States.

By 1990, aromatherapy had sparked a nationwide boom in the sale of incense, scented candles, and bath oils and became a popular adjunct of massage and stress-management programs. Today, Egyptian, ayurvedic, Chinese, and Native American practices are all being studied with a view toward scientific adaptation. Drug-free treatments for shingles and herpes have already been developed, and there are indications essential oils can also be helpful in treating colds and similar airborne infectious diseases, arthritis, and muscle disorders.

The Power of Fragrance

Aromatherapy is based on the belief that plants, particularly flowers and herbs, have healing properties that can be concentrated when the plants are distilled into fragrant oils. The aroma of the oils is by no means simply an attractive extra, like the candy coating on a bitter pill. The limbic system of the brain is highly sensitive to odors and routinely encodes them into patterns of associations and

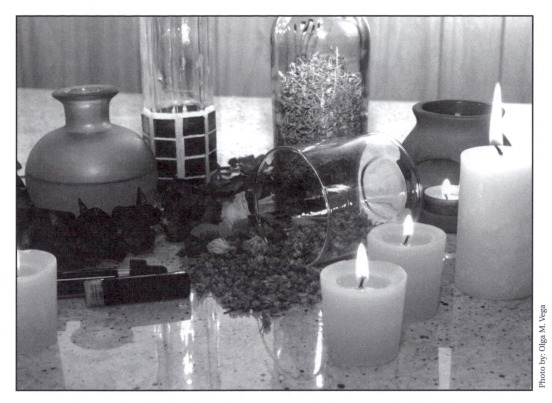

Photo by: Olga M. Vega

Aromatherapy, a branch of herbal medicine, uses aromatic plant extracts in oils and fragrant candles to awaken memories that alter basic physical functions, such as heart and breath rate.

memories that are ever present within the unconscious. Because the limbic system is also a "switchboard" controlling heart rate, blood pressure, breathing, and hormone levels, aroma provides a subtle yet effective way to induce beneficial changes in the vital functions of the organism.

When essential oils are rubbed into the skin, the power of their fragrance is thought to be increased by their ability to penetrate bodily tissue and make swift entry into the bloodstream. In the case of eucalyptus, for example, the action is said to be anti-inflammatory in nature. Other oils are believed to have antiviral, antibacterial, or detoxifying powers.

Approximately three dozen essential oils are now in common use among Aromatherapists. Though the oils can be administered separately, a typical treatment entails a blend of oils made to suit the physiological and psychological needs of the individual. It is for this reason

that aromatherapy is often described as an art and a science. The rules governing the mixing and application of the plant extracts have to be interpreted in a way that is sensitive to the person's inner and outer condition.

Using Aromatherapy

Aromatherapy can be performed by either a practitioner who is likely to specialize in both aromatherapy and traditional herbal medicine or a massage therapist who includes aromatherapy in his or her regimen. It is also possible to approach aromatherapy as home care, using products bought at a holistic health center or ordered from an aromatherapy institute. Generally speaking, beginners are advised to consult an expert before embarking on aromatherapy.

Once the appropriate essential oils have been acquired, they are either inhaled or applied to the skin through one of several methods. The oil can be put on a piece of cotton that is held close to the nose and sniffed. Diffusers that disperse the oil into the air are equally effective.

The manner in which the oils are applied to the skin depends in part on the nature of the problem being treated. Herpes lesions respond to direct application of oil, whereas relief from stress customarily requires soaking in bath water containing some essential oil. When the oils are incorporated into massage, they are always mixed with a carrier lotion such as jojoba.

An Effective Treatment

Aromatherapy can bring relief from stress and promote a sense of well-being that activates the organism's capacity for self-healing. It has also been used effectively in the treatment of burns, insect bites, bruises, disorders of the skin ranging from acne to herpes, indigestion, colds, flu, and immune deficiencies.

As a caution, no aromatherapy treatment should ever involve more than a few drops of essential oil. Overdosage may cause a severe toxic reaction. A physician's guidance is required if the oil is to be placed on the tongue or swallowed.

Resources:

Aromatherapy Seminars
3379 S. Robertson Boulevard
Los Angeles, CA 90034
Tel: (800) 677-2368
Offers a variety of educational services in aromatherapy, including introductory and advanced training programs, correspondence courses, and videotapes.

National Association for Holistic Aromatherapy
P.O. Box 17622
Boulder, CO 80398-0622
Tel: (303) 258-3791
Provides courses in aromatherapy and a nationwide referral service for aromatherapists.

The Pacific Institute of Aromatherapy
P.O. Box 6842
San Rafael, CA 94903
Tel: (415) 479-9121
A research and teaching institute that offers individual and group courses in aromatherapy.

Further Reading:

Lavabre, Marcel. *Aromatherapy Workbook.* Rochester, VT: Healing Arts Press, 1990.

Rose, Jeanne. *The Aromatherapy Book: Applications and Inhalations.* Berkeley, CA: North Atlantic Books, 1992.

Tisserand, Robert. *Aromatherapy to Heal and Tend the Body.* Santa Fe, NM: Lotus Light Press, 1988.

Valnet, Jean. *The Practice of Aromatherapy.* Rochester, VT: Inner Traditions, 1990 (first published 1977).

BATES METHOD

The Bates method is a system of holistic eye care that uses mental and physical exercises, rather than corrective lenses, to improve chronic problems of vision. It is named after its founder, the American ophthalmologist William Bates (1860–1931), who challenged the medical establishment by ascribing poor sight to habitual misuse of eye muscles caused ultimately by emotional stress. Bates believed the damaging habits could be unlearned through application of a daily routine of exercises designed to relieve tension in the eye muscles and teach the eyes to function in a relaxed, natural way. Contemporary vision training makes extensive use of these exercises.

A Controversial Treatment

Bates was a prominent ophthalmologist in New York City when he began to doubt the fundamental principles of his profession. Problems of vision were generally considered hereditary or part of the aging process and treated with prescription glasses, which did little to halt, let alone reverse, the weakening of vision.

After several years of research, Bates published a controversial book, *Better*

Eyesight Without Glasses (1920), in which he argued that the standard treatment was not only based on false premises but actually damaged patients' ability to recover. Glasses, Bates reasoned, reinforced bad use of eye muscles, caused initially by psychological tension, and destined their wearers to a lifetime of impaired vision. The remedial exercises recommended by Bates proved to be as controversial as his attack upon prescription glasses and found little support in professional circles.

Nonetheless, the Bates method did attract followers and had some notable successes. One of these success stories was the British writer Aldous Huxley. In an essay about his experiences with the treatment, Huxley contended that questions concerning the "orthodoxy" of the Bates method were misinformed. It is, he explained, "a method of education, fundamentally similar to the method of education devised and successfully used by all the teachers of psycho-physical skills for the last several thousand years."

Practitioners believe that the Bates method is a pioneering form of biofeedback and stress-reduction training. In addition, Bates is notable as one of the first doctors to recognize the relationship between vision and emotional disturbance, an insight of vast significance to fields ranging from special education to sports to the study of art.

Reeducating the Eye

According to Bates, "we see very largely with the mind and only partly with the eyes." This hypothesis led Bates to regard vision as inherently individual and variable: mood, memory, health, and circumstances play a role in what and how a person sees.

His primary concern was the functioning of the six muscles controlling the shape of the eye. In his opinion, they determine the eye's ability to focus and, therefore, constitute the all-important link between mind and vision. Accumulated tension in any of these small muscles could gradually weaken vision, producing nearsightedness, farsightedness, astigmatism, or a condition such as "lazy eye." Conversely, Bates argued, releasing the tension and encouraging the muscles to regain their innate flexibility and strength could repair poor vision.

Bates's understanding of vision is based on the behavioral model of health, also crucial to the Alexander technique, which credits the organism with the ability to heal itself once "blocks" in its natural operation are removed. To this end, he formulated a set of eye exercises, commonly referred to as the Bates method, which he believed could "reeducate" the muscles of the eye.

No doubt, the most surprising of Bates's training exercises is one that turns the vision test chart into a memory device. By memorizing the letters and numbers on the chart, trainees simultaneously sharpen their acuity of vision and assume mastery of a source of anxiety. Most of the exercises were designed to stop the habitual staring Bates identified as a prime symptom of "blocked" vision. In "shifting," the trainee learns to look "through" objects, while in "swinging," they move their eyes in accordance with a rhythmic side-to-side swaying of the body.

A Flexible and Demanding Treatment

Treatment with the Bates method is available from optometrists who have

Though contemporary vision training incorporates many new techniques, it is based on Bates's approach and makes extensive use of the exercises he devised. These have also been an important resource for airline pilots and athletes seeking to strengthen their eye-brain coordination.

specialized in vision training. Programs of therapy are adjusted to meet the individual's need and are likely to include recently developed techniques or updated versions of the Bates exercises. In most cases, therapy entails several months of weekly training sessions and faithful performance of a routine of daily exercises at home, school, or work.

Benefits and Risks

The Bates method is credited with dramatic improvement in the vision of many people required to wear corrective lenses because of a common vision problem. By relieving a key pocket of stress, it is also thought to enhance the individual's sense of well-being and sometimes can speed recovery from other disorders.

But the Bates method, with or without a comprehensive vision training program, should not be considered an appropriate treatment for cataracts, glaucoma, or other diseases of the eye. Anyone with these or related problems is advised to consult a licensed ophthalmologist.

Resources:

College of Optometrists in Vision Development
P.O. Box 285
Chula Vista, CA 91912
Tel: (619)425-6191
Fax: (619)425-0733
A professional organization for optometrists specializing in the Bates method and other techniques of vision training.

Further Reading:

Bates, W. *The Bates Method for Better Eyesight Without Glasses.* New York: Henry Holt & Co., 1987 (first published 1920).

Cheney, E. *The Eyes Have It: A Self-Help Manual for Better Vision.* York Beach, ME: Samuel Weiser, Inc., 1987.

BEHAVIORAL VISION THERAPY

Behavioral vision therapy is an optometric specialty that uses a visual training regimen to improve vision by strengthening the vital link between the mind and the eye complex. In contrast, surgery for eye-muscle problems targets the physical structure of the eye while neglecting the mental aspects of seeing and therefore may produce less-than-desirable results. Behavioral optometrists consider environmental factors that affect vision as well as psychological and physiological factors that may contribute to—and result from—vision difficulties. With vision training, significant improvements in social, academic, and athletic skills can be achieved.

The History of Behavioral Vision Therapy

In the mid-1800s, the French ophthalmologist Emile Javal developed a scientific and nonsurgical method of visual rehabilitation known as orthoptics after witnessing the horrible outcomes of eye surgery for both his father and sister. Orthoptics was designed to treat improper eye alignment, specifically crossed eyes (inward turn), wall eyes (outward turn), and lazy eyes (visual impairment not correctable by glasses). Modern vision therapy, an advanced form of the orthoptic eye exercises developed by Dr. Javal, deals with a much wider variety of visual and perceptual problems while also considering their effects on behavior and performance. By the twentieth century the practice of orthoptics had progressed significantly in England and France.

The dawn of orthoptics in the United States occurred in 1912. This was the result of the publication of a comprehensive text on stereoscopic, or three-dimensional (3-D), eye exercises by Dr. David Wells, an ophthalmologist at Boston University Medical School. A large part of this classic text is devoted to the treatment of eye-muscle problems that are harder to diagnose because they are not as easily recognized as crossed or wall eyes, which have a definite observable cosmetic component. Wells believed that subtle eye problems were more common than the visibly obvious eye turns. Wells proposed the idea that having a single unified vision of the world through two eyes is an important and complex psychic ability, and that "its inefficiency could result in an inability to fix one's mind on study and reading." Wells also strongly felt that the clinical significance of common eye problems was largely ignored by practicing ophthalmologists. Many modern practitioners of vision therapy feel that this is still a problem among ophthalmologists.

The Optometric Extension Program (OEP), postgraduate study dedicated to education and research in vision, was established in 1928. OEP represented the earliest organized approach to orthoptics within the optometric profession, and it is still a vital force in the field of behavioral vision care today. A leading figure in OEP, Dr. A. M. Skeffington, broadened the orthoptic approach, giving it a much more holistic base. He introduced the idea that eye-muscle and focusing deficiencies, rather than developing spontaneously, may evolve as a person grows and adapts to the environment. Skeffington and other behavioral optometrists also introduced the revolutionary concepts of reducing and controlling nearsightedness and improving focusing ability through vision training.

A Humanistic Approach to Vision

Modern vision therapy is based on the concept that vision is a dynamic process made up of numerous skills that can be learned through training. In addition, vision is a process influenced by emotions, intellect, posture, breathing, physiology, visual working habits, lighting conditions, diet, and by our own style of visual perception. An expanded, humanistic approach to vision further maintains that total visual performance cannot be adequately reduced to a single measurement such as 20/20. More traditional methods measure visual performance by reading charts at a distance of twenty feet, assessing the ability to focus on stationary images directly ahead. The rating 20/20 is equated as "perfect vision." It has never been scientifically or clinically validated that 20/20 endows us with the ability to see with comfort, efficiency, meaning, or while in motion. As the educational consultant Sally Brockett has written, "When we speak of vision, we are referring to the ability of the brain to organize and interpret information seen so it becomes understandable or meaningful. Even individuals with good eyesight (20/20 acuity) can have undiagnosed vision problems that make it difficult to correctly comprehend the visual message." Although testing for 20/20 is clinically valid, this measurement is only a partial assessment of an extremely complex process. According to behavioral optometrists, traditional eye-care methods—those represented by the simple chart test—need to be supplemented by more dynamic approaches to testing and enhancing visual performance.

The "Eye Gym": Experiencing Behavioral Vision Therapy

Participants in a behavioral vision therapy program have all aspects of their visual performance tested and trained in an "eye gym," which has an almost carnival-like appearance. It consists of walking rails, balance boards, trampolines, eye-exercise equipment, metronomes, focusing charts, special training lenses and prisms, strobe lights, and other light-therapy devices. This equipment is used to improve visual comfort, efficiency, and performance. Exercises vary in difficulty and frequently involve several different kinds of sensory information

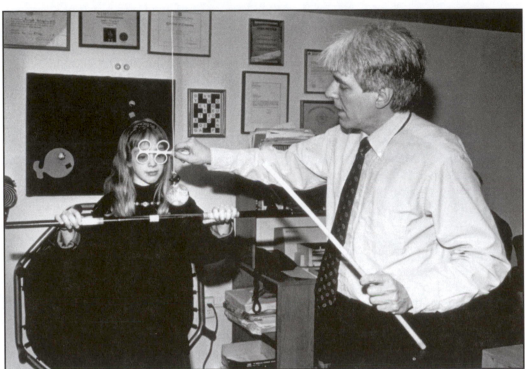

Photo by: Jonathan Gutlib

Optometrist Dr. Joseph Shapiro uses physical behavioral vision therapy exercises to help a young girl improve her vision.

presented simultaneously to the patient. For example, an individual may stand on a balance board and attempt eye-hand coordination tasks while trying to perform in time with a metronome. The exercises are repeated and, over time, they increase in difficulty until the individual gradually enhances neurological response related to vision and establishes good habits.

Visual biofeedback is commonly incorporated into treatment, giving the individual a physiological readout of current performance levels. Often people are unaware of the extent, nature, or even presence of eye problems. Feedback indicators show blurring, doubling, or vanishing of an image. Training techniques are designed to isolate and highlight symptoms of eye dysfunction, enabling the individual to better recognize, understand, and respond to the specific features of his or her vision problems. The individual is taught to send a conscious message to the eyes to restore the clarity, singleness of vision, or presence of the image. This practice

strengthens the eye and brain connection and can improve performance in most cases. An example of an optical device used for a biofeedback session might be a pair of glasses with one red lens and one green lens. An individual wearing these glasses and looking at a beam of light should perceive only a single light that is a red-green mixture that results from the brain's combination of sensory input received through the red lens and the green lens. In contrast, an individual who perceives two separate lights, one red and one green, has double vision. Alternatively, the person who perceives only one colored light, either red or green, is relying primarily on one eye to see. Now the individual has concrete, understandable feedback that something is wrong, and can start working on consciously changing the incorrect response. Through practice, the proper response may become naturally and unconsciously incorporated into the individual's daily performance. Depending on the individual's level of performance during a treatment session, home exercises are usually prescribed.

Conditions Helped by Behavioral Vision Therapy

Conditions that might bring you to a behavioral optometrist include persistent eye strain, blurring or double vision, headaches, short attention span, learning problems or reading discomfort, lazy eye at any age, eye-muscle problems, depth-perception difficulties, or worsening eyesight. Behavioral optometrists can offer alternative therapies if you are having eye or vision problems and the only solution offered by other doctors is another pair of glasses, or you are told that you have 20/20 vision and thus there is nothing wrong with your eyes. Behavioral optometrists cite examples in which proper assessment and treatment of vision problems have helped children with behavior problems participate productively in the classroom; improved the performance of top athletes; and given children the confidence to take part in social activities that previously might have drawn attention to their vision difficulties.

—*Dr. Joseph Shapiro, Optometrist*

Resources:

American Optometric Association
243 N. Lindbergh Blvd.
St. Louis, MO 63141
Tel: (314) 991-4100
Fax: (314) 991-4101
Professional society of optometrists. The association will provide referrals to behavioral optometrists upon request.

College of Optometrists in Vision Development (COVD)
P.O. Box 285
Chula Vista, CA 91912
Tel: (619) 425-6191
Fax: (619) 425-0733
Organization for optometrists involved in orthoptics and optometric vision therapy. It publishes the Journal of Optometric Vision Development *quarterly.*

Optometric Extension Program Foundation
1921 E. Carnegie, Suite 3L
Santa Ana, CA 92705
Tel: (714) 250-8070
Fax: (714) 250-8157
Arranges conferences and seminars as well as publishes the Journal of Behavioral Optometry *bimonthly.*

Further Reading:

Beverstock, Caroline. *Your Child's Vision Is Important.* Newark, DE: The International Reading Association, 1990.

Brockett, Sally. *"Vision Therapy: A Beneficial Intervention for Developmental Disabilities."* Web site: www.autism.org/visual/htm

Cohen, Neville S., and Joseph L. Shapiro. *Out of Sight and into Vision.* New York: Simon & Schuster, 1977.

Dawkins, Hazel Richmond, et al. *The Suddenly Successful Student: A Guide to Overcoming Learning and Behavioral Problems.* Second revised edition. Santa Ana, CA: Optometric Extension Program, 1990.

Flax, Nathan, ed. *Vision Therapy and Insurance: A Position Statement.* New York: State University of New York/State College of Optometry, 1986.

The study of developmental vision, that is, of the development of the faculty of sight, emerged in the 1950s. The Gesell Institute of Child Development in New Haven, Connecticut, sponsored controlled studies of children and served as a training ground for optometrists in applied research. Working on the premise that newborn children do not have the visual abilities of adults, researchers at the Gesell Institute tested the eyesight of infants over a period of time in order to identify the components involved in the development of vision.

Keogh, Barbara, and Michelle Pelland. "Vision Training Revisited." *Journal of Learning Disabilities*, Vol. 18, No. 4, April, 1985.

Marcus, Steven E., and Arthur S. Seiderman. *20/20 Is Not Enough: The New World of Vision*. New York: Knopf, 1989.

Toufexis, Anastasia. "Workouts for the Eyes." *Time*, February 13, 1989.

Wells, David Washburn. *Stereoscopic Treatment of Heterophoria and Heterotropia*. New York: E. B. Meyrowitz, 1912.

EYE MOVEMENT DESENSITIZATION AND REPROCESSING

Eye movement desensitization and reprocessing (EMDR) speeds recovery from a traumatic event by separating upsetting memories into basic parts. The therapy typically involves simple exercises such as using the eyes to track a rapidly moving object. While discussing the upsetting events, these movements in the body create a reaction in the mind, desensitizing the brain to the disturbing sensory and emotional aspects of a memory and allowing the sufferer to begin reprocessing that trauma in the present. Traditional psychotherapy is then used to help the client digest the trauma and store it. While the mechanics of EMDR are not fully understood, it has gained particular respect for its application in cases of post-traumatic stress disorder (PTSD), a common condition among Vietnam veterans and rape victims. It can also be used to help process less acute traumas such as negative childhood experiences, which can lead to poor self-esteem and unhappiness.

A History of EMDR

EMDR emerged from the experiences of Francine Shapiro, Ph.D. While taking a walk in 1987, Dr. Shapiro noticed that disturbing thoughts that she was having sometimes disappeared suddenly. When she consciously brought these thoughts back, they held none of the previous "hot" or negative weight. She later realized that at the time of her original thoughts, her eyes had spontaneously begun a rapid back-and-forth motion. Dr. Shapiro theorized that the removal of the upset from the memory might be linked to that movement, and tested her theory as treatment for post-traumatic stress disorder. Initial success in small, controlled studies encouraged her to pursue research further and to found the EMDR Institute. Since 1990, more than 22,000 therapists worldwide have been trained in this method.

The Theory of EMDR

EMDR helps to reprocess memories that were not properly handled by the brain when they initially occurred. EMDR theory asserts that the brain handles "memory" as a package of five distinct information components: the picture or image, the thought or auditory bundle, an emotional feeling, a physical sensation, and the belief about oneself that results from the event. This information is perceived via the senses as what we see, hear, smell, touch, and taste. Under normal circumstances, the brain metabolizes, or processes, these five types of information by talking, thinking, and dreaming about them. Through these activities, the brain sorts the information, storing the valuable aspects for easy retrieval and discarding smaller, insignificant bits of data.

In traumatic situations, however, this natural process does not always function properly. A malfunction may leave the information in a distressing, "undigested" state. In such cases, the mind locks all five types of information together, surrounding the resulting lump with negative emotional energy. The event thus becomes a blockage in the mental storage system. Any attempt to access information from the event stirs the negative energy surrounding it. In severe cases, this negative energy overwhelms and debilitates the sufferer. In these situations, the normal processes of thinking, talking, and dreaming are inadequate ways of handling these blockages. Just as a cut will not properly heal as long as a splinter is still in it, the body's normal processes can, at best, only work around a damaged memory bundle.

EMDR may act as a more intense version of rapid eye movement (REM) sleep, harnessing the body to effect a change in the mind. The mechanics of the EMDR and REM sleep are similar. During REM sleep, a dreamer's eyes move rapidly from side to side. Dr. Shapiro believes that this eye movement stimulates links between the two sides of the brain. Because each side of the brain serves a different role—the left side is the positive, analytical side, while the right side is the less linear, more sensory-oriented side—this link through REM seems to help information pass between the two sides and be processed. Hence, REM is one catalyst for natural memory "digestion."

Yet normal REM sleep cannot penetrate some particularly severe hurts. As the patient's unconscious seeks to access the memory through REM sleep, the sleeper's mind re-creates the painful negative sensations that occurred at the time of the hurt. Once awake, the right and left sides of the brain are no longer able to continue their information processing. The hurt remains locked in the body and mind.

Just as a car engine must be properly warmed up to tackle steep hills, an activity of the body—eye movement—warms the brain to the task of unraveling even the most dense ball of hurt. It is believed that the conscious rapid eye movement powerfully ignites one side of the brain, then the other in rapid succession, until finally both sides churn together. Once warmed like this, the subconscious is empowered to process the hurt without undue discomfort to the patient. The splinter being thus removed, normal healing begins.

Following the Baton

A typical EMDR session lasts ninety minutes. The patient is asked to think about the disturbing event. The practitioner then asks the patient to follow the therapist's fingers or a light bar with his or her eyes. The patient continues thinking of the memory as the practitioner moves the fingers or pointer rapidly from side to side. The participants then stop and discuss any information or revelations that occurred while the patient's eyes were moving. For most people, the traumatic event feels unexplainably less traumatic and more clear or more distant. The sufferer can finally talk with some detachment about the event, which enables the beginning of the healing process.

Risks and Benefits

In many case studies, EMDR has helped victims of PTSD and other anxiety-ridden conditions cope with their conditions. The therapy is still largely unproved, however, and does not work with all patients. Ideally it should be performed in comfortable, stress-free situations and does not affect all people in the same way. Additionally, EMDR should be performed only by a trained and licensed/certified psychotherapist. While the therapy may reduce the emotional attachment surrounding an event, the patient is still left with factual memories of the unpleasant event, which are best processed through the therapeutic skills of a trained professional.

—*Barbara Parrett, RN, M.S.*

Resources:

EMDR Institute, Inc.
P.O. Box 51010
Pacific Grove, CA 93950-6010
Tel: (408)372-3900
Web site: www.emdr.com
Provides information on EMDR.

Further Reading:

Parnell, Laurel. *EMDR : The Revolutionary New Therapy for Freeing the Mind, Clearing the Body, and Opening the Heart.* New York : W. W. Norton & Co., 1997.

Shapiro, Francine, M.D. *EMDR: Breakthrough Therapy for Overcoming Anxiety, Stress, and Trauma.* New York: Basic Books, 1997.

———. *Eye Movement Desensitization and Reprocessing: Basic Principles, Protocols, and Procedures.* Guilford, NC: Guilford Press, 1995.

FLOWER REMEDIES

Flower remedies are liquid preparations made from the flowering heads of plants and trees that are used to deal with emotional and psychological difficulties. These difficulties include fear, lack of self-confidence, jealousy, anger, and resentment, and are believed by alternative health-care professionals to be one of the root causes of physical disorder.

Flower remedies are not chosen according to physical ailments but instead are selected based on emotional and psychological difficulties, which include information on personality and behavioral traits. Once administered, it is believed that flower remedies trigger a mechanism within the brain that stimulates the body's internal healing processes, eventually resulting in a healthier emotional, psychological, and physical state. Flower remedies have been used successfully not only on humans but also to deal with negative emotional and behavioral traits in animals.

Nature's Remedies
In the early 1930s Dr. Edward Bach, a young British physician, discovered that many of his patients displayed various emotional and psychological difficulties prior to the onset of physical disease. He also found these same difficulties would complicate disease once it manifested, thereby making it more difficult to treat. The doctor's prior experience with pharmaceutical drugs and their side effects convinced him the answer to this dilemma could be found in nature, not in the laboratory. Bach left his practice and decided to research his theories. Leaving his practice to research his theories, he began experimenting with various species of plants.

Thirty-Eight Remedies
Believing the greatest healing value resides in the flowering heads of plants and trees, the doctor began developing ways to prepare and administer them. Flowers were picked at various times in their blooming cycle and floated in a bowl of freshly obtained spring water, in direct sunlight. Other flowers were gathered and prepared by boiling them in water. These preparations were then administered in minute doses according to the emotional and psychological profile of the patient. After years of research, thirty-eight flowering plants, trees, and special waters were discovered, preparations that were found to have a profound positive effect in a wide range of emotional and psychological difficulties.

In the last few decades several companies and researchers have produced these same thirty-eight flower remedy preparations under different brand names, and have also produced other flower remedy preparations from newly discovered flowering plants found in other parts of the world.

Deeply visionary, Dr. Bach wrote: "All emotional, psychological, and physical disorder grows out of a conflict between our personality and our Soul," and he believed we should regard illness as a signal that we are out of harmony within ourselves.

Over the past number of years scientists have begun to look at just how negative thoughts and emotions affect our health. Their studies show that if an emotional difficulty is not resolved within a reasonable period of time, generally from six months to a year, serious internal problems and eventually physical disease can develop.

In early stages we may see the development of functional difficulties, which include predisposition to colds and

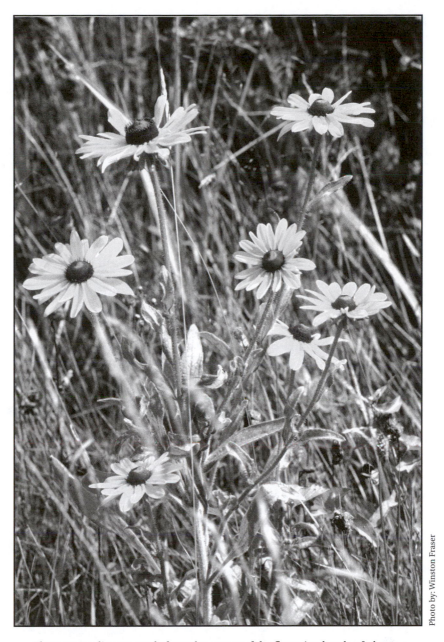

Photo by: Winston Fraser

Flower remedies are made from the extract of the flowering heads of plants, picked in various points in their blooming cycles, with different types of spring water and a small percentage of alcohol.

other infections, sexual dysfunction, headaches, fatigue, allergies, and digestive problems. These problems, among others, are the first physical warning signs that we are out of harmony within. And if underlying psycho-emotional and spiritual conflicts are not resolved, physical disease might result. It is here the physician is generally consulted. To this

Bach wrote: "The main reason for the failure of modern medicine is that it is dealing with results, not causes. . . . Disease will never be cured or eradicated by present materialistic methods for the simple reason that disease in its origin is not material, [but the] ultimate result produced in the body, the end product of deep and long-acting forces. . ."

Using Flower Remedies

Flower remedies are easy to choose and use. Ellon, Inc., a major international supplier of these flower remedies, provides a free self-help questionnaire on choosing and applying the remedies.

Once chosen, remedies may be taken any number of ways—directly from the concentrate bottles under the tongue, by mixing several drops of each remedy in a drink and sipping at intervals, or by mixing several drops of each remedy in a one-ounce dropper bottle with water and consuming it over a period of time. For people with alcohol sensitivities (most flower remedy preparations contain some alcohol as a preservative), these remedies can also be applied directly from the concentrate bottle to the temples, wrists, behind the ears, or under the arms. This can also be an effective way of administering flower remedies to infants and small children.

Flower remedies are known to have a unique and personal effect on each person taking them. Remedies are taken until difficulties are resolved, when there is a lifting of the negative emotional state, or a stabilizing of overreactive personality traits. In general, most people can resolve difficulties within one to twelve weeks, although some may take longer. Once these difficulties are resolved, the remedies may be discontinued. Often, however, one can experience a "peeling" effect, where one or more emotional difficulties are resolved and other underlying emotions emerge. In these and other instances, new remedies may be chosen, as needed, by consulting the self-help questionnaire.

The Benefits of Flower Remedies

Since the mid-1930s, the thirty-eight flower preparations have been used successfully by countless physicians and others to deal with a wide range of difficulties that include, but are not limited to, fear, anxiety, uncertainty, indecisiveness, envy, jealousy, and lack of self-confidence. They've also been used to deal with the stress associated with everyday problems, such as financial difficulties, relationship problems,

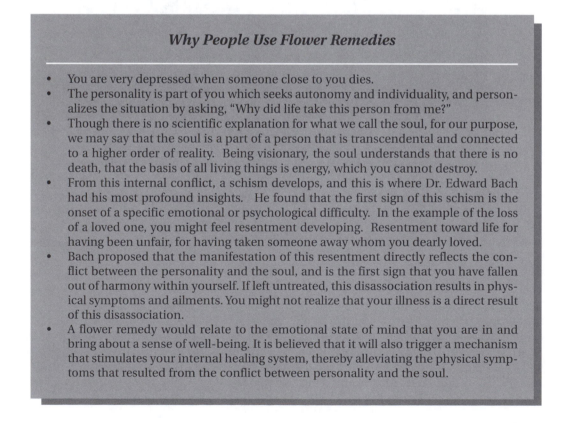

Why People Use Flower Remedies

- You are very depressed when someone close to you dies.
- The personality is part of you which seeks autonomy and individuality, and personalizes the situation by asking, "Why did life take this person from me?"
- Though there is no scientific explanation for what we call the soul, for our purpose, we may say that the soul is a part of a person that is transcendental and connected to a higher order of reality. Being visionary, the soul understands that there is no death, that the basis of all living things is energy, which you cannot destroy.
- From this internal conflict, a schism develops, and this is where Dr. Edward Bach had his most profound insights. He found that the first sign of this schism is the onset of a specific emotional or psychological difficulty. In the example of the loss of a loved one, you might feel resentment developing. Resentment toward life for having been unfair, for having taken someone away whom you dearly loved.
- Bach proposed that the manifestation of this resentment directly reflects the conflict between the personality and the soul, and is the first sign that you have fallen out of harmony within yourself. If left untreated, this disassociation results in physical symptoms and ailments. You might not realize that your illness is a direct result of this disassociation.
- A flower remedy would relate to the emotional state of mind that you are in and bring about a sense of well-being. It is believed that it will also trigger a mechanism that stimulates your internal healing system, thereby alleviating the physical symptoms that resulted from the conflict between personality and the soul.

day-to-day worries, periods of transition, and job-related tensions. Additionally, preparations of these flowers have proven effective in dealing with stress-related hyperactivity in children, dieting and eating problems, learning difficulties, sleeping problems, and to help ease the trauma of divorce and other loss.

—Leslie J. Kaslof

Resources:

Ellon, Inc.
193 Middle St. Ste. 201
Portland, ME 04101
Tel: (800) 423-2256
Produces and distributes worldwide the thirty-eight flower preparations. Carries a full line of flower remedy product information. Also provides an extremely useful self-help questionnaire for choosing the thirty-eight flower remedies.

Flower Essence Society
P.O. Box 459
Nevada City, CA 95959
Tel: (916) 263-9162
Disseminates various information about flower remedies. Sells its own line of flower essences and imports and distributes other lines of flower remedies.

Further Reading:

Bach, Edward, and F.J. Wheeler. *Bach Flower Remedies.* New Canaan, CT: Keats, 1979.

Kaslof, Leslie J. *The Traditional Flower Remedies of Dr. Edward Bach: A Self-Help Guide.* New Canaan, CT: Keats, 1993.

Vlamis, Gregory. *Flowers to the Rescue.* New York: Thorsons, 1986.

HYDROTHERAPY

Hydrotherapy is the treatment of injury or disease with the application of water in one of its three forms—steam, liquid, or ice. It may be used as hot or cold applications alone, or it may be applied one after the other in contrasting applications. Hydrotherapy exerts its effects both locally and at sites away from its application. Its distant effects are mediated through a reflex arc that is a normal function of the nervous system. An example of this reflex action would be the effect of hydrotherapy on the liver. An application of heat over the liver will not heat the liver itself, but through the reflex arc, there will be vasodilation of the liver as if it were heated directly.

Hydrotherapy may be used to aid in the treatment of addiction through detoxification treatments or to aid in the general mental and physical health of a person by encouraging relaxation, increasing energy level or vitality, and strengthening the immune and other total body systems.

The Ancient and Modern History of Hydrotherapy

Hydrotherapy has been employed throughout the world, from earliest recorded history to the present. The Egyptians, Babylonians, Greeks, Chinese, Native Americans, and numerous other cultures have used water for therapeutic purposes. Baths, saunas, mineral soaks, flushes, irrigations, steams, and compresses are just some of the ways water has been used for healing purposes. The Greek physician Hippocrates employed hydrotherapy in the treatment of fevers, ulcers, hemorrhages, and other medical and surgical conditions. The Roman baths are a prime example of the social, hygienic, and medical uses of hydrotherapy.

Modern hydrotherapy owes much to several practitioners of the art. Some were trained physicians, while others were lay practitioners who learned more by experience than training. A nineteenth-century Austrian peasant, Vincent Priessnitz (1799–1852), is said to have treated his own broken ribs with cold water applications, and soon began treating others with great success. German priest Father Sebastian

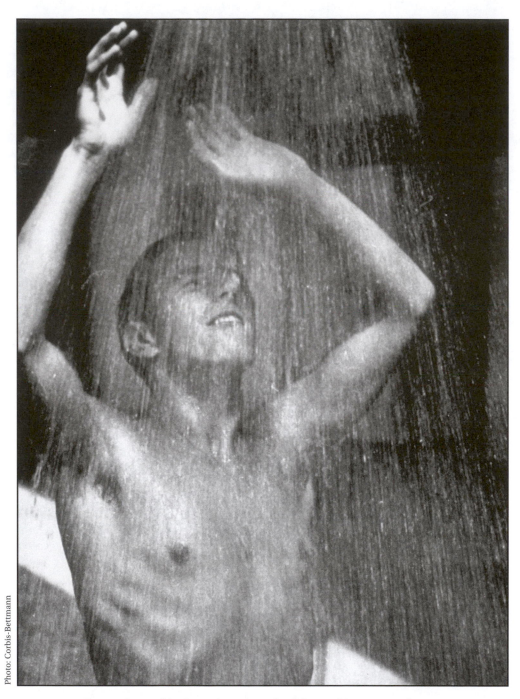

Photo: Corbis-Bettmann

Even a pleasurable shower is an example of the soothing powers of water.

Kneipp (1821–1897) was cured of tuberculosis after he had begun immersing himself in cold water a few times a week. His book *My Water Cure* (1890) is a classic in the field of hydrotherapy. William Winternitz (1834–1912) was a prominent physician who was the first to demonstrate that hydrotherapy exerts its greatest influence on the nervous system. John Harvey Kellogg (1852–1943) established the Battle Creek Sanitorium in Michigan, where hundreds of patients were treated with hydrotherapy, diet, and exercise. Dr. Kellogg wrote *Rational Hydrotherapy* (1900), which remains the most comprehensive text

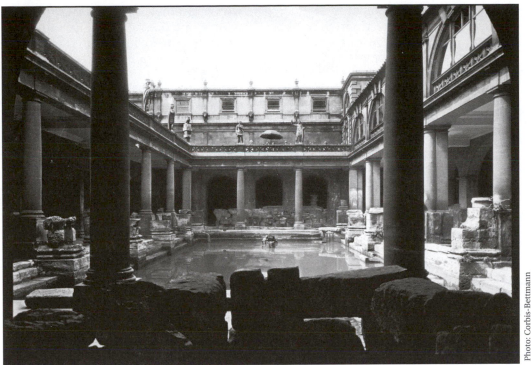

Photo: Corbis-Bettmann

In Bath, England, the same hot springs discovered by Romans in the first century C.E. are still enjoyed for their therapeutic value.

ever written on the subject of hydrotherapy. It includes more than 1,100 pages of text and illustrations.

Today hydrotherapy is used as either a primary or supplemental therapy by a number of physicians, physical therapists, and psychologists to treat a wide range of conditions, including stress, AIDS, addictions, and allergies.

The Theory Behind Hydrotherapy

Hydrotherapy recognizes the interrelatedness of the mind and body. Although most hydrotherapy treatments aim to relieve a physical condition, the theory supporting the treatment is always based on the knowledge that the state of the body affects the state of the mind. The chemicals, nutrients, or toxins that affect both the mind and body are messengers that communicate vital information connecting the major organs and systems of the whole person. Hydrotherapy directly stimulates these messengers.

External hydrotherapy—the application of water to the outside of the body—is divided into three types: hot water, cold water, or contrast. Hot water stimulates the immune system to release white blood cells that remove toxins from the blood. It also relaxes muscles and soothes nerves. The nerves are responsible for sending all messages from the brain to other areas of the body and, therefore, play an important role in our emotional and mental as well as physical condition. Cold water counteracts swelling and inflammation by constricting the blood vessels. Contrasting applications of hot and cold water stimulate the endocrine and adrenal glands, reduce congestion, and improve organ functioning.

Water with a high content of certain minerals can provide additional benefits. Water high in sulfur, for example, can help ease the effects of arthritis, rheumatism, and skin diseases. Bicarbonated spring water has been used in the treatment of allergies.

Internal applications of hydrotherapy may also be made. These may be as simple as drinking water to relieve dehydration or as complex as the application of internal irrigations. Internal irrigations of hydrotherapy are frequently used to dislodge unwanted material from the area being irrigated. Ear lavage is used to clean earwax from the external ear canal, whereas enema or colonic irrigation is used to eliminate dry, hard fecal material from the colon. It is, therefore, possible, using internal application, to take advantage of the thermal, chemical, and/or mechanical properties of water.

Making Use of the Different Properties of Water

There are countless forms of hydrotherapy, including baths and soaks, steams and saunas, irrigations and flushes, and wraps and compresses. The chemical properties of water allow it to be used to dissolve and remove unwanted materials from the body. This might be done by immersion in a tank of hot water, allowing water-soluble substances to dissolve from the skin. It may also be used in irrigations applied to the body. The chemical properties of water are also helpful in dissolving and applying desirable compounds, such as Epsom salts, to the body. Both internal and external applications may be made using herbal teas and other infusions, such as echinacea or goldenseal.

The thermal properties of water make it useful for adding heat to or removing heat from the body. It can be used to raise a low body temperature or reduce a fever. Hydrotherapy can also aid in relieving the heat from inflammations, such as those that might occur with a sprained ankle, or to add heat to relieve muscle spasms. In addition, water has been found to alleviate the stresses and strains of everyday life, as well as treating emotional and mental disturbances by soothing the nervous system.

The mechanical properties of water, in the form of sprays and showers, can be stimulating to various parts of the body. The mechanical action of immersion in water can exert pressure to help relieve swelling, provide buoyancy to counteract the effects of gravity—easing pain and improving movement, and provide resistance for exercise. For people whose general body condition is so poor that "on-land" exercise programs prove impossible, hydrotherapy can create the physical environment where progress can be made, thus stimulating the patient's motivation—an important emotional component of the healing process.

The Benefits and Contraindications of Hydrotherapy

Hydrotherapy treatments strengthen the body's own functions and defense mechanisms. They work with the body and the mind, enabling them to restore balance and let healing occur.

When applying hydrotherapy treatments, care must be taken with the elderly and the very young. People of these ages often have a diminished ability to maintain their body temperature and, therefore, can be heated or chilled too much. Persons with diminished sensation or poor circulation should also be treated with great care since it is possible to burn or freeze tissue without their being aware.

—*Douglas C. Lewis, ND*

Hydrotherapy is a holistic approach to healing. It holds that the body-mind has its own self-regulating and healing processes and mechanisms. By its gentle, noninvasive techniques, it aims to stimulate these innate healing capacities.

Resources:

American Association of Naturopathic Physicians
2366 Eastlake Avenue., Ste. 322
Seattle, WA 98102
Tel: (206) 323-7610
Provides referrals nationwide to health care professionals who practice hydrotherapy.

Bastyr University Natural Health Clinic
1307 North 45th St., Ste. 200
Seattle, WA 98103
Tel: (206) 632-0354
A teaching and treatment clinic for the use of hydrotherapy.

National College of Naturopathic Medicine
11231 Southeast Market St.
Portland, OR 97216
Tel: (503) 255-4860
Offers referrals to naturopathic doctors as well as training in naturopathic medicine.

Further Reading:

Boyle, Wade, and Andre Saine. *Lectures in Naturo-pathic Hydrotherapy.* East Palestine, OH: Buck-eye Naturopathic Press, 1988.

Croutier, Alev Lytle. *Taking the Waters.* New York: Abbeville Press, 1992.

Moor, Fred B., et al. *Manual of Hydrotherapy and Massage.* Boise: Pacific Press Publishing Associ-ation, 1964.

Ruoti, Richard, David Morris, and Andrew Cole. *Aquatic Rehabilitation.* Philadelphia: Lippin-cott, 1997.

Thrash, Agatha, and Calvin Thrash. *Home Reme-dies.* Seale, AL: Thrash Publications, 1981.

LIGHT THERAPY

Light therapy is a general term for therapies that use the entire electromagnetic spectrum or specific wavelengths of light to treat physical and emotional problems. While light therapy draws upon ancient ideas about the healing powers of sunlight, it is in many ways a new field still in the process of conducting clinical research and determining therapeutic applications. There are many variations of light therapy. A therapist may direct solid or strobing flashes of light into a client's eyes or onto parts of the body. Different types of light, including full-spectrum, ultraviolet, infrared, colored, and laser, are being tested for their abil-ity to treat a wide range of conditions, including depression, insomnia, fatigue, premenstrual syndrome, psori-asis, jaundice, learning difficulties, and addictions.

The History of Light Therapy

From ancient to modern times, sunlight has played a central role in the cure of disease. The use of light in modern med-icine began in the early eighteenth and nineteenth centuries as scientists dis-covered the component frequencies of sunlight and observed its effects on ani-mals and humans. In 1703 English physi-cist Sir Isaac Newton chronicled his pioneering experiments with sunlight in his book *Optiks*. He was the first to show that sunshine's white light, when passed through a prism, divides into seven wavelengths of the visible color spec-trum—red, orange, yellow, green, blue, indigo, and violet. In the early 1800s two German physicists, John Herschel and Johann Ritter, discovered that sunlight also contained components of the elec-tromagnetic spectrum not visible to the unaided eye—the longer, slower infrared rays and shorter, faster ultraviolet rays. In 1870, scientists proved that sunlight kills bacteria and other microorganisms. The first surgical theaters used ultravio-let lights to effectively and inexpensively reduce airborne microorganisms by 50 percent. In 1905 Danish physician Dr. Niels R. Finsen received the Nobel Prize in medicine for establishing that visible wavelengths of blue-violet and invisible

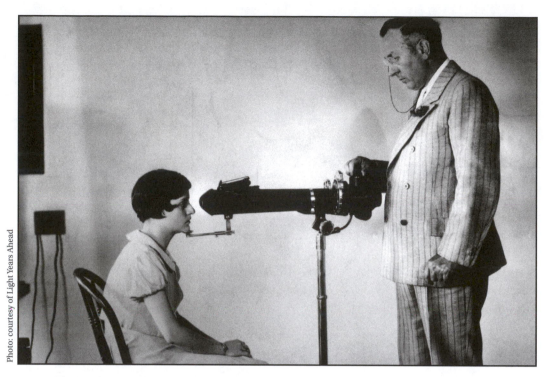

Photo: courtesy of Light Years Ahead

The Cameron-Spitler syntonizer, circa 1935, was one of the early syntonic optometry phototherapy devices.

ultraviolet, when isolated and focused on the body, could cure tuberculosis of the skin and other infectious conditions, such as measles and scarlet fever. Finsen also effectively treated smallpox by using red light (filtered sunlight or artificial light that excludes the heating rays of infrared and the burning rays of blue-violet and ultraviolet). Psychiatric applications of light therapy began in the 1880s, when mental hospitals in Europe and South America routinely calmed agitated patients with artificial blue light and energized depressed and unresponsive patients with red light applied through the eyes and on the body.

Throughout the opening decades of the twentieth century, therapeutic sun-bathing, a method known as the "sun cure," was a widely prescribed medical treatment for tuberculosis, cholera, viral pneumonia, bronchial asthma, gout, jaundice, and severe wounds. At the same time, advances in the design of electric lighting made it possible for hospitals in America and Europe to have "heliotherapy wards" that used artificial light for the treatment of cardiovascular and degenerative disorders.

After the development of the first antibiotics in 1938, interest in light therapy and other natural healing methods waned. However, in the 1940s Harry Spitler, a medical doctor and an optometrist, contributed to the development of light therapy with his investigation of syntonic optometry. The term *syntonic* comes from a Greek word meaning "to bring into balance." Spitler's treatment used rhythmic flashing of colored light into the eyes to improve visual acuity and coordination as well as energize and relax the autonomic nervous system. The patient's response varies with different flash rates and colors. He found that warm colors—red, orange, and yellow—were invigorating, while cool colors—green, blue, and violet—were relaxing. Spitler's pioneering work demonstrated that light entering the eyes profoundly impacts the autonomic nervous system and the endocrine system, balancing important hormones and brain chemistry.

Current investigations into therapeutic potentials of light were touched off in 1983 by psychiatrist Norman Rosenthal's study of winter depression, or seasonal affective disorder (SAD). He and his coworkers at the National Institute of Mental Health and more than 200 medical colleges around the world showed that regular exposure to full-spectrum (artificial lighting that has all the colors of sunlight) fluorescent light alleviates the symptoms of SAD in 80 percent of people. People with SAD begin to experience symptoms at the onset of winter, usually in September, as the days become shorter and darker. Rosenthal's technique is called bright light therapy, as it uses therapeutic doses of light more than twenty times brighter than typical indoor lighting. Bright light therapy has been used by NASA to adjust the daily rhythms of space shuttle astronauts and by mental health professionals to help people cope with shift work, jet lag, addictions, and various psychiatric conditions.

The Effects of Light on the Body

Major physiological processes in the brain and body are switched on and off by the presence or absence of natural or artificial light. Biochemical processes triggered by light include the production of vitamin D, the inhibition of melatonin (a hormone that affects mood), and the stimulation of serotonin and norepinephrine (brain chemicals that influence mental alertness and well-being). Light-sensitive cells in the eyes called photoreceptors convert sunlight into electrochemical impulses, which are transmitted through the optic nerve to brain centers that affect vision and activate the endocrine system. Many functions necessary to growth and well-being—breathing, sleeping, blood pressure, body temperature, appetite, moods, mental acuity, and the immune system—are governed by the endocrine system and hence are affected by natural light.

There is also evidence suggesting that proper quantities of visually perceived light are needed for healthy functioning of the cerebral cortex, the part of the brain that controls motivation, learning, and creativity; the limbic system, the part of the brain that stores emotional impressions of the world; and the motor cortex and the brain stem, the parts of the brain that coordinate body movement and the maintenance of life.

Types of Light Therapy

There are many different ways that light may be used in therapy. Goals and techniques will differ with each procedure. A therapist may direct the light into a person's eyes or on other body parts, and the light shown may be in strobing flashes or as solid light. The benefits may be both physical and psychological. There are several common forms of light therapy using full-spectrum or specific frequencies of colored light.

Neurosensory Development. For the last twenty-five years, optometrist Dr. John Downing has researched, applied, and extended Spitler's theories and formulated a form of light therapy called neurosensory development. Like Spitler, Downing promoted the therapeutic use of strobing colored light. A typical session begins with a discussion of the participant's medical and optometric history to determine the program and therapy. Light is administered with a device that Downing invented, the photron ocular light stimulator. It uses a combination of twelve colored-glass filters, from red to violet, placed in front of a special full-spectrum xenon light with an adjustable strobe capable of flashing from one to sixty cycles per second.

To determine a program of therapy, the patient is classified as either a slow or fast neurological type, and then the colors and flash rates on the photron are adjusted to counteract and balance the person's neurological tendencies. For example, blue, indigo, and violet, which tend to slow down and relax, are flashed slowly (six to twelve times a minute) into the eyes of a fast neurological individual. Conversely, a slow neurological individual is treated with rapid flashes (thirteen to sixty times per minute) of red, orange, and yellow. The typical course of treatment entails twenty or more half-hour sessions of light therapy.

These techniques lead to an increase in the patient's visual field and to a reduction of his or her blind spot, indicating that more light energy is reaching the visual cortex and other key brain structures. Besides visual enhancement, the types of individuals who appear to be helped by neurosensory development are those with chronic fatigue, menstrual difficulties, thyroid problems, insomnia, depression, and mental inefficiency.

Brief Strobic Phototherapy. Like neurosensory development, this method also uses the photron. However, the treatment goal is different. It is used to help the client access his or her thoughts and feelings and work on the emotional components of physical illness. Brief strobic phototherapy (BSP) was pioneered by Dr. Jacob Liberman, an optometrist, and Dr. Steven Vazquez, a medical psychotherapist. In this system the psychotherapist uses strobing colored light to facilitate awareness and resolution of the client's thoughts, feelings, and memories.

Generally the therapist chooses a color and flash rate that is emotionally evocative and uncomfortable to the client. Various colors tend to access different psychological content and are selected according to the client's objectives. This stimulation is used to facilitate a participant's awareness of unresolved, unconscious thoughts, feelings, and sensations. At the start of a typical session, the therapist uses flashes of colored light to put a person into a trancelike state. Then the client engages in a variety of psychological techniques to help facilitate emotional processing, such as talking, deep breathing, eye movement, awareness of physical sensations, and recollection of dreams. The rhythmic colored lights stimulate brain wave patterns that evoke different states of consciousness. Clients look into the light and can easily and rapidly see their unconscious material projected before them. By selecting specific colors and specific strobe rates, desired results can be targeted. BSP seeks to release repressed traumas or other memories and emotions that may be the root cause of illness. It may be part of treatment for various psychological problems, including depression, anxiety, panic attacks, obsessive compulsive disorder, addiction, eating disorders, closed brain injuries, and dissociative identity disorder.

Bright Light Therapy. This common form of light therapy was developed in the 1980s to treat the condition known as winter depression, or seasonal affective disorder (SAD). More recently this therapy has been successfully applied to a wide variety of psychiatric conditions, including sleep difficulties, food and substance addictions, jet lag, Alzheimer's disease, and attention deficit disorder in children.

The treatment itself is used either under professional guidance or for self-care applications for less serious stress symptoms. The light is usually viewed at home using a portable light box designed to fit on a desk or table. The participant sits with his or her head and upper body facing about three feet from the light box and focuses his or her eyes upon a surface illuminated by the light, not the light itself.

The full-spectrum fluorescent light may be as much as twenty times stronger than normal room light and is usually the most effective when it replicates the quality of natural light just before dawn or sunset. The intensity of the light and the scheduling and length of exposure are determined on a case-by-case basis. Daily exposure in the early morning for thirty minutes to several hours is often recommended, and an additional late-afternoon session may be prescribed. Bright light therapy is usually confined to the fall and winter months, when SAD patients experience severe depression, lethargy, fatigue, decreased energy and activity level, anxiety, irritability, lowered sex drive, avoidance of social activities, sadness,

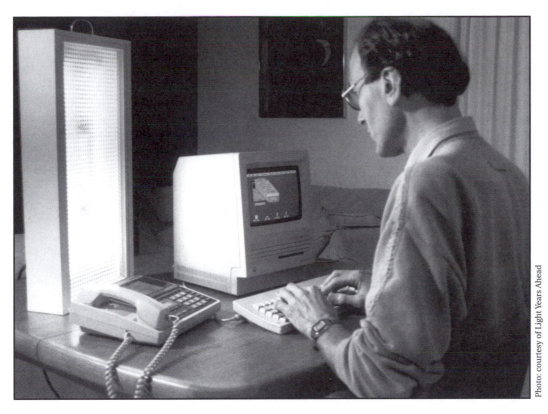

Illumination from a full-spectrum light box helps alleviate the symptoms of seasonal affective disorder (SAD).

concentration and sleep difficulties, interpersonal difficulties, carbohydrate and sweet cravings, and weight gain. Bright light therapy is usually discontinued in the spring as the days get longer and brighter. Once a satisfactory regimen is established, it must be maintained to receive maximum benefits. Bright light therapy relieves the symptoms of SAD; it does not cure the disorder.

Colorpuncture. This discipline uses a light pen to apply different frequencies of visible light on the acupoints and meridians, where needles are placed in a traditional acupuncture treatment. This procedure was developed by German naturopath Peter Mandel in the early 1970s. A colorpuncture therapist balances one's vital energy by either stimulating or sedating it with light. Different colors have different effects. Warm colors, such as red and yellow, are used to add energy while cool colors, such as green and blue, are used to subtract energy. A therapist may monitor the status of a client's energy flow before and after treatments by taking his or her pulse or by examining a kirlian photograph, a black-and-white image in which the body's radiating energy appears. Colorpuncture is often used in place of acupuncture, especially among children or adults who are frightened by needles. It has the same applications as acupuncture, including the treatment of respiratory and gastrointestinal infections, neurological and muscular difficulties, visual and learning problems, and pain. It may be used for stimulation of the immune system and as adjunctive therapy for those with mental disorders and addictions.

There are many other medical applications of light, including ultraviolet (UV) sterilization of human blood (photoluminesence) and the UV treatment of psoriasis and infant jaundice. The photodynamic treatment of cancer uses light to activate cancer medications and guide them to diseased tissue. Some types of light therapy, such as bright light therapy, are becoming more popular in the medical community and may be used either alone or in combination with psychiatric medication. Others, such as syntonic optometry, neurosensory development, and brief strobic photostimulation, are gaining acceptance as research accumulates.

Cautions

In over two decades of experimental trials, Bright light therapy, neurosensory development, brief strobic phototherapy, and colorpuncture have been consistently found to be safe and effective when used under the supervision of a competent and licensed health professional. However, an overexposure to bright full-spectrum light can produce negative side effects, including eye irritation, headaches, insomnia, and agitation. These can be decreased by reducing exposure time and by sitting farther from the light source. Strobic colored light stimulation can temporarily stimulate a "healing crisis," a temporary exacerbation of old emotional conflicts or physical difficulties in the process of releasing old traumas.

Each individual's reaction to light through the eyes and on the body is unique. One in three thousand people can experience photosensitive seizures, brought on by flashing lights such as those found in video games, televisions, and nightclubs. Individuals with a history of severe emotional difficulties or visual pathology should not begin phototherapy without consulting their licensed health care professional.

—*Dr. Brian J. Breiling*

Resources:

College of Syntonic Optometry
Betsy Hancock, DO
21 East 5th St.
Bloomsburg, PA 17815
Tel: (717) 784-2131
Organization of optometrists who incorporate syntonic light therapy into their work; offers a referral service.

Health Institute of North Texas
P.O. Box 820963
North Richland Hills, TX 76182
Tel: (817) 268-7050
Fax: (817) 285-7729
e-mail: Vazquez@txcc.net
Holistic treatment center, founded by psychologist Dr. Steven Vazquez, offering treatment and education on brief strobic phototherapy (BSP).

Society for Light Treatment and Biological Rhythms
10200 West 44th Avenue, # 302
Wheatridge, CO 80033-2840
Tel: (303) 424-3697
Fax: (303) 422-8894
e-mail: sltbr@resourcenter.com
Web site: www.websciences.org/sltbr
Publishes newsletter on medical research on the use of full-spectrum and colored light.

Universal Light Technologies
P.O. Box 520
Carbondale, CO 81623
Toll-free: (800) 81 LIGHT
Fax: (303) 927-0101
Web site: www.ulight.com
Organization founded by optometrist Dr. Jacob Liberman that offers treatment and education with strobic colored light and other modes of light therapy.

Winter Depression Program
Columbia Presbyterian Medical Center
722 W. 168th Street
New York, NY 10032
Tel: (212) 960-5714
Web site: www.cet.org/cet1996
Clinical program for treatment of SAD headed by Dr. Michael Terman, pioneer bright light researcher; also provides information and referrals for light therapy.

Further Reading:

Breiling, Brian, ed. *Light Years Ahead: The Illustrated Guide to Full Spectrum and Colored Light in Mindbody Healing.* Berkeley, CA: Celestial Arts Press, 1996.

Liberman, Jacob. *Light: Medicine of the Future.* Santa Fe, NM: Bear & Co, 1991.

Mandel, Peter. *Practical Compendium of Color-puncture*. Bruchal, Germany: Energetik Verlag, 1986.

Rosenthal, Norman. *Winter Blues: Seasonal Affective Disorder: What It Is and How to Overcome It*. New York, NY: Guilford, 1993.

SOUNDING

Sounding, originally known as toning, is a discipline that developed from the belief that being heard is one of the greatest needs of all people. No matter what our age, it is important that we are heard. Often we do not have the right words that allow others to understand exactly what we mean. Sounding strives to improve how people use their own voice and listening abilities in order to help them release many things that are not spoken and keep us from feeling as if we are in real communication with the world.

Discovering the Power of the Voice

Sounding was developed by Don Campbell as a result of nearly fifteen years of studying voice. Focused on how sound and music affect learning and health, he created a series of exercises meant to improve how people communicate with themselves and the world around them. In 1988, he founded the Institute for Music, Health, and Education in Boulder, Colorado, and served as the Executive Director until 1995. Campbell has written several books and produced cassette tapes that describe his theories and outline a program of sounding exercises. He has traveled to forty countries teaching musicians, teachers, physicians, therapists, and business trainers the basic principles and exercises of sounding. Sounding is now being used in hospitals, schools, and educational centers throughout the world to release stress.

What is Sounding?

According to Campbell, the voice is the first real tool we ever have to bring attention to ourselves, tell the world we need something, or even show how happy we are. The first sounds we make as infants are "coos" and "woos." There are hums and giggles, slides and wild curves that our voice projects to let our parents know that we are experiencing pain, pleasure, or even self-discovery. A lot of sounds that little children make are actually pleasurable sounds, although that squeak and wreak may drive others in the room crazy. Once we get to school, we are told to sit down, be quiet, and earn our education. To sit down and not be able to express our thoughts freely with the safety of being understood and heard is inhibiting to our minds, bodies, and emotions.

Campbell believes that one of the great purposes of education is that we learn to express our thoughts. Sometimes our thoughts come out in creative art forms like music, dance, and painting. Other times our expression comes in writing, and not speech. But it is our speech that allows the world community and our social peers to immediately know what we are thinking.

Yet, says Campbell, we are taught that we do not want the world to know everything we are thinking. And so we put on a mask, a persona, or a personality that keeps our inner thoughts from going to the outside world. Yet often when we do not learn to express ourselves and sound our minds and bodies, by the time we are finished with college, we spend a life in tension, repression, and actually harm our body by the stress of not releasing our sounds and our inner thoughts.

Learning to speak our mind, to become aware of our body, and to let our emotions tell the truth is a lifelong education. Learning to speak involves learning to listen. Listening is not just hearing. It is the ability to focus on outer information and attend and reach out into the world. By improving our own listening to the point that we genuinely realize that other people may not have the right words or the right timing to best communicate with us, we develop a little more patience.

Sounding: A Complementary Therapy

Sounding is a way in which you can bring about changes in your vocal production, self-expression, and listening abilities by spending just five to eight minutes releasing sounds from your body. It is important to remember that just a gentle hum while driving the car, or even while reading and studying, is used to provide an enormous release of energy. Toning, which actually means elongating vowel sounds with a relaxed chin and jaw, relaxes the whole body and mind. In six weeks of humming or toning, Campbell believes that a person can awaken to a new world of inner massage and vibration.

As a clinician, Campbell has worked with thousands of people to release their voice by toning. As Campbell states: "The left brain may think this is overly simple and perhaps trivial. But the rest of the brain and the body enjoys the vibration and expression."

Sounding is used as a complementary therapy to a variety of different physical and emotional therapies. Because the exercises can be fitted to the participant's schedule of treatment, sounding is often used as a warm-up exercise in schools, clinics, and hospitals for other activities or therapies.

Everyone Can Benefit from Sounding

Sounding practitioners believe that one of the strengths of this therapy is that everyone can use it with just a relaxed jaw. Whether you are a nurse, doctor, therapist, or teacher, going back to our primal, natural sound can tap elegant, natural pathways to enlighten our mind and body.

—From an interview with Don Campbell

Resources:

Mozart Effect Center
P.O. Box 4179
Boulder, CO 80306
Tel: (303) 440-8046
Web site: www.mozarteffect.com

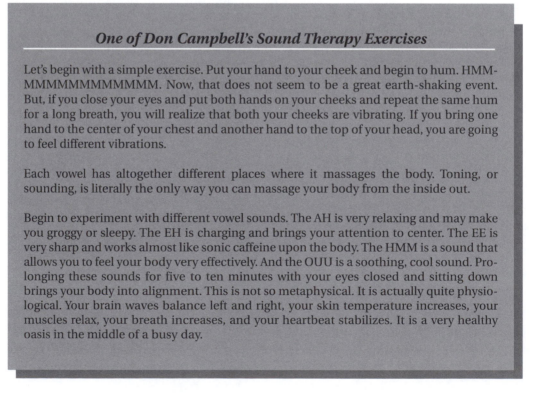

One of Don Campbell's Sound Therapy Exercises

Let's begin with a simple exercise. Put your hand to your cheek and begin to hum. HMM-MMMMMMMMMMMM. Now, that does not seem to be a great earth-shaking event. But, if you close your eyes and put both hands on your cheeks and repeat the same hum for a long breath, you will realize that both your cheeks are vibrating. If you bring one hand to the center of your chest and another hand to the top of your head, you are going to feel different vibrations.

Each vowel has altogether different places where it massages the body. Toning, or sounding, is literally the only way you can massage your body from the inside out.

Begin to experiment with different vowel sounds. The AH is very relaxing and may make you groggy or sleepy. The EH is charging and brings your attention to center. The EE is very sharp and works almost like sonic caffeine upon the body. The HMM is a sound that allows you to feel your body very effectively. And the OUU is a soothing, cool sound. Prolonging these sounds for five to ten minutes with your eyes closed and sitting down brings your body into alignment. This is not so metaphysical. It is actually quite physiological. Your brain waves balance left and right, your skin temperature increases, your muscles relax, your breath increases, and your heartbeat stabilizes. It is a very healthy oasis in the middle of a busy day.

Provides information on Sounding, including the cassette sets Heal Yourself with Your Own Voice *(Sounds True, 1991) and* The Power of Music *(5 tapes, Nightingale Conant, 1995).*

Further Reading:

Campbell, Don G. *Introduction to the Musical Brain.* St. Louis, MO: MMB Music, Inc., 1983.

———. *The Roar of Silence.* Wheaton, IL: Quest Books, 1989.

———. *100 Ways to Improve Teaching Using Your Voice and Music.* Tucson: Zephyr Press, 1992.

———. *The Mozart Effect™.* New York: Avon Books, 1997.

Campbell, Don G., and Chris Brewer. *Rhythms of Learning.* Tucson: Zephyr Press, 1991.

TOMATIS METHOD

The Tomatis method is a form of sound therapy discovered by Dr. Alfred Tomatis in the early 1950s. The Tomatis method is not a therapy for individuals who are severely hearing-impaired; instead, it is meant for individuals who have lost the ability to listen clearly to the world around them. The therapy works to overcome various health problems that can affect an individual's ability to listen and communicate with others, such as childhood ear infections, stress, accidents or traumas, or major lifestyle disruptions. Considered listening training, Tomatis therapy is accomplished with the aid of an electronic ear, which is a specialized device that trains the ear to block out disorder and static. The Tomatis method is also used to improve vocal ability, heighten creativity and concentration, improve reading levels, and lessen stress in both children and adults.

The Development of the Tomatis Method

Alfred Tomatis was born in 1920 in Nice, France. He studied to be a doctor of medicine specializing in troubles of the ear and language. During his early twenties, he worked for the French Ministries of Labour and War and the French Air Force. As one of his duties, he investigated hearing loss among factory workers constructing aircraft. At the same time, he treated a European opera singer who had lost the ability to sing in tune. When Tomatis compared the test results for both the laborers and the singer, he found the same kind of hearing loss. From those results, he realized that the ear and voice are connected. "The voice can produce only what the ear can hear," Tomatis said.

From his experiments, Tomatis developed a device called the electronic ear, which improves listening, learning, and language by reeducating the ear. The electronic ear exercises the muscles of the middle ear. Special headphones make it possible to sense vibrations through bones and increase the ear's frequency ranges to sound.

Tomatis then developed a new discipline he called audio-psycho-phonology, or APP. It is a science that acknowledges the connection between ear, voice, and psychology. It deals with the functional, social, and psychological factors that impact listening, communication, language, motor control, learning, and health.

Tomatis has published fourteen books and more than fifty articles that document his research and the neurophysiology and psychology of listening. Three of his books have been translated into English: *The Conscious Ear, The Ear and Language,* and *Education and Dyslexia.*

The Philosophy of the Tomatis Method

The Tomatis method makes a crucial distinction between listening and hearing. *Listening* is defined as the active

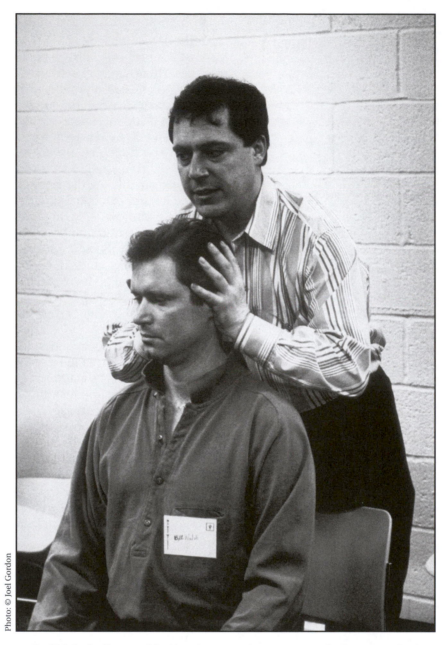

Photo: © Joel Gordon

Paul Madaule, director of the Listening Centre in Toronto, uses the Tomatis method
to help a client adjust his posture to improve listening and speaking abilities.

ability, intention, and desire to focus on sounds we want to analyze and to reject the ones we do not want. *Hearing*, on the other hand, is simply the passive reception of sound. Listening is a skill that can be both lost and recovered. Our ability and desire to listen can be poorly developed, diminished, or even halted at any stage of our lives. If a person has difficulty listening to the world around him or her, this dysfunction could result from a health problem like childhood ear infections, accident, trauma, a major lifestyle disruption, or stress. With the help of the electronic ear, the ability (or disability) to listen is something that can be identified, improved, and/or corrected.

By training the ear and the mind to listen, the Tomatis method is expected to improve one's motivation to communicate and learn.

Experiencing the Tomatis Method

The program begins with an initial assessment. That is followed by a consultation to review the results and the recommendation of a specific program. Once the listening training begins, the individual listens for two hours each day. A typical program includes intensive sessions (one session per day for fifteen days, eight days, and eight days with breaks of three to six weeks separating the intensives). Longer programs are recommended when severe or long-standing problems exist.

The Tomatis method is provided over an intense but relatively short time span. Sounds are presented through special headsets with bone and air conduction. First, the listener does passive sessions of hearing sounds modified by the electronic ear. The types of sounds used in this phase may include Mozart, Gregorian chant, and the filtered voice of the patient's mother. As soon as the foundation and desire for language and learning appear, active sessions of repeating sounds (humming, words, phrases, and sentences) and reading aloud begin. A microphone connected to the electronic ear allows the patient to listen to his or her own voice. While listening, children and adults are encouraged to draw or paint, work puzzles, play games, and relax.

Each listener receives a reassessment and consultation at the start and end of each intensive. These monitor changes and allow for the program to be adjusted based on the listener's progress. Parents report on the changes they observe in their children. Adults provide reports on changes they observe in their own voices, listening, stress levels, creativity, attention, organization, spatial awareness, posture, ability to tune out distractions, desire to express themselves, musical ability, and reading ability. Other structured and unstructured behavioral observations during the program provide feedback, as do the reports of any other professionals working with the individual, such as speech pathologists, psychologists, teachers, physicians, and occupational therapists.

The Benefits of the Tomatis Method

The Tomatis method can be helpful for people of all ages and with many types of problems, including those involving learning, language, social interaction, attention deficit, voice, speech, motor control, dyslexia, balance, posture, rhythm, and low motivation. Tomatis found that these types of disorders are almost always affected by sound stimulation.

—Dr. Billie Thompson

Resources:

Sound Listening and Learning Center (Tomatis Center)
2701 E. Camelback Rd., Suite 205
Phoenix, AZ 85016
Tel: (602) 381-0086
Fax: (602) 957-6741
e-mail: drbthmpsn@aol.com
Provides information on Tomatis training and practitioners.

Tomatis in Practice

One of Tomatis's experiments dealt with children who had learning disabilities. During these tests, he recreated for these children the sound of a mother's voice to her unborn child. One autistic child who hadn't spoken since he was four began to babble like a ten-month-old infant. Tomatis realized how important his method was.

Sound Listening and Learning Center
200 E. Del Mar, Suite 208
Pasadena, CA 91105
Tel: (626) 405-2386
Fax: (626) 405-2387
Refers practitioners and disseminates information regarding the Tomatis method.

Further Reading:

Tomatis, A. A. *The Conscious Ear.* Rhinebeck: Station Hill Press, 1991.

———. *The Ear and Language.* Norval, Ontario: Moulin Publishing, 1996.

PART VI: SUBTLE ENERGY PRACTICES

Do-In • Feng Shui • Magnet Therapy • Polarity Therapy • Qigong • Reiki • SHEN® • Therapeutic Touch

Subtle energy therapies are bodywork methods that share a belief that our physical bodies are surrounded by and imbued with an energetic essence that is invisible to the naked eye. Nevertheless, the state of this essence is thought to be the primary cause of health and disease. Practitioners of subtle energy therapies use a variety of techniques to perceive blocks in the flow of this energy and work to alleviate them.

Subtle energy therapies are part of a larger group of practices that have come to be known collectively as bodywork, a term describing a wide variety of methods that use touch to improve awareness of feelings and sensations in the body, improve physical functioning, relieve pain, and encourage relaxation. There are many disciplines

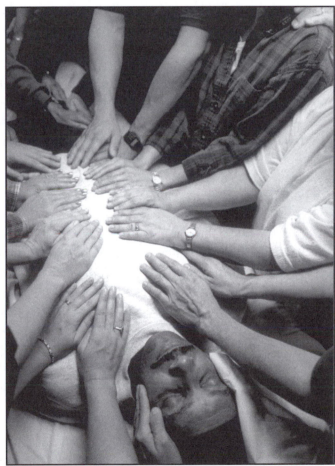

Photo: © Joel Gordon

Many subtle energy practices use the palms of hands to move subtle energy through the body.

in this book that may be included in the category Bodywork. They can be found in the sections entitled Massage, Skeletal Manipulation Methods, Acupuncture and Asian Bodywork, Movement Therapy Methods, and Body-Oriented Psychotherapies.

In addition to the energetic bodywork practices traditionally associated with the title "subtle energy therapy," this section also includes non-bodywork practices such as feng shui and magnet therapy. Feng shui is based on observation of subtle energy in one's environment. Magnet therapy focuses on electromagnetic energy surrounding and infusing the body and works with this energy in much the same way as subtle energy practices work with subtle energy.

Subtle Energy Is Known by Many Names

The concept of an energetic life force has a long and honored tradition throughout the world. It is the basis of ayurvedic, Asian, Western esoteric, and many modern therapeutic health care practices.

The energetic life force has been known by many different names around the world and throughout time. The Sanskrit word *prana* means "breath," and refers to both the material air taken into the lungs and the metaphorical breath or energy of life. In this way *prana* is similar to the Judeo-Christian concept of "breath" as the essence of life described in the Hebrew Bible. God breathes life into Adam, thereby changing him from inert clay into the first living man.

Chi or *qi* is the Chinese word used to describe the subtle energy permeating the body. In the Chinese model *chi* moves through the body in a series of invisible channels known as meridians. The meridians touch every organ of the body, regulating the flow of *chi*. *Ki* is the Japanese name for *chi*.

The energetic life force has also been known by many names in Western scientific health models. The Greek physician Hippocrates (c. 460–377 BCE), known as the father of orthodox or allopathic medicine, recognized an invisible life force, which he described as the body's own internal healing and balancing mechanism. He believed that the proper role of the physician is to do only what is necessary to aid this invisible healing energy.

From the first through the fourth century CE Gnostic Christian sects in Greece and the Roman Empire practiced religious healing rituals based on the belief that the divine spirit of Christ existed literally in each person. Variations of these practices, relying on touch methods of healing, survive to this day and have been incorporated into contemporary subtle energy therapies such as reiki and therapeutic touch.

Samuel Hahnemann (1755–1843), a German physician working in the latter part of the eighteenth century, developed the health care modality called homeopathy based on his belief in a dynamis, or vital force. Like Hippocrates, Hahnemann believed that this invisible energy was the primary healing and life-giving agent of the body.

Another German physician, Wilhelm Reich (1897–1957), working in the early nineteenth century in Europe and the United States, combined elements of Sigmund Freud's groundbreaking psychological theory with his own research into the nature of neuroses and other diseases to create medical orgonomy. Reich believed that the entire universe was pulsating with an invisible life energy, which he called orgone, that was to some extent the cause of all health or disease. Contemporary subtle energy therapies such as SHEN® and polarity combine various cultural and historical beliefs about the energetic life force with Western psychological and physical modalities to improve and maintain the physical, psychological, and spiritual dimensions of life.

How Practitioners Locate and Alleviate Blockages

The techniques developed to encourage the balance and flow of subtle energy throughout the body are as numerous and creative as the human imagination. They include physical exercises and breathing practices such as those found in yoga and t'ai chi, meditation methods, herbal remedies such as those used in ayurvedic and traditional Chinese medicine and homeopathy, and massage techniques such as those used in acupressure and shiatsu. Most of the specific subtle energy therapies included in this section use techniques similar to forms of massage or bodywork except that they generally rely less on physical manipulation and more on very light touch, which is used to perceive and reorganize the body's internal and external energy fields. Some methods such as qigong or do-in use many methods of manipulating subtle energy, including self-massage, massage by others, dietary and herbal practices, and movement exercises. Magnet therapy, a Western approach to manipulating electromagnetic energy, considered by some to be the physical explanation of subtle energy, doesn't use touch at all, but relies on the force of the positive and negative pulls of strategically placed magnets. Feng shui, the ancient Chinese method of environmental and spatial design, harmonizes the flow of subtle energy within a person with the flow of that energy in the environment by carefully attending to the various shapes and materials in a landscape, house, or room.

Subtle Energy and Western Science

Advanced scientific research on the effects of subtle energy is taking place at the Menninger Foundation. Researchers there have observed and witnessed seemingly miraculous feats attributed to subtle energy but have yet to prove the existence of subtle energy within the known physical field as Western science understands it. The Institute of Noetic Sciences also studies subtle energy and is working toward explaining it in Western scientific terms. Advanced research by many physicists suggests similarities between Western scientific wave/particle and energy theories of the nature of matter and the ancient subtle energy theories. Therefore, subtle energy therapies may require a leap of faith for some, but for others they may represent the cutting edge of body-mind-spirit healing today.

—Nancy Allison, CMA

Resources:

Institute of Noetic Science (IONS)
P.O. Box 909
Sausalito, CA 94966
Tel: (415) 331-5650
Organization that studies the mind, consciousness, and human potential. IONS also organizes lectures and conferences, publishes books and journals, and offers research grants.

Menninger Foundation
PO Box 829
Topeka, KS 66601-0829
Tel: (913) 273-7500

Training and research center for mental health professionals. The foundation studies conventional and unconventional methods of treating mental illnesses.

Further Reading:

Manning, Clark A., and Louis J. Vanrenen, eds. *Bioenergetic Medicines East and West: Acupuncture and Homeopathy.* Berkeley, CA: North Atlantic Books, 1988.

Claire, Thomas. *Bodywork: What Type of Massage to Get and How to Make the Most of It.* New York: William Morrow and Company, Inc., 1995.

Do-In

Do-in is the Japanese name for an ancient exercise system that brings the mind and body into concert with the inherent, natural rhythms of human life. This self-help program, which includes self-acupressure, massage, breathing techniques, and physical exercise, enhances the flow of vital life energy in the body. Do-in, however, is more than just relearning ancient lessons. It is the art of unlearning the artificial habits that we are taught in modern life and a return to an earlier, more instinctual life.

The Return to Ancient Habits

The first mention of do-in appears in the most famous medical treatise of ancient China, *The Yellow Emperor's Classic*, or *Nei Ching*. This third-century BCE book alludes to a legend in which men and women lived as gods, enjoying a healthy, long life with incredible physical, mental, and spiritual powers. According to the medical sage Chi Po, the people of this time lived in a balance typified by the two complementary energies of life, yin and yang. Through mental discipline and careful attention to diet and other bodily needs, these people were able to live in harmony with nature and thus attain health and longevity.

As men and women moved into civilized communities, these natural ways of eating and living were forgotten. The special powers that do-in exercises (which resemble yoga postures, breathing, and meditative practices) were believed to have brought—extra-long life and the ability to raise the dead, walk on water, foresee the future, communicate telepathically, and control the weather, among others—were lost as well.

According to do-in lore, Taoist sages in the mountains of India, China, Korea, and Japan preserved the ancient forgotten movements and practices. These sages, or sen-nin, developed systematic teachings and exercise routines to help regain, develop, and maintain good physical health and sharp, quick minds. These regimens, known as do-in in Japan and tao-yin in China, were then written or told to others. New forms developed in response to the changing needs of the people. Chi kung and t'ai chi ch'üan, which share many similarities to the original do-in routines, can be viewed as later forms of do-in. Many other Asian disciplines, including yoga, karate, judo, aikido, and kung fu, also make use of basic theories of do-in.

Michio Kushi, a leading pioneer of the American natural foods movements, first introduced do-in to the United States. As part of "Macrobiotics," Dr. Kushi's system for practicing a more natural and balanced lifestyle, do-in exercises are used to complement a natural diet of grains, beans, vegetables, and other natural foods.

The Theory of Do-In

Several years ago, researchers filmed the movements of sleepers at night. Afterward, when the tapes were sped up, the tossings and turnings of sleepers in fact resembled a carefully choreographed dance. Practitioners of do-in describe this "dance" as an instinctual version of do-in, carried out by the subconscious mind during sleep.

The movement of humankind toward civilization was a movement away from a more natural life. As people were forced to live according to a "civilized" schedule and ignore their body's urges to eat, sleep, and exercise at will, the visceral, instinctual nature of people was suppressed and weakened. Natural movements were suppressed and forgotten. Still, practitioners of do-in believe that they remain in all of us. Thus, do-in movements do not need to be taught so much as released.

Experiencing Do-In

Do-in comprises a regimen of many different exercises. Do-in practices include self-massage and self-acupressure techniques; stretching and twisting movements; breathing exercises; meditation and visualization techniques; dancelike movements and routines to ease specific ailments; the use of special sounds; and healing with the palms.

These practices can be done at any time of the day. Certain exercises are suggested for morning or evening practice. Loose, cotton clothing is preferred. It is best to practice in a well-ventilated and well-lit room. When possible, practice outdoors is recommended.

Benefits of Do-In

In do-in and other Eastern healing arts, the body is viewed as having antenna. It picks up energy and vibration from its surroundings. Do-in helps "tune" these antenna. By practicing the various techniques of do-in, the body is able to pick up, circulate, and accumulate more energy from the environment. Once collected, this subtle energy flows throughout the body, rejuvenating and enlivening the organs, tissues, cells, and systems. Thus, do-in is doubly beneficial. Even as the body becomes more healthy through this newly collected energy, a healthier body is better equipped to perform do-in.

Do-in movements mimic the body's own rhythms such that all people will recognize them. Still, instruction is encouraged to achieve proper technique and emphasis.

—*John Kozinski*

Resources:

John Kozinski Seminars
P.O. Box 526
Becket, MA 01223
Tel: (413) 623-5925
e-mail: kozinski@berkshire.net
Provides information about "Energy Healing," a seminar that features do-in.

Kushi Institute
P.O. Box 7
Becket, Massachusetts 01223
Tel: (413) 623-5925
Do-in forms are an integral part of seminars at this macrobiotics center. The Kushi Institute can also help locate do-in courses at other macrobiotics centers throughout the United States and Canada.

Further Reading:

Hua Ching, Ni. *Attune Your Body with Dao-In*. Santa Monica: SevenStar Communications, 1994.

Kushi, Michio. *The Book of Do-In*. Tokyo: Japan Publications, 1986.

——. *Forgotten Worlds*. Becket, MA: One Peaceful World Press, 1992.

FENG SHUI

Feng shui is an ancient Chinese philosophy and spiritual practice of arranging environments, based on the idea that all living things in the

The Japanese Sen-Nin

For the sen-nin, do-in involved eight to ten hours daily of rigorous exercise under the guidance of an experienced teacher. In order to follow this extreme lifestyle, the sen-nin lived in the mountain regions, and followed a special diet consisting of wild plants, such as grains, seeds, fruits and bark. Later, aspects of the practice were incorporated into Chinese t'ai chi ch'üan, as well as acupuncture and acupressure.

universe are affected by the forces of nature in their environments. Feng shui practitioners believe that by properly designing certain environments, they can direct the energy in all living things, known as *chi,* in a way that promotes harmony, prosperity, and good health.

The History of Feng Shui

The practice of feng shui began in China more than 3,000 years ago. It was first used to locate grave sites that would bring good luck for the spirit of the deceased and descendants who believed that their ancestors' spirits continued to affect them. Then farmers used it to find the best locations to plant crops and build homes. They studied the land to observe how the forces of nature, particularly those of wind and water, interacted. By observing the natural properties of the land and how it was shaped by the forces of nature, they tried to discern how the *chi* was flowing in that area and how they could interact with it to achieve favorable results for their crops. Later, villages, towns, and cities were built using these principles. Europeans first learned about feng shui practices in the nineteenth century through British missionaries' accounts of Chinese society and beliefs.

In early Chinese societies, feng shui was practiced by experts in astrology, numerology, and supernatural forces. These respected individuals came to be known as "geomancers." When a person wanted to build a home, farm, road, temple, or find a grave site, a geomancer was consulted for his understanding of feng shui. He would make important decisions about the proper location and design to ensure the most beneficial flow of *chi.*

The social importance of feng shui persisted in China until the late 1960s, when China began its Cultural Revolution, which abolished many elements of traditional culture, including feng shui. Although it has remained popular in Hong Kong, its practice in China is only recently being restored. However, many

people in China have been hesitant to accept its principles and practices. The suppression of feng shui in China prevented it from being integrated with contemporary beliefs and needs, making it appear archaic and superstitious. However, as a growing number of designers and architects in Asia and in the United States discover these traditional practices, the popularity of feng shui is being renewed and spread worldwide.

Principles of Feng Shui

According to traditional Chinese philosophy, the earth emanates an energy called *chi,* which if weakened or interfered with could be devastating to a person or community. According to this philosophy, *chi* moves through every object, creature, and space like the flow of blood through the body or a river through a landscape. Feng shui is used to ensure that buildings are placed and interior environments are designed in a way that does not aggravate or disrupt this flow of energy.

This view of the relationship between human beings, vital life energy, and their environments is based primarily on two Chinese concepts: the Tao and yin and yang. The Tao, which may be translated as "the path" or "the way," refers to the ever constant patterns of change in the basic elements of nature, of which human beings are an intrinsic part. This concept is the core of Taoism, a religion characterized by its reverence for nature. According to Taoism, human beings should seek to observe patterns of nature, such as the changing seasons or transitions between night and day, and put their lives in a harmonious relationship with these patterns. Resisting the natural course of the Tao will only cause difficulties and misfortune.

The movement of the Tao is imaged as a constant dance between yin and yang, the two basic complementary energies in nature. Yin energy is characterized by its dark, cool, caring, and receptive properties. Taoists observe

The Ba-Gua in Feng Shui

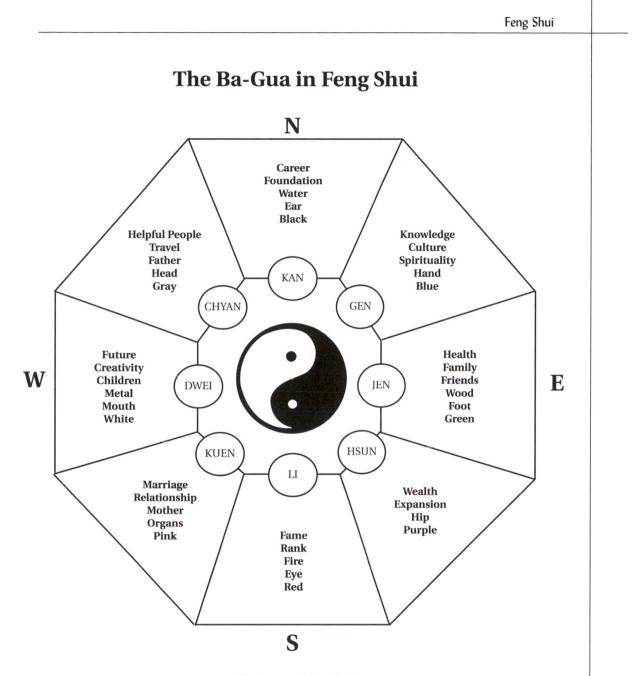

The ba-gua in feng shui.

yin energy in water; soft, flowing fabrics such as silk; and cool colors such as blues and purples. Yang energy is characterized by its light, warm, straight, and active qualities. Wind, wood, straight objects such as knives or swords, and vibrant saturated colors such as reds and yellows exhibit higher degrees of yang energy.

According to the principles of feng shui, a healthy environment will acknowledge the Tao by a harmonious balance of yin and yang energy and unobstructed pathways for the *chi* to flow between them. The building will be situated in the landscape with respect to the flow of wind and water. Interiors will be created by the careful selection and placement of walls, doorways, and windows in order to respect the flow of *chi* and the balance of yin and yang in the building materials. Finally, the colors and materials of the objects in a room will also be selected with respect for the balance, harmony, and flow of the forces of nature.

The Ba-Gua and Feng Shui Cures

To design a home or office properly according to the principles of feng shui, the design, materials, and function of every area should be adjusted to match the occupants' needs with the ba-gua. The ba-gua is an eight-sided "compass" that matches a specific color and human need or desire with each of the eight directions according to principles derived from ancient Chinese astrology, geometry, and mathematics. The ba-gua is used to identify areas where the flow of *chi* or the balance of yin and yang creates favorable or unfavorable conditions. Yang is most concentrated in the south, and yin is most concentrated in the north. The eight directions of the ba-gua and the associated colors and human needs are:

South (*Li*): fame, red
Southeast (*Hsun*): wealth, purple
East (*Jen*): family, green
Northeast (*Gen*): knowledge, blue
North (*Kan*): career, black
Northwest (*Chyan*): helpful people/travel, gray
West (*Dwei*): children/future/creativity, white
Southwest (*Kuen*): marriage/relationship, pink

However, for spaces that do not easily align with the ba-gua, feng shui details a set of "cures" to remedy disturbances to the flow of *chi*. There are eight basic cures:

- *Light*—In addition to electric lights, this category consists of objects capable of light reflection and refraction, including mirrors, leaded glass, and crystals. Mirrors are frequently used in rooms designed according to feng shui. They may be aimed to deflect the flow of *chi* away from an area or used to enhance *chi* by reflecting a pleasing image.
- *Sound*— Sound is thought to set static *chi* in motion. A room is filled with sound to radiate the *chi* throughout the space. Sound may be produced

by wind chimes, bells, or recorded music. Wind chimes are often used by feng shui to draw good *chi* from outside into a home.

- *Living items*—These include plants, trees or flowers (real or realistic), aquariums, or fishbowls. Plants are used to generate *chi*. Fish symbolize money and fishbowls are often used in homes and businesses settings to bring wealth.
- *Moving objects*—Moving objects are used to stimulate *chi*. Motion may be produced by mobiles, fountains, windmills, whirligigs, or windsocks. Objects that are naturally powered, such as these, are preferred.
- *Heavy objects*—Heavy objects have the opposite effect from moving objects. They are used to introduce stillness in areas where *chi* moves too quickly. These may be large stones, heavy furniture, or statues.
- *Electrically powered objects*—The electricity that powers televisions, computers, stereos, or air conditioners affects the flow of *chi*. Since the energies may conflict, a space designed according to feng shui will proportion the use of electricity to balance the two energies. When properly distributed, electricity may also stimulate *chi*.
- *Straight lines*—These are usually bamboo flutes but may also include swords, scrolls, and fans. The straight lines in these objects are used to direct *chi* to a desired location. Flutes are popular cures because they may be arranged to resemble the octagonal shape of the ba-gua.
- *Colors*—Colors are used for their symbolic value within the ba-gua. When designing a room, a person may emphasize the colors that correspond to a desired direction.

Practicing Feng Shui

Feng shui may be used to develop the proper placement of a building in a landscape or to design the interior and exterior walls, doors, and windows of a building. It is also often used to design individual rooms in a way that will benefit the people who use them. The ba-gua is used to identify the direction that represents a principle, such as knowledge or fame, that a person wants to change. Then, feng shui cures are used to stimulate the flow of *chi* in that area. For example, a person who wants to design a room to benefit his or her family will see that "family" is located in the east on the ba-gua. He or she will see if any barriers are cutting off the flow of *chi* to the east in the room. The *ba-gua* associates the color green with the family, so the room will be designed with green objects. A plant may be placed next to the east wall to further stimulate the *chi*.

A person may be able to use feng shui without hiring a consultant. There are a number of how-to books on feng shui that offer some basic lessons. However, a person who wants to employ more complex aspects of feng shui may consult an expert. When people consult feng shui experts to design their homes, they may be asked about their lives and what they would like to enhance or change. The practitioner and client will go through each of the client's rooms and discuss positioning of important objects in the room such as the bed, desk, couch, artworks, plants, and colors to create the best possible environment to enhance or change the desired aspect.

Benefits

Although feng shui can be used simply to bring beauty and serenity to an environment, it is also used to bring benefits to many aspects of a person's life. A person who wants to improve his or her fortune in business, relationships, or family may use feng shui to be sure that *chi* is flowing properly in the corresponding directions of his or her home or business environment.

Today, feng shui is used in both personal and professional settings. Several companies in the United States and Asia use feng shui to design office spaces, hoping to increase their fortune in business. Service industries, like restaurants and hotels, have used feng shui to make clients feel more comfortable and willing to spend more money. As its popularity grows, feng shui is changing the

According to feng shui, it is very important that furniture and objects are properly placed in each room. There are specific guidelines for essential parts of a home, including the entrance, the bed, and the kitchen.

- Entrance—Designing a house with feng shui requires careful consideration of the entrance, since it is where *chi* enters the building. Traditionally, homes designed with feng shui will have southern entrances, since that is the direction in which the most favorable energy is thought to flow. One should be careful that the *chi* is not hindered by an obstacle blocking the front door, such as a tree or another building.

- Bed—One of the most significant placements in a home designed with feng shui is the location of a bed. The location of one's bed is thought to affect one's health and marriage. A properly positioned bed will give a person "command" of the bedroom door. A person is never to have his or her back to the entrance. When a person is in bed, he or she should face the doorway, but should not be in direct line of it. The ba-gua is often used to help determine the proper location of a bed.

- Kitchen—Homes designed with feng shui often have kitchens in the southern or eastern side of the house, since these directions represent fire and wood on the ba-gua. Small spaces and sharp corners should be avoided since they inhibit the flow of *chi*. A proper kitchen will be designed to allow the chef to see the kitchen's entrance and be prepared when a person arrives.

way that many people view the relationship between a person and his or her
surroundings.

—*Marilyn Saltzman*

Resources:

Yun Lin Temple
2959 Russell Street
Berkeley, CA 94705
Tel: (510) 841-2347
This organization offers courses in feng shui
throughout the United States.

Further Reading:

Rossbach, Sarah. *Feng Shui, the Chinese Art of*
Placement. London: Century Hutchenson, 1987.

———. *Living Color—Master Lin Yun's Guide to Feng*
Shui. New York: Kodansha International, 1994.

Skinner, Stephen. *The Living Earth Manual of*
Feng Shui. London: Arkana, 1989.

Spear, William. *Feng Shui Made Easy.* San Francisco: Harper San Francisco, 1995.

MAGNET THERAPY

Magnet therapy, which is also called
magnetotherapy, refers to the
practice of applying a magnetic
field to the body for the treatment of physical and emotional disorders. It can relieve
discomfort, pain, or swelling, and it has
been used to treat both acute injuries,
such as cuts and burns, and many chronic
conditions, most notably arthritis. Some
experts say that magnet therapy is useful
in treating depression and such mental
disorders as hallucinations and delusions.
Experts are not clear about why magnet
therapy works, but most agree that it has
been used effectively to treat diseases and
ailments such as arthritis, sprains, torn ligaments, headaches, certain types of

insomnia, and environmental stress. Placing the magnets directly over the area of
pain can help diminish the pain from
these afflictions.

The Development of Magnetic Therapy

Several books have been published over
the last few decades, in which the
authors make reference to magnet therapy being used in times prior even to the
development of acupuncture. If true,
this would make the use of magnets for
healing purposes one of the very oldest
of all therapies. Some advocates of magnet therapy believe that magnets have
been used to treat pain as far back as the
ancient Egyptians, Hebrews, Arabs,
Indians, and Chinese. There are even
reports of a natural magnetic material
called lodestone being ground up and
used as a potion as far back as 100,000
years ago. Whether these modern-day
historical accounts of ancient magnet
therapy are true or not, it does not
diminish the fact that, at the present
time, the use of magnets for therapeutic
purposes is enjoying a renewed interest
and an increase in popularity.

The Philosophy of Magnet Therapy

There are many theories about the
mechanism of magnet therapy, but no
one knows for certain how it works.
Some theorists speculate that the local
application of magnetic fields increases
blood flow through the capillaries,
which brings more oxygen and nutrients to the tissues. Others have suggested that the magnetic fields alter nerve
function, muting the transmission of
pain impulses from an area of the body
that hurts. Some practitioners insist
that the biomagnetic north pole, or negative pole of the magnet, somehow
changes the acid-base balance of certain fluids in the tissues, making the
area under the north pole magnets
more alkaline. One expert theorizes that
the "vector potential" and "curl" of the
magnetic field may have important
effects on enzyme function.

Magnets have both a negative, or
north, and a positive, or south, pole.

There are two different ways of naming the poles of the magnet. For purposes of what some people call biomagnetic therapy, the poles should be named as follows: the north pole of a magnet is the one that will attract the arrowhead; the south pole repels the arrowhead or pointer of a compass. Many magnetotherapists believe that the negative pole has a calming effect on the body, whereas the positive pole causes stress. Being exposed to the positive pole for too long can have a deleterious effect upon an individual. Proponents of so-called unipolar magnetic therapy believe that it is primarily the biomagnetic north pole, or negative pole, that should be oriented to face the body, so that the south pole always faces away from the body. Other magnet therapists think that bipolar therapy, which exposes the body to both north and south magnetic poles, arranged in some sort of spatial pattern, helps to heal the body better than unipolar magnet therapy.

Magnet Therapy in Practice

The magnetic field can be produced by permanent magnets, or electromagnets utilizing pulsed or alternating electrical currents going through a coil of wire. The permanent magnet-type devices come in a large variety of shapes and sizes. They can be as simple as a single, large, flat magnet, or as complex as a custom-fitted, contoured, cloth-covered pouch containing many small, flat, circular, or rectangular magnets. A common method of magnetotherapy is simply placing magnets over, near, under, or on an area of the body that hurts. In most types of magnetic products, many small, flat, circular or rectangular magnets are placed so that all the magnets are oriented with the north pole facing toward the body and the south pole facing away from the body. (The north pole is the one that will attract the arrowhead of the compass.)

These devices produce a magnetic field of several dozen to several hundred gauss at the surface of the body where they are applied. A gauss is a unit of magnetic flux density or magnetic field strength. For comparison purposes, the magnetic field of the Earth that causes a compass arrow to point north is about half a gauss. In contrast, the magnets used in most permanent magnet devices are usually about 700 gauss or more.

Depending on the condition of the individual, the magnets may be applied several times a day or for days or weeks at a time. Some people may prefer to sleep on a magnetic bed or mattress pad. For others, magnet therapy may involve hours of treatment at a magnetic therapist's office usually using pulsed-magnetic fields.

Benefits of Magnetic Field Therapy

Most people who have tried magnet therapy have experienced positive results from it, though they agree that more research is needed to understand how magnet therapy works. There have been tens of thousands of anecdotal reports that either bipolar or unipolar magnet therapy has relieved the pain or discomfort of such conditions as arthritis, fibromyalgia, rheumatism, gout, back pain, shoulder pain, carpal tunnel syndrome, bed sores, ulcers, diabetic neuropathy, trigeminal neuralgia, and toothaches. In addition, there are thousands of reports of magnetic field therapy being used for acute injuries such as sprains, strains, torn ligaments, and soft tissue injuries, such as a smashed thumb, pinched finger, insect bite, burn, scrape, cut, or bruise.

One of the benefits of magnet therapy is that foreign substances are not introduced into the body. In the long run, this form of therapy might prove safer than over-the-counter medications and other treatments.

—Dr. John Zimmerman

Resources:

Bio-Electro-Magnetics Institute (BEMI)
Dr. John Zimmerman, President
2490 West Moana Lane
Reno, NV 89509-7801
Tel: (702) 827-9099 (best time to call is 8:00-10:00

AM Pacific time)
Offers resources and information on magnet therapy.

North American Academy of Magnetic Therapy
Cindy Kornspan, National Secretary
28240 Agoura Rd, Suite 202
Agoura, California 91301
Tel: (818) 991-5277 or (800) 457-1853
Professional organization for practitioners of magnet therapy.

Further Reading:

Becker, Robert O., and Andrew A. Marino. *Electromagnetism and Life.* Albany: State University of New York Press, 1982.

Becker, Robert O., and Gary Seldon. *The Body Electric: Electromagnetism and the Foundation of Life.* New York: William Morrow & Company, 1985.

Burke, Abott George. *Magnetic Therapy.* Oklahoma City, OK: Saint George Press, 1980.

Hanneman, Holger. *Magnet Therapy.* New York: Sterling Publishing Company, 1983.

Philpott, William H. *Biomagnetic Handbook.* Choctaw, OK: Enviro-Tech Publisher, 1990.

Washnis, George J., and Richard Z. Hirack. *Discovery of Magnetic Health.* Rockville, MD: Nova Publishing Co., 1993.

POLARITY THERAPY

Polarity therapy is a holistic method of healing that acts upon the field of bipolar energy surrounding and animating the body. It assumes that illness is caused by an imbalance or block in the field, and through touch, diet, exercise, and counseling attempts to realign balance and recharge the overall level of energy. While the principles of polarity therapy were formulated in the twentieth century, they incorporate the teachings of several ancient traditions of medicine, particularly the ayurvedic tradition of India. Proponents of polarity therapy view it as a means of alleviating chronic physical problems, forming healthy habits in everyday life, and enhancing other modes of medical treatment.

The History of Polarity Therapy

Polarity therapy was developed by Randolph Stone (1890–1981), an American who was initially trained as a chiropractor and later as an osteopathic physician and naturopath. During the 1920s Stone realized that modern Western medicine could not explain the health benefits resulting from chiropractic techniques of applying direct manual pressure to parts of the body. With chiropractic techniques as a basis, he embarked on a global study of medicine that entailed voluminous reading and campaigns of travel to observe healers at work preparing medications and treating patients. Attempts to gather knowledge into universal systems were common in the twenties.

The Swiss psychoanalyst C. G. Jung was integrating the world's symbols into a system of psychology, and Stone endeavored to make a comparable grand synthesis of healing traditions. He studied ayurvedic medicine in India, acupuncture, acupressure, and herbal medicine in China, and the modes of healing used in the West prior to the scientific revolution. By the 1940s he was convinced that medicine did have a central universal principle, the concept of a bipolar life force, and could be unified into one coherent system of precepts and techniques.

The final work of defining the system was carried out in Stone's private practice in Chicago and in a writing project that he started in 1948 and completed in 1970. Even staunch advocates of polarity therapy acknowledge that *Health Building* and *Polarity Therapy*, Stone's major treatises, are difficult reading and have numerous inconsistencies and ambiguities. This has left his teachings open to wide interpretation, which results in polarity therapists varying in their approach to treatment.

Nonetheless, Stone is recognized as an important pioneer in holistic medicine. His principles and techniques have been a catalyst for research into non-Western medicine as well as an effective therapy in their own right. polarity therapy is now available throughout the United States and is offered by polarity practitioners required to meet standards for practice established by the American Polarity Therapy Association in 1987.

The Theory of Polarity Therapy

Stone believed the body is animated by a three-dimensional field of pulsating energy called *chi* in Chinese tradition and *prana* in ayurvedic medicine. When the energy flows outward, it is considered positive and when it contracts backward, it is considered negative. There is no moral connotation to the distinction, but Stone followed ayurvedic teaching that maintains that complex, dynamic interplay of the positive and negative currents determine the particular character of every portion of the human organism. Further, he held that the polarized energy pervades the cosmos, pulsating in patterns that can be correlated with the patterns it assumes in the human body. Like the ayurvedic masters, Stone approached the human being as a microcosm of the larger macrocosm, the universe. "As within, so without," was one of his favorite sayings.

Polarity therapy focuses upon the connection between the energy structures of the five elements distinguished in ayurvedic tradition: ether, air, fire, water, and earth, and five of the energy centers in the body known as chakras in Eastern thought. Each element-chakra unit is associated with a quality of energy, an organ of the body, and a bodily function. The entire element-chakra series is found acting together in every human being, usually in a way that features some imbalance.

The imbalance is regarded as the key to unlocking the mysteries of individual personality and health. If, for example, the air-chakra correspondence is dominant, mental activity is presumed to be the person's great strength and potential weakness. She or he will have unusual intellectual powers that pose no problem so long as efforts to redress the imbalance are made. Otherwise, the excess air energy will disrupt the flow of energy and cause an illness to occur in the upper chest and lungs, where the air-chakra is located.

Microcosmic energy movement is the main diagnostic and therapeutic tool of polarity therapy. Through observation and touch, the practitioner assesses the functioning of the element-chakra system, then proceeds to correct any dangerous disequilibrium. Manual pressure is applied on or around the chakras in order to balance the energy flow, and often a regimen of corrective exercises and diet is prescribed. Because the person's entire being, mind and body, is at stake, Stone believed polarity therapy should also address troublesome personality traits.

Experiencing Polarity Therapy

A polarity therapy session lasts an hour to an hour and a half. It generally begins with a discussion of the patient's health history, lifestyle, and therapy goals. During the course of the interview, the practitioner pays close attention to vocal changes, gestures, and aspects of posture indicative of the patient's element-chakra system. The assessment continues after the patient, still fully dressed, lies on a treatment table and bodywork starts. The practitioner is trained to use her or his hands as a type of magnetic transmitter of energy.

In the opening phase of the bodywork, the hands cradle the patient's head, then move to other sites in the body, all the while picking up various qualities of pulsation. After contact, a diagnosis is made and the practitioner uses more touching to harmonize the positive and negative charges of energy throughout the body.

A polarity therapy practitioner always employs both hands for treatment and draws upon a repertory of more than twenty movements that include gentle to vigorous holding, vibrating, and rocking motions. A session may include stretch releases of the neck and spine, cranial balancing, work on reflex points in the ears, hands, and feet, connective tissue strokes, and strokes that connect the chakras. During these movements the type of touch may vary from light and balancing to stimulating to deep and dispersing. No two sessions are ever alike because ongoing energy assessment of the patient determines the sequence of movements and type of touch.

As the bodywork proceeds, the patient may become deeply relaxed, see dreamlike images, or feel a release of emotion and the need to talk about past traumas and current problems. The conclusion of the session depends on the practitioner's view of Stone's teachings. Some focus primarily upon the bodywork, while others emphasize the importance of supporting the bodywork with diet, exercise, and psychological counseling.

The diet prescribed is usually vegetarian and may include a preliminary regimen to detoxify and cleanse the body. The exercises, based on yoga routines, involve squats, stretches, rhythmic movements, deep breathing, and utterance of the sound "Ha!" Like the other components in polarity therapy, the counseling is designed to promote freedom and balance in the patient's energy field.

The Benefits of Polarity Therapy
Polarity therapy acts as a tonic that brings relief from specific problems such as digestion problems and produces an overall sense of well-being, increased energy, and serenity in the patient. Though it should not be regarded as a substitute for medical diagnosis and therapy, it can accelerate the effects of conventional treatments for major illnesses and promote recovery from surgery. As a holistic system of health care, polarity therapy can also provide

Polarity Practitioners

The standards of practice established by the American Polarity Therapy Association require training of a polarity practitioner in over 615 hours of study in bodywork, exercise, nutrition, anatomy, communication skills, professional ethics, and energy evaluation. Practitioners are registered at two levels: associate polarity practitioner (APP) and registered polarity practitioner (RPP). The American Polarity Therapy Association publishes a directory of registered polarity practitioners and trainers .

Choosing a polarity practitioner should be based on your personal needs and practitioner qualification. The polarity practitioner you choose should be nationally registered with APTA. Registered polarity practitioners are required to meet basic standards after which their training may vary, based on school emphasis, postgraduate training, and additional degrees/specialties in other fields. Many polarity practitioners are qualified in other disciplines such as medicine; chiropractic, osteopathic, and naturopathic practice; nursing; massage; psychology; and social work. Many polarity practitioners work for one hour and charge between $50 and $100 per session. Practitioners with additional training and degrees may work differently and charge more based on their expertise.

guidelines for regulating everyday habits so as to strengthen the body's resistance and achieve inner harmony with one's sense of self and one's feelings.

—John Beaulieu, ND, Ph.D.

Resources:

American Polarity Association
2888 Bluff Street, Suite 149
Boulder, CO 80301
Tel: (303) 545-2080
Fax: (303) 545-2161
Sets standards for certification in polarity therapy, maintains a list of certified polarity therapy practitioners, and provides information about the theory and practice of polarity therapy.

Further Reading:

Beaulieu, John. *Polarity Therapy Workbook.* New York: BioSonic Enterprises, 1994.

Stills, Franklyn. *The Polarity Process: Energy as a Healing Art.* Dorset, England: Element Books, 1990.

Stone, Randolph. *Health Building: The Conscious Art of Living Well.* Sebastopol, CA: CRCS Publications, 1987.

———. *Polarity Therapy.* 2 vols. Sebastopol, CA: CRCS Publications, 1987.

QIGONG

Qigong is the most popular method of disease prevention in China. It means, literally, "energy cultivation," and is an ancient system of exercise, breathing techniques, self-massage, and meditation designed to purify, gather, and circulate life energy, called *qi*. Many studies in China and the United States have shown that practicing qigong improves health, increases vitality, and can reduce pain, anxiety, and depression. Qigong emphasizes strengthening the immune system and treating problems when they are *subclinical*—that is, before they produce obvious symptoms. However, qigong is also a method of disease treatment. It has been found effective for disorders such as hypertension, headaches, bronchitis, asthma, ulcers, arthritis, chronic pain, and some forms of cancer. The patient learns self-healing skills and how to take greater charge of his or her own health. Instead of shifting all responsibility into the hands of a physician, the qigong patient cooperates in the healing process.

Chinese Energy Medicine
The Chinese word *qi*, pronounced "chee," means "vital breath" or "life energy." According to Chinese medicine, health is the result of an abundance of clear flowing *qi*. Disease is caused when the body's reserves of *qi* are depleted through physical, emotional, or environmental stress or when the *qi* is stuck and unable to flow. Stagnant *qi*, like stagnant water, is a breeding ground for disease. When *qi* flow is blocked, some areas of the body have too much energy or a yang condition, creating tension, congestion, and inflammation. Other areas have too little energy or a yin condition, creating weakness and conditions such as poor digestion and anemia. When the *qi* is completely gone, the body is dead.

The History of Qigong
Qigong began many thousands of years ago with healing dances of ancient Chinese shamans. For instance, in the third millennium BCE, a bear-masked shaman would lead a dance to cleanse a village before the New Year. This developed into the philosophy that movement and exercise could also cleanse and refresh the body. According the Chinese doctor Hua Tuo (110–207 CE), "A door hinge won't rust as long as it is used." Similarly, physical movement stimulates internal movement of the healing energy called *qi*.

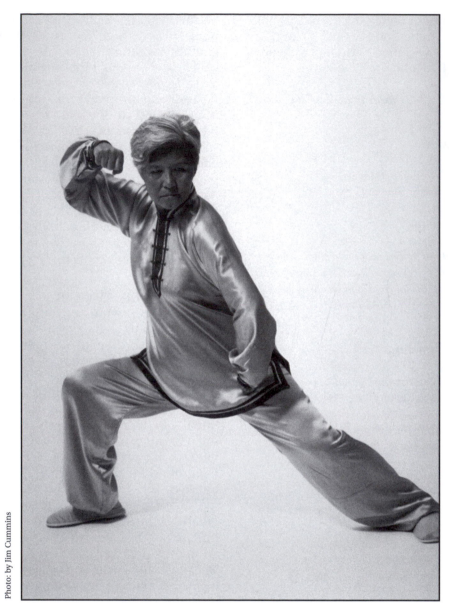

Photo: by Jim Cummins

Madame Gao Fu of Beijing, seventy-six-year-old master of Chen-style taiji quan (t'ai chi ch'uän), one of China's most popular qigong systems, noted for its fluidity and dynamic, coiling movements.

The practice of controlling *qi* through movement and exercise was originally called *dao-yin*, which means "leading and guiding the *qi*." In 1973, archaeologists discovered the first written record of these exercises in a text called *Dao-yin Tu*, "Dao-yin Illustrated," in a tomb near the city of Changsha. The *Dao-yin Tu*, dated approximately 168 BCE, shows forty-four seated and standing figures in various qigong postures.

There are short captions under several of the figures indicating the disease that the particular posture or exercise was designed to treat. The figures are from all walks of life—rich and poor, farmer and bureaucrat, man and woman, young and old.

By the second century CE, qigong was a popular healing therapy practiced by a very broad segment of Chinese society. Later centuries produced a

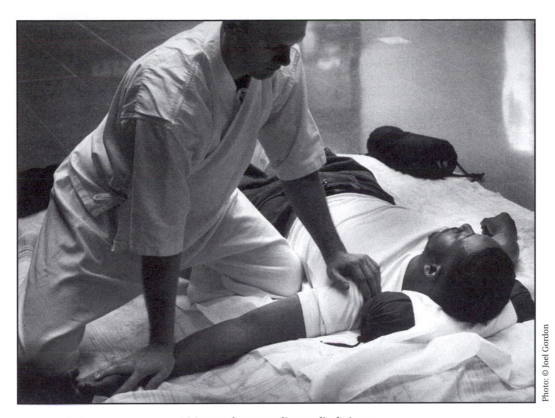

Photo: © Joel Gordon

A Western doctor applies medical qigong.

wealth of practical and philosophical literature on qigong. Most early texts are found in the *Taoist Canon,* the 1,120-volume collection of Taoist religious works. Taoists had a great interest in qigong because it includes meditation techniques that cultivate tranquil self-awareness and a feeling of harmony with nature and the cosmos. Most modern qigong texts are written by doctors rather than Taoists. In this century, the practice of qigong was not encouraged by the Communist regime in China until the late 1980s, when it was adopted as a sanctioned method of disease prevention. Throughout the 1990s qigong has experienced a huge resurgence in popularity, with over 90 million practitioners in China and several thousand in the United States.

Applications and Styles of Qigong

Qigong has three principal applications. Medical qigong is qigong for improving health. This is further divided into self-healing qigong, made up of exercises and meditations, and a method of healing patients called external *qi* healing. An external *qi* healer attempts to transmit healing energy by holding his or her hands either a few inches above or lightly on a diseased area. This method is similar to therapeutic touch, practiced by many nurses in the West. Spiritual qigong, the second major application of qigong, uses meditative practices, such as abdominal respiration and mental quiet, to develop a serene and hardy spirit, immune to stress and worry. Martial arts qigong, the third application, emphasizes dynamic qigong exercises that improve balance, coordination, strength, and stamina and that make the body more resistant to injury. Martial arts qigong can improve performance in any sport, increasing power in a tennis serve, a swimmer's stroke, or a boxer's punch.

There are thousands of qigong styles. Some are named after legendary or actual founders; others are named after animals that the exercises imitate (e.g., crane style, five animal frolics, turtle breathing); some describe health benefits (inner nourishing, tendon strengthening, relaxation qigong, improving vision); and many are identified by philosophical principles: wisdom (*zhi-neng*) qigong, primordial (*hun yuan*) qigong, inner elixir qigong, etc. Most qigong exercises are gentle, fluid, and graceful. Some styles, such as taiji quan (t'ai chi ch'üan), look like dance, consisting of many postures linked one to the next, like a flowing stream. In the past, many styles were taught to only a small, select number of students or to family members. Today, several qigong schools have millions of followers each, with branches in major Chinese cities. Students generally select one or two qigong styles according to their interests, health needs, and teacher availability.

The Qigong Posture

The foundation of all qigong practices is correct posture. Practicing the qigong posture is, of itself, good qigong. Stand with the feet parallel, shoulder width apart. Your knees should be slightly bent. Feel the weight of your body dropping down through the feet and into the ground. You are like a tree with deep roots. The abdomen is relaxed rather than unnaturally held in. The chest is also open and relaxed, neither depressed nor distended. The back is straight. Imagine that your tailbone is being pulled slightly down and your head lifted up, as though held like a puppet on a string. The entire spine feels stretched open. Your shoulders are relaxed rather than lifted in an "uptight" posture. The shoulders drop straight down, neither pulled back nor slouched forward. The fingers are gently extended, as if water were streaming out the fingertips. The mouth is lightly closed. Your eyes are open, gazing softly into the distance. The whole body is as relaxed as possible. If you need only five ounces of strength to stand, do not use six! The extra ounce is unnecessary effort and stress.

While holding this stance for a comfortable length of time—generally about five to ten minutes—observe your breath. The most natural and healthiest way of breathing is to allow the abdomen to gently expand as you inhale and retract as you exhale. Think to yourself, "My breath is slow, long, deep, smooth, and even." Let the breath move at its own pace. Do not pull the breath in; do not push it out. Let nature's wisdom work without interference. As you continue standing, notice how the fingers begin to tingle from improved circulation. You may also feel a pleasant sensation of warmth, stability, and inner strength. These are signs that the *qi* is both gathering and circulating.

The Qigong Prescription

It is recommended that qigong be practiced daily before breakfast. The morning is called the "springtime of the day," the best time to plant seeds of new growth. The guiding principles in qigong are practice, patience, and moderation. Qigong is a lifetime discipline. It is possible to reap benefits after only a

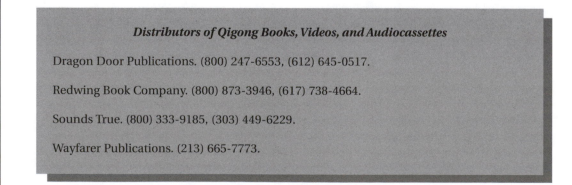

Distributors of Qigong Books, Videos, and Audiocassettes

Dragon Door Publications. (800) 247-6553, (612) 645-0517.

Redwing Book Company. (800) 873-3946, (617) 738-4664.

Sounds True. (800) 333-9185, (303) 449-6229.

Wayfarer Publications. (213) 665-7773.

few lessons or to continue gathering *qi* for a lifetime. Practice, but not to excess. If there is pain, there is no gain, because pain inhibits learning and personal growth. Qigong students should not seek quick results but rather slow, steady progress. The body is an energy garden that must be tended and nurtured daily. According to the ancient Chinese philosopher Mencius, you cannot make wheat grow more quickly by pulling on the stalks!

—*Kenneth S. Cohen, M.A.*

Resources:

American Foundation of Traditional Chinese
   Medicine
505 Beach St.
San Francisco, CA 94133
Tel: (415) 776-0502
Publishes a quarterly newsletter titled Gateways; *offers a referral service and international listing of classes, and sponsors continuing education programs.*

The Qigong Institute
561 Berkley Ave.
Menlo Park, CA 94025
Promotes education, research, and clinical work. Offers lectures and demonstrations and sponsors a qigong science program.

The Qigong Research and Practice Center
P.O. Box 1727
Nederland, CO 80466
Tel: (303) 258-0971
Offers training classes and conducts research into the efficacy of qigong.

Further Reading:

Cohen, Kenneth S. *The Way of Qigong.* New York: Ballantine Books, 1997.

Eisenberg, David, M.D. *Encounters with Qi.* New York: W.W. Norton & Co., 1985.

Jiao Guorui. *Qigong Essentials for Health Promotion.* Beijing: China Reconstructs Press, 1988.

Wang, Simon, M.D., Ph.D., and Julius L. Liu, M.D. *Qi Gong for Health and Longevity.* Tustin, CA: The East Health Development Group, 1994.

Qi: The Journal of Traditional Eastern Health & Fitness. Anaheim Hills, CA: Insight Publishing. 800-787-2600. (Lists many qigong schools).

REIKI

Reiki is a mode of healing, based on ancient Buddhist teachings, that uses hands-on touch to strengthen energy on the physical, intellectual, emotional, and spiritual planes. Reiki (pronounced "ray-key") combines two Japanese words, *rei* referring to the vital force that pervades the entire cosmos, and ki, referring to the life force that animates every individual being. In reiki treatment, universal and individual energy are aligned and balanced through the application of gentle hands-on touch to energy pathways of the body. Since no medication is ever prescribed, reiki is widely regarded as one of the most natural of all holistic systems of healing. Advocates of reiki credit it with benefits ranging from reduction of stress to quantum healing, including recovery from acute, chronic conditions. It is often used as an adjunct to medical treatment in order to gain relief from the trauma of illness and to accelerate healing.

The Rediscovery of Reiki
Until recently reiki has been taught as an oral tradition, making it difficult to be precise about either the early development of reiki or many of its tenets. It may be the world's oldest system of healing, with origins that reach back to the dawn of civilization. There is agreement that after antiquity, knowledge of the original system was lost until it was rediscovered in the second half of the nineteenth century by a Japanese man, Mikao Usui.

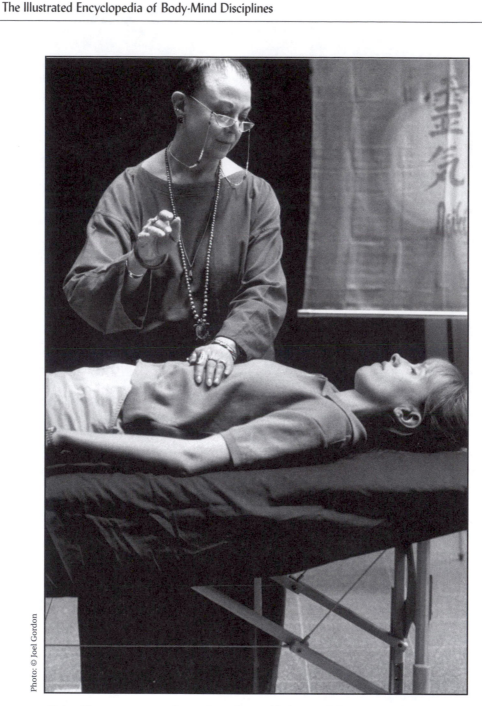

Elaine Abrams uses a gentle touch to align and balance subtle energy within a person.

Mikao Usui transcends the categories Buddhist, Christian, scholar of theology, teacher, holy man, and charismatic healer. Oral tradition holds that the path that led him to reiki started at a Christian seminary in Kyoto, sometime around 1850, when a student asked Usui why he was willing to explain Christ's spiritual teachings but said nothing about his miraculous powers of healing. Though simple, the question raised fundamental problems about the relationship of body, mind, and spirit in Western and Eastern religion. To resolve the question, Usui resigned his post in Kyoto and embarked on a quest that took him to the graduate school of the University of Chicago and eventually back to Kyoto to a Zen Buddhist monastery. By this time his research was concentrated on the earliest records of Hindu and Buddhist belief, and at the monastery he came upon ancient sutras (Buddhist teachings written in Sanskrit) that gave him an insight into the principles he had been pursuing.

A deeply spiritual man, Usui knew that his understanding of the sutras would be incomplete so long as it remained on the intellectual level. After studying the texts, he ascended the sacred mountain Kuriyama and fasted and meditated for twenty-one days. Very early on the morning of the twenty-first day, he had a vision in which a brilliant light struck him between the eyes, exploded into tiny colored bubbles, then gave way to a number of gleaming Sanskrit characters. Usui believed that this vision initiated him into the ancient system of reiki and empowered him to revive its methods of healing. Upon return to Kyoto, he brought about cures that were considered miraculous. He traveled throughout Japan and attracted a devoted following.

Shortly before Usui's death he passed the reiki teachings to Chijuro Hayashi, who founded the first reiki clinic. One of the patients cured in Hayashi's clinic during the 1930s was Hawayo Takata, a Japanese-American woman. She studied reiki with Hayashi, became his successor in 1941, and in the 1970s traveled throughout North America, offering reiki treatment and the combination of training and initiation needed to become a reiki practitioner. Takata is responsible for transforming reiki into an internationally known mode of healing with a network of professional organizations. Many advanced reiki practitioners are now qualified to provide treatment. In addition, a number of massage therapists, nurses, and other health care professionals incorporate aspects of reiki into their repertory of techniques. Today many reiki master-instructors are qualified to provide instruction in the Usui system of natural healing as well as offer treatment.

The Philosophy and Methods of Reiki

Reiki is based on a belief that the individual is animated by a vital energy emanating from the life force of the universe and falls ill if the flow of energy is weakened. Further, it is believed that everyone is born with the ability to access this universal energy. Opening pathways of healing using universal energy is reiki's central objective. To learn the procedures for self-treatment and treating others using the Usui system, a would-be practitioner must herself or himself receive an "attunement," in order to become attuned to the energy-transfer system. This attunement can be given only by an experienced reiki master instructor in a ceremony of initiation. Though no religious dogma is involved in reiki, Usui's teachings require that it be administered in a sacred manner. Sanskrit symbols from Usui's vision on Mount Kuriyama serve as the formulaic key to knowledge. Hands-on touch is the key component in the opening of an individual's energy transfer ability.

Reiki's attunements/initiations and symbols may confound rational explanation, but practitioners and masters are content simply to trust in their beneficial workings. Most practitioners and masters emphasize that hands-on touch of energy pathways in the body has been a means of therapy used around the world for millennia. They deliver reiki through hand patterns and positions that relate to the major organs and systems of the body, assisting the flow of energy through these systems. It follows that if reiki normalizes the flow of energy to the entire system, it would generate profound physical and emotional benefits, improving the entire organism's resistance to stress and disease.

Experiencing Reiki

While reiki treatment may vary, based on the practitioner's level of experience and the recipient's needs, it generally takes the form of a bodywork session that lasts from an hour to an hour and a half. During the bodywork the recipient remains fully clothed and lies on a massage table, first in a supine, then in a prone position. Sometimes ambient sound of a relaxing type, music or recordings of pleasant sounds in a natural environment such as a stream of water, is provided. The recipient may express preferences for such things.

Reiki bodywork should not be confused with massage. The hands-on touch is gentle and aims not to manipulate tissue, but rather to transmit universal life force to the recipient. The practitioner uses both hands, palms down, fingers held together, and proceeds in a pattern over the recipient's body. After the front surface has been treated, the client turns and treatment continues on the back. Each positioning of the hands is maintained for three to five minutes without any movement of the fingers or change in the initial gentle touch. Practitioners may use twenty or more hand positions in any single session.

Experience of reiki bodywork differs from person to person; each client's perception of how the energy transfer feels will vary. A slight warmth or tingling coming from the hands of the practitioner may be felt, or his or her hands may feel cool. In some instances recipients doze or go into a threshold condition between sleep and full consciousness. Most find reiki relaxing and refreshing. The full effects of treatment

may be experienced immediately or not until several days after a session.

It is recommended that first-time recipients receive three or four treatments as close together as the recipient can manage in order to deepen the process of healing. The number and timing of subsequent treatments depends on the nature of the recipient's condition.

Hands-on bodywork has become standard in reiki practice, but touch is not necessary to the healing process. According to Usui, the channeling of the universal life force can be achieved through mental and manual focus that is effective even over long distances, which is learned as an advanced technique. After attunement/initiation, it is suggested that reiki be used as a mode of self-care as well as care for others.

The Benefits of Reiki

Practitioners believe reiki gives recipients a sense of trust and overall well-being. It is particularly beneficial in the treatment of stress and stress-related illnesses. Reiki is also considered helpful in debilitating disease because it supplies energy and strengthens the immune system. While reiki is not a religious system, it often becomes a potent stimulus to self-healing and spiritual growth.

—*Elaine J. Abrams, Reiki Master-Instructor*

Reiki Training

Reiki instruction has three degrees or levels. In first degree, or level I, training, the participant receives attunement from a reiki master. He or she also learns techniques for administering self-care. In second degree, or level II, training, the participant receives further attunements of energy from a reiki master. He or she also embarks on study of the ancient symbols and sounds Dr. Usui recovered from the sutras, learning to apply them to the healing process. Third degree, or level III, provides the participant with yet another attunement and final study of the ancient symbols and sounds used in reiki. Practitioners with third degree training are called reiki masters, and are the only ones able to offer level I and II instruction.

Resources:

The Reiki Alliance
PO Box 41
Cataldo, ID 83810
Tel: (208) 682-3535
Fax: (208) 682-4848
A professional organization comprised of credentialed usui system reiki masters.

The Reiki Alliance Europe
Honthorststraat 40 II 1071 DG
Amsterdam, Netherlands
Tel: (20) 6719276
Fax: (20) 6711736
The European headquarters of the Reiki Alliance.

Further Reading:

Brown, Fran. *Living Reiki: Takata's Teachings.* Mendicino, CA: LifeRhythm, 1992.

Haberly, Helen J. *Reiki: Hawayo Takata's Story.* Salem, OR: Blue Mountain Publications, 1990.

Sharamon, Shalila, and Baginski, Bodo. *Reiki: Universal Life Energy.* Transl. Baker, Christopher, and Harrison, Judith. Mendocino, CA: Life Rhythm, 1988.

SHEN®

SHEN®, which stands for specific human energy nexus, is a relatively recent approach to body-mind health and wellness that is concerned with how the body deals with repressed emotion. SHEN techniques release trapped emotional trauma from specific areas by focusing energy on the biofield that surrounds and permeates the human body. The release and resolution of these emotions are meant to reestablish normal functioning of the affected organs and balance emotional and physical forces in the body.

How SHEN® Developed

SHEN's basic concepts were developed by scientist Richard R. Pavek after he retired from a career in business in order to start a new career as an alternative medical and health practitioner. In 1977 he began formulating his original concepts about emotions and their effects on the body and the mind from observations made during his own experimentation with the hands-on healing techniques he was developing.

It was apparent to him that emotions were far more significant in determining our health than was then presented in the medical and psychological textbooks. While the textbooks were teaching that emotions occurred in the brain and were unimportant by-products of mental activity, he, along with many other scientists, physicians, and psychologists, believed that emotions were far more complex and often played a dominant role in our lives. Pavek theorized that when we have an emotion, we feel it in our bodies, our bodies react to it, and our minds cannot easily make it go away. It seemed to him that since emotions were not readily controlled by the brain, they were not directly produced by the brain. It followed that emotional empowerment is as important to how we live our lives as intellectual development.

As he began to determine the effects emotions had on the body, Pavek noticed a relationship between the locations of painful emotions and the physical disorders with which they were associated. For example, he realized that anger and fear, emotions that are associated with eating disorders, are experienced in the same region of the body that contains the digestive organs. This relationship of the emotions being felt in the body where related disorders occur is the same for long-term grief and heart disorders, and for shame, guilt, and the dysfunctions they produce. He conceived that the organs in that region of our bodies must be adversely affected by those emotions *because they are experienced there.* Somehow, emotions were controlling the body.

The last part of the puzzle fell into place when he noticed that if we felt painful emotions, such as fear, grief, and shame, our bodies would clench around the locations where they are felt. Subsequently, the emotion would be trapped inside that location. He reasoned that the physical tension that trapped the emotion would interfere with normal flow of blood and other nutrients and prevent the physical organs in the region from functioning normally. With these principles established, Pavek began developing the SHEN techniques now being used to release trapped emotional trauma within the recipient's body. He demonstrated that release and resolution of these emotions does reestablish normal functioning of the organs.

How SHEN® Works

SHEN is a unique hands-on process that does not use physical pressure or manipulation. Instead, it uses the biofield that surrounds and permeates the human body. This field was first identified in ancient times and has been in use in healing ever since. In some forms of biofield treatment the *qi* (pronounced *chee;* it is the Chinese name for the energy that makes up the biofield) from the practitioner's hands is applied to the body, either in direct contact with the skin or through clothing. In other forms the hands are placed close to, but not touching, the body. SHEN practitioners use both forms, but most of the time their hands are in contact with the body through regular clothing.

Typical Session of SHEN®

During the SHEN session the recipient reclines fully clothed on a hammock-like frame or a table similar to a massage table, but with twice as much padding. The recipient is encouraged to relax while the practitioner places his or her hands in a rationally planned sequence of several positions around the regions in the body where, according to Pavek's theories, we mainly experience or feel the individual emotions. These are the heart, the upper abdomen, the lower abdomen, and the groin. The recipient often feels tingles or warmth as the *qi* between the practitioner's hands flows through his or her body. Often the client drifts into a light sleep state, similar to what one experiences just before falling fully asleep or just before becoming fully awake.

While in this state, emotionally charged, dreamlike images often emerge. Sometimes memories of forgotten, painful emotional events from earlier portions of one's life come to the surface and are relived. Whenever emotions come to the surface in a SHEN session they are experienced in a different way than we usually experience them. Instead of being driven to physically respond to, or act out the effects of the emotion, the person strongly feels the emotion in one of the emotion regions. This occurs in a way the person can handle and absorb. Very often these feelings are understood and resolved when they are recalled in a SHEN

SHEN Physics

SHEN's singular techniques are unusually effective because they are based on conventional physics rather than on the metaphysical principles used in the past. Through a series of careful experiments, Dr. Pavek has been able to show that the biofield is regulated by the same patterns of arrangement that oversee all other moving fields in nature; electricity, magnetism, oceanic currents, and weather currents. SHEN practitioners learn to apply the *qi* between their hands to the recipient according to these patterns in ways that produce the greatest effect.

session. Recall of previous emotional states and the resolution of troubling emotions are the hallmarks of the SHEN session; emotional empowerment is its intent.

There are certified SHEN practitioners and interns throughout the United States, Canada, and many European countries. More are being trained in a comprehensive professional training program that is currently available in several countries.

Benefits of SHEN®

SHEN is greatly beneficial with all physical conditions where unpleasant or painful emotions are major factors. These include conditions that have often been slow to respond to conventional medical or psychological treatment methods. Among these are anorexia, bulimia, compulsive behaviors, disturbed childhood sleep patterns, emotional depression, emotionally upset digestion, migraines, panic attacks, severe premenstrual and menstrual distress, all types of post-traumatic stress disorders, and recurrent nightmares.

Besides being instrumental in causing physio-emotional disorders, our emotions often interfere with our thoughts and we find ourselves unable to think clearly, often ending up at cross purposes with our best and most desired interests. SHEN has proven to be a safe and reliable process that is extremely beneficial in resolving unpleasant and detrimental emotional states that undermine rational thinking and normal psychological development. By clearing out the old, crippling, and injurious emotional energy, SHEN paves the way for emotional empowerment.

SHEN is very helpful in dealing with grief, feelings of humiliation, and with resolving troublesome dreams. In addition, it has been extremely beneficial in promoting and accelerating recovery from alcohol and drug addictions and from childhood and adult physical, sexual and/or emotional abuse. It is often very successful where more conventional methods and approaches have failed to foster psychological and behavioral

change, or real emotional empowerment and true personal growth.

—*Richard Pavek*

Resources:

The SHEN Therapy Institute
20 YFH Gate 6 Road
Sausalito, CA 94965
Tel: (415) 332-2593
Fax: (415) 331-2455
Provides information about research and development, and training in the United States and Canada.

The International SHEN Therapy Association
3213 West Wheeler, No. 202
Seattle, WA 98199
Tel: (206) 298-9468
Fax: (206) 283-1256
A not-for-profit corporation founded in 1990 with the goal of expanding and promoting SHEN throughout the world. ISTA is charged with the responsibility of maintaining and administering uniform worldwide standards for Certified SHEN Practitioners, for maintaining an internship training program, and for examining and granting certification to interns.

SHEN Therapy Centre
26 Inverleith Row
Edinburgh, EH3 5QH
Tel/fax: 0131-551-5091
Scotland
Information about practitioners and training in the United Kingdom.

SHEN Therapy Centre
73 Claremont Park, Circular Rd.
Galway, Ireland
Tel: 91-525-941
Fax: 91-529-807
Provides information about practitioners and training in Ireland.

THERAPEUTIC TOUCH

Therapeutic touch is an approach to healing that assesses and balances the energy field that surrounds and penetrates the body with the goal of supporting an individual's own potential for self-healing. Therapeutic touch, or TT, as it is affectionately known to practitioners and devotees, is a contemporary interpretation of a number of very ancient healing practices, one of which is the laying on of hands.

Finding the Common Denominator

TT was developed in the 1970s by a nurse healer and research scientist at New York University, Dolores Krieger, Ph.D., RN, in collaboration with a clairvoyant, Dora Kunz. They were interested in studying various healers to see if there were any underlying principles that might form a common basis for healing. They also wanted to know if there were any basic principles that might be taught to other people for use in healing. They did indeed find certain fundamental principles at work in healing, and therapeutic touch developed from their research. Dr. Krieger maintains that healing is a natural human potential that can be learned by virtually anyone.

Clearing Areas of Imbalances

The practice of TT is based on the assumption that the human being represents an open energy system, and that this system is bilaterally symmetrical. The practitioner feels for areas of imbalance in the receiver's field, such as areas of temperature difference (hot or cold), pressure, tingling, or other sensations. These sensations are cues that an area is out of balance. Once the practitioner has gained a snapshot "feel" for the client's energy field, he or she then works to rebalance the field.

The therapeutic touch practitioner clears areas of imbalance by gently brushing away any places of congestion, in a movement known as "unruffling." The movement looks almost as though the practitioner is using his or her hands to iron out wrinkles in the space around the receiver's body. The practitioner then transfers energy to any areas in the receiver's field that may feel as though they lack energy. The practitioner does this by holding his or her hands a few inches from the receiver's body, and sending energy through the palms to the receiver until the receiver's energy field feels as though it has "filled up."

While some people may think that therapeutic touch sounds a little like hocus-pocus, this practice has, in fact, been the subject of intense scientific scrutiny. One of Dr. Krieger's most important contributions to the field of healing has been her commitment to subjecting TT to academic research. Therapeutic touch has been the subject of no less than 27 doctoral studies, 15 postdoctoral studies, and innumerable Master's theses—plus 2 National Institutes of Health (NIH) grants and 83 articles in 5 countries. TT is taught at more than eighty colleges in the United States and in seventy foreign countries.

Therapeutic touch is practiced by a large and devoted following, many of whom are nurse healers. As the practice grows, however, many other health professionals and laypersons are discovering the many benefits of TT. It is one bodywork practice that is very easy for laypersons to learn to use with family members and friends. In fact, the foundational techniques can be learned in a one-day workshop. Even children can be taught to do TT.

Centering

A typical TT treatment lasts about twenty to thirty minutes. The receiver remains dressed in street clothes, generally seated on a stool or straight-backed chair, facing sideways, so that the back is exposed for treatment. If this position is uncomfortable, or unsuitable because an individual has difficulty sitting, treatment can be performed with the receiver lying on a comfortable padded surface.

The TT practitioner begins treatment by quietly centering, or focusing his or her thoughts, while requesting that the receiver do the same. Centering calms the mind, and enables both practitioner and receiver to access deep inner resources that are powerful forces in healing. While centered and attuned to the receiver, the practitioner assesses the receiver's field. The practitioner does this by gently, rhythmically, and rapidly passing his or her hands, palms facing the receiver, about four to six inches over the receiver's body. The practitioner then proceeds to clear areas of imbalance and transfer energy as needed to the receiver's field.

A Safe Practice

Studies have shown that TT is effective at inducing relaxation, diminishing pain, alleviating anxiety, and accelerating healing. Receivers report various sensations during treatment, such as tingling, heat, and other effects. They often say they feel both relaxed and energized. Therapeutic touch is especially recommended for acute conditions, such as infections, wounds, and sprains.

Because therapeutic touch is gentle, and the practitioner often does not even touch the body, there are very few situations where it cannot be used. Treatments should be shorter and gentler for infants, the elderly, women who are pregnant, seriously ill people, and individuals with head injuries.

—Thomas Claire

Resources:

Nurse Healers–Professional Associates, Inc.
P.O. Box 444
Allison Park, PA 15101-0444
Nurse Healers-Professional Associates is the organization to which Dr. Krieger gave all her original TT materials. They can help you find more information on therapeutic touch.

Pumpkin Hollow Foundation
RR#1, Box 135
Craryville, NY 12521
Tel: (518) 325-3583, or (518) 325-7105
Offers the only year-round setting where a full program of TT classes from beginning to advanced is offered.

The Therapeutic Touch Network (Ontario)
P.O. Box 85551
875 Eglinton Avenue West
Toronto, ON M6C 4A8
Canada
Tel: (416) 65 TOUCH
Provides information about Canadian programs and practitioners.

Further Reading:

Claire, Thomas, M.S., LMT. *Bodywork: What Type of Massage to Get—and How to Make the Most of It.* New York: William Morrow, 1995.

Krieger, Dolores, Ph.D., RN. *Accepting Your Power to Heal: The Personal Practice of Therapeutic Touch.* Santa Fe, NM: Bear & Co., 1993.

——. *The Therapeutic Touch: How to Use Your Hands to Help or to Heal.* New York: Prentice-Hall, 1979.

Macrae, Janet, Ph.D., RN. *Therapeutic Touch: A Practical Guide.* New York: Knopf, 1987.

PART VII: MASSAGE

Bowen Technique • Connective Tissue Therapy℠ • CORE Structural Integrative Therapy • Infant Massage • Muscular Therapy • Myofascial Release • Myofascial Trigger Point Therapy • Reflexology • Rolfing® • Rosen Method • St. John Method of Neuromuscular Therapy • Swedish Massage

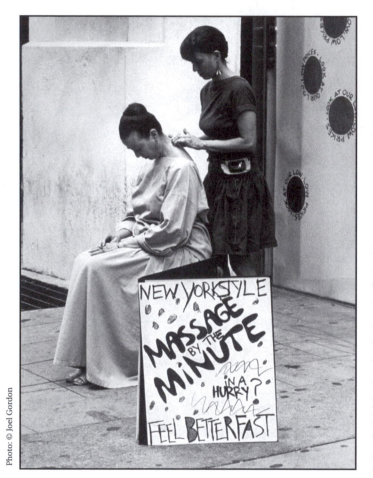

Photo: © Joel Gordon

Massage is one of the most widely available body-mind therapies.

Massage is one of the oldest methods of healing the body, mind, and spirit. The instinct to console one another through touch is perhaps as old as humanity itself. According to the seminal study *Healing Massage Techniques: Holistic, Classic, and Emerging Methods* (1988), the first cave dwellers probably rubbed their bruises and aches by instinct, the same way many other animals touch and groom each other. Humans recognized the therapeutic power of touch very early on by observing its physical and psychological benefits. Many different massage techniques have grown out of that instinct—known today under the broad umbrella called massage therapy.

How Massage Therapy Developed

The use of massage as a therapeutic tool has been documented throughout history. In the Americas, massage and joint manipulation was used by the Maya, Inca, and other native peoples. Traditional African and Eastern cultures used sharp stones to scratch the skin's surface in a healing practice similar to Chinese acupuncture. Indigenous peoples of the South Pacific have their own forms of massage as well.

Although touch has been used as a method of folk healing in many cultures, the development of formal therapeutic massage is strongly rooted in China. Evidence for this can be found in *The Yellow Emperor's Classic of Internal Medicine*, which, according to legend, was written by the Yellow Emperor Huang-ti, who died in 2598 BCE. Two descriptive names were used in China for massage: *anmo,* meaning press-rub, and *tui-na,* meaning push-pull. According to *Fundamentals of Therapeutic Massage* by Sandy Fritz (1995), these methods involved kneading and rubbing down the entire body with the hands and using a gentle pressure and traction on all the joints. Acupressure, the ancient practice of applying hand and finger pressure to specific points on the body, developed out of Chinese acupuncture—the practice of stimulating certain points along the body by inserting tiny needles.

Chinese massage techniques spread along trade routes to Japan and other Asian countries, including India, where they have enjoyed respect for their therapeutic value to this day. There is evidence in medical literature that massage was used as a respected element in ancient Egyptian and Persian medical practices. The "laying on of hands" and "anointing with oils" has been recorded in the writings of the early Hebrews and Christians; in fact, there is reference to these practices in Isaiah of the Bible.

Massage was considered an integral part of ayurvedic medicine in ancient India. Alexander the Great (356–323 BCE) was one of those responsible for bringing massage to the West. When conquering India, his troops were ravaged by fatal snake bites. The Indian physicians had developed advanced surgical techniques to treat these snake bites, so Alexander replaced all of his Greek physicians with Indian physicians, and massage was incorporated into Greek medicine. Tschanpua—eventually known as shampooing—was a technique initially employed by Alexander's officers; it survived until the 1800s. Last used by the British Colonial Army, it was incorporated as a part of a greater health regimen that also involved bathing and the use of scented oils.

The ancient Greeks built great bathhouses, called thurmae, where exercise, massage, baths, and scholastic studies were available, much like modern-day health spas. Citizens visited the thurmae daily as a part of the "duty of health." Socrates, Plato, and Aristotle were all teachers at thurmae and also received massage there. The Greeks employed massage especially in conjunction with athletics; for example, an athlete would be massaged before taking part in the Olympic Games.

Hippocrates, often referred to as the father of modern medicine, lived in ancient Greece from 460 to 377 BCE. He learned massage and gymnastics and developed his own method of medicine. He wrote prescriptions for massage and exercise. Many of his techniques have survived to this day.

The Romans learned massage from the Greeks. Massage and baths were used extensively throughout the Roman Empire (27 BCE–476 CE), which covered most of Europe. Cicero wrote about receiving massage and attributed his health to it. Even Julius Caesar (100–44 BCE) had himself "pinched all over" daily for relief of nerve pain and to treat epilepsy, a severe nervous disorder.

After the fall of Rome and the barbarian invasions, the rise of monasticism helped to preserve written accounts of the use of massage in the West. The monks were both scribes and physicians. Although they were not medically trained as Roman physicians were, they carried on the practice of massage, exercise, and anointing with oils as a part of folk medicine. Eventually the monks abandoned the practice of medicine as well as massage, and as a result massage faded in Europe.

During the Middle Ages, invasions and wars caused great political and social chaos in Europe. Communication among countries was lost. This contributed to the decline of medicine, massage, and medical advancements. At this time, supernatural occurrences were often associated with massage, and it has been reported in some sources that many healers were persecuted by the church for having evil powers.

Change occurred once again after the Black Plague, which destroyed large populations in Europe. A time period known as the Renaissance (fourteenth to sixteenth centuries CE) followed. Travel increased and communications were restored. People started learning about Arabic and Persian culture, where the Greco-Roman traditions of massage had thrived.

In the late fourteenth century, massage was first used in postsurgical recovery, and was even considered a noninvasive type of surgery. Formal two-year medical training programs were established at universities all across Europe, similar to the old Roman schools. A well-known French physician, Ambroise Paré (1517–1590), began using massage for postsurgical healing of wounds and joint stiffness. His ideas helped to make massage better accepted by the medical community of the West and were passed on to other European physicians.

Massage was finally popularized in the West by the work of a Swede named Per Henrik Ling (1776–1839). A fencing master and gymnastics instructor, Ling is credited with the development of Swedish massage. After curing himself of rheumatism in his arm by the use of massage techniques, he began a study of the art and developed a system that included massage and exercise. He based his system on the new science of physiology.

Because of his continual study and dedication, Ling's method eventually became accepted and known as "the Ling system" or the "Swedish movement treatment." In 1813 he established the Royal Gymnastic Central Institute, the first college to have massage a part of the curriculum. It was popular internationally. Even the czar of Russia sent someone to study at the school. Through the writings and practice of Ling's students, his system became well known throughout Europe. Many new forms of massage are based on this standard form.

From 1813 to 1918 massage became quite popular as a medical treatment. Many spas were built all over Europe for the rheumatoid "cure." In the mid-1800s two Vermont physicians, Charles Faytte Taylor and George Henry Taylor brought massage to the United States from Europe. However, after World War I the popularity of massage in orthodox Western medicine declined once again with the rise in pharmaceutical drugs and new medical technologies.

This decline lasted through World War II, and massage did not appear again in medical literature until the late 1970s. After the reopening of China to the West during President Richard Nixon's administration, American physicians traveled there to learn acupuncture and returned with the basics of acupressure and other Chinese massage. Massage began to reappear in American popular culture in the 1960s after President John Kennedy began to emphasize physical fitness as important to preventative medicine.

Massage was a part of the new age movement that began with the hippies in the United States, but it was not really taken seriously by the medical community until the 1980s, when studies were published describing the benefits of Eastern techniques for certain conditions. It gained popularity as a method of managing pain. On-site massage at the workplace became popular for work-related pain and stress management.

Sports massage has also flourished with the popularity of athletics. Practitioners in the twentieth century began to innovate the practice of massage by combining techniques and adding their own insights. This synthesis of old and new methods contributed to the resurgence of therapeutic massage in the United States and throughout the world.

Basic Systems of Massage

Today there have grown several systems, or modalities, of massage. They can be divided into three different approaches:

- Mechanical approaches attempt to change the quality of muscles, tendons, and ligaments or blood and lymph flow by the direct application of force. Connective Tissue Therapy™, myofascial release, Rolfing, and manual lymph drainage are some of the popular forms that fall in this category.
- Movement approaches focus on passively repatterning habits of moving the body for greater ease and relief. Neuromuscular facilitation and trigger-point myotherapy are good examples.
- Energetic approaches deal with influencing reflexes in the nervous system and balancing energy in the body. Shiatsu and many Eastern forms of massage, as well as polarity, therapeutic touch, reiki, and Zero Balancing® deal with this approach. Because these methods use substantially different techniques from the first two approaches, they are dealt with in separate sections of this encyclopedia.

Many modalities, including medical and sports massage, may integrate all three approaches.

Massage aims to bring the participant's body, mind, and spirit into balance by encouraging the body's own healing potential. The body has the amazing ability to bring itself back to equilibrium through many built-in balancing mechanisms. For example, when a harmful microorganism enters the body, one's temperature rises to kill the germ and then eventually returns to normal temperature (98.6° F). Using a mechanical or movement approach, massage therapists determine where imbalances may lie in the structure of the body (perhaps very tight muscles) and support the body's return to a more balanced state (i.e., encouraging the nervous system and musculature to let go of excess tension in overcontracted muscles). This is done by manipulating the soft tissues of the body—mainly muscles, tendons, and ligaments.

Because the body and its systems are quite complex, a certain level of understanding of energy-flow patterns, knowledge of anatomy and physiology, and competence is required in order to give an effective massage. Thus, many states in the United States require massage therapists to be licensed professionals who have a certain number of hours of specialized training in a certified school and abide by certain rules and ethical guidelines. This ensures the public a safe, quality service and is similar to other professions in the field of health science such as physical therapists, doctors, and chiropractors, who must also be licensed.

The requirements for licensure vary from state to state in the United States. Some states do not require a license at all; most states require between 500 and 1,000 hours of training in anatomy and physiology as well as massage technique. Ontario, Canada, requires very extensive training of 2,200 hours, while British Columbia has a 3,000-hour curriculum, and massage has become a more recognized profession there, more integrated into the medical community. Recently in the United States, standards for national certification have been established to require at least 500 hours of training and the successful completion of a national exam.

Licensure has also helped to distinguish massage therapy from the business of prostitution, which sometimes shrouds itself under the veil of "massage." Therapeutic massage is a nonsexual health practice.

The Power of Touch

Massage is usually done with the hands, but elbows, forearms, knees, or feet may be used. The client may be clothed, as is the custom with Japanese shiatsu, which is done on the floor or a mat with the practitioner kneeling alongside the client and crawling along different parts of the body to administer pressure. Touch may also be administered directly to the skin and underlying muscles of unclothed clients as with Swedish massage. Usually in these cases the client lies on a massage table and is draped with sheets and/or towels so that only the part of the body being worked on is exposed, and most often a cream, oil, or some form of lubricant is used on the skin.

A typical treatment session lasts about one hour. If one is going for medical massage for a specific injury, it may last only thirty to forty minutes. Thai massage sessions, which involve many elaborate stretches that the practitioner does for the participant, may last for two hours.

Benefits and Risks

There are many benefits to massage therapy. Above all, it is used to relieve pain. Psychologically, touch gives a message of caring, compassion, and support to a participant and can thereby help reduce stress and aid healing. Mechanically, it can alleviate muscle spasm and help increase flexibility. Physiologically, circulation of blood and lymph is increased, which helps deliver nutrients to all the cells of the body and also helps to remove the waste products of cells. Studies with AIDS patients have shown that massage therapy can help activate the immune system. Touch can have a soothing or stimulating effect on the nervous system. Furthermore, it heightens awareness of the body and its sensations, which supports the connection of body, mind, and spirit. Scientific research is currently being done at the Touch Research Institute in Florida to further investigate the effects of touch and therapeutic massage.

Despite all of these healing effects, there are times when massage therapy is not appropriate. Massage should not be administered if either the client or the practitioner is under the influence of certain types of drugs, such as cortisone treatments or mind-altering drugs. It should also be avoided if the client or the practitioner has a fever or a communicable disease such as the measles or influenza.

Cancer is another major contraindication for massage. Many forms of massage therapy, especially Swedish, involve moving lymph fluid, which may cause the cancer to spread. If the participant has been diagnosed with any form of inflammation of the blood vessels (especially phlebitis) or with having a blood clot, massage should not be done for fear of moving the blood clot where it may damage the heart or cause a stroke. Massage should be avoided locally if the participant has varicose veins, bruises, or open wounds. Liver problems and other inflammations of internal organs should be investigated with the client's doctor before massage is administered.

—Katie Scoville , with information from an interview with Richard van Why, publisher of The Bodywork Knowledgebase.

Resources:

American Massage Therapy Association (AMTA)
820 Davis St., Suite 100
Evanston, IL 60201
Tel: (847) 864-0123
Fax: (847) 864-1178
Web site: www.amtamassage.org
An organization that provides information and resources on massage therapy. Publishes the Massage Therapy Journal.

The American Oriental Bodywork Therapy
   Association (AOBTA)
Glendale Executive Campus, Ste. 510
1000 White Horse Rd.
Vorhees, NJ 08043
Tel: (609) 782-1616
Fax: (516) 364-5559
Web site: www.healthy.net/pan/pa/bodywork
The AOBTA is a national organization of bodyworkers in eleven different styles. They certify practitioners, teachers, and schools throughout the United States. The organization enforces minimum entry-level standards (500 hours) for all types of Oriental bodyworkers. Currently represents about 1,200 members.

College of Massage Therapists of Ontario
1867 Yonge Street, Ste. 810
Toronto, ON M451Y5
Canada
Organization that promotes the therapeutic use of massage in Canada.

National Certification Board for Therapeutic
   Massage and Bodywork
8201 Greensboro Dr.
Suite 300
MacLean, VA 22102
Tel: (800) 296-0664
Fax: (703) 610-9015
Web site: www.ncbtmb.com
Establishes and implements certification standards for massage therapists.

Further Reading:

Fritz, Sandy. *Mosby's Fundamentals of Therapeutic Massage.* St. Louis, MO: Mosby-Year Book, Inc., 1995.

Lidell, Lucinda. *The Book of Massage.* New York: Fireside, 1984.

Tappan, F. M. *Healing Massage Techniques: Holistic, Classic, and Emerging Methods.* Norwalk, CT: Appleton & Lange, 1988.

BOWEN TECHNIQUE

Bowen technique or Bowtech© is a system of muscle and connective tissue movements used to stimulate energy flow and restore the body's self-healing resources. A Bowtech specialist uses a series of gently rolling movements to manipulate a client's connective tissue, including muscles, tendons, and ligaments. With the goal of stimulating, balancing, and realigning the body's energy flows, the Bowen technique is used by many health care professionals as an adjunct to their work; however, it is increasingly used as a stand-alone therapy, with many Bowen practitioners maintaining their own clinics.

The Bowen technique was developed in Australia by Thomas A. Bowen (1903–1982). He began his professional training with a year of medical school, followed by service in the Australian army during World War II. After the war, while working in an industrial plant, he gained a reputation for being able to help his coworkers with their aches and pains. Because he was able to help so many people, he decided to open a clinic using his method of muscle manipulation. By 1975 he was seeing 13,000 patients per year. After his death, Bowen's work was continued by his colleagues Oswald and Elaine Rentsch. The Rentsches had previously documented Bowen's technique and since his death they have introduced it throughout Australia, North America, and Europe. More than 6,000 people worldwide have been trained to practice or administer the Bowen technique.

The Bowtech therapist uses two or four fingers to gently roll muscles from side to side. Known as the Golgi tendon reflex, this movement triggers muscles to relax. This movement appears to affect the body's autonomic nervous system and creates balance on a cellular level. Some believe that Bowtech sets up vibrational patterns that correspond to particular areas of the body. The body

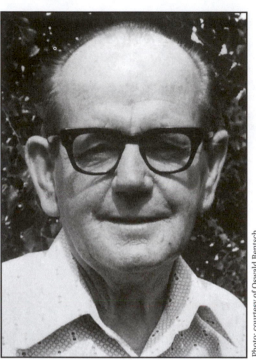

Thomas A. Bowen, founder of the Bowen technique.

Photo: courtesy of Oswald Rentsch

then attempts to alter its usual vibrations to match those ideal vibrational patterns and in so doing, brings itself into harmony.

A typical treatment lasts between twenty and forty minutes. It is usually done on a massage table or bed, where a client will lie comfortably and fully clothed on his or her back or abdomen. The therapist relaxes a muscle, tendon, or ligament by gently rolling it back and forth with his or her fingers. Each session includes a series of waiting periods when the therapist will pause to allow the recipient's body to integrate the changes to the area being treated. Generally an increase in blood supply and lymphatic drainage results in the release of tension and reduced muscle spasms. Unlike traditional Swedish massage, the technique is gentle and contacts only muscles on the surface of the body, with no deep rubbing.

The Bowen technique may be performed on anyone, from newborn infants to seniors. It may be incorporated into the treatment of the disabled or patients with chronic illnesses, including multiple

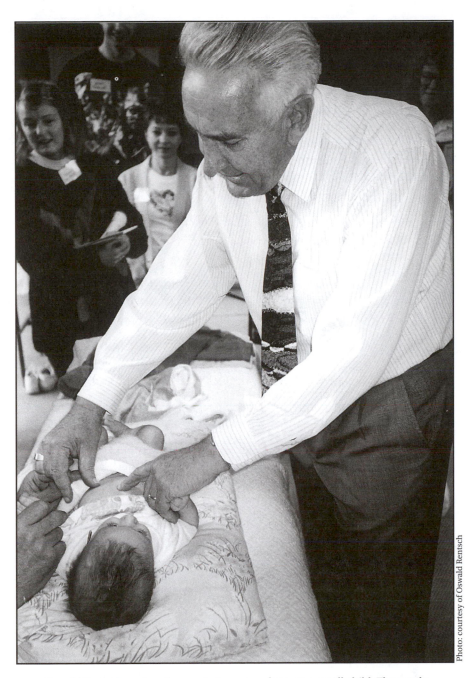

Photo: courtesy of Oswald Rentsch

Oswald Rentsch performing respiratory procedures on a small child. The gentle moves relax the diaphragm, easing gastrointestinal tract and breathing dysfunction.

sclerosis, cerebral palsy, muscular dystrophy, acute and chronic fatigue, and stress disorders. It has also been used to speed rehabilitation of sports injuries and accidents, regardless of how old or recent the injuries may be.

—*Oswald Rentsch*

Resources:

Bowtech©
P.O. Box 733
Hamilton, Victoria 3300
Australia
Tel: 011 61 3 55 723000
e-mail: bowtech©h140.aone.net.au
Promotes the study and use of the Bowen technique.

Connective Tissue Therapy℠

Connective Tissue Therapy℠ is a form of bodywork, sometimes called *binde* or *bindegewebsmassage*, that stimulates the tissue between skin and muscle in order to relieve pain and promote mental, emotional, and physical well-being. Developed by a German physiotherapist, Elizabeth Dicke, it posits a powerful association between particular areas of connective tissue and specific paths of the nervous system and internal organs. Following Dicke's teachings, Connective Tissue Therapy plots treatment so as to activate relays between areas of tissue and different parts of the body. Connective Tissue Therapy can help restore balance to the neuromuscular and organ systems after illness and has a relaxing effect beneficial to self-healing and health maintenance.

Discovering *Bindegewebsmassage*

Dicke discovered the basic principle of Connective Tissue Therapy in 1929, when she was incapacitated by toxemia of the right leg so severe that doctors recommended amputation. While touching an area of her lower back, she came across abnormally thick, tense layers of tissue and realized she felt sensations of warmth and tingling in her infected leg whenever she stroked the area of abnormal tissue in a pulling manner. Though recovery required three months and the help of a physiotherapist who followed Dicke's specific instructions, the transmission of energy from the lower back became the means by which Dicke saved her leg.

After she resumed activity as a physiotherapist, Dicke began to explore the ramifications of her discovery. She noticed, for example, correspondences between malfunction in various organs and changes in tension on specific areas of the body's surface, named "Head zones" after Henry Head, the nineteenth-century English neurologist who first studied them. According to Head, the nerves, organs, and their correlated "Head zones" of skin are rooted in the same segment of the spinal cord. Dicke built on Head's work, using the "zones" as a guide for locating pathways of connective tissue that could be manipulated to improve organ function.

By 1938 Dicke had formulated the system of bodywork she called *bindegewebsmassage*, literally connective tissue massage, and started to search out ways to introduce it to the medical community and the general public. She collaborated with a number of scientists in publishing the material in article and book form and became active as a teacher.

The Theory of Connective Tissue Therapy℠

Connective Tissue Therapy concentrates upon the subcutaneous sheaths of tissue, known as fascia, that are found throughout the body surrounding, supporting, and connecting the nerves, blood vessels, muscles, and organs. While distinct from muscles, fascia is an important determinant of strength and range of motion and in a healthy person is usually robust and

The Popularity of Connective Tissue Therapy™

The Elizabeth Dicke Society was founded in 1954 to preserve and expand her legacy. Bindegewebsmassage is a widely accepted physical therapy in Germany and in many countries it is regarded as a medical treatment for organ and circulatory disease. In the United States Connective Tissue Therapy remains less well known than many other types of bodywork, but it is taught at various massage schools, and the technique is part of the repertory of many massage therapists.

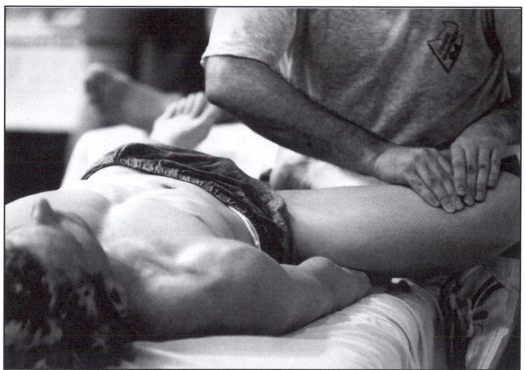

Connective Tissue Therapy^{SM} being given to a swimmer.

flexible. Conversely, tension in the fascia, evident in a thickening of tissue and loss of ease in movement, is a sign of dysfunction caused by disease or by an imbalance likely to cause disease if it is not corrected.

Through massage, Connective Tissue Therapy attempts to restore suppleness and vitality to fascia that has tightened and become numbed or painful. It is postulated that the massage is effective because it activates the parasympathetic nervous system, which controls relaxation as well as pain relief and healing in the vital organs and all other parts of the body.

Experiencing Connective Tissue Therapy^{SM}

Length and frequency of sessions in Connective Tissue Therapy vary according to the needs of the receiver. Since the benefits increase with each additional session, a series of ten to twenty sessions may be recommended for a receiver with a severe problem or one interested in learning about the body's potential for health. During treatment,

done without oils or lotions, the receiver sits on a chair or lies flat. The treatment starts at the pelvic area, then proceeds over the body, using a technique in which the therapist hooks his or her fingers into the skin and upper layer of fascia while performing a pulling stroke. The strokes cause temporary marks on the skin and sensations ranging from dull to sharp. As the treatment continues the receiver may experience a desire to sleep, excessive perspiration, deepened breathing, or a drop in body temperature. Benefits from the session may last for months following a series of treatments.

The Benefits of Connective Tissue Therapy^{SM}

Connective Tissue Therapy brings about a relaxation of the fascia that is particularly helpful in restoring function and range of motion and in stimulating bone and muscle repair of damage suffered from injuries, arthritis, and other degenerative disorders. It has a tonic effect upon the circulatory and nervous systems that can aid the elimination of toxins; the healing of wounds in a way that prevents the formation of scar tissue; promote recovery from kidney and other organ malfunction; and lessen stress and anxiety. It can also be an effective adjunct to other forms of treatment.

—*Jackie Hand*

Resources:

Theresa Lamb (CTT^{SM})
2140 Lower Smith Gap Rd.
Kunkletown, PA 18058
Tel: (610) 826-5957
Provides training in CTT^{SM}.

Wholistic Pathway
152 North Wellwood Avenue, Suite 5
Lindenurst, NY 11757
Tel: (516) 226-3898
Offers training in bindegewebsmassage.

Further Reading:

Dicke, Elizabeth, et al. *A Manual of Reflexive Therapy of the Connective Tissue (Connective Tissue Massage) 'Bindegewebsmassage'.* Scarsdale, NY: Sidney S. Simon, 1978.

Ebner, Maria. *Connective Tissue Massage: Theory and Therapeutic Application.* Huntington, NY: Robert E. Krieger Publishing Co., 1980.

Tappan, Frances. *Healing Massage Techniques: Holistic, Classic, and Emerging Techniques.* Norwalk, CT: Appleton & Lang, 1988.

CORE STRUCTURAL INTEGRATIVE THERAPY

CORE structural integrative therapy is a system of bodywork that seeks to improve the structure and function of the musculoskeletal system and connective tissues of the human body.

CORE practitioners utilize client-assisted movement while applying massage techniques, which brings heightened awareness of the body and allows the client to participate in releasing tension and pain. This system was originated by George P. Kousaleos, founder of the CORE Institute School of Massage Therapy and Structural Bodywork.

A typical session of CORE structural integrative therapy includes an analysis of the client's structural alignment and movement patterns, the application of full-body or regional bodywork techniques that stretch and tone the body's myofascial network, and instruction of corrective and postural exercises. CORE bodywork techniques vary from moderate to deep pressure, and sessions can be organized for specific ailments or for general benefit.

CORE structural integrative therapy usually involves ten sessions of bodywork, but also includes introductory and maintenance sessions that support a lifelong system of improved alignment and optimal performance. The CORE system includes CORE myofascial therapy, a full-body session that introduces the client to the concepts and benefits of structural alignment; CORE extrinsic therapy, a three-session series that aligns the superficial musculature, which allows for greater freedom of movement; CORE intrinsic therapy, a four-session series that aligns the deepest musculature, which supports the pelvis, spine, and cranium; and CORE integration therapy, the final three-session series, which provides integrated movement patterns throughout the body.

A person will experience the physical benefits of CORE structural integrative therapy immediately. Clients may feel a lighter, longer, and looser relationship of muscles and joints. Some people who receive CORE therapy often perceive that they are using less energy to produce all physical activities, and that they sleep and rest at a deeper level. Some clients will also experience a release of emotional memories and trauma, often resulting in a greater sense of self-reliance.

While CORE structural integrative therapy can be beneficial for every age group and activity level, the positive aspects are greater for those who are actively engaged in rigorous physical or mental endeavors. Many clients report immediate improvement in their physical and psychological stress levels, resulting in a higher state of clarity and focus. From 1994 to 1996 CORE practitioners have worked with British Olympic athletes who were in training for the 1996 Atlanta Olympics. It is estimated that more than 300 Olympic athletes and coaches have received CORE techniques.

—*George Kousaleos and Gary Genna*

Resources:

The CORE Institute
223 West Carolina Street
Tallahassee, FL 32308
Tel: (904) 222-8673
Fax: (904) 561-6160
Offers training for CORE practitioners. All CORE practitioners have been trained though the faculty of the CORE Institute and are nationally certified in therapeutic massage and bodywork. Training in CORE structural integrative therapy is offered throughout North America.

INFANT MASSAGE

Infant massage is an ancient tradition in many cultures throughout the world. Since the 1970s this art has been enjoying a renaissance in the West. Traditional infant massage strokes, like those practiced in India, are used in the United States as a way for parents and other caregivers to communicate their love, caring, and respect for their babies and children. Studies seem to indicate that the positive effects of practicing infant massage are just as profound on the parent's physical, mental, and emotional well-being as they are on the child's.

The History of Infant Massage

Vimala McClure was one of the first individuals to bring the practice of massaging babies to the United States. While living in India in the early seventies, McClure observed the beneficial effects of daily massage on infants. She returned to the United States and put together a curriculum for parent-infant classes. McClure wrote a book on the subject, *Infant Massage: A Handbook for Loving Parents*, developed an instructor training program, and in 1981 founded the International Association for Infant Massage (IAIM). The purpose of IAIM is to integrate the art of infant massage into the parenting traditions of Western cultures. IAIM offers courses for parents and other caregivers and, according to its mission statement, works to "promote nurturing touch and communication through training, education, and research so that parents, caregivers, and children are loved, valued, and respected throughout the world community." There are presently more than 1,500 active certified infant massage instructors (CIMI) throughout the world.

How Infant Massage Works

Infant massage includes the critical elements of bonding: eye-to-eye and skin-to-skin contact, smiling, soothing sounds, cuddling, and sound and smell reciprocity. "Touch communication" provides a common language for parent/child communication. Babies communicate through many types of nonverbal cues such as rubbing their eyes when tired, sucking their hands when hungry, smiling when happy, crying when hungry, wet, or in need of attention. By learning to read the nonverbal cues that babies use to express a full range of emotions in response to the massage, caregivers develop a tangible

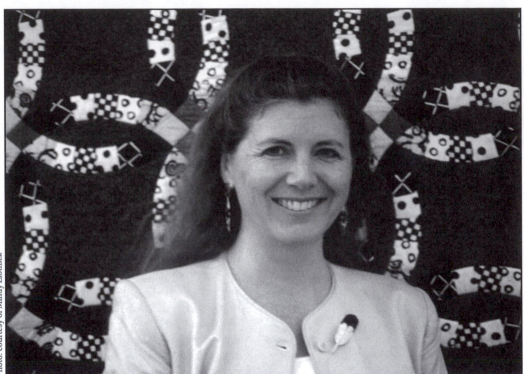

Photo: courtesy of Mindy Zlotnick

Vimala McClure brought infant massage techniques from India to the United States.

sense of their own powers to help soothe, comfort, and nurture their babies.

Renowned British anthropologist Ashley Montague points out in his book *Touching* that all mammals except human beings lick their young. This licking process serves to stimulate the physiological systems and aids in the bonding process. Montague postulates that the massage tradition, found in most countries of the world, is the human equivalent of mammals licking their young for health and well-being.

Clinical evidence shows that loving, touching, and nurturing contact between caregiver and infant has a positive impact on subsequent physical, mental, and emotional development of the child. Many studies suggest the benefits of positive, interactive contact as an integral part of early life. They also suggest that a lack of early interactive touch can have a negative impact on a child's development.

Research on the Positive Effects of Infant Massage

Research conducted over the years in regard to human touch has indicated that it is particularly beneficial for vulnerable babies. One landmark study by F. A. Scafidi shows that premature babies who were massaged daily developed more rapidly both physically, with greater weight gain, and neurologically. In 1987 researcher K. J. Ottenbacker analyzed nineteen separate infant stimulation studies and found that 72 percent of the infants receiving some form of tactile stimulation were positively affected. Most of the investigators of the nineteen separate studies reported greater weight gain and better outcomes on developmental assessments compared to those infants who did not receive as much stimulation.

Studies conducted at the Touch Research Institute (TRI) at the University of Miami Medical Center since its inception in 1992 affirm the effectiveness of

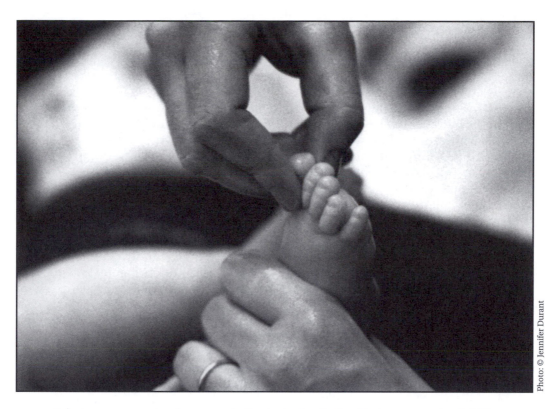

Infant massage uses touch communication to develop the bond between parent and child.

the techniques outlined in Vimala McClure's book. TRI studies have shown that massage improves cardiac and respiratory output, promotes longer and deeper sleeping patterns, and develops immunological factors. In one TRI study conducted by researcher Tiffany Field, babies of depressed adolescent mothers were massaged by their mothers. These babies fell asleep faster and became more vocal, mother-baby interactions improved, and the mothers perceived that the babies were easier to soothe. Field has also identified other positive effects that providing massage can have on the caregiver, including improved mood and a reduction in anxiety. In addition, their stress levels decreased and they reported improved self-esteem.

Infant Massage Classes
Certified infant massage instructors (CIMI) conduct parent education classes in a variety of settings, usually in small groups to facilitate communication and support among the caregivers in the group. Instructors teach a series of classes over a four- to five-week period. It usually takes about a month for a healthy baby to learn to accept a full-body massage.

Parents are encouraged to massage their baby on a regular basis, every day if possible. Since the premise of the work is that parents are teachers of relaxation, parents are also encouraged to set up relaxed environments for themselves, so that they can pass on this sense of relaxation to their babies. Infant massage's precepts also encourage self-care for parents as a means of caring for one's child.

Practicing Infant Massage
An important tenet of the massage is learning to show respect for the baby. It is very important that caregivers learn to use tactile, auditory, and visual cues to ask the baby's permission to massage.

This can be done by rubbing small circles around the hairline, holding their baby's hands together, or placing the baby's hands on his or her chest and then waiting for a response from the baby. Learning to understand and respect the baby's answer, which is given with the same kinds of nonverbal cues, is part of learning to communicate through appropriate touch. By asking permission in this way, parents also teach their children to discern touch that is loving and appropriate. Asking permission is also a way of demonstrating respect for the baby. By giving the baby respect, the caregiver helps the baby develop self-respect.

Babies are massaged without clothes, using edible oils that are absorbed by the skin, such as sunflower or almond oil, so that the baby will not be harmed if he or she swallows any oil. A massage lasts as long as the baby gives permission and the caregiver is available. This can be as short as two minutes or as long as an hour. Most massages are twenty to twenty-five minutes long.

Massaging a baby is a tactile expression of love and security. Experience and clinical research show that babies enjoy and benefit from firm, confident touch as opposed to light, feathery touch. Babies typically move, kick, and talk throughout the massage. They are not quiet recipients like adults. Parents are encouraged to actively listen to their babies' responses to the touch of the massage. This type of interaction teaches parents to talk with their hands and listen with their hearts.

Massage is a dance between the parent and baby. The techniques taught in classes or learned from a book or video are the basic choreography. Once a parent is comfortable with the massage, improvisation begins. Parents use the same strokes that generations of parents all over the world have used, yet each parent and child develop a "duet" that is their own unique expression of love.

The Benefits of Infant Massage

The practice of infant massage enhances the parent-baby bond, helping create loving and respectful relationships among family members. The massage time offers parents an opportunity to explore and develop their responses to the baby's sounds, movements, and facial expressions. Babies are taught that they are aware human beings who deserve respect, tenderness, warmth, and above all, a listening heart. This type of interaction serves as a model for the child as he or she grows and for the parent as well, encouraging them to develop respectful, loving relationships with an ever-widening circle of people.

—Mindy Zlotnick

Resources:

IAIM (International Association of Infant Massage)
1720 Willow Creek Circle Suite #516
Eugene, OR 97402
Toll-free: (800) 248-5432
Fax: (541) 485-7372
e-mail: iaimus@aol.com
Organization that trains and certifies instructors.

IAIM trains and certifies individuals to teach parents and caregivers to massage their babies. Many CIMIs are branching out to work with special-needs populations, such as physically challenged infants, infants who are drug-exposed or HIV-positive, medically fragile infants, as well as teen moms, incarcerated moms, homeless families, and women recovering from drug and alcohol addiction.

Further Reading:

Books:

Kennel, J., and M. Klaus. *Parent-Infant Bonding*, 2nd edition. St. Louis: CV Mosby, 1982.

McClure, Vimala. *Infant Massage: A Handbook for Loving Parents*. New York: Bantam Books, 1989.

Montague, Ashley. *Touching*. New York: Harper and Row, 1978.

Journals:

Field, Tiffany. "The Benefits of Infant Massage on Growth and Development." *Pediatric Basics*, Volume 71, 1996.

Ottenbacher, K. J., et al. "The Effectiveness of Tactile Stimulation as an Early Intervention: A Quantitative Evaluation." *Journal of Developmental Behavioral Pediatrics*, 8: 68–76, 1987.

Scafidi, F. A., T. Field, and S. M. Schanberg, et al. "Effects of Kinesthetic Stimulation on the Clinical Course and the Sleep/Wake Behaviors of Pre-term Neonates." *Infant Behavior and Development*, 1986: 9:91–105.

Scafidi, F .A., et al. "Massage Stimulates Growth in Preterm Infants, a Replication." *Infant Behavior and Development*, 1990 13:167–68.

MUSCULAR THERAPY

Muscular therapy, also referred to as the Benjamin system of muscular therapy, consists of a series of techniques and exercises designed to promote physical health and reduce muscular tension and stress caused by physical injury. It is also an educational process in which the client learns to understand the cause of his or her physical symptoms and what needs to be done to alleviate them.

Muscular therapy was developed by Dr. Ben Benjamin from a synthesis of several approaches to working with the body. Dr. Benjamin's interest in the field began in 1958, when he sustained a serious injury.

After several frustrating failed attempts to obtain relief, his injury was successfully treated by Alfred Kagan, a well-known French practitioner who had developed original techniques for the treatment of muscular tension and injury. During the course of his treatment, Dr. Benjamin became interested in Kagan's method and studied with him after his recovery. He observed and analyzed Kagan's complex technique. From his observation Dr. Benjamin created a series of more than 700 discrete muscular manipulations.

Following his work with Kagan, Dr. Benjamin spent several years studying the origins of physical tension and learning ways that people could care for themselves without requiring continual treatment from a physician or therapist. He became particularly interested in the work of Dr. Wilhelm Reich, F. M. Alexander, and Dr. James Cyriax and sought ways of incorporating some of their ideas into his approach to tension reduction. In Reich's work, Benjamin learned of the emotional component of muscular tension. Dr. Benjamin realized that this understanding of the physical manifestation of emotional distress could help the practitioner distinguish between emotional distress in the body and mechanical or injury-related tension. In his study of the Alexander technique, Dr. Benjamin discovered a method for establishing proper movement habits. He felt that by using these techniques, practitioners could learn to use their bodies more effectively and avoid movement habits that cause pain, tension, and injury. The third influence was the injury evaluation and deep friction treatment developed by Dr. Cyriax.

These three approaches combined with Benjamin's original treatment techniques provide a comprehensive understanding of the nature and treatment of physical tension. They enable the practitioner to determine if an injury has been caused primarily by overuse, an alignment problem, or by emotional stress. Using these techniques, Benjamin was able to distinguish between a serious injury, which requires a physician's attention, and one that is relatively minor and could be safely handled with muscular therapy techniques. Benjamin's techniques are not designed to treat muscular tension caused by emotional stress.

A therapist works with the client by performing deep massage, including a variety of area-specific strokes, pressure, and rhythms to reduce chronic tension and pain. In a typical session, therapists may educate clients about the causes and effects of tension. Clients learn techniques designed to prevent the buildup of new tension. These may include basic exercises for warming up, stretching, and building strength.

—Ben Benjamin, Ph.D., and
Mary Ann di Roberts

Resources:

Muscular Therapy Institute
122 Rindge Avenue
Cambridge, MA 02140
Tel: (617) 576-1300
The Muscular Therapy Institute offers a two-year training program in massage therapy that emphasizes physical technique, clear professional boundaries, and good communication skills.

Further Reading:

Benjamin, Ben E. *Are You Tense? The Benjamin System of Muscular Therapy.* New York: Pantheon, 1978.

———. *Exercise Without Injury.* New York: Summit Books, 1979.

———.*Listen to Your Pain: The Active Person's Guide to Understanding, Identifying and Treating Pain and Injury.* New York: Viking/Penguin, 1984.

MYOFASCIAL RELEASE

Myofascial release is a gentle, hands-on form of therapy that involves applying an extremely mild and gentle form of pressure to the body in order to relieve tension in the soft connective tissue called fascia. Myofascial release is the release of the connective tissue, or fascia. The therapist applies a stretching technique to the body that exerts a small amount of pressure to the fascia. Myofascial release experts have shown that fascia will soften and begin to release tension when the pressure is sustained over time. It is used to relieve chronic pain, especially in areas such as the neck, jaw, and back. With the release of physical pain, patients report that there is often a release of emotions that were formerly buried deep in the subconscious. Myofascial release uncovers "secrets" stored in the body.

How Myofascial Release Developed

Myofascial release was developed by John F. Barnes, PT. Barnes graduated from the University of Pennsylvania in 1960 with a degree in physical therapy. He started his own practice in 1966.

Barnes's first experience with what we now know as myofascial release began when he was seventeen. He accidentally injured his back while lifting weights. He initially ignored the pain of this injury but eventually, in his own work as a therapist, came to the realization that he was in worse shape than most of his patients. The pain grew so bad that, from age twenty-five to thirty, he could not sit for more than two to three minutes at a time. Finally, Barnes went to see a neurologist and an orthopedist, who diagnosed him with a crushed disc. They removed the disc, which took the intensity out of his pain and allowed him to function. However, he still had problems with his back, and through his frustration in trying to help himself before and after his surgery, he developed techniques that relieved the symptoms. This injury also gave Barnes an understanding of what it is really like to be "trapped" in pain.

Barnes began trying these techniques on his patients. Despite the fact he did not know why these techniques worked, he noticed that patients were responding consistently. While attending a course about the connective tissue system, he realized that his therapy dealt directly with the body's fascia. The soft tissue mobilization techniques he learned at this course were basically an old form of myofascial release. He used these techniques to control his own pain, but because of the difficulty moving, he tended to hold each position for an extended period. This extended time factor turned out to be what was so important in releasing the total myofascial complex. Older forms of myofascial release were too superficial to give complete release.

The Theory of Myofascial Release

Fascia extends from the head of the body to the feet. In a normal, healthy state, the fascia is relaxed and wavy in configuration. It has the ability to stretch and move without restriction. When we experience physical trauma, such as inflammation, a fall, whiplash, surgery, or even just habitual poor posture over time, the fascia loses its flexibility. It becomes tight, restricted, and a source of tension to the rest of the body. The changes these traumas cause in the fascial system influence the skeletal framework for our posture, and the fascia can exert excessive pressure, producing pain, headaches, or restricted motion.

Because fascia permeates all regions of the body and is all interconnected, when it scars and hardens in one area following a trauma, it can put tension on adjacent pain-sensitive structures as well as on structures in far-away areas. Thus a restriction in one region can theoretically put a "drag" on the fascia in any other direction. Because all muscle is enveloped by and ingrained with fascia, *myofascial release* is the term that has been given to the techniques that are used to relieve soft tissue from the abnormal grip of tight fascia.

Fascia is made up of a fibrous, soft, gel-like substance, which can be softened when released. Myofascial release allows therapists to become sculptors with their fingers, hands, and elbows. By steadily releasing the fascia, they can remold the body back into a more healthful, functional, and comfortable position. This is because the pressure stretches the connective tissue, and removes the tightness that causes the pain.

Experiencing Myofascial Release

A myofascial release session usually lasts thirty to ninety minutes. The client undresses down to his or her underwear and lies on a massage table. Unlike massage, no oil is used. The therapist uses his or her fingers, palms, elbows, and forearms to warm and stretch the fascia. The pressure is gentle but firm and is used for at least 90 to 120 seconds with each therapeutic stroke. When an individual first begins this form of treatment, therapists recommend the patient have several sessions a week. As his or her condition gradually progresses, the patient begins to need less treatment.

The Benefits of Myofascial Release

Barnes has seen consistent, positive results using myofascial release to treat acute pain, chronic pain, fibromyalgia, headaches, scoliosis, chronic fatigue syndrome, birth injuries, cerebral palsy, geriatric problems, pediatric problems, and movement dysfunction.

Myofascial release experts say that this form of therapy works especially well for individuals seeking long-term relief for chronic pain and immobility that are caused by extreme tightness of the muscles. Common areas of treatment in the body include the neck, jaw, and back. Myofascial release can also reduce muscle tension and treat recurring injuries and other stress-related problems.

—Tara Welch for Myofascial Release Treatment Centers and Seminars

Resources:

MFR Treatment Centers and Seminars
Routes 30 and 252
10 South Leopard Road, Suite 1
Paoli, PA 19301
Tel: (610) 644-0136 or (800) FASCIAL
Web site: www.vll.com/mfr
Provides information on MFR, organizes seminars and training programs, offers treatment programs, and refers patients to qualified practitioners.

Further Reading:

John F. Barnes, PT. *Myofascial Release: The Search for Excellence, a Comprehensive Evaluatory and Treatment Approach.* Paoli, PA: Rehabilitation Services Inc. T/A, Myofascial Release Seminars, 1990.

MYOFASCIAL TRIGGER POINT THERAPY

Myofascial trigger point therapy (MTPT) is a physical, therapeutic discipline for treating myofascial, or muscular and connective tissue pain in muscles and joints by focusing on trigger points, which are defined as sensitive areas in the muscle that are very tender to the touch. MTPT therapists apply pressure, among other techniques, to trigger points in order to release these areas of constriction and pain. It is intended to provide the client with a greater awareness of his or her body, and to release stress and tension.

The History of MTPT

While many people contributed to the development and spread of MTPT, the person most responsible for its birth was Dr. Janet Travell. Born in New York City in 1901, Dr. Travell began practicing medicine in 1926. Her concentration was in the areas of internal medicine, cardiovascular disease, neurology, pharmacology, and musculoskeletal pain. In 1961 she was appointed physician to the president of the United States, serving both presidents John F. Kennedy and Lyndon B. Johnson. Her major interest over the last forty years was the mechanism and management of chronic pain syndromes, especially those related to myofascial trigger points.

She initially reported on the phenomenon of trigger points in 1942, determining that these points of tenderness could limit a person's range of motion and produce pain in other parts of the body. She also noted that sustained pressure applied directly to trigger points could be an efficient treatment technique. Over the next forty-seven years, Dr. Travell continued her research and mapped out the locations of common trigger points, their pain patterns, and methods of treating them.

She coauthored the textbook *Myofascial Pain and Dysfunction: The Trigger Point Manual* with David Simons, M.D. It is considered the most comprehensive work available on the subject of myofascial pain. Dr. Travell died in 1997.

In 1979, Bonnie Prudden founded the Bonnie Prudden School for Physical Fitness and Myotherapy, based on the trigger point principles described by Dr. Travell. The school teaches the treatment of muscle pain through pressure applied to trigger points.

Defining Myofascial Trigger Point Therapy

MTPT is a noninvasive therapeutic program for the relief and control of myofascial pain and dysfunction. The goal of treatment is the client's recovery to a normal or as near normal function as possible with either complete recovery from or significant reduction in pain.

This is achieved through a systematized approach, which consists of ischemic compression (direct pressure) applied to trigger points, spray and stretch

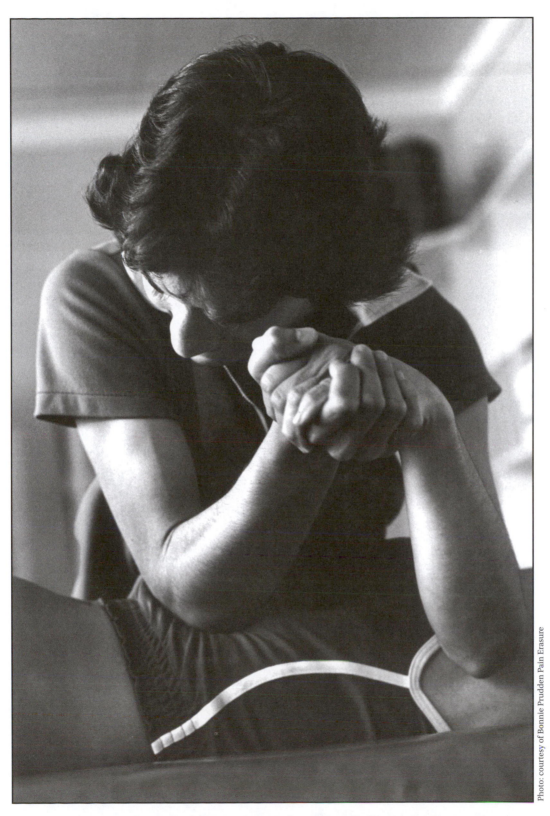

Photo: courtesy of Bonnie Prudden Pain Erasure

Using elbows, knuckles, or fingers, Lori Drummond, master certified Bonnie Prudden myother-
apist, releases a trigger point that causes pain in the lower back.

technique (spraying a vapocoolant along the muscle while simultaneously stretching it), passive stretch, and a specifically designed stretch and corrective exercise program. The exercise program requires the client to be very aware of his or her body to avoid future pain.

Factors that aggravate trigger points must be eliminated or modified to achieve lasting results. For example, if a client is having neck and shoulder pain, and his or her job involves working at a computer, the therapist will make suggestions for ways of doing the activity with less stress on the muscles. Clients' posture, sleep positions, daily activities, and nutrition may also be addressed.

Success of therapy is measured by the level of pain reduction experienced by the client and increased range of motion, strength, endurance, and other measures of improved function.

MTPT is part of an interdisciplinary approach to myofascial pain and dysfunction. Although myofascial trigger point therapists are knowledgeable in the areas of myofascial pain and dysfunction, they are not diagnosticians. They must, therefore, rely on medical clearance (prescription) and support by a licensed doctor of medicine, chiropractic, osteopathy, or dentist before beginning a treatment plan. This protects the client from delayed diagnosis, delayed treatment, or treatment that might conflict with some other aspect of the healing process.

Description of a MTPT Session

An MTPT session is usually an hour in length. At the initial visit a complete medical history is taken. Muscles are palpated or touched to determine the exact locations of trigger points. Range of motion, or how far the client can move a particular limb or joint, is also noted.

As patients are palpated for trigger points, they are also treated. Treatment consists of the application of sustained direct pressure to the trigger point and/or the use of spray and stretch technique.

The muscle is then passively stretched. Moist heat may be applied to the muscle to further induce relaxation. The patient is given exercises, usually in the form of stretching, in order to maintain the effects of therapy and retrain the muscle to function at its normal resting length. Perpetuating factors may also be discussed at this time, such as eliminating or modifying certain activities that may aggravate the muscles, alternate sleeping positions, correct posture, etc. Progress is checked by monitoring the client's pain levels and periodic evaluations of range of motion.

The Benefits and Risks

The benefits of MTPT are as follows: the decrease or elimination of pain; increased movement and flexibility; increased energy and activity level. Common problems that are helped by therapy are lower back, neck, shoulder, face, arm, hand, knee, leg, and foot pain; temporal mandibular joint disorder (TMJD); sciatica; carpal tunnel syndrome; whiplash; fibromyalgia; tennis elbow; plantar fasciitis; and headaches.

People with any of the following conditions should not engage in myofascial trigger point therapy: systemic or localized infection; acute ciculatory condition; aneurysm; obstructive edema; acute healing fracture; advanced diabetes; and hypersensitivity of the skin.

—*Elliot Shratter*

Resources:

Academy of Myofascial Trigger Point Therapy
Richard Finn, Director
1312 East Carson St.
Pittsburgh, PA 15203
Tel: (412) 481-2553
Offers training in myofascial trigger point therapy leading to national certification.

National Association of Myofascial Trigger Point Therapists
Web site: www.frontiernet/painrel/index.shtml

Further Reading:

Travell, Janet, and David Simons. *Myofascial Pain and Dysfunction: The Trigger Point Manual.* Volumes I and II. New York: William & Wilkins Co., 1992.

Reflexology

Reflexology is both an ancient and modern "hands-on" therapeutic technique that activates and facilitates the natural healing powers of the body. This is accomplished by applying noninvasive, penetrating pressure to specific reflex points and areas on the feet, hands, and ears. In most instances this pressure work is focused on the feet because of the accessibility and larger size of the reflex points, the sensitivity of the feet, and their physical and energetic connection with the earth. Reflexology has been found to be most effective in stimulating and balancing the energy flow to specific organs, glands, and other physiological systems of the body that correspond to these reflex points, so that the body can utilize this energy to begin healing, or to maintain optimal function.

History of Reflexology

Reflexology was practiced in many ancient cultures, including Asian, Chinese, Egyptian, Greek, Japanese, and Native North American. The rediscovery and promotion of this technique in the West is attributed largely to Eunice Ingham, an American masseuse, who formulated her own unique "pressure technique" for the feet after many years of working with patients with various complaints and illnesses. She synthesized different popular theories with her own personal explorations and experiences to create what is recognized as modern reflexology.

Basic Principles of Reflexology

Reflexology works through the nervous system, the circulatory system, and through correspondences of subtle energy currents. As in Fitsgerald's principles of zone therapy, the body is divided into ten vertical zones that run the entire length of the body from head to foot. The ten zones on the feet (five on each foot) contain the reflex points that are worked in a session. The theory is that the whole body is superimposed upon a zone grid on the feet (also hands and ears). Therapeutically working a reflex point on the foot will result in the stimulation of all the body parts relating to that zone. In this way a practitioner can release blocked energy in any part of the body by applying systematic pressure to the corresponding reflex point on the feet.

Like acupuncture, reflexology is still not completely understood. The feet are extremely sensitive, with more than 7,200 nerves, and no doubt the stimulation of these nerve endings partially accounts for the beneficial results. However, there are also less easily discernible energy currents and relationships in the body that also contribute to the healing power of this technique. In addition, the skill of the practitioner, enhanced by his or her personal sensitivity, awareness, empathy, intention, and integrity, contributes to the effectiveness of reflexology.

Reflexology in Practice

How a client experiences a session depends upon the style or method of reflexology being employed as well as the quality of resonance between the practitioner and client. Depending upon the style of the practitioner, some clients may share thoughts and feelings, what is referred to as "verbally unwinding," as the practitioner applies pressure to the reflex points. Others may maintain an interior focus, as in a meditative state, while others may relax into a deep, restful sleep. It is important for the client to be in communication with the practitioner with regard to the

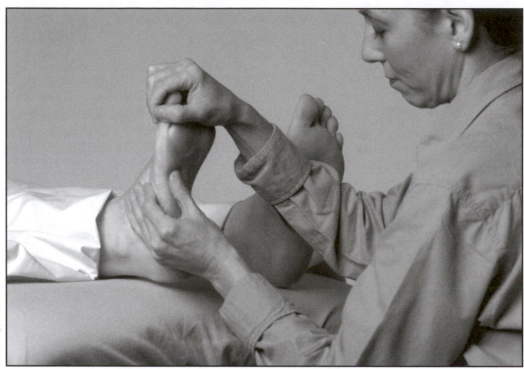

Photo: © Joel Gordon

A reflexologist treats all parts of the body by massaging the feet.

degree of pressure being applied, which could be described as a "good hurt," but which still allows the client to feel relaxed. Many people express feelings and sensations of tingling, warmth, expansiveness, electrical currents, pleasant numbness in certain areas, and overall euphoria. The effects of reflexology are cumulative, producing subtle, long-term results, although dramatic and immediate results are also quite common.

Benefits and Risks

As with any type of therapeutic bodywork, personal health habits, genetic factors, emotional and mental attitudes, and amount of physical activity all play a part in one's personal health. Reflexology is not recommended for those suffering from the following conditions: hemorrhaging; intense pain of an unknown origin; any break in the skin; severe swelling characterized by red-hot pain with loss of motion; contagious or infectious disease of the foot (such as ulcerations); burns; chronic inflammations; neoplasms/tumors; varicose veins; severe sprain of the ankle or foot; severe bruises; hematomas; and in some instances, recent surgery. When the foot is too painful to work, the corresponding points on the hand can be worked instead.

Reflexology reduces and alleviates the debilitating effects of stress, the prime cause of many ailments. It provides a natural way of promoting balance within and between all the systems of the body by affecting all the organs, glands, and body parts. Added benefits include a deep feeling of groundedness. It also assists in detoxification by breaking up crystallized deposits of uric acid that lodge in the feet. It contributes to relief from nervous disorders, intestinal disorders, poor circulation, digestive problems, glandular disorders, headaches, fatigue, post-menstrual syndrome, back spasms, infertility disorders, sinusitis, eye problems, emotional shock and grief, and a great variety of sports injuries. In extreme chronic conditions, it is best used in conjunction with other therapies and under the supervision or awareness of a medical doctor.

—*Laura Norman*

Resources:

American Reflexology Certification Board (ARCB)
P.O. Box 620607
Littleton, CO 80162
Tel: (303) 933-6921
Web site: www.ns.net/quantum/arcb
Offers information regarding certification requirements and testing, and provides certification for qualified practitioners.

Laura Norman & Associates
Reflexology Center
41 Park Avenue, Suite 8A
New York, NY 10016
Tel: (212) 532-4404
Offers services and certification training in reflexology.

Reflexology Association of America
4012 S. Rainbow Blvd.
Las Vegas, NV 89103-2059
Provides information about educational programs and recommends certified practitioners.

Further Reading:

Grinberg, Avi. *Holistic Reflexology.* London: Thorsons Publishing, 1989.

Ingham, Eunice. *The Original Works of Eunice P. Ingham: Stories the Feet Can Tell Through Reflexology: Stories the Feet Have Told Through Reflexology.* With revisions by Dwight C. Byars. St. Petersburg, FL: Ingham Publishing, Inc., 1984.

Kunz, Kevin, and Barbara Kunz. *The Practitioner's Guide to Reflexology.* Englewood Cliffs, NJ: Prentice-Hall, Inc., 1985.

——. *Hand Reflexology Workbook.* Englewood Cliffs, NJ: Prentice-Hall, Inc., 1985.

Norman, Laura. *Feet First: A Guide to Foot Reflexology.* New York: Simon & Schuster, 1988.

ROLFING®

Rolfing® is an original methodology of structural integration of the body through the use of fascial (also known as connective tissue) massage. Structural integration is a holistic approach that seeks to align a person's body in order to improve physiological and psychological functioning. It starts with the body's relationship to gravity; in fact, one of its primary objectives is to reeducate the body to move more efficiently and without tension and pain.

The Development of Rolfing®
Rolfing was developed by Dr. Ida P. Rolf, an American biochemist who studied the flexibility of proteins in connective

---

Reflexology

Reflexology has been found to be most effective in stimulating and balancing energy flow to specific organs, glands, and other physiological systems of the body that correspond to these reflex points, so that the body can utilize this energy to begin healing, or to maintain optimal function. Clients are fully clothed during sessions with only their feet exposed, and are usually most comfortable reclining on a padded bodywork table or bed. The practitioner applies pressure to the feet in a systematic fashion to induce deep relaxation (one of the hallmarks of reflexology), which facilitates the flow of energy.

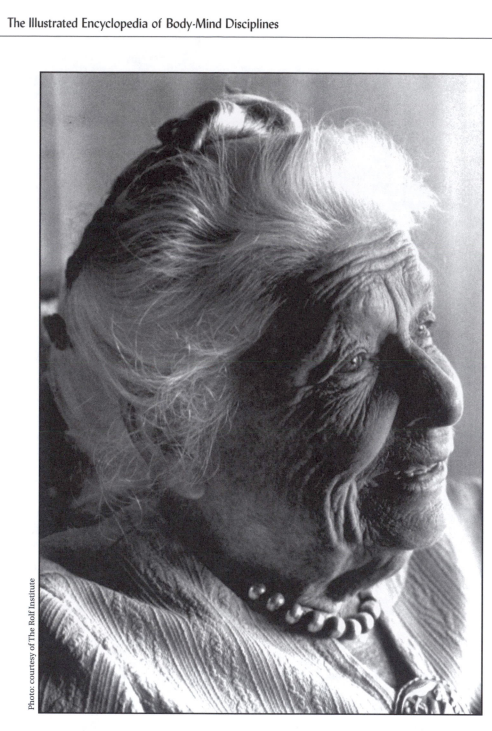

Photo: courtesy of The Rolf Institute

Dr. Ida P. Rolf, developer of Rolfing, a seminal method of connective tissue massage.

tissue in the 1930s and 1940s. Dr. Rolf was a young research biochemist at the Rockefeller Institute in New York City studying connective tissue (a network of tissue beneath the skin that links other tissues and forms ligaments, tendons, and aponeuroses), particularly its plasticity, or capacity for being molded or altered.

Along with other researchers, Dr. Rolf discovered that connective tissue is the organ of structure of the human body and that its shape, elasticity, even its length, can be altered with the application of appropriate pressure. She spent the next fifty or so years traveling widely—studying and eventually teaching a systematic way to go about organizing human structure. She called her method structural integration, and eventually, in the late 1960s, it became more widely known as Rolfing.

Basic Principles of Rolfing®

Rolfing is based on the following three ideas: First, the human body is affected by gravity, and when the body's major segments (head, shoulders, chest, pelvis, legs) are properly aligned, gravity works to uplift the body rather than pull it down.

Second, connective tissue, or the myofascial network of the body—a continuous bandage that ensheathes the whole body and all parts of the body, even individual muscle fibers—can be molded and changed.

Third, the key to aligning the body in gravity is systematically releasing the connective tissue network. This will allow the muscles to return to a balanced relationship with each other. It will also free the body of many chronic tensions and aches.

"When the body gets working appropriately," Ida Rolf said, "the force of gravity can flow through. Rolfers make a life study of relating bodies and their fields to the earth and its gravity field, and we organize the body so that the gravity field can reinforce the body's energy field. This is our primary concept."

When a body is properly aligned it can release the physical tensions and holding patterns resulting from years of compensation resulting in impaired balance and movement. It can also release the emotional stress that accompanies the physical symptoms.

After many years of searching, Dr. Rolf discovered that Rolfing works best in a ten-session format. The ten sessions are designed to slowly and methodically get the body—probably stuck from many years of poor compensation from accidents and injuries and from poor postural habits, along with a multitude of other possibilities—to lengthen, widen, deepen, or just let go.

Rolfing® in Practice

The first session of Rolfing begins after a thorough interview and structural analysis, usually using Polaroid pictures. Rolfers attempt to identify the main structural issue in a person's body, or the reason a person remains stuck and unable to find the ease or support he or she needs.

For example, in a person who has been slumping with the head forward for a number of years, the tissue of the upper chest has been responding by getting shorter; the muscles of the upper back (now assigned the task of holding the head on) have become more rigid. The person is unable to voluntarily get his or her head back over the shoulders where it belongs. The pelvis will very likely be tipped forward, unable to provide support for the shoulders and head. In turn the pelvis is probably not getting the support it needs from having the legs and feet under it. Rolfing examines the relationships between body parts—left and right, back and front, lower and upper, core and limb.

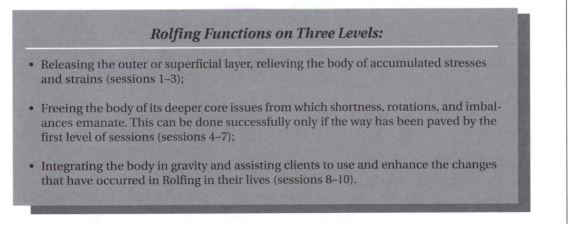

Rolfing Functions on Three Levels:

- Releasing the outer or superficial layer, relieving the body of accumulated stresses and strains (sessions 1–3);

- Freeing the body of its deeper core issues from which shortness, rotations, and imbalances emanate. This can be done successfully only if the way has been paved by the first level of sessions (sessions 4–7);

- Integrating the body in gravity and assisting clients to use and enhance the changes that have occurred in Rolfing in their lives (sessions 8–10).

During Rolfing sessions the client either lies on a low table, or occasionally, sits or stands. The Rolfer begins to release tension from the outer layers of the tissue with the application of pressure, using the fingers and hands as primary tools. The first session begins on the torso to release the outer wrapping (superficial fascia) and free up the breath. The work is done slowly and with the cooperation of the client, usually through specific feedback to help the Rolfer relax the fascial tissue. There is some pressure—the proper application of pressure is what makes the tissue release and change.

Although some clients find the degree of pressure painful, most clients find it acceptable, at times even pleasurable. Rolfers ask their clients to guide them and to participate in their process of harmonizing body parts. At various times, the client may be asked to stand and move about so that the results of the work can be felt and assessed by both the client and the Rolfer.

Sessions are cumulative and work progressively deeper into the body's structural issues. An important goal of Rolfing is not just to get the body to change, but to get the whole system to incorporate and use that change. Rolfing sessions generally last an hour and are usually spaced about a week apart

Benefits and Risks of Rolfing®

The primary objective of Rolfing is the release of the body's chronic and limiting holding patterns. After Rolfing sessions, people have reported freer movement and breathing, increased flexibility, release of chronic muscular tension and pain, psychological growth, and most important, continuous and progressive change.

Not everybody is an ideal candidate for Rolfing. Rolfing is designed to get at the underlying roots of chronic body issues or for people who want to feel and understand their bodies. In general, Rolfing deals with chronic rather than

acute problems. People seeking immediate pain relief would be better served by a wide range of body therapies that would better address these issues.

—*Allan Davidson*

Resources:

The Rolf Institute
205 Canyon Blvd.
Boulder, CO 80302
Tel: (800) 530-8875 or (303) 449-5903
Web site: www.rolfinst.com
Founded in 1971, the institute trains Rolfers and Rolfing movement integration teachers, conducts research, and provides information to the public.

Further Reading:

Anson, Briah. *Rolfing: Stories of Personal Empowerment*. Kansas City, MO: Heartland Personal Growth Press, 1991.

Fahey, Brian. *The Power of Balance: A Rolfing View of Health*. Portland, OR: Metamorphous Press, 1989.

Feitus, Rosemary, ed. *Ida Rolf Talks About Rolfing and Physical Reality*. Rochester, VT: Healing Arts Press, 1990.

Rolf, Ida. *Rolfing: Reestablishing the Natural Alignment*. Rochester, VT: Healing Arts Press, 1989.

Schultz, R. Louis, and Rosemary Feitus. *The Endless Web*. Berkeley, CA: North Atlantic Books, 1997.

ROSEN METHOD

The Rosen method is a form of therapeutic bodywork that uses gentle touch and supportive words to bring about a release of muscular and breathing constrictions, called "holdings," that limit our physical, emotional, and spiritual well-being. Developed by Marion Rosen, this method enables the mind and body to work together for optimal healing and growth, by facilitating awareness and integration of repressed emotional experiences that underlie and sustain physical holdings. The Rosen method is often used as an adjunct to psychotherapy and to physical therapy, for it is considered a preventative practice that enables people to alter their predispositions to psychological and physical illness.

Two Discoveries

Marion Rosen trained in Munich in the 1930s with Lucy Heyer, herself a student of Elsa Gindler, the "grandmother" of today's breathing and relaxation techniques. Rosen apprenticed with Heyer's group of therapists, giving breathwork instruction and massage to the psychoanalytic patients of Carl Jung. Rosen studied physical therapy further in Stockholm and at the Mayo Clinic in the United States. She became a physical therapist and has conducted a private practice in Oakland, California, since 1950. During this time she developed the Rosen method of bodywork and the Rosen method of movement.

Over several years, Rosen made two intriguing discoveries. The first was that some of her clients would improve, only to relapse, while other clients maintained their improvements. Rosen wondered: The body likes to feel well, but if the body feels better after treatments, why do the same problems recur?

Her second discovery was that when she worked with some clients, they began to tell her deeply emotional things that they had never before told to anyone. Why, Rosen wondered, were they telling me these things? She observed that those clients who talked with such openness were the clients who made lasting changes. The intriguing question became: What is the link between a client's spontaneous verbalizations and his or her physical healing? Perhaps, thought Rosen, there is some-

thing behind recurring dysfunction and chronic pain that is revealing itself via these spontaneous verbalizations.

Following this line of inquiry, Rosen thus discovered a route to lasting physical improvements that involves touching the body in such a way that the mind, via memories, images, and emotions, becomes an active participant in the body's healing.

The Importance of Self-Awareness

Current memory research supports that the sensory modalities (visual, emotional, kinesthetic, verbal, etc.) store information in different parts of the brain, forming interactive networks throughout the brain. Rosen believes that memories can be accessed by the restimulation of any of these senses. Rosen's touch stimulates the kinesthetic area to release memories, emotions, and associated images, also known as *body-memory*.

Body-memory includes emotional states because emotions are patterns of brief physiological responses whose function may be to move us to act. Every emotion has its own biological signature; for example, fear makes our sensory circuits more sensitive and activates our autonomic nervous system. Each emotional state has its own repertoire of physical reactions, thoughts, and memories.

We are mentally and physically equipped to suppress and override our emotions and their programs of action. This is called *inhibition* and takes place in the prefrontal cortex of our brain. The physical equivalent of this is muscular tightening.

Rosen method practitioners believe that from infancy on, when events give rise to feelings that are overwhelming, threatening, or unacceptable, we inhibit them neurologically and physiologically. These responses, becoming automatic, may assume a life of their own over time. We forget, or we have never consciously known, their original purposes and meanings, yet they live on in our bodies as muscular holding and affect our current physical and emotional well-being.

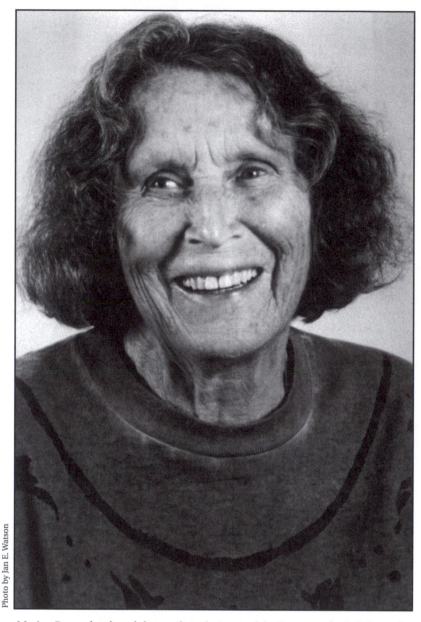

Photo by Jan E. Watson

Marion Rosen developed the gentle techniques of the Rosen method while work-ing with the patients of the Swiss psychologist Carl Jung.

We usually are not aware that we are restricting our muscles and our breath until these holdings create dysfunction and pain. When the body and the breath are chronically held, all of our emotions, whether they be happy or sad, are dimin-ished, leaving us with the experience of inner deadness or emptiness.

When a Rosen method practitioner attends to these muscular holdings, he or she believes that he or she is contacting the body's "barriers to self-awareness." As the practitioner's touch and verbal encouragement elicit memories from the body, information that had been uncon-scious moves into conscious awareness. This is of great importance, for now the traumatic memories—events, emotions—can be acknowledged and accepted.

Rosen method practitioners believe that as participants discover clues to the origin and meaning of their holdings,

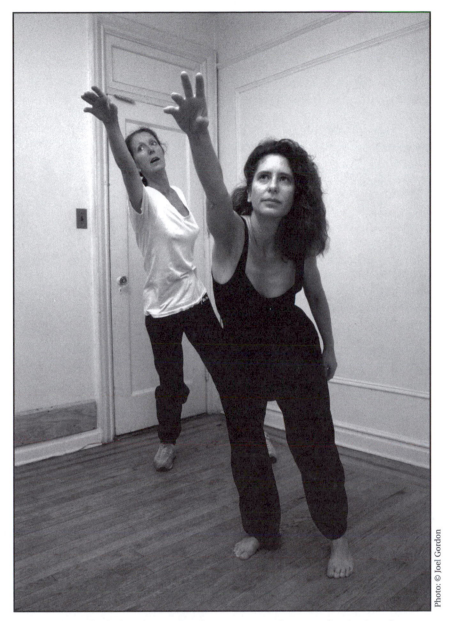

Photo: © Joel Gordon

The Rosen method of movement involves movement therapy style exercises that can be used in conjunction with the Rosen method of bodywork.

and as they experience their suppressed emotions, they come to a greater acceptance and appreciation of who they actually are. In finding these components of themselves that were forgotten, or never known, they gain a larger view of themselves in which living life more fully becomes possible.

Perhaps the greatest benefit of the Rosen method is its ability to bring people to the point of choosing different ways of expressing themselves and of being in the world: different ways of interacting, moving, looking, and feeling. The Rosen practitioner intends to be a midwife in the client's process of self-discovery. Rosen quotes Jesus from the Book of Thomas: "If you bring forth what is within you, what you bring forth will save you. If you do not bring forth what is in you, what you do not bring forth will destroy you."

The Power of Touch

A Rosen session is one hour. The participant lies on a massage table, removing as much outer clothing as he or she is comfortable with, always keeping on undergarments or wearing a swimsuit. Sessions are conducted with the client lying both face-up and face-down, so that the entire body can be contacted. No oils are used.

Practitioners, with gentle, noninvasive touch and supportive, encouraging words, direct the client's awareness to shifts in muscle tension and breathing patterns. The Rosen touch is an open, soft, listening hand, but with the quality of curiosity. A Rosen method practitioner asks through touch, "How is this person, really?" The practitioner's hands do not attempt to fix or change the client's body, for the intent is that the client experience what his or her body feels like, and what it is doing, in this moment. Through an open hand, the Rosen practitioner attempts to communicate acceptance, appreciation, and engagement. In this environment of safety and support, the participant's body seems to relax and open to healing itself.

A Rosen method practitioner focuses on a muscular tightness until it relaxes. It is a basic premise of the Rosen method that these shifts in the quality of the breath indicate and mirror changes in the quality of the client's emotions and associated images, memories, and thoughts. The Rosen method aims to increase the client's awareness of these shifts by asking, "What just happened?" "Can you say more about that?" or by simply saying, "Yes." Rosen method practitioners do not reinforce thoughts and emotions that are not echoed in the body and the breath. Marion Rosen calls this "one's body supporting the truth of one's words."

Benefits and Risks

Rosen method practitioners believe that the Rosen method's greatest contribution to health is preventative: enabling people to recognize tendencies or predispositions toward illness and then to reverse those tendencies. It can provide relief from symptoms caused by stress, injury, and fatigue. It has been shown to be an effective adjunct to psychotherapy, shortening the treatment process. People who are at appropriate stages of recovery from trauma, physical and sexual abuse, eating disorders, and addictions may benefit from adding the Rosen method to their treatment programs.

The Rosen method is not recommended for individuals suffering from severe emotional disturbance or acute physical pain.

—*Ivy Green*

THE ST. JOHN METHOD OF NEUROMUSCULAR THERAPY

The St. John method of neuromuscular therapy combines bodywork and physical rehabilitation techniques to alleviate chronic pain related to stress or injury. Although recently developed, it rests on the assumption, formulated in a number of much earlier holistic therapies, that pain can be traced to a block or distortion in the flow of messages from the nervous system to the rest of the body's structures.

What distinguishes the St. John method from such forerunners as chiropractic is its hybrid approach to treatment. Through massage as well as analysis of a client's posture and gait, it seeks to free the transmission of nerve impulses and restore harmony to the entire organism.

Relieving Pain

Paul St. John, the founder of the St. John method, began to study the phenomenon of pain in 1974 after a devastating automobile accident. Noticing that firm pressure on his neck and shoulders brought temporary relief from the constant aches caused by his injuries, he undertook research that started with massage and led to the disciplines of chiropractic and neurology.

By 1978, St. John had cured himself and put together a method of bodywork aimed specifically at the problem of persistent pain arising from trauma rather than disease. Convinced of its efficacy, he set up a clinical practice and eventually established an information and teaching center, the St. John Neuromuscular Pain Relief Institute.

Today, his treatment is widely acclaimed as an important addition to the repertory of physical and massage therapists specializing in pain management. They receive their training in a series of four seminars available only through the St. John Neuromuscular Pain Relief Institute.

Homeostasis

While the St. John method incorporates Eastern and Scandinavian techniques of massage, its approach to the diagnosis of pain derives from the concept of homeostasis first popularized by American chiropractic teaching. Homeostasis (meaning human equilibrium) refers to the belief that the human organism functions perfectly so long as it exists in a state of ease and harmony, free from mental or physical disturbance. With this idea as its foundation, the St. John method views chronic pain as a symptom of a trauma that lingers on in the form of a block or imbalance in the organism's mechanisms of response.

Further, the St. John method posits that such old injuries are often neglected because they manifest themselves in an indirect fashion. They may appear healed yet be the cause of acute pain in another, apparently unrelated part of the body. For the St. John method, chronic pain is thus a systemic, not a localized problem and cannot be understood or cured unless the totality of the organism's neuromuscular activity is examined.

Instead of X rays, the St. John method directly observes the nervous system's capacity to maintain the equilibrium of the body. These symptoms have been codified into the five so-called principles of pain: tissue with an insufficient blood supply; imbalance in the muscle and skeletal system; habitual distortion of posture and gait; "trigger points" of pain explicable only by reference to another region of the body; and "nerve compression" by soft tissue, cartilage, or bone.

By means of the five "principles of pain," the St. John method charts chronic pain's pathway from the nervous system through the bones, muscles, and blood vessels to soft tissue and the experience of distress. Since the pain is habitual, successful treatment is believed to require bodywork that goes beyond relaxation to disruption of the unhealthy pathways and reeducation of the neuromuscular system. A type of therapeutic massage that exerts strong pressure on tissue is accordingly a standard feature of the St. John method.

The St. John Method in Practice

Treatment with the St. John method is usually received from a physical or massage therapist who has completed the seminar program of the St. John Neuromuscular Pain Relief Institute. A first office visit will include a conversation about the patient's needs and a physical examination based on the five "principles of pain."

The patient's posture, gait, and the tone of body tissue are analyzed through visual observation. Additional information about "trigger points" and thickened, unhealthy areas of tissue is obtained by palpating the body. Once a diagnosis has been reached, the therapist and patient agree upon a plan of treatment, which varies according to individual need but generally comprises a series of office visits for therapeutic bodywork.

173

The form of massage used in the St. John method is designed to interrupt dysfunctional responses in the neuro-muscular system and stimulate healthy blood circulation. Manual pressure is exerted upon selected portions of the patient's body in a rhythmic series of eight- to twelve-second applications.

Though the therapist will be sensitive to the patient's condition, the pressure is supposed to be strong enough to produce moderate discomfort. The discomfort is regarded as crucial evidence that the bodywork is affecting receptors in the nervous system and initiating the desired balancing of the body's structures.

Many Benefits

The St. John method has gained recognition for its success in relieving soft-tissue pain without the use of drugs or costly laboratory tests. Advocates also claim that it can help rebuild injured tissue; eliminate spasms and hyper contractions, enhance the flow of blood and lymphatic fluids, restore alignment to posture, and free the individual from the aftermath of severe stress and trauma.

Resources:

American Pain Association
1615 L Street, NW, Suite 925
Washington, DC 20036
Tel: (202) 296-9200
Provides information about techniques for the relief of chronic pain.

SWEDISH MASSAGE

Swedish massage, also known as traditional massage, is a type of massage characterized by its use of five distinct stroke techniques. Developed by Per Henrik Ling, these techniques are applied by Swedish massage therapists to improve blood flow to the heart. The combination of these strokes is believed to be an extremely effective tool to bring about relaxation, stress reduction, better circulation, and a general sense of well-being.

How Swedish Massage Developed

Swedish massage has its origins in the dedicated work of Swedish fencing master and gymnastic instructor Per Henrik Ling (1776–1839). Ling suffered from a form of rheumatism that affected his fencing arm. As a result, he began to use anatomical and physiological principles as a basis of a systematic method of massage in order to relieve his symptoms. His method became known as the "Ling system." In 1813, the Royal Gymnastic Central Institute of Stockholm introduced the Ling system of massage to its curriculum, where it became known as Swedish massage.

Basic Techniques of Swedish Massage

There are five stroke techniques used in Swedish massage: effleurage, petrissage, friction, tapotement, and vibration. As a general rule, the majority of strokes in a Swedish massage move toward the heart in order to facilitate blood flow back to the heart. For example, an effleurage stroke may begin at the foot and travel toward the pelvis.

The most often used technique of these five strokes is effleurage. Effleurage strokes are long, gliding strokes that may be deep or superficial. They are used to initiate the massage in order to disperse a lubricant over the body part being massaged, to accustom the person to being massaged to the touch of the therapist, and to allow the therapist to discover areas of spasm and tenderness. It is also used as a transitional stroke interspersed with other strokes. Deep effleurage may be used to passively stretch a muscle group.

Petrissage is a kneading stroke that gently lifts the muscle mass and rhythmically rolls, squeezes, or wrings it. This stroke has a stimulating effect on the muscles, deeper blood vessels, and lymphatics. It helps to break down adhesions in the soft tissues and relieves the muscles of metabolic wastes while increasing blood supply to the area.

Friction is most often performed in small circular motions with the tips of the fingers or the thumb. It is a deeper stroke used around the joints, bony prominences, or scar tissue. This stroke should be followed by effleurage to promote absorption of localized blockages or swelling.

Tapotement, or percussion, is the stereotyped, often misrepresented, Swedish massage stroke commonly portrayed in motion pictures. This stroke is done with the hand rapidly alternating in hacking, clapping, or cupping movement. Tapotement has a stimulating effect on the muscles as well as on the nerves if done for brief periods, and a sedating effect on the nerves if prolonged. If, however, a stimulating effect is desired, tapotement renders a slight sense of stimulation and well-being.

Vibration is performed in a rhythmical vibrating motion coming from the whole arm, with the elbow, wrist, and fingers kept stiff in a slightly flexed position. The pressure applied with this stroke should be very light, to impart a smoothing effect.

How Swedish Massage Is Practiced

Swedish massage begins with the person being massaged lying on his or her back, fully draped with a sheet or towels so that only the part being massaged is exposed. A full-body massage follows a general order of right arm, left arm, right leg, left leg, chest, abdomen; the person then rolls over and the massage continues with the back of the left leg, back of the right leg, and lastly the back. A typical massage ranges from thirty minutes to one hour depending on the person's needs.

For maximum comfort of the person being massaged, the room should be warm but not stuffy. The person should be positioned in a comfortable, relaxed position, with the part of the body being massaged properly supported. Massage strokes should begin at a moderate intensity and increase in intensity based on the tolerance of the person being massaged. The massage should end as gently as it was begun.

Benefits and Cautions

There are many beneficial effects of Swedish massage. The most discernible effect is its analgesic, soothing effect upon sensory nerve endings in the skin. Depending upon the type of strokes used, and the length of the massage treatment, this may produce a sense of relaxation, stimulation, or even exhaustion on the nervous system. These effects are useful in eliminating many painful muscular, neurological, and arthritic conditions.

Swedish massage also improves circulation and increases nutrition to the joints and soft tissues while easing the demand on the heart by assisting the heart's ability to move blood through the circulatory system. Massage improves nutrition to the tissues of the body by facilitating a cellular exchange of oxygen and nutrients in the blood with carbon dioxide and cellular metabolic wastes as circulation is increased. This is essential for people who have been incapacitated by injury or disease.

It should be noted, however, that not everyone should be massaged. Massage enhances circulation, therefore anything that can be spread via the circulatory system should not be massaged. These include cancer, acute febrile conditions, jaundice conditions, bacterial infections, pain associated with infections, and areas of acute inflammation. Massage should not be given to fracture sites, as it may cause a separation of bony fragments.

Hemorrhages, acute phlebitis, thrombosis, and varicose veins should not be massaged due to the risk of dislodging a clot in the blood vessels. Persons with cardiovascular problems should be carefully screened and massaged only with a physician's recommendation.

Care should be taken in areas of abnormal or decreased sensation due to stroke, diabetes, or people using medications such as muscle relaxants. The person receiving the massage may have an abnormal vasomotor response to massage or may not be able to give accurate sensory feedback on the depth of the massage.

—*Janie McGee*

Further Reading:

Tappan, F. M. *Healing Massage Techniques: Holistic, Classic, and Emerging Methods.* 2nd ed. Norwalk, CT: Appleton & Lange, 1988.

PART VIII: ACUPUNCTURE AND ASIAN BODYWORK

Acupressure • Acupuncture • Jin Shin Do® Bodymind Acupressure™ • Jin Shin Jyutsu® Physio-Philosophy • Process Acupressure • Shiatsu • Tui Na

Acupuncture and Asian bodywork are holistic methods of healing, health maintenance, and human development based on the principles of traditional Chinese medicine (TCM). Asian bodywork is formally referred to as Oriental bodywork by many professionals in the field and, in the United States, the professional organization of Asian bodyworkers is called the American Oriental Bodywork Therapy Association (AOBTA). All Asian bodywork practices are part of a larger group of methods that have come to be known collectively as bodywork, a general term describing a wide variety of methods that use touch to improve awareness of feelings and sensations in the body and improve physical functioning. They are also used to relieve pain and encourage

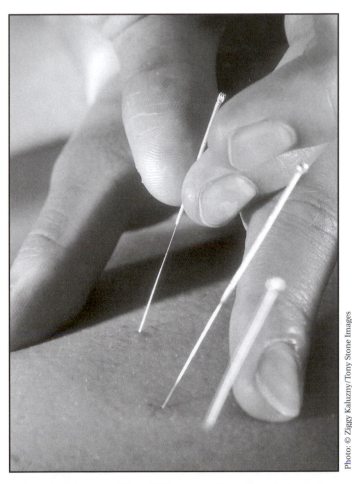

Photo: © Ziggy Kaluzny/Tony Stone Images

The principles of traditional Chinese medicine form the basis for acupuncture and forms of Asian bodywork.

relaxation. There are many disciplines in this book that are included in the bodywork category. They may be found in this volume in the sections entitled Body-Oriented Psychotherapies, Massage, Movement Therapy Methods, Skeletal Manipulation Methods, Somatic Practices, and Subtle Energy Therapies.

All acupuncture and Asian bodywork practices view the physical, mental, and emotional states of a person to be the result of *chi*—an invisible life energy. As water

177

flows through canyons and riverbeds, *chi* travels through the body in channels called meridians. All the methods described in this section are based on observing and manipulating the flow of *chi* through twelve major meridians, each of which corresponds to organs and systems in the physical body.

According to TCM theory, when *chi* is flowing freely through the meridians, an individual will be healthy, well-balanced, and able to adapt quickly and easily to changes in his or her internal and external environment. When the *chi* is blocked, it will produce uncomfortable physical and emotional conditions that will eventually produce debilitating diseases.

Different Approaches to Manipulating *Chi*

Each of the methods included in this section employs different techniques to manipulate the flow of *chi* through the body. Acupuncturists insert thin, stainless steel needles at specific points along the meridians known as acupoints. Acupressure and tui na, the ancient Chinese forms of massage, use many different techniques from gentle stroking to firm grasping and pinching of the acupoints. In shiatsu massage the practitioner uses his or her arms, elbows, knees, and feet to create the many different pressing, stroking, stretching, and percussive movements applied to the acupoints. Jin Shin Jyutsu®, revived in Japan in the early part of this century from ancient Chinese and Tibetan sources, is characterized by its technique of applying pressure to two points simultaneously. Contemporary methods such as Jin Shin Do® and process acupressure combine the ancient techniques with others developed by Western body-oriented psychotherapies in order to affect the flow of *chi*.

While all these methods work to alleviate physical pain, they all recognize the many different causes of illness and imbalance. Since every aspect of life, from inner emotions to external environment, is seen as interdependent with the others, an acupuncturist or Asian bodyworker may also suggest changes in diet, exercise, or lifestyle to help an individual find and maintain a harmonic relationship with the constant flux of the forces of nature.

Since TCM theory believes that no two people have exactly the same physical, mental, or emotional methods for coping with nature's flux, all changes will be recommended according to the particular needs of the individual and his or her symptoms and energy patterns. All methods stress the need for moderation to achieve balance and harmony with nature. Some methods of Oriental bodywork stress the importance of self-applied bodywork, as the responsibility associated with self-care is seen as a necessary part of the process of strengthening *chi*.

A Multitude of Benefits

Acupuncture and the various forms of Asian bodywork have been used by millions to heal hundreds of physical problems. They are useful for acute muscle and soft tissue problems such as sprains and strains as well as conditions resulting from overwork. These techniques have also been shown to be effective with many chronic problems related to stress, such as headaches, insomnia, stomach disorders, asthma, and arthritis. Other complex chronic problems that combine emotional and physical attributes, such as alcohol, tobacco, and drug addictions, have been treated successfully with these methods. On a physical level, acupuncture and Asian bodywork aid circulation of all body fluids, removing harmful toxins from the system. By clearing blockages on the physical level, these practices tone and balance the interdependent organs and systems, opening neurochemical lines of communication in the body. But it is by clearing away blockages on the energetic level, and by treating every individual as a unique image of nature that they teach awareness and respect for the inner and outer needs of each person at each stage of life, providing a means for living a long, healthy, happy, productive life.

—Nancy Allison, CMA

Resources:

American Association of Acupuncture and Oriental Medicine (AAAOM)
4101 Lake Boone Trail, Suite 201
Raleigh, NC 27607
Tel: (919) 787-5181
Offers information about traditional Chinese medicine.

The American Oriental Bodywork Therapy Association (AOBTA)
Glendale Executive Campus, Suite 510
1000 White Horse Rd.
Vorhees, NJ 08043
Tel: (609) 782-1616
Fax: (516) 364-5559
A professional organization that has determined and enforces minimum entry-level standards (500 hours) for all types of Asian bodywork. Currently represents about 1,200 members.

Further Reading:

Claire, Thomas. *Bodywork: What Type of Massage to Get—And How to Make the Most of It.* New York: William Morrow, 1995.

Knaster, Mirka. *Discovering the Body's Wisdom.* New York: Bantam Books, 1996.

ACUPRESSURE

Acupressure is an ancient practice of applying hand and finger pressure to specific points on the body in order to control the flow of *chi*, or vital energy, which, according to traditional Chinese medical theory, courses through the body at all times. It is believed that doing this helps alleviate tension, pain, and other discomforting symptoms, and to prevent harmful toxins and disease from spreading throughout the body. According to recorded history, acupressure, as a formal and defined therapeutic practice, originated in China more than 2,000 years ago. Oral tradition suggests that the practice is even older than that, up to 5,000 years old.

Acupressure is a part of traditional Chinese medicine, the system of holistic medicine that relates all of the parts of the body to each other through the flow of *chi*. Further, it relates the health of the human body to a person's genetic background, psychological conditions, and to exterior conditions of nature, such as climate and the changes of the seasons.

How the Ancient Art of Acupressure Developed

It is hard to know the exact date of acupressure's origin since it is known to predate existing written records. It is thought to derive from the instinctive practice of people rubbing, holding, or kneading painful places on the body for relief. Through experimentation and close observation, early healers developed an understanding of certain places on the body that could assist in the recovery from illness and promote wellness. Over many years of practice and experience with acupressure, healers came to identify the points on the body, called acupoints, where stimulation produced maximum effects. They found that stimulation of these points cured numbness, stiffness, and chills in afflicted areas. The use of acupoints was refined and tested through study of the body, experience with patients, and contemplation over a period of at least 2,000 years. It is still practiced in Asia today.

Though traditional Chinese medicine was overshadowed somewhat during the last century by the introduction of Western medicine, it has now come back into widespread use. At present both Eastern and Western medical practices are often used together in order to provide maximum relief to patients. Since the "opening" of China to the West in the 1960s, the principles and methods of traditional Chinese medicine are now being disseminated throughout the West, in acupuncture, acupressure, and herbal medicine programs where Westerners are able to study these ancient methods with traditional Eastern practitioners. Training for acupressure specialists begins with a basic 150-hour certification program and can range up to 850 hours for advanced training programs.

Other Forms of Bodywork Based on the Acupressure Model

Various styles of acupressure were developed over time, although they all rely on the basic traditional model of energy flow through the meridians, acupoints, and whole person. Tui na is the Chinese massage method of using acupoints to regulate energy flow. Amma was the name used in Japan for a similar method. Shiatsu, meaning "finger pressure" in Japanese, is a vigorous form of acupressure that uses firm and rhythmic pressure on acupoints over the whole body for three to ten seconds each. Jin shin jyutsu is the practice of holding two-point combinations at the same time until a release of energy and tension is felt. It was developed by Jiro Murai in Japan in the twentieth century and has been taught throughout the world. Contemporary American progressions from jin shin jyutsu are: Jin Shin Do®, developed by Iona Marsaa Teeguarden, which combines gentle yet

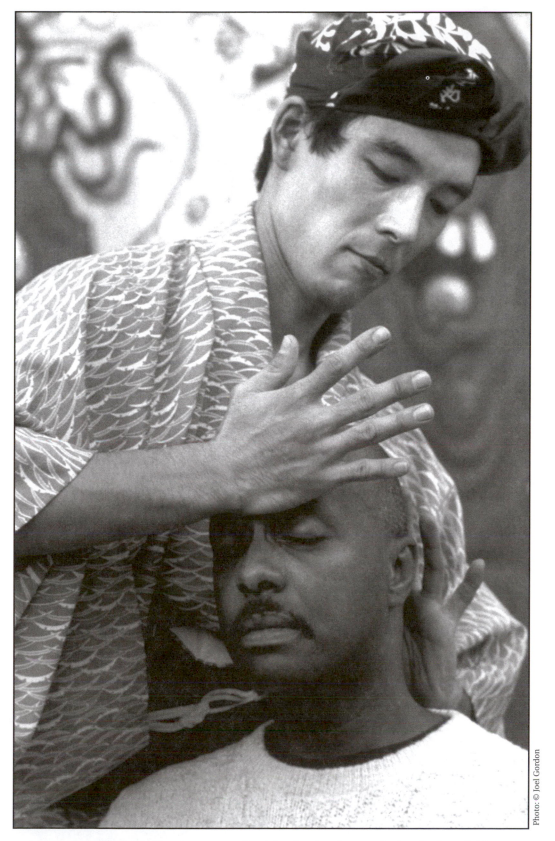

An acupressurist applies pressure to a client's head and neck to manipulate the flow of *chi*.

Photo: © Joel Gordon

deep finger pressure on acupoints with simple verbal techniques that heighten awareness of the connection between the body and the mind; and process acupressure, developed by Aminah Raheem, which combines psychological and spiritual work in consciousness with acupressure. In addition, self-acupressure techniques such as acu-yoga, developed by Michael Reed Gach in America, teach people how to find their acupoints and to release energy and relieve tension through self-massage.

Meridians and Acupoints

The Chinese holistic system is postulated on the premise that when the energy system and the internal organs of the body are functioning normally, a person will be in good health. Conversely, if either the energy or the organs are out of balance or distressed, illness will eventually occur. Therefore, the therapeutic approach is to locate any site of congestion, tension, or imbalance, in either energy or organs, and then to apply the method that will release this obstruction, thereby returning the body to its own internal regulation processes and health.

The energy system of the body was mapped during ancient times. It is defined by explicit energy pathways (called meridians) that flow up and down the body, from head to toe. Twelve of these pathways are linked to internal organs and are said to help regulate the health of these organs. The pathways are accessed by acupoints, or "windows," into the pathways, which can be stimulated to affect energy flow. Originally 361 acupoints were located on the surface of the body. These are still the

primary acupoints today. Through the centuries more acupoints have been added to the map so that there are now some 2,000 points in the contemporary Chinese system.

The Importance of Open Communication

In initial meetings with an acupressure therapist, open communication is established between patient and therapist. A therapist will determine a patient's total body symptoms, and establish a thorough family and childhood history to uncover genetic or environmental reasons that could cause or contribute to a patient's disorder. Once the patient and therapist are satisfied that all significant issues have been discussed, the patient is encouraged to relax and pressure is applied to predetermined pressure points. During the session, acupressure should result in lessened muscle tension, increased blood circulation, as well as a release of endorphins and subsequent pain relief. Toxins are also released and purged from the body. Length and frequency of the sessions are determined by the therapist and patient and depend on the severity of the problem.

A Powerful Tool

Acupressure is particularly beneficial for those who suffer with severe back pain, arthritis, nonarticular rheumatism, or chronic muscle aches. It can aid in relieving the pain of headaches. It is also credited with balancing the different systems of the body and eliminating harmful toxins. In this sense it is considered a powerful preventive tool against

In acupressure, pressure is applied to the body by an acupressure specialist using his or her hand, knuckle, finger, or a blunt-tipped instrument called a tei shin, which causes the body to release endorphins, an important neurochemical that is credited with effective pain relief. Various styles of acupressure have been developed over time, although they all rely on the use of acupoints to control energy flow through the meridians and regulate the whole person—body, mind, and spirit.

the onslaught of illness and disease as it purifies and strengthens the body's resistance, resulting in a healthy, vital existence.

As a caution, self-acupressure requires no special tools but instruction is encouraged in order to effectively determine pressure points.

—*Aminah Raheem, Ph.D.*

Resources:

Acupressure Institute
1533 Shattuck Avenue
Berkeley, CA 94709
Tel: (510) 845-1059
Offers certification programs from basic to advanced, including specialized classes and an 850-hour program.

The American Oriental Bodywork Therapy Association (AOBTA)
Glendale Executive Campus, Ste. 510
1000 White Horse Rd.
Vorhees, NJ 08043
Tel: (609) 782-1616
Fax: (516) 364-5559
Web site: www.healthy.net/pan/pa/bodywork
A professional organization that has determined and enforces minimum entry-level standards (500 hours) for all types of Oriental bodywork. Currently represents about 1,200 members.

Jin Shin Do Foundation for Bodymind Acupressure
366 California Avenue, Ste. 16
Palo Alto, CA 94306
Tel: (408) 763-7702
Provides a myriad of information on Jin Shin Do acupressure, including a list of registered practitioners, newsletters, books, videotapes, and training courses.

Further Reading:

The Academy of Traditional Chinese Medicine. *An Outline of Chinese Acupuncture.* Peking: Foreign Languages Press, 1975.

Raheem, Aminah. *Soul Return: Integrating Body, Psyche and Spirit.* Santa Cruz: Aslan, 1991.

(Available from author at Process Acupressure Unlimited, P.O. Box 1096, Capitola, CA 95010.)

Serizawa, Katsusuke. *Tsubo: Vital Points for Oriental Therapy.* Tokyo: Japan Publications, Inc., 1976.

Steinfeld, Alan. *Careers in Alternative Medicine.* New York: Rosen Publishing, 1997.

Teeguarden, Iona Marsaa. *Acupressure Way of Health: Jin Shin Do.* Tokyo: Japan Publications, Inc., 1978.

——. *A Complete Guide to Acupressure.* Tokyo: Japan Publications, Inc., 1996.

ACUPUNCTURE

Acupuncture is one of the ancient healing practices recommended by traditional Chinese medicine to cure disease, relieve pain, and maintain health. Acupuncture is a holistic medicine, that is, it stresses the interconnectedness of one's body, mind, and spirit. An acupuncturist understands that physical ailments can affect one's emotional or psychological state and equally, emotional, spiritual, or psychological difficulties can lead to disease. According to Chinese philosophy, energy—called *chi* or *qi* (pronounced *chee* or *key*)—circulates through all things, including our bodies. The proper flow of *chi* is essential to good health. The practice of acupuncture involves placing needles into specific points on the body in order to control the flow of this energy.

Origins and Development of Acupuncture

There is evidence suggesting that acupuncture has been practiced for more than 5,000 years. It is mentioned in one of the first written records of traditional Chinese medicine practices, called the

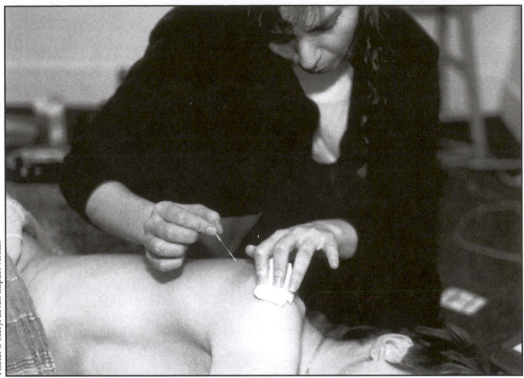

Photo: © Meryl Levin/Impact Visuals

A practitioner of traditional Chinese medicine works with herbs and oils to administer acupuncture. Here she removes the needles used in acupuncture.

Huang-ti Nei Ching (The Yellow Emperor's Classic of Internal Medicine). This text was compiled sometime between 213 BCE and 240 CE, and is reputed to document practices used during the legendary reign of the Yellow Emperor in China (2697–2595 BCE). Acupuncture started spreading throughout Asia around 1000 CE and reached Europe by around 1700 CE.

Until recently in the United States, acupuncture has been used mostly for anesthesia and for the treatment of alcohol, tobacco, and drug addictions. These are very limited uses of acupuncture that may be of help in some situations but do not embrace the underlying holistic philosophy of acupuncture. As more studies reinforce the benefits of acupuncture, its use as a method of health care and health maintenance seems to be increasing in the West.

The Philosophy of Acupuncture

Acupuncture is based on the belief that our body, mind, and spirit are fully integrated aspects of our being. They cannot be separated from one another. They must be balanced in order for us to be healthy. *Chi* is the energy of our lives, what motivates us, our life essence—it affects our whole being. It is believed that when the energy flows we feel generally well, and when it is impeded we feel out of balance and begin to develop the symptoms of disease. *Chi* is thought to travel in channels, called meridians, deep inside the body. Acupuncture points are the places where these meridians come close to the surface and where the *chi* can then be influenced.

Acupuncture, like all aspects of traditional Chinese medicine, is firmly rooted in Chinese philosophy. The Tao, yin and yang, the five elements, and the twelve meridians or officials provide the foundations for acupuncture's origin, development, and procedures.

Tao. The principle of the Tao comes from the book *Tao Teh Ching (Book of the Way of Life)*, written by the philosopher

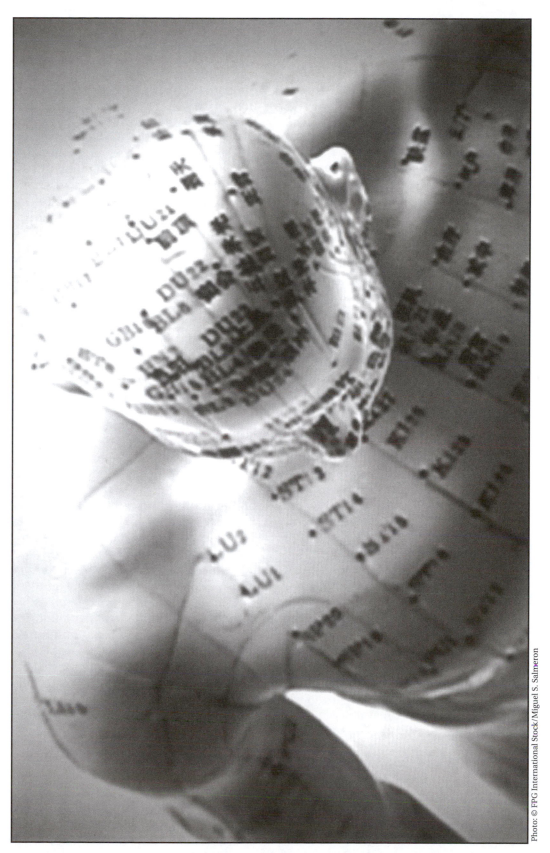

A three-dimensional acupuncture model shows the meridians and acupoints.

Lao-tzu. Like the Taoist principles that Lao-tzu described in this classic book, acupuncture emphasizes the importance of balance and harmony, change and growth, and ever-flowing energy of one's life.

Yin-Yang. The terms yin and yang represent polar opposites that according to Taoism are continually merging into, and creating balance with, each other. Yin and yang create balance in the world and in ourselves. Yin is the cool, nighttime, reflective energy that takes things to completion; yang is the hot, daytime, active energy that starts things into motion. Yin is often considered representative of female energy and yang of the male energy.

Five Elements. Chinese philosophy sees individuals as an integral part of nature, a microcosm reflecting the macrocosm. In nature we have elements such as fire, earth, metal, water, and wood. In acupuncture we envision these elements within us. We can feel all fired up or burned out; dry and stiff as dried wood or flexible and supple as a willow shoot; hard and cold as steel or hot and flowing as molten gold; fresh and pure as a freshwater stream or stagnant and dank like a polluted well. An acupuncturist uses these and many, many more images to conceptualize a person's state of well-being.

Meridians. The twelve meridians, or officials, are seen as channels within our bodies that act as conduits for the *chi* to flow through, to animate and nourish us. The meridians have names akin to Western medical terms for organs but are much broader in their scope. For example, the lung meridian is thought of as the receiver of *chi*. It takes energy in and lets it go. In addition to breathing, the lung meridian has the capacity for inspiration on an emotional and spiritual level. The small intestine meridian is in charge of "separation of pure from impure." On a physical level this determines which nutrients to absorb or to discard. On an emotional and spiritual level it determines which aspects of ourselves we will keep and which we will let go.

Experiencing an Acupuncture Session

Today, a session with an acupuncturist is conducted in much the same way it was thousands of years ago. Talking to the patient, hearing his or her description of the illness, is very important. The practitioner wants to hear the patient describe the problem in his or her own words rather than a standard medical definition or diagnosis. The practitioner will want to know about the patient's background, including family history and his or her childhood. According to traditional Chinese medicine, no two people ever have exactly the same illness, even if the Western diagnosis would be the same. One's individuality affects how and why one becomes ill and must be taken into consideration when deciding on a treatment. Listening to the sound of the patient's voice, seeing subtle face color, palpating (touching), noticing any unusual breath or body odor, examining the tongue and taking the pulse at the wrist are all very important methods of diagnosis and aid in formulating a treatment plan. There are several hundred acupuncture points, and the practitioner chooses which will be used in a session by using these diagnostic methods.

The goal, simply stated, is to restore the flow and balance of *chi*. The acupuncturist accomplishes this by inserting very thin, solid, sterile stainless steel needles into acupuncture points in order to open blockages and manipulate the *chi*. Needles are placed and either taken out quickly or left to stay in for up to thirty to forty minutes, depending on what the acupuncturist wants to accomplish. On occasion the acupuncturist will warm or energize the *chi* by burning an herb called *Artemesia vulgaris* (mugwort, moxa) on the skin. This technique is called moxibustion. The practitioner may check the patient's pulse again and will decide whether or not to treat more points. An acupuncturist may also recommend herbal remedies, dietary and/or lifestyle changes, or exercises, to assist in recovery.

Benefits

The World Health Organization accepts acupuncture as a treatment for more than 100 health problems, including migraines, bronchitis, back pain, sinusitis, high blood pressure, ulcers, arthritis, PMS, hay fever, and the common cold. Also, various studies in China, Europe, and the United States have shown acupuncture to be a useful tool in treating drug and alcohol addictions, mental disorders, depression, anxiety, insomnia, and stress.

Theories from the Western Perspective

From a Western perspective, two theories as to how acupuncture works have been put forth. One by researchers Melzack and Wall is called the double gate theory of pain. This theory suggests that acupuncture stimulates certain nerves that close a neurological "gate" in the spinal column, inhibiting pain fibers from ascending to higher cognitive levels. The other theory, suggested by the studies of several different researchers, suggests that acupuncture stimulates opiate-like substances called endorphins and enkephalins that account for its pain-relieving effects. These theories are enlightening but, acupuncturists contend, do not account fully for the far-reaching and long-lasting effects that acupuncture can have on a patient's body, mind, and spirit.

—*Dr. Robert J. Abramson*

Resources:

American Association of Acupuncture and Oriental Medicine
4101 Lake Boone Trail, 201
Raleigh, NC 27607
Tel: (919) 787-5181
Works to improve awareness and acceptance of acupuncture as a form of complementary medicine.

National Acupuncture and Oriental Medicine Alliance (NAOMA)
638 Prospect Ave.

Hartford, CT 06105-4298
Professional organization with a membership of individual practitioners and medical colleges. The group lobbies to integrate acupuncture into American health care.

Worsley Institute of Classical Acupuncture, Inc.
6175 N.W. 153rd Street, Suite 324
Miami Lakes, FL 33014
Offers information, resources, and training in five-element acupuncture.

Further Reading:

Mann, Felix. *Acupuncture: The Ancient Chinese Art of Healing.* Magnolia, MA: Peter Smith, 1990.

——. *Acupuncture: Cure of Many Diseases.* Second Edition. Oxford, UK: Butterworth-Heinemann Ltd., 1992.

Melzack, Ronald. *The Puzzle of Pain.* New York: Basic Books, Inc., 1973.

Mitchell, Ellinor R. *Plain Talk About Acupuncture.* New York: Whalehall, Inc., 1987.

Worsley, J.R. *Traditional Acupuncture, Volume II.* Warwickshire, U.K.: College of Traditional Acupuncture, U.K., 1990.

JIN SHIN DO® BODYMIND ACUPRESSURE™

Jin Shin Do® Bodymind Acupressure™ is a form of Asian bodywork that was developed by Iona Marsaa Teeguarden. It combines gentle yet deep finger pressure on specific points on the the body (acupoints) with simple verbal techniques to release tension and heighten the connection between body and mind. Jin Shin Do is effective in helping to relieve muscular pain and stress-related problems such as headaches, backaches, anxiety, fatigue,

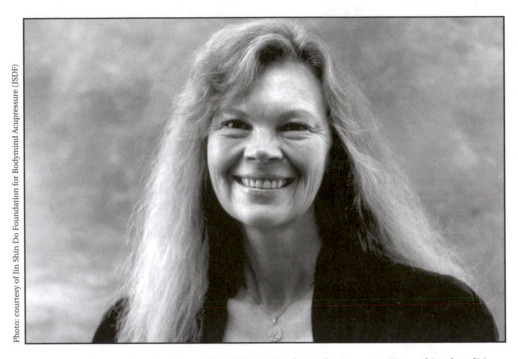

Iona Marsaa Teeguarden, developer of Jin Shin Do® Bodymind Acupressure™, combined traditional Asian bodywork practices with the theories of body-oriented psychotherapist Wilhelm Reich.

insomnia, eye strain, menstrual and menopausal discomfort, digestive distress, joint pain, urogenital problems, sinus pain, and allergies.

The Recent Development of Jin Shin Do®

Iona Marsaa Teeguarden was born in 1949 in Rugby, North Dakota. She studied piano performance and philosophy at the University of Michigan, but was still in search of a profession when she met Mary Burmeister, who practiced Jin Shin Jyutsu®, a Japanese acupressure technique developed in the twentieth century by Jiro Murai. Teeguarden turned to Burmeister in 1971 for relief of back pain due to scoliosis. The improvement that Teeguarden experienced motivated her to study acupressure and, two years later, she began to treat clients in her home, working mainly with patients suffering from pain. She subsequently studied with Chinese, Korean, and Japanese acupuncture and acupressure specialists.

In 1979, to better understand how to respond to emotions released by her patients during sessions, Teeguarden returned to school, receiving an M.A. in psychology from Antioch University in 1980 and a license to practice psychotherapy in 1982. Integrating Western and Eastern theories, she developed the emotional kaleidoscope, a detailed map of body-mind connections identifying acupoints that have an effect on specific emotions.

In 1982 Teeguarden began to develop a new teaching approach, including a color-coded system that illustrates where the forty-five basic points are on the body and how to combine them in a simple way. She also established the Jin Shin Do Foundation, and began offering teacher training programs. There are now about eighty authorized Jin Shin Do teachers, and more than 300 registered Jin Shin Do acupressurists throughout the world.

A Synthesis of Techniques

The energy system of the body was mapped in ancient times by practitioners of traditional Chinese medicine. It is defined by energy pathways (called meridians) that flow up and down the body, from head to toe. Practitioners believe these meridians help regulate the health of internal organs as well the physical and psychological processes that these organs control.

In developing Jin Shin Do, Teeguarden connected four main energy flows taught by Jiro Murai with the eight "strange flows," or "extraordinary meridians," of acupuncture. The strange flows are a primary self-regulating system that, when functioning correctly, move energy around the body, continually adjusting and moderating the balance of the twelve organ meridians. They also store and release energy for the meridians.

To this already rich therapeutic heritage, Teeguarden added a Western component—Dr. Wilhelm Reich's view of the body as a series of segments that contain muscular tension related to specific emotional experiences. Reich stated that the health of human beings depends upon proper flow of energy within the body. He believed that a stoppage of energy flow is unhealthy and results in both character armoring and muscular armoring.

Character armor is evident in the attitudes of people and the makeup of their personalities. For example, a common type of character armor is aloofness stemming from guilt and shame. Muscular armor is apparent in muscular tensions and contractions, which are physical barriers to the flow of energy. Both forms of armoring eventually lead to pain. Reich contended that they are unconscious techniques used by the body-mind complex to cope with early traumatic experiences and that the character armoring and muscular armoring are just different aspects of the same defense.

Teeguarden related classic Chinese theories of the emotions and acupoints with Reichian theories of character and muscular armoring. She found that armoring could be released by holding "local points," or acupoints in the area of

tension, with "distal points," which are far away from the area of tension but enhance the effectiveness of local-point pressure. At the same time, she uses psychotherapeutic techniques, verbally encouraging the individual to remain open to emotions and thoughts that arise when muscular armor begins to dissolve.

Achieving Relaxation

A typical session lasts between sixty and ninety minutes, with the client clothed and lying on his or her back on a massage table. The practitioner evaluates the tension pattern in the body by asking the client and through pulse reading and inquiring touch, or "point palpation." After identifying main points of muscular contraction, the practitioner holds combinations of acupoints to release tensions and rebalance energy. The individual being treated initially will feel sensitivity at the point of pressure, but that is quickly replaced by a pleasurable feeling of tension being discharged. The general effect is a state of deep relaxation in which the individual achieves a peaceful mental state and a deeper awareness of his or her body. After a session, clients typically feel relaxed and rejuvenated. Over a series of sessions, armoring is progressively released in the head, neck, shoulders, arms, back, chest, diaphragm, abdomen, pelvis, and legs.

The Way of the Compassionate Spirit

Teeguarden, like Reich, believes that when we are not allowed to express an emotion, we hold it back by tightening the muscles that would normally express it. This tension can become chronic, with the muscles involved becoming rigid and incapable of expression. Teeguarden believes that when we hold our emotions back with muscular tension, we also impede the flow of the Oriental energy pathways.

At its basic level, Jin Shin Do is a relaxation method that helps release physical and emotional tension, and so is named "The Way of the Compassionate Spirit." In the hands of a trained psychotherapist, it appears to help ease the effects of childhood abuse and other trauma trapped by the body in the form of physical tension. Treatment can have the intensity of catharsis, but is generally characterized by gentleness. JSD acupressurists avoid pressing on open sores and rashes, and pressing too hard in cases of phlebitis (inflammation of a vein), varicosities (swollen veins), broken blood vessels, or extensive bruising. Certain points are forbidden during pregnancy. Of course, clients should first consult their medical doctor, particularly in the case of chronic or acute conditions.

—*Iona Marsaa Teeguarden*

Resources:

American Oriental Bodywork Therapy Association
Glendale Executive Campus, 510
1000 White Horse Rd.
Vorhees, NJ 08043
Tel: (609) 782-1616
Fax: (609) 782-1653
Founded in 1984, this organization represents practitioners and teachers of all types of Oriental bodywork, including acupressure, shiatsu, and AMMA. The American Oriental Bodywork Therapy Association Council of Schools and Programs includes the JSDF among its members.

Jin Shin Do Foundation for Bodymind Acupressure (JSDF)
P.O. Box 1097
Felton, CA 95018
or
1084G San Miguel Canyon Rd.
Watsonville, CA 95076
Tel: (408) 763-7702
Fax: (408) 763-1551
Founded in 1982, the Jin Shin Do Foundation is a network of Jin Shin Do teachers and acupressurists throughout the United States, Canada, Europe, and elsewhere. Write for a free newsletter, which includes a list of books, charts, and audio and video tapes available as well as a description of the

Jin Shin Do training program. An international directory is also available.

Further Reading:

Teeguarden, Iona Marsaa. *The Acupressure Way of Health: Jin Shin Do.* New York: Japan Publication, 1978.

———. *Color-Coded Strange Flows Chart.* Watsonville, CA: Jin Shin Do Foundation, 1981.

———. *A Complete Guide to Acupressure.* New York: Japan Publication, 1996.

———. *Fundamentals of Self-Acupressure.* Watsonville, CA: Jin Shin Do Foundation, 1989.

———. *The Joy of Feeling: Bodymind Acupressure.* New York: Japan Publication, 1987.

Jin Shin Jyutsu® Physio-Philosophy

Jin Shin Jyutsu® Physio-Philosophy is an ancient art that uses the hands on specific areas of the body to harmonize the flow of life-giving energy throughout the body. It can be utilized either as a "self-help" tool or received from a practitioner. Jin Shin Jyutsu provides the body with an excellent opportunity to restore and maintain healthy physical, mental, emotional, and spiritual well-being.

An Ancient Discipline

According to records in the Imperial Archives of Japan, the principles of Jin Shin Jyutsu date back to ancient times. This understanding was passed down in the oral tradition from generation to generation, until many of the principles became distorted and the art was nearly lost.

Near the turn of the twentieth century this art was rediscovered by Master Jiro Murai, the second son born into a family of medical professionals. Faced with a life-threatening illness, considered terminal by traditional medicine, Jiro Murai turned to the wisdom of the great sages for his salvation. Jiro healed himself through the application of hand mudras and through breathing exercises.

Upon his healing, Master Murai vowed to dedicate his life to the study and development of the art he eventually named Jin Shin Jyutsu, which translates as "the art of the Creator through man of compassion and knowing."

In the late 1940s, Jiro met Mary Burmeister, an American-born Japanese, working in the U.S. diplomatic corps. Upon their first meeting, Jiro asked Mary if she would like to bring a gift from Japan back to America. Without knowing what Jiro was referring to, Mary accepted his offer, and became Jiro's first student. Mary studied with him for the next six years, and then for another six years of correspondence after she returned to the United States until Jiro's death.

Mary spent the next several years deepening her understanding of the art of Jin Shin Jyutsu. It wasn't until the early 1960s that Mary was approached by the doctor of a neighbor she had been helping. Having noted positive change in the neighbor, this doctor wanted to learn more about what had helped so much and became Mary's first student. Mary continued to teach until 1990, sharing her awareness and understanding of this profound art with thousands of students across the United

States and western Europe. Mary has since selected eight instructors whom she has certified to continue her teachings and those of Jiro Murai.

Safety-Energy Locks

Jin Shin Jyutsu employs twenty-six safety-energy locks throughout the body. These are found along the various pathways through which the universal energy travels. This energy flow creates and supports life, and all the functions of the body, including organ function. For many reasons—hereditary, character, stress, accidents, tension of daily lifestyle, etc.—these pathways may become blocked, causing symptoms and illnesses. By placing our hands (jumper cables) on these safety-energy locks in specific sequences (flows), practitioners can unlock these areas to restore harmony, balance, and the proper functioning of the body. There are many different sequences that can be used, and these sequences are determined by listening to the pulse and reading the conformation of the body. These show where attention is required.

To apply Jin Shin Jyutsu, the hands are placed on a clothed body. There is no massage or manipulation. Practitioners only wait to feel the rhythmic pulsation in the safety-energy lock to know that area is in harmony with the universal energy. Then they move on to the next area of the sequence. Upon completion of this sequence, they will have become aware of the harmony restored to this

Studying Jin Shin Jyutsu®

For those interested in studying Jin Shin Jyutsu, the basic five-day course is offered in the United States, Canada, Brazil, and throughout Europe. The number of locations expands each year as interest grows. At this point, there are only eight instructors authorized by Jin Shin Jyutsu®, Inc., the sole organization offering instruction in this discipline. The class includes lecture, material, and a good deal of hands-on experience. It is broken down into two parts. Part I is the first three days and covers the safety-energy locks. Part II is the remaining two days, and covers the seventeen "individualized" body function energy flows. Anyone is welcome to attend, and there is no prerequisite.

particular flow of energy. Symptoms will disappear over time or, in some cases, immediately.

These sequences can be applied by a practitioner to another person, or by an individual utilizing them for self-help. This self-help is an important aspect of Jin Shin Jyutsu as self-awareness, or "now know myself," helps us to maintain balance and harmony, or to simply feel relaxed and peaceful. In order to find the proper techniques and sequences for self-help, people can consult their practitioner or self-help books.

Jin Shin Jyutsu is an art, not merely a technique. A technique is a mechanical application whereas an art is a skillful creation. This art is supported strongly by its underlying philosophy, which emphasizes an awareness of ourselves and of our connection to the universal energy. By maintaining this, we remain in harmony—happy and healthy. When we forget the philosophy, we can utilize our "jumper cables" to recharge our batteries and restore the proper functioning of our body. As Mary has said, "Philosophy is the richness of Jin Shin Jyutsu, and the technique is for when we don't live the philosophy. It's a tool to get us out of trouble."

Achieving Harmony

A Jin Shin Jyutsu session lasts about an hour. The recipient lies face-up on a table or any available comfortable surface. The practitioner will "listen" to the pulse not for diagnosis, but to determine which energy function flows might be utilized to bring the body to its natural state of harmony. At this point, the practitioner uses the hands in specific sequences to restore energy flow. By the end of the session, the pulse should be even and balanced.

The practitioner often provides information during or after the session. The actual experience and results may vary from person to person. The recipient may feel a sense of relaxation and deeper breathing as the energy flow is restored. The immediate effects of the

session will continue for eight hours, as the circulation pattern is completed.

—Ian Kraut

Resources:

Jin Shin Jyutsu®, Inc.
8719 E. San Alberto
Scottsdale, AZ 85257
Tel: (602) 998-9331
Fax: (602) 998-9335
Web site: www.inficad.com/*.010jsjinc
Offers information on seminars, books and materials, and practitioner referrals.

Further Reading:

Burmeister, Alice. *The Touch of Healing: Energizing Body, Mind, and Spirit with the Art of Jin Shin Jyutsu.* New York: Bantam Books, 1997.

PROCESS ACUPRESSURE

Process acupressure (PA) was developed as a single modality for addressing and supporting all parts of an individual. According to PA, touch is able to release tension stored in a person's body, allowing him or her to develop more balance, strength, and clarity to understand and handle problems better. As in traditional acupressure, gentle pressure is applied to the body to strengthen, release, and balance the body's energy systems. PA also is concerned with revealing a person's soul, or inner wisdom. This deep inner knowing is accessed as a guiding influence over one's healing and development.

PA grew out of Dr. Aminah Raheem's search for ways to support a person's wellness and growth in body, mind, emotions, and soul simultaneously. In PA, she combined traditional acupressure methods with the unique touch of Zero Balancing®. It also uses skills developed from

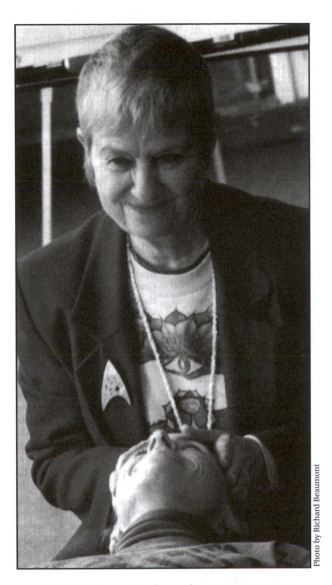

Photo by Richard Beaumont

Aminah Raheem, developer of process acupressure.

transpersonal psychology, which includes Carl Jung's analytical psychology, Roberto Assagioli's psychosynthesis, and Arnold Mindell's process oriented psychotherapy. It took six years for Dr. Raheem to test and develop her theoretical framework into a hands-on application. PA premiered in Zurich, Switzerland, in 1986. Since then it has been continuously taught there and in the United States and England to body-workers, psychologists, and laypersons.

According to PA, energy offers the most natural access to the whole person because it integrates the body, mind, emotions, and soul. Two energy systems—meridians and chakras—are referenced in PA. While the meridians comprise the network of energy pathways used in Chinese acupuncture, chakras are an ancient Hindu system of energy vortices along the central midline of the body. Both of these systems are directly connected and intermingled, with the meridians feeding energy into and out of the chakras.

By allowing personal history to surface from the body during bodywork, PA is able to process directly the most relevant psychological material for the person's growth at the time. For example, if memories or traumas from the past arise during the bodywork, the PA practitioner knows how to help a person bring feelings and images to consciousness, allowing him or her to reach a resolution. Or if feelings, images, or issues come to mind during the bodywork they can be explored and furthered in consciousness for the client's health and well-being.

Typically a PA session takes from one to one and one-half hours. In a typical PA session the client lies on a massage table, fully clothed, and relaxes deeply while the practitioner applies custom-designed acupressure techniques. Physical, psychological, or spiritual issues are addressed in a team approach by both practitioner and client. In some cases a problem is clarified and resolved in one session. More commonly, several sessions are required to resolve a condition and prevent recurrence.

PA has been used to address a variety of physical symptoms, including back problems, headaches, respiratory, digestive, and systemic problems as well as colds, flus, allergies, and healing from injuries. Advocates also recommend PA to help relieve stress-related conditions, including post-traumatic stress. PA is promoted as a method of furthering and empowering development in the well person who wishes to grow toward his or her full potential.

PA should not be used to treat severe medical problems and does not supplant medical care. It should not be used for psychotics or people during severe psychotic episodes because it uncovers and releases unconscious material that may be overwhelming for a person in a weakened ego state.

—Aminah Raheem

Resources:

Process Acupressure Unlimited
P.O. Box 1096
Capitola, CA 95010
Certifies health care professionals as PA practitioners after progressive levels of training, supervised

experience, and examination. PA does not give licensure, therefore practitioners must be licensed in a professional health care modality, such as massage, medicine, or osteopathy; or in a psychological field, such as marriage and family counseling, psychology, or psychiatry, before they can be certified in PA.

Further Reading:

Raheem, Aminah. *Process Acupressure I.* Palm Beach Gardens, FL: The Upledger Institute, Inc., 1994.

———. *Process Acupressure II: Releases for the Whole Being.* Palm Beach Gardens, FL: The Upledger Institute, Inc., 1994.

———. *Process Acupressure III: The Hologram.* Aptos, CA: Process Acupressure Association, 1996.

———. *Soul Return: Integrating Body, Psyche and Spirit.* Santa Rosa, CA: Aslan Publishing, 1991.

SHIATSU

Shiatsu is a method of Japanese bodywork derived from ancient healing practices. In shiatsu, practitioners apply pressure using the fingers, palms, elbows, forearms, knees, and even feet, to pressure points (called *tsubos* in Japanese) along a receiver's body. This practice encourages the proper flow of *qi*, or life energy, which, according to traditional Chinese medicine, is necessary for the optimum health of one's body and mind. Primarily, shiatsu is recommended as a preventative technique, that is, to be practiced even when you are healthy in order to maintain good health. It is also practiced for the relief of pain, to improve mental functioning, and to relieve a variety of ailments, including chronic stress, digestive problems, and lower back pain.

Shiatsu: A Practice with Ancient Roots
The use of bodywork and massage for

curing disease and improving health has ancient origins in China. Massage is one of the treatment principles of traditional Chinese medicine, the basic tenets of which are thought to date back to the legendary reign of the Yellow Emperor in China from 2697–2595 BCE. Although the principles of traditional Chinese medicine were not written down until some time between 213 BCE and 240 CE, people believe that the practices had been passed from generation to generation for thousands of years before that.

The various practices of traditional Chinese medicine spread throughout Asia, making their way to Japan in about 500 to 600 CE. In Japan, massage became known as amma, which literally means rubdown. By the early 1900s amma was still being practiced in Japan but had earned a reputation as folk medicine and became associated more with pleasure, relaxation, and sensuality than with medicine. As a result, some practitioners who wanted to continue practicing therapeutic massage began calling their practice shiatsu. These practitioners worked to raise public awareness of the healing aspects of massage. Today shiatsu is one of the most popular forms of massage in Japan.

Balancing and Fortifying Life Energy

Shiatsu is a holistic form of bodywork. This means that the body and mind are viewed as connected to each other, as well as to the external environment. Practitioners of shiatsu believe that a vital life energy, called *qi,* surrounds and interpenetrates the physical body. *Qi* flows through the body through invisible channels called meridians. Practitioners of shiatsu are trained to manipulate pressure points that lie along these channels of energy in order to balance a receiver's energy. According to the traditional Asian worldview, illness or disease (including emotional and psychological problems) is the result of an imbalance in the flow of *qi.* By balancing and fortifying vital life energy, the shiatsu therapist can help a client maintain and improve his or her health. Shiatsu is thought to help prevent the onset of illness. If illness or disease has already set in, shiatsu is used to encourage the body's healing process.

Experiencing Shiatsu Massage

Shiatsu emphasizes the physical manipulation of the body. It aims to work with both the physical body and the energy that surrounds and interpenetrates it. As the number of practitioners grows, the variety of styles of shiatsu also grows. A shiatsu session may be a vigorous massage or it may employ only gentle touch, depending on the practitioner. Some people find the more vigorous method painful. One should seek a shiatsu therapist that best meets his or her own personal needs. Increasingly, Western shiatsu practice is gentle and less invasive than the traditional Japanese approach. The most well known and representative form of this style of shiatsu is Ohashiatsu®. Ohashiatsu® was developed by a Japanese man named Wataru Ohashi. Ohashi probably did more than any other person to introduce and popularize shiatsu in the West. Ohashi's style of shiatsu is taught and practiced at the Ohashi Institute.

Traditionally, someone receiving shiatsu dresses in loose, comfortable clothing and lies on a comfortable futon—a kind of Japanese mattress—or cushioned space on the floor. The practitioner kneels and

Shiatsu therapy is widely available, so anyone interested in experiencing this rejuvenating form of treatment should have no trouble finding an experienced practitioner. Many spas, health clubs, and resorts offer shiatsu as one of their treatments. As the training of practitioners can vary widely, you should check the educational background and experience of any practitioner you are considering visiting.

crawls around the person he or she is massaging. Because there are different approaches to shiatsu, however, some practitioners have receivers disrobe to their level of comfort and lie on a padded massage table rather than on the floor. A typical shiatsu session lasts from a half hour to an hour and a half. Pressure can be light or deep depending upon the style of shiatsu practiced and what is best for the receiver.

Practitioners may also gently stretch the receiver's body. They may also act as a kind of coach or teacher to the receiver in order to help him or her achieve better energy balance. For instance, a shiatsu therapist might recommend a more nutritional diet, getting more exercise, or other helpful suggestions regarding lifestyle.

Benefits for the Body and Mind

People who receive shiatsu often say they feel both energized and relaxed at the same time. They may also feel calm and peaceful, lighter in spirit, and physical aches and pains may diminish. Shiatsu is considered by many to be a wonderful healing practice for individuals seeking physical relief of muscle aches and soft tissue pains. It is also a useful practice for exploring the energetic aspects of bodywork.

Shiatsu can be an important part of an ongoing health maintenance program. By taking time to be more aware of our bodies, we may be able to spot physical and emotional problems before they have a chance to make us sick. In addition to helping relieve aches and pains, shiatsu can fortify the functioning of the immune system, which protects us from illness; stimulate circulation, which is vital to life; provide massage to the internal organs; and encourage proper functioning of the nervous and endocrine systems. People who receive shiatsu often report relief from a variety of complaints, including low back pain, sinus problems, constipation, and premenstrual syndrome.

When to Avoid Shiatsu

Shiatsu therapy can be used by nearly anyone. However, there are some instances in which it should be avoided, or caution should be exercised in its use. You should not receive shiatsu if you have cancer. It should also be avoided if you suffer from brittle bones or are on cortisone treatment, which weakens the bones. Shiatsu should not be practiced under the influence of alcohol or by anyone with a fever or contagious disease. If you have high blood pressure, you should not receive shiatsu to the abdomen; pregnant women should consult with their doctor before treatment.

—*Thomas Claire*

Resources:

American Oriental Bodywork Therapy Association (AOBTA)
Glendale Executive Campus, Suite 510
1000 White Horse Road
Vorhees, NJ 08043
Tel: (609) 782-1616
Fax: (609) 782-1653
The AOBTA is a professional organization that represents practitioners of a number of different styles of Asian bodywork, including shiatsu.

The Ohashi Institute
P.O. Box 505
Wallace Rd.
Kinderhook, NY 12106
Tel: (800) 810-4190
Fax: (518) 758-6809
The Ohashi Institute has twelve locations in the United States and Europe. It is the leading worldwide educational institute devoted to the teaching and practice of shiatsu, and serves as a bridge between Western and Eastern healing arts.

Further Reading:

Bienfield, Harriet, LAc, and Efrem Korngold, LAc, OMD. *Between Heaven and Earth: A Guide to Chinese Medicine.* New York: Ballantine Books, 1991.

Claire, Thomas, M.A., LMT. *BodyWork: What Type of Massage to Get—and How to Make the Most of It.* New York: William Morrow, 1995.

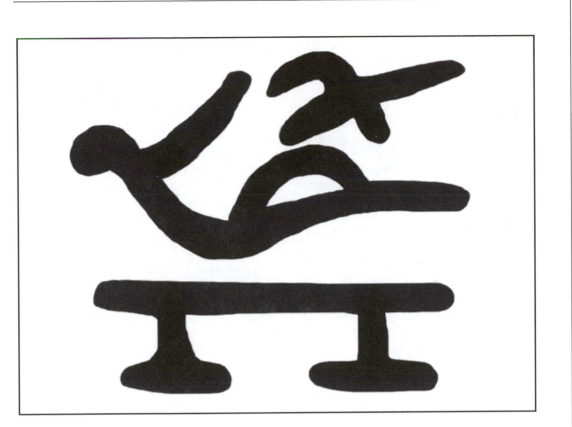

The oldest mention of bodywork in Chinese texts is more than 4,000 years old and looks like this.

Connelly, Dianne M., Ph.D., MAc. *Traditional Acupuncture: The Law of the Five Elements.* Columbia, MD: The Centre for Traditional Acupuncture, 1989.

Haas, Elson M., M.D. *Staying Healthy with the Seasons.* Berkeley, CA: Celestial Arts, 1981.

Ohashi, Wataru. *Do-It-Yourself Shiatsu: How to Perform the Ancient Japanese Art of "Acupuncture Without Needles."* New York: E. P. Dutton, 1976.

Ohashi, Wataru, with Tom Monte. *Reading the Body: Ohashi's Book of Oriental Diagnosis.* New York: Arkana, 1991.

Tui Na

Tui na is an ancient form of massage used for maintaining and improving health, to cure disease, and to relieve pain. It is one of several methods recommended by traditional Chinese medical philosophy, now commonly referred to as traditional Chinese medicine. The philosophy of traditional Chinese medicine and the methods that it recommends are holistic in nature, viewing the health of an individual as affected by three equally important and interconnected aspects of our being: body, mind, and spirit. Practitioners of tui na manipulate the physical body by pushing, pulling, pinching, and tapping on it. The goal is to affect the flow and balance of the vital energy called *qi*, which according to Chinese philosophy flows through our bodies and affects the health of mind, body, and spirit.

The History of Tui Na
Chinese massage can be dated as far back as 4,000 years ago. Archaeologists have discovered an early form of Chinese writing dating to this time that looks more like pictograms than the

sophisticated characters used today. In this early form of writing they have found what they believe are mentions of massage.

Some experts have concluded from this evidence that massage was developed to an extent that it was used and discussed at the court of the emperor, where all writing took place.

Massage is also mentioned in the oldest existing medical text, *Huang-ti Nei Ching (The Yellow Emperor's Classic of Internal Medicine)*. This text was compiled during the Han Dynasty in China, which spanned 206 BCE to 240 CE. Some experts believe that the *Huang-ti Nei Ching* documents practices that had been handed down verbally for thousands of years, from the time of the legendary reign of the Yellow Emperor in China (2697–2595 BCE), suggesting that medical massage may be up to 5,000 years old.

Massage evolved to such a point that in the fifth century CE, a doctoral degree was created for it at the Imperial College of Medicine in Xian, the ancient capital of the Tang Dynasty. Massage was originally called *moshou*, which means "hand rubbing," then became known as *anmo* which means "press and rub," and by the Ming Dynasty (1368–1644) the name *tui na*, meaning "push and grasp," was used.

During the Republican period (1911–1949) in China all forms of traditional medicine were overshadowed by Western allopathic medicine. Traditional medical practices gained a reputation as folk medicine, and more and more young people began to study and practice Western medicine. With the establishment of the People's Republic in 1949, the government made an effort to gather and systematize traditional medical practices under the heading Traditional Chinese Medicine and to integrate Chinese and Western healing methods. Today in China clinics are available for both styles of healing, and patients can choose where they want to go. In addition, many hospitals use a combination of Western allopathic and traditional practices to create the most effective treatment.

How Tui Na Works

All of the treatment methods of traditional Chinese medicine, including tui na, take a holistic view of humans as composed of inseparable components of body, mind, and spirit. The principles of traditional Chinese medicine are influenced by the naturalist school of Taoism, which emphasizes a lifestyle based on moderation and harmony with natural cycles. According to Taoism, the highest ideals of human attainment—wisdom, serenity, and compassion—come with age. So this medical system seeks to maintain health and vitality into old age. There is a strong focus on preventing disease.

According to the traditional Chinese medical theory, a major component of life is called *qi*, a vital life energy that is in constant motion through channels in our bodies. If *qi* is deficient, excessive, or stagnant we feel dis-ease, which can eventually lead to disease. Tui na uses a variety of hand techniques—massaging the body, applying pressure to specific points that affect the *qi*, and holding the body in certain poses. These techniques act on the *qi* to move and invigorate it and restore balance in the individual's whole self.

Experiencing Tui Na

In a typical session, a tui na practitioner will use traditional Chinese medicine's

Physicians in traditional Chinese medicine have always been required to demonstrate a mastery of bodywork to increase their digital sensitivity for competent palpatory and assessment skills. Today in China, massage is a doctoral study that takes five to six years to complete.

four methods of evaluation—looking, listening/smelling, asking, and touching to gather information about the patient. Practitioners believe that interior disharmonies can appear in the exterior of the self and that exterior stresses can affect the interior of the self. Since all aspects of life and behavior reflect the other, all are important to the therapist, including specific complaints, pain, movement patterns, sleep and dietary patterns, lifestyle, etc. The massage therapist will seek to weave all the data together to see the entire tapestry of the patient's energetic landscape. That is, to determine how the *qi* is flowing, where it may be blocked or stagnant, and how this is affecting the individual as a whole.

After the assessment, the therapist will choose specific points, pathways, and hand techniques to create a massage that is specifically helpful for that patient on that day. The hand techniques can vary from gentle stroking to firm grasping and pinching with innumerable combinations and possibilities. The session can last for thirty to sixty minutes. The therapist's intention during this session is to see some immediate change and lay the groundwork for long-term progress.

Benefits and Risks

In China tui na is used as a health maintenance program, to treat chronic stress-related problems, such as headaches, insomnia, and stomach disorders; illnesses, such as asthma and arthritis; and injuries, such as sprains. Patients often feel an increase in energy, relief from pain, diminished fevers, improvements in digestion and sleep, and a regulation of the processes of the internal organs. Tui na is not recommended for fractures, in the case of infections, or when there are open wounds or lesions on the body.

Tui na is a quickly growing therapy in the United States, with licensed practitioners available throughout the country.

Because tui na is considered a complementary therapy to Western scientific medicine, each state regulates it differently. Always check to see if your practitioner is state licensed and/or nationally certified. This will ensure that he or she is adequately trained and familiar with pathologies and conditions that make this treatment inadvisable.

—*Gina Martin*

Resources:

The American Oriental Bodywork Therapy Association (AOBTA)
Glendale Executive Campus, Ste. 510
1000 White Horse Rd.
Vorhees, NJ 08043
Tel: (609) 782-1616
Fax: (516) 364-5559
Web site: www.healthy.net/pan/pa/bodywork
The AOBTA is a national organization of bodyworkers in eleven different styles. They certify practitioners, teachers, and schools throughout the United States. The organization enforces minimum entry-level standards (500 hours) for all types of Oriental bodyworkers. Currently represents about 1,200 members.

The Swedish Institute of Massage Therapy and Allied Health Sciences
226 W. 26th St.
New York, NY 10010
Tel: (212) 924-5900
Master Jeffrey Yuen, and licensed massage therapists Reggie Crosan, Alix Kasat, Paula Chin, Tom Banaciak, and Gina Martin offer classes and sessions.

Further Reading:

Chengnan, S., ed. *Chinese Bodywork: A Complete Manual of Chinese Therapeutic Massage.* Berkeley, CA: Pacific View Press, 1990.

Eisenberg, D., and T. L. Wright. *Encounters with Qi: Exploring Chinese Medicine.* Rev. ed., New York: W. W. Norton, 1995.

PART IX: MOVEMENT THERAPY METHODS

Alexander Technique • Aston-Patterning® • Bartenieff Fundamentals • Body-Mind Centering® • Feldenkrais Method® • Hanna Somatic Education® • Hellerwork • Ideokinesis • Kinetic Awareness • Meir Schneider Self-Healing Method • Sensory Awareness • Soma Neuromuscular Integration • Somato Respiratory Integration • Trager Psychophysical Integration

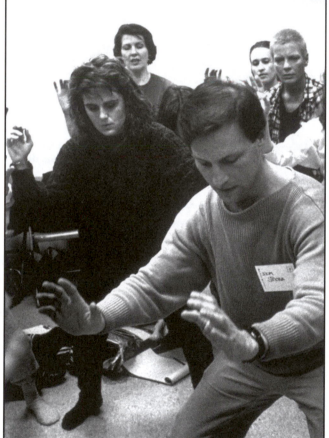

Photo: © Joel Gordon

Movement therapies enhance the whole person by expanding his or her ability to move.

Movement therapy methods are disciplines that seek to relieve pain, improve physical performance, and increase the potential for emotional and creative expression by developing awareness of body movement and repatterning it. These methods are part of a larger group of methods that have come to be known collectively as bodywork, a general term describing a wide variety of methods that use touch and movement to improve awareness of feelings and sensations in the body and improve physical functioning. Bodywork methods are also used to relieve pain and encourage relaxation.

There are many disciplines in this book that are included in the bodywork category. They can be found in the sections entitled Acupuncture and Asian Bodywork, Body-Oriented Psychotherapies, Massage, Skeletal Manipulation Methods, Somatic Practices, and Subtle Energy Therapies. Movement therapy methods are distinguished from other bodywork methods by their use of the process of movement itself as their primary diagnostic and therapeutic tool.

In addition to believing in the primacy of the curative and life-enhancing value of movement, these disciplines share certain common origins. They were all developed in the West in the twentieth century. Many of the originators of these disciplines were driven by the urgent need to solve their own physical health problems. In doing so they each recognized a lack of mental awareness of body movement patterns as a root cause of their symptoms. Eventually each found a way to teach his or her unique path of discovery to others.

Pioneers in Movement Therapy

There is no single figure who can be credited with the start of the field of movement therapy. Like the invention of the telephone, movement therapy is an idea that was developed simultaneously by several people working separately in different parts of the world. At the turn of the century F. M. Alexander (1869–1955), an Australian actor, developed a method for freeing the body of excess tension and changing inefficient movement patterns while searching for a cure for his own recurring loss of voice. He named his method the Alexander technique.

Working just a little later in time and several continents away, a young German woman, Elsa Gindler (1885–1961), developed her method of "restorative observation" as a cure for her own life-threatening bout with tuberculosis. Later, while working as a young movement educator, Gindler met the musician and teacher Heinrich Jacoby (1889–1964). He was exploring teaching methods that addressed the effects of mental attitudes on performance. They combined their ideas and methods to create sensory awareness, a practice designed to "free people from conditioned habits, fears, and tensions."

At about the same time that Gindler was curing herself of tuberculosis, an American teenager, Mable Elsworth Todd (?–1956), was teaching herself to walk and move normally after a severe back injury. The methods she discovered became the basis of her private dance education practice and eventually the method known as ideokinesis. All three of these tireless educators introduced thousands of people, many of whom were performers, to a whole new way of integrating their bodies and minds for optimum efficiency and expressiveness performance.

A second wave of movement therapy methods occurred in the 1940s and 1950s. At this time performing artists such as Irmgard Bartenieff (1900–1981) were exploring the ways in which body and mind interact in the process of movement. But people from other fields also turned their attention to the connection between movement and health, such as Milton Trager, an athlete, and Moshe Feldenkrais, a physicist and engineer. While some of these pioneers continued to be driven by self-healing needs, others were responding to mass healing crises, such as the polio epidemic of the 1940s. This helped take movement therapy beyond the performing arts, directly into the world of health care.

In the 1960s and 1970s a third wave of movement therapy methods was developed by performing artists, engineers, a philosopher, healers, and people from the established medical profession. Most of these explorers were students of second-wave founders, and the new disciplines they created were firmly rooted in the principles and theories of their teachers. Many individuals developing new methods were deeply influenced by Dr. Ida Rolf, making use of Rolf's method of physically manipulating the tissue covering the muscles (see entry on Rolfing for more information on this discipline). For example, Joseph Heller, the founder of Hellerwork, and Drs. Bill and Ellen Williams, the founders of soma neuromuscular integration, combined Rolf's methods with movement exercises and psychological processing techniques to bring greater levels of body-mind integration to the process of healing and maintaining health through movement.

In the late 1990s many of the organizations that support the teaching and professional activities of the various methods described in this section banded together under the umbrella of the International Somatic Movement Therapy and Education Association (ISMTEA). ISMTEA aims to increase public awareness of the value of movement therapy in health and education and to insure quality among movement therapists. Recently ISMTEA petitioned and won the right from the U.S. government to include the title Registered Movement Therapist® among the official U.S. Department of Labor occupational titles. This step integrates movement therapy methods further into the mainstream of American health care practices.

Unifying Principles of Movement Therapy

Movement therapists stress the fact that the living body is in constant motion. From the subtle expanding and contracting motions of breathing to the more obvious exertion of muscles during strenuous activity, efficient movement is believed by movement therapists to be crucial for human health. And since movement therapists see the human being as an integrated combination of physical, mental, and emotional aspects, all body movement is seen as related to the emotional life of the mover.

Inefficient and painful movement patterns are seen as creative coping mechanisms that our body and mind develop to deal with traumatic experiences or chronically stressful physical or emotional situations. Learning to move painlessly or more freely and expressively is often an "unlearning" process by which our individual, intuitive coping strategies can be relinquished in favor of patterns that work more harmoniously with natural forces such as gravity and with the physical realities of our bodies.

The first step in this educational process is to become aware of habitual movement patterns that are restrictive and counterproductive. Some of these may be very deep and subtle such as holding our breath when we want to exert our strength. Since oxygen is essential to the functioning of our muscles, holding our breath will only frustrate our efforts. Most methods use some form of touch to help develop awareness of counterproductive patterns. Many employ forms of manipulation that have grown out of specific bodywork, or massage practices.

The second stage in the movement therapy education process is described by ISMTEA as "gaining increased awareness and control over basic psycho-physiological processes which can begin to correct restrictive habit patterns and can lead toward optimal body-mind performance." For instance, as you continue to explore your ability to exert force in a powerful tennis serve, for example, you may become aware of a buried psychological reason that causes you to hold your breath and prevents you from releasing all your power into the serve.

While all the methods described in this section of the encyclopedia believe that human beings have all the internal self-healing mechanisms they need to develop the increased awareness of the second stage of the movement therapy education process, different methods will approach this stage of movement education in different ways. Some methods, like sensory awareness, believe that solely developing consciousness of your physical sensations without taking any subsequent action will stimulate the self-correcting mechanisms. Most methods, however, teach that a conscious control over movement patterns is necessary to achieve a complete change and healing. In most methods it is believed that this conscious control will eventually function on an unconscious level. This occurs through a repatterning of the messages your brain sends to your muscles via your nervous system.

The third level of learning in the movement therapy model is to be able to express these new movement patterns in all your daily activities. To help you do this, movement therapists might recommend certain exercises that you practice at home. They might help you find visual images that will help you perform particular movements more efficiently. They may help you evaluate lifestyle practices such as the kind of shoes you wear, or the arrangement of your study area, which could also be negatively affecting your performance.

Finally it is the goal of all movement therapists to help you learn to be self-reliant so that you can continue developing without their help. Mastering the three preceding levels of learning can help you develop new physical and mental awareness, along with newly ingrained neuromuscular reflex patterns that allow you greater freedom, ease, and pleasure living in your moving body.

—Nancy Allison, CMA

Resources:

International Somatic Movement Education and
  Therapy Association
148 W. 23rd Street, #1H
New York, NY 10011
Tel: (212) 229-7666

The Somatics Society
1516 Grant Avenue, Suite 212
Novato, CA 94945
Tel: (415) 892-0617
Fax: (415) 892-4388
Organization offering seminars and information
for all movement therapy educators. Publishes the
biannual magazine-journal Somatics.

Further Reading:

Claire, Thomas. *Bodywork: What Type of Massage to Get—And How to Make the Most of It.* New York: William Morrow, 1995.

Knaster, Mirka. *Discovering the Body's Wisdom.* New York: Bantam Books, 1996.

ALEXANDER TECHNIQUE

The Alexander technique is a method used to help people illuminate their unconscious patterns of body tension and correct habits that cause physical and emotional problems. It is used to allow a person to pattern his or her body's movement, inhibiting habits that cause tension or pain and replacing them with those that help his or her body to function more efficiently. Teachers of the Alexander technique believe that people can gain greater control over the way they use their bodies once these habitual movements are brought to consciousness. An individual may then apply new and healthier ways of using his or her body to improve the performance of activities in his or her life. For almost a century this technique has been used to help people find relief from many chronic painful conditions and to help performing artists and athletes expand their potential.

The History of the Alexander Technique

The Alexander technique was developed by Frederick Matthias Alexander (1869–1955), an Australian actor who experienced a recurring loss of his voice. Through ten years of self-observation and experimentation with the aid of a three-way mirror, he observed that the manner in which he was breathing and holding his head was the source of his difficulties. He was able to correct his voice problems by altering his posture, muscular reaction patterns, and behavior. In addition, he observed that these changes improved his physical health, emotional outlook, and the balance throughout his body. Pursuing his findings further, Alexander began to study the way the body functioned during various activities, looking for signs of misalignment or misuse of his own muscular-skeletal system. He discerned that mental and physical habits, acquired early in life, often control one's everyday movements. Over time, Alexander developed a technique for breaking inefficient and counterproductive habits and replacing them with conscious, constructive control. Throughout the rest of his life, Alexander taught his technique in England. Today there are more than 3,000 certified Alexander teachers worldwide, teaching privately or in schools, institutions, and corporations.

The Theory of the Alexander Technique

Alexander believed that the alignment of the head, neck, and spine was the most important relationship within the body, affecting the functioning of the entire body and mind. He called the relationship of head to neck the "primary control" and found it to be the integrating force for all movement. Alexander believed that from an early age constant stress and accommodation to both physical and emotional environments caused people to distrust the natural alignment and integration of the head and neck. According to Alexander's theories, by the time a person is fully grown he or she establishes patterns of postural and muscular-skeletal distortion that give him or her uniquely identifiable movement characteristics, but also contribute greatly to his or her individual physical and emotional problems.

Through his extensive self-examination process, Alexander found that proper positioning of the head creates a reflexive lengthening of the spine, which stimulates a gentle upward release, relieving forces of compression throughout the entire body. Compression can be responsible for tight muscles, poor breathing, tightness or constriction around the joints, and for poor communication throughout the nervous system. Because the nervous system, which consists of the brain, the spinal cord, and the nerves, is the communication system for the whole self, poor communication can lead to disorders including headaches, backaches, stomachaches, and even low self-esteem.

Alexander believed that all people could develop conscious awareness of their distorted muscular-skeletal patterns.

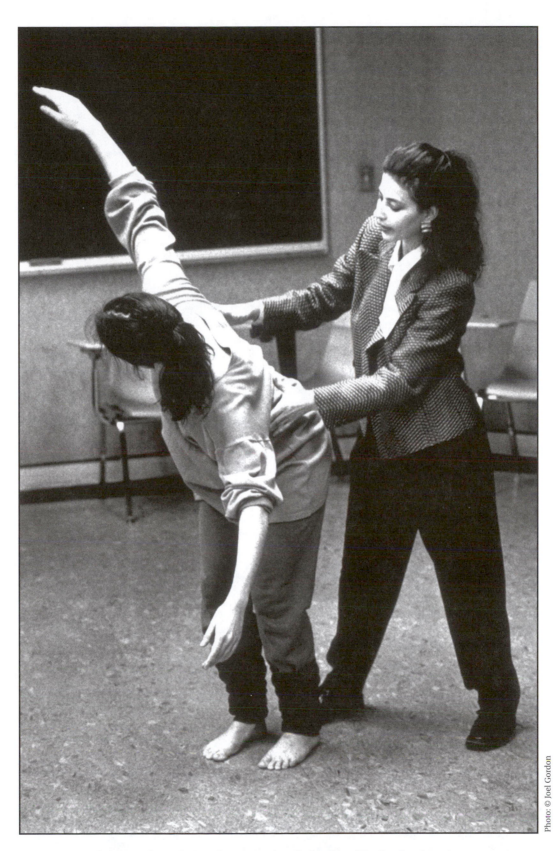

The Alexander technique focuses on the relationship of the head to the spine.

By developing that awareness, people could learn to resist or inhibit old, restrictive, or dysfunctional patterns and thereby allow the body to function and develop effectively and effortlessly.

The Alexander Technique in Practice

Experts in the Alexander technique are called teachers, since the process of therapy is considered a reeducation of the body. A teacher seeks to equip students with the skills to recognize and modify movement patterns used in basic activities. During a session the student is led through a sequence of simple exercises such as sitting, walking, bending, or even crawling to help him or her become aware of the body's movement. The student receives both verbal and hands-on instruction. A teacher may use touch to place a student's body in proper alignment. At the same time, a teacher may verbally reinforce a student and direct him or her toward better posture and movement. These activities are gentle and painless. The teacher's goal is to familiarize a student with proper body alignment and patterns of motion, allowing him or her to use the lessons independently. The specific exercises that a person experiences in a session will be designed according to the activities that he or she wants to improve. For example, athletes, actors, singers, or musicians will want to focus on motions and parts of the body that are used in each activity. The emphasis throughout is on self-awareness and improved control.

The Benefits of the Alexander Technique

The result of Alexander lessons is often a sense of greater lightness, vitality, and well-being. Participants commonly report greater ease of motion, greater flexibility, and relief of pain. The technique is frequently used by people with chronic neck and spinal injuries and disorders, including scoliosis. Athletes, dancers, and other performing artists have found that it enhances physical functioning and creativity.

—*Diane Young*

Resources:

The American Center for the Alexander Technique, Inc.
129 West 67th Street
New York, NY 10023
Tel: (212) 799-0468
The oldest Alexander technique training center in the United States.

North American Society of Teachers of the Alexander Technique (NASTAT)
3010 Hennepin Avenue South, Suite 10
Minneapolis, MN 55408
Tel: (800) 473-0620
Fax: (612) 822-7224
e-mail: nastat@ix.netcom.com
Offers information on practitioners, training programs, reading lists, and other materials.

Further Reading:

Alexander, F. M. *Constructive Conscious Control of the Individual.* 1923. Reprint. Long Beach, CA: Centerline Press, 1985.

———. *The Alexander Technique: The Essential Writings of F. Matthias Alexander,* ed. Edward Maisel. New York: Lyle Stuart, 1990.

A session in the Alexander technique generally lasts from thirty minutes to an hour. A series of twenty to thirty sessions, conducted once or twice a week, is typically recommended. People who have a poorly developed kinesthetic sense, or sense of movement, may take a longer time to become aware of their body movement.

Barlow, Wilfred. *The Alexander Technique: How to Use Your Body Without Stress.* Rochester, VT: Healing Arts Press, 1990.

Caplan, Deborah. *Back Trouble: A New Approach to Prevention and Recovery.* Gainesville, FL: Triad Publishing. 1987.

Gray, John. *Your Guide to the Alexander Technique.* New York: St. Martin's Press, 1990.

ASTON-PATTERNING®

Aston-Patterning® (A-P) is an educational system developed by Judith Aston based on more than thirty years of teaching and life experience. The Aston process combines bodywork, movement education, fitness, and ergonomics. Ergonomics is a method of arranging living and work areas so that they are used most efficiently and safely. A-P may be used as a rehabilitative process for those seeking relief from acute or chronic pain, and it is also used to assist people who wish to improve posture, athletic performance, or overall efficiency in daily living activities.

The Theory of Aston-Patterning®

Aston-Patterning practitioners look at the alignment of your body, the ways that you move, and areas of tension and discomfort in your movements. They believe that everyday activities—at work, school, and home—athletics, injuries, and emotional history all work together to develop patterns of movement in your body. Some of these patterns are easy on the body and some are not. They may be caused by reactions to injuries, by physical reactions to emotional distress, or by physical environments that are improperly designed. By understanding individual patterns, A-P practitioners provide sessions that are highly individualized and produce positive changes in posture and movement habits that are long-lasting.

Traditionally, medical understanding of body alignment has been based on a linear model. Lines are drawn up and down or side to side to define alignment. Movement is traditionally perceived as symmetrical—that is, balanced equally on each side. In contrast, Aston models of the body have volume—they are three-dimensional. When looking at alignment and movement, consideration is given to the unique length, width, and depth of each body. Aston concepts also consider the body's internal structure, which is naturally asymmetrical. It has the heart on the left, the liver on the right, and although there are paired organs (i.e., lungs), each has its own shape and size. Therefore, A-P practitioners believe that since we are naturally asymmetrical, movement needs to be slightly asymmetrical in response to this internal design. A-P practitioners use this information to help individuals find their body's natural alignment and to recommend efficient, tension-free ways to move.

What Happens in an Aston-Patterning® Session?

Aston-Patterning sessions are customized to individuals' interests, taking into account their own unique patterns created by their histories. This method requires that each client take an active role in his or her process of change. Throughout a session, one wears comfortable clothing and may be asked to perform a variety of movements—sitting, standing, or lying down—as the A-P practitioner assesses his or her three-dimensional body shape, movement, and muscular tensions. This information is used to design a program of therapy to release the muscular tension and reeducate the body for a new, efficient movement pattern. These new patterns are practiced, and once learned, are applied to the person's goals and interests.

Each well-rounded session includes a blend of pain-free bodywork, movement coaching, fitness training, and ergonomics. Massage tables, padded stools, and lotions are used for releasing patterns of

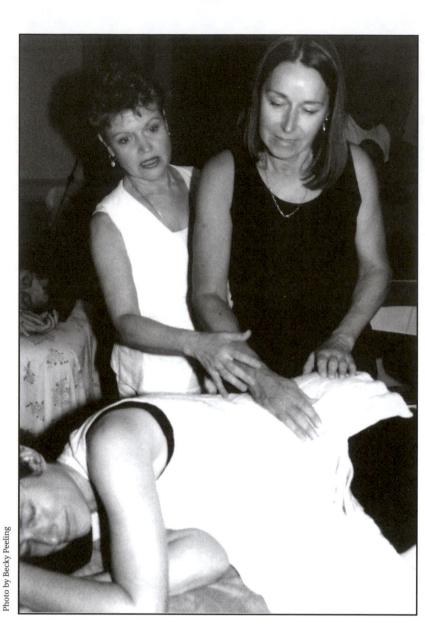

Photo by Becky Peeling

Through touch, Judith Aston teaches the bodywork techniques used in Aston-Patterning.

muscle tension. Stools, stretch cords, toning platforms, and exercise and ergonomic equipment are used to help clients be more aware of where their body is in space. This equipment is also used to improve alignment and body mechanics and increase overall fitness. Mirrors and skeleton models play a part in the visual education and explanation during a client session. Special foam wedges (designed by Aston) help clients modify their environment (car seat backs, office chairs, etc.) to support the new, more efficient alignment.

Private A-P sessions are normally one and a half to two hours long. Though sessions are most effective when offered as a series, they may also be beneficial on a one-time basis. Group lessons or clinics are also available, offered for a wide variety of applications from athletics to daily activities.

How Aston-Patterning® Developed

Aston-Patterning is named after its founder, Judith Aston. She earned a bachelor's degree in fine arts at UCLA, with a specialization in dance therapy. She completed her master's degree at UCLA in 1965, with emphasis in theater, psychology, and dance. During this time Aston also earned a lifetime teaching credential in secondary education. Her teachings focused on the relationship between dance movement and the movements encountered in everyday life.

Aston believed that "there must be a better way" to teach movement. On one occasion Aston had a student, a track athlete, who had reluctantly enrolled in her ballroom dancing course to meet college requirements. Though the young man was consistently able to post record times on the track, he had two left feet on the dance floor. When traditional teaching methods failed, Aston tried a very different approach. She took the student out to the track, where she carefully observed his running style and his movement patterns. Aston asked him to sprint, then jog—also requesting that he run forward, then backward, and to run left, then right. She used her creative skills to integrate the young man's individual running patterns into dance patterns. Before long, they were dancing the foxtrot right on the running track. This and similar success stories led Judith Aston to focus on the "how-tos" of teaching. By understanding that "what you teach" is not as important as "how you teach it," Aston realized incredible results.

In 1966 Aston was in a car accident that caused severe whiplash and significant tissue injuries to her neck and back. Another accident the following year made her condition worse. Doctors recommended that she undergo surgery but Aston looked for an alternative solution. One doctor suggested Aston get in touch with Dr. Ida Rolf, who was at the Esalen Institute in Big Sur, California. Rolf, founder of the Rolfing system, was a respected expert in the field of soft-tissue mobilization. Rolf was interested in Aston's education background, and at Rolf's request, Aston developed the first movement education system to be used at the Rolf Institute.

In the late 1960s, Aston expanded her knowledge of movement therapy by completing massage training and Rolfing studies. As she continued to practice her own theories, she began to move away from traditional Rolfing principles, especially in regard to her perception of the body and movement as asymmetrical rather than symmetrical. By 1977, Judith Aston had developed her own basic classes in movement and bodywork and trademarked the title "Aston-Patterning."

The Benefits of Aston-Patterning®

Aston-Patterning can help individuals use their bodies more efficiently and become aware of stressful movements that can be harmful to the body. Because it focuses on relearning how to use the body more efficiently, it is used as a rehabilitative therapy for those seeking relief from acute or chronic pain. It is also used to assist people who wish to improve posture, athletic performance, or overall efficiency of movement in activities of daily living. Many people who have been through Aston-Patterning have reported that sessions help them to "better understand their own bodies." As a result, these people seem to enjoy long-lasting benefits.

—*Allison Funk,*
Certified Aston-Patterning Practitioner

Resources:

The Aston Training Center (ATC)
P.O. Box 3568
Incline Village, NV 89450-3568
Tel: (702) 831-8228
Fax: (702) 831-8955
Provides printed material and course descriptions upon request. Courses include two- to five-day options. A twenty-one-week practitioner training is

offered every two years. Also offers information about A-P practitioners or classes in specific areas of the country.

Further Reading:

Aston, Judith. "Your Ideal Body." *Physical Therapy Today*, Summer 1991, Vol. 14, No. 2, pp. 30, 32, 34, 36.

Aston, Judith, and Jeff Low. "Your Three-Dimensional Body: The Aston System of Body Usage, Movement, and Fitness." *Physical Therapy Today*, Fall 1993, Vol. 16, No. 3, pp. 50–59.

Brody, Liz. "Axling: A New Spin on Fitness." *Shape*, April 1993, Vol. 12, No. 8, pp. 80–84.

Calvert, Robert. "Exclusive Interview with Judith Aston, Developer of Aston-Patterning Bodywork." *Massage.* Issue 16, October-November, 1988, pp. 12–13, 15, 17–19.

Cook, Jennifer. "Body Ease." *Self.* December 1985, p. 146.

Low, Jeffrey. "The Modern Body Therapies." *Massage*, Issue 16, October-November, 1988, pp. 48–50, 52, 54–55.

Richardson, Nancy, R.P.T. "Aston-Patterning," *Physical Therapy Forum*, October 28, 1987, Vol. VI, No. 43, pp. 1, 3.

Servid, Laura. "Aston-Patterning: Accessing the Power of the Ground." *P.T. and O.T. Today*, July 21, 1997, pp. 18–22.

Woods, Jenna. "Forces of Nature in the Aston Paradigm: Key Concepts of Aston-Patterning." *Massage and Bodywork*, Spring 1997, pp. 123–25.

——. "A Patterns Tale: Moving into Aston-Patterning." *Massage and Bodywork*, Fall, 1996, pp. 95–97.

BARTENIEFF FUNDAMENTALS^{SM}

Bartenieff Fundamentals[SM] are a set of movements that reinforce efficient communication between the mind and body as the body moves. The Fundamentals were developed by Irmgard Bartenieff, a German dancer, choreographer, and physical therapist. A person trained in Bartenieff Fundamentals is able to observe an individual's movement style and diagnose what makes that individual struggle or succeed with certain movements. Fundamentals are used by people who are recovering from injuries or coping with physical limitations caused by illness. Athletes, dancers, and people involved in fitness training use the Fundamentals to improve their coordination and overall performance.

The History of Bartenieff Fundamentals^{SM}

Bartenieff (1900–1981) studied biology, art, and dance before beginning her diploma studies in Berlin with Rudolf Laban in 1925. Laban was a Hungarian movement theorist, choreographer, and teacher responsible for introducing several influential theories about the nature of movement. Laban created a system to observe, record, and analyze all types of movement including dance, the martial arts, and everyday actions. Bartenieff emigrated to America in 1936 and began applying her knowledge of human movement to help the ill and the injured. She studied physical therapy at New York University and began working in that field. She also explored the therapeutic possibilities of dance, helping to found the field of dance therapy.

Bartenieff is known for the innovations in physical therapy she developed in the 1940s and 1950s while she worked as chief physical therapist for the Polio Service of New York City at Willard Parker Hospital and later at an orthopedic hospital for children. An epidemic of polio had swept America, crippling many children and adults. To help these physically challenged individuals, Bartenieff drew from her knowledge of physical therapy and what she had learned from Laban about the dynamics of movement and how the mover can interact with the full circumference of space that surrounds him. She developed the Fundamentals to help polio patients regain their full range of movement. In traditional physical therapy, the therapist manipulates the limbs of a patient who remains, for the most part, passive. Bartenieff insisted that her patients take an active role mentally, physically, and emotionally in the movement sequences she designed to increase their mobility. Her methods were successful, and her patients progressed more rapidly than those treated by traditional physical therapy.

Bartenieff first called her method "Correctives," a term doctors used to describe orthopedic exercises for correcting posture and the alignment of the spine. But the movement sequences Bartenieff perfected were more than isolated exercises. She renamed them Bartenieff Fundamentals because she saw them as the building blocks of all human movement. She referred to the movements as "sequences" rather than "exercises" because she wanted to emphasize that a mover should always be thinking about each movement and its connection to the next; never should a mover simply count the number of repetitions. Doing the Fundamentals properly, she believed, helps the mover restore efficient neuromuscular pathways, the communication channels between muscle, nerve, bone and breath within the body.

To promote her method and the theories of Laban, Bartenieff founded the Laban Institute of Movement Studies in New York City. Since the 1960s, Bartenieff and other Laban movement analysts, who are the only certified Bartenieff Fundamentals practitioners, have helped athletes, actors, dancers, musicians, children, and adults. Some use the Fundamentals to recover from injuries, others to improve or polish their performance in a sport or specialized movement skill. Today there are more than 800 certified Laban movement analysts (CMAs) practicing throughout the world.

The Theory of Bartenieff Fundamentals^{SM}

Like Laban, Bartenieff approached movement as requiring a person's commitment on a physical, an emotional, and a mental level. Through his observation of people engaged in such varied activities as t'ai chi ch'üan, folk dancing, and factory assembly line work, Laban developed a system for analyzing movement known as Laban movement analysis (LMA). Laban's system breaks movement into four primary components: body, space, effort (dynamics), and shape. Although Bartenieff Fundamentals promote awareness of all four components, the Fundamentals primarily emphasize the body.

The Fundamentals are developmentally based; that is, they mirror the stages of development of the brain and motor skills that babies and toddlers progress through on their way to mastering mature movement patterns. Practicing the Fundamentals strengthens the body's internal support for both everyday and highly skilled movement. The Fundamentals require the use of deep muscles, close to the core of the body, and the use of breath support to increase the power and flow of movement. They also require a clear spatial intent: an understanding of where movement initiates in the body and how it sequences through the body from one part to another. Practicing Bartenieff Fundamentals helps a mover understand how to initiate and complete a movement efficiently.

By watching a mover perform the Fundamentals, a CMA can identify which body parts do or do not function together smoothly and where movement does or does not flow in the body. Astute observation skills allow a CMA to tailor movement sequences specifically for an individual who wants to address problem areas and meet goals for improvement.

Experiencing Bartenieff Fundamentals^{SM}

Fundamentals are taught in groups or in one-on-one sessions that usually take place in a studio with a wooden floor. Participants should wear clothing that allows freedom of movement. The Fundamentals are usually done lying on the floor. There the individual more easily becomes aware of the body's parts, the center of weight, and how it relates to the initiation of action. Without the struggle against gravity or interaction with the environment or other people, the individual can focus mentally on what is going on in the body. In addition to demonstrating the movement sequences clearly, CMAs often use imagery to help students understand movement qualities or to sense more readily how the movement should flow through the body. Using a hands-on technique, CMAs also guide students in performing the movement sequences correctly, drawing attention to where in the body the movement begins.

Although there are many variations of Bartenieff Fundamentals, the most commonly known are "the basic six." They are thigh lift (hip flexion), pelvic forward shift, pelvic lateral shift, vertical body half, knee drop, and arm circle. All practitioners use these six sequences to analyze movement. They also develop variations based on the principles of Bartenieff Fundamentals to address specific problems. Because the Fundamentals provide the foundation for so many other actions, they look simple. However, once people begin to study them, they find that moving from the core of the body without excess tension is not easy. Most people tend to move inefficiently. Often they don't notice their inefficient habit until a teacher, a coach, or an injury brings it to their attention.

Benefits

Studying Bartenieff Fundamentals helps an individual learn to move more easily and more expressively. Athletes from many sports have improved their performance and reduced the risk of injury after incorporating Bartenieff Fundamentals into their training. Dancers,

actors, and musicians have found that practice of the Fundamentals brings greater clarity and expression to their performances. People rehabilitating from injuries and other conditions that limit mobility have used the Fundamentals to regain functional and expressive movements. Others practice the Fundamentals simply for the joy they experience from moving more fluidly and with greater ease.

—Janet Hamburg, CMA

Resources:

Laban/Bartenieff Institute of Movement Studies
234 Fifth Avenue
New York, NY 10001
Tel: (212) 477-4299
Offers classes in Bartenieff Fundamentals and certification programs in Laban movement analysis.

Further Reading:

Bartenieff, Irmgard, and Dori Lewis. *Body Movement: Coping with the Environment.* New York: Gordon and Breach Science Publishers, Inc., 1980.

Laban, Rudolf. *The Mastery of Movement.* Rev. and enlarged by Lisa Ullman. Boston: Plays, Inc., 1971.

———. *The Language of Movement: A Guidebook to Choreutics.* Lisa Ullman, ed. Boston: Plays, Inc., 1974.

BODY-MIND CENTERING®

Body-Mind Centering® is a therapeutic and educational system combining movement, vocal, perceptual, and hands-on work with the study of life's physiological, psychological, and developmental processes.

Body-Mind Centering can help one to balance one's inner and outer experience in the context of one's environment. While the work itself does not directly treat symptoms, by creating new options for listening and responding to one's own body and the external environment, Body-Mind Centering promotes self-healing and enhances one's quality of life.

The Founding of Body-Mind Centering®

Body-Mind Centering was developed during the 1960s by American Bonnie Bainbridge Cohen, who studied occupational therapy at Ohio State University. She continued her studies in England, where she was certified as a neurodevelopmental therapist. She was also certified as a Laban movement analyst and as a Kestenberg movement profiler. Bainbridge Cohen's professional background and her interests in dance, martial arts, and yoga are reflected in her work, which combines Eastern and Western approaches to relating mind and body. By the late 1960s her work had begun to influence the fields of dance and body and movement therapies. In 1973 she founded the School for Body-Mind Centering to train and certify practitioners and teachers.

Integration of Mind and Body

Bainbridge Cohen has compared the relationship of mind and body to wind blowing sand. She said, "The mind is like the wind and the body is like the sand. If you want to know how the wind is blowing, look at the sand." (Bainbridge Cohen, *Program Guide for Body-Mind Centering Certification Program*, 1994). This kind of interrelationship is at the heart of Body-Mind Centering. Relationship is a key and multilayered principle in this work, where the mind and body are engaged in a dynamic, interactive process that shapes the development of the organism. Fundamental to this process is the interaction between the systems of the body and one's movement development.

Body-Mind Centering identifies seven body systems (skeletal, ligamentous, muscular, organ, endocrine, fluids, and nervous), each contributing independently to the expression of the body-mind, and at the same time balancing and interacting with all the other systems, creating a unique expressive quality for each individual.

Although a Body-Mind Centering approach to study of the systems of the body may entail lessons in anatomy through pictures, models, and movement, it does not view the body as an object to be brought under the control of the intellect. This approach is based on the premise that the body has a wisdom of its own, and Body-Mind Centering seeks to mobilize and support this wisdom. This inner knowing is manifested in both a new awareness of the body-mind and a greater vitality and coherence among its various parts. The resonance of the voice, for example, is used to reach down into the torso to arouse the visceral organs and to promote integration of the inner and outer structures of the body—a key for gaining awareness of and healing the body.

The bones of the skeletal system are studied by means of illustrations and models and by tracing, or palpating, their forms through the skin with the hands. The learning process in Body-Mind Centering interweaves abstract and sensory knowledge of the body's structure, moving toward the goal of enhancing the body's functioning and range of expression.

Body-Mind Centering considers movement the expression of "inner learning" accumulated since infancy, as basic skills (such as breathing, nursing, rolling, crawling, and walking) are acquired and the structure of the organism takes form. How a person moves or even holds his or her body is a reflection of a process of personal evolution. Further, Body-Mind Centering assumes that each stage in human growth underlies and supports the next and must be fully realized if the individual is to achieve the balance and ease needed to withstand

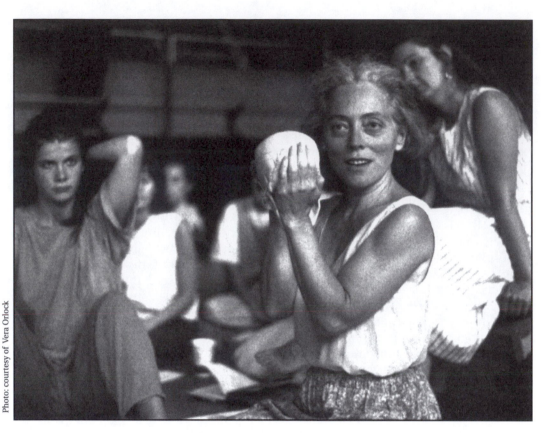

Bonnie Bainbridge Cohen, founder of Body-Mind Centering.

stress and interact with the world in satisfying ways. Conversely, skipped or unintegrated patterns can lead to alignment/movement problems, systems imbalance, and problems in perception, organization, memory, and creativity.

Body-Mind Centering developmental movement sessions can help infants, children, or adults identify developmental gaps and facilitate the learning of any absent patterns, allowing them to realize new potential. These "repatterning" sequences involve exploring the anatomical and psychological ramifications of basic movements, such as breathing, pushing the hands against a surface, or reaching out for what one desires.

A Class in Body-Mind Centering®

Group classes or private sessions in Body-Mind Centering are directed toward the individual's self-discovery and transformation. They may be organized around the specific concerns and goals of the participants, or they may present principles of the work for exploration. A typical class may involve movement or hands-on bodywork to heighten the student's awareness of a specific system or area of his or her body.

The class may also include "repatterning" exercises, study of anatomical illustrations and models, and experiential explorations to increase sensory awareness and integrate that awareness with one's intention and action. The number and frequency of private sessions are determined by the client in consultation with the practitioner. The work is designed to supply insights and skills that can be incorporated into daily experiences.

The Benefits of Body-Mind Centering®

By creating new options for how one senses, feels, and acts in the world,

Body-Mind Centering can help individuals change limiting patterns or attitudes. It can be used to address problems such as headaches, chronic pain, sports injuries, hypertension, eating disorders, and perceptual and learning difficulties. It can also be used as a means to improving flexibility, coordination, creative expression, communication, and sense of self-identity and well-being.

—Vera Orlock

Resources:

The Body-Mind Centering® Association
16 Center St., Suite 530
Northampton, MA 01060
Tel: (413) 582-3617
Organization that promotes the study and use of Body-Mind Centering.

Videotapes:

Bainbridge Cohen, Bonnie (1996). "Experiential Anatomy in the Training of Young Dancers." (Set of two videos on the foot and the pelvis with an accompanying text. Available from SBMC, 189 Pondview Dr., Amherst, MA, 01002.)

Stokes, Beverly. (1995). "Amazing Babies: Moving in the First Year." (Available from Beverly Stokes, 418 St. Claire Ave., E. Toronto, ON, Canada M47 1P5.)

Further Reading:

Bainbridge Cohen, B. *Sensing, Feeling and Action: The Experiential Anatomy of Body-Mind Centering.* Northampton, MA: Contact Editions, 1993.

Grossinger, Richard. *Planet Medicine.* (2 Vols.). Berkeley, CA: North Atlantic Books, 1995.

Hartley, Linda. *The Wisdom of the Body Moving: An Introduction to BodyMind Centering®.* Barrytown, NY: Station Hill Press, 1993.

Johnson, Don Hanlon. *Body, Spirit and Democracy.* Berkeley, CA: North Atlantic Books, 1993.

——. *Bone, Breath and Gesture: Practices of Embodiment.* D. H. Jonson, ed. Berkeley, CA: North Atlantic Books, 1995.

——. *Groundworks: Narratives of Embodiment.* D. H. Jonson, ed. Berkeley, CA: North Atlantic Books, 1997.

Olsen, Andrea, in collaboration with Caryn McHose. *Body Stories: A Guide to Experiential Anatomy.* Barrytown, NY: Station Hill Press, 1991.

FELDENKRAIS METHOD®

The Feldenkrais Method® is an approach for improving both physical and mental functioning through the exploration of body movement patterns and the use of attention. It is based on the brain's innate capacity for learning and the potential for lifelong development and growth. Movement is used as the medium toward understanding our habits and

Body-Mind Centering® strives to give the individual access to the totality of his or her development by enabling him or her to explore the body's structure through movement, sensory awareness, and imagery. First the cells, next the systems of the body, then movement and action in the world are examined as elements in a progressive formation of self. Participation in this review enables the individual to bring consciousness to bear on strengthening and focusing his or her own body-mind interaction.

identifying, learning, and acquiring alternatives that promote ease and well-being. The applications of the Feldenkrais Method range from reducing pain, improving neurologically based difficulties and learning disabilities, and increasing mobility to enhancing performance of professional athletes, dancers, musicians, and actors. People who come to do Feldenkrais are referred to as students, rather than patients, because learning underlies the basis of the method.

Origins and Development of the Feldenkrais Method®

The Feldenkrais Method was developed by Dr. Moshe Feldenkrais. Born in Russia, Feldenkrais emigrated to Israel at the age of thirteen. After receiving degrees in mechanical and electrical engineering, he earned his D.Sc. in physics at the Sorbonne in Paris. He subsequently worked for a number of years in the French nuclear research program. Physically active, Feldenkrais played soccer and practiced the martial arts. He studied with Kano Jigoro, the originator of judo, and in 1936 became one of the first Europeans to earn a black belt in that discipline. A chronic knee injury prompted him to apply his knowledge of physics, body mechanics, neurology, learning theory, and psychology to the body and mind. His investigations resulted in the formulation of a unique synthesis of science and aesthetics, known as the Feldenkrais Method.

The Process of Movement

A lesson could begin with a practitioner saying, "As you're sitting, what are you aware of about your sitting? Perhaps it's your back against the chair, or your feet on the floor, or your buttocks on the seat. Now bring your attention to what the back of your neck is doing; to what your chest is doing; to what your shins are doing."

A student's reply might be, "It is doing this." Yet most often, it is "I have

no idea what those parts are doing." This answer indicates that we give little or no attention to certain parts of ourselves or we tend to notice the same parts habitually. The fact is our *whole self* is involved in everything we do, but we sense only certain parts of ourselves in our actions and it generally tends to be the same parts. Through a more complete self-image in our actions and a more even distribution of effort and force throughout our whole self, an overall enhancement of movement, action, and thought results.

The practitioner might continue, "While seated, *without changing the placement of your feet*, notice where you have placed your feet. Slowly come to standing. (You may find that it is impossible to get up without changing where your feet are placed.) Sit again, move your feet an inch closer together and come to standing. Move your feet back to where you started and then move them an inch further apart and come to standing. Can you observe that a different placement of your feet influences your ability to come to standing? You may notice the effects of this in your breathing, your jaw, your neck, your balance, or in the amount of effort required in each action. Slowly get up to standing as you look down. As you slowly get up, look up. Then get up looking right. Next get up looking left. Can you sense that the different placement of your eyes affects how you come to standing?" This process would continue with more variations in order to help the student clarify, inform, and understand how one goes from sitting to standing.

The foundation of this kind of exploration is not the kind of learning based solely on information; rather it involves learning that can lead to a change in action, a change in thinking and feeling. The introduction of new variations awakens curiosity and teaches adaptation for continually altering circumstances. Rather than attempting to learn the "right way" of doing something, or "correcting" or "fixing," a student can explore choices, options, and different ways of using

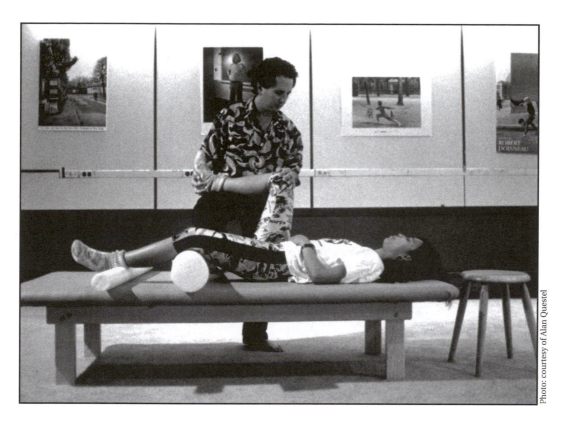

Alan Questel guides a client in a Functional Integration® exercise.

himself. Thus, he can act more effectively and efficiently depending on the context and the intention in that moment.

The Feldenkrais Method utilizes attention in a learning environment that is safe, easy, and geared toward an appropriate degree of challenge. In this context, he can discover and shift habitual patterns that interfere with functioning. He becomes his own laboratory for developing understanding and awareness of his daily actions.

The Two Modalities of the Feldenkrais Method®

There are two main modalities of learning in the Feldenkrais Method: Awareness Through Movement® and Functional Integration®. Awareness Through Movement lessons are group sessions. Participants are verbally led through a series of structured movement sequences that utilize attention, perception, and imagination. Designed to evoke a more synergistic use of oneself, the lessons establish new patterns of movement. As the lessons progress, participants become more aware of their movement habits, affording new patterns of behavior. There are more than a thousand different lessons with movements ranging from developmentally based patterns to innovative configurations. The movements are usually done lying down or sitting, and in a manner that recognizes each participant's own pace and range of motion. Comfort, ease, and the quality of movement are the main criteria used as one is developing more inner authority.

The other modality, Functional Integration, is a one-to-one, hands-on interaction specifically designed to meet the needs of an individual. Practitioners, primarily through the use of their hands, guide students to a new and more varied use of themselves. The quality of touch is noninvasive, informative, and interactive in nature. Students usually lie or sit and are comfortably dressed. As with Awareness Through Movement group lessons, these individualized sessions use movement as the means to promote changes in patterns of thinking, sensing, feeling, and interacting with others.

Benefits of the Feldenkrais Method®

The Feldenkrais Method aims to improve physical and mental functioning. It is applicable to anyone wanting to enhance the quality of his or her everyday life and activities. People from many different walks of life do Feldenkrais. They report results of increased vitality, enhancement of self-image, better breathing and posture, greater flexibility and range of motion, and reduction of pain. By bringing attention to the process of movement, students usually feel lighter and more graceful, and have greater ease and effectiveness in turning their intentions into actions.

—Alan S. Questel

Resources:

The Feldenkrais Guild of North America
P.O. Box 489
Albany, OR 97321
Tel: (800) 775-2118
Fax: (503) 926-0572
e-mail: fldgld@aol.com
Offers information regarding practitioners in your area, training programs, and other services.

Feldenkrais Resources
830 Bancroft Way, Suite 112
Berkeley, CA 94710
Tel: (800) 765-1907

Fax: (510) 540-7683
e-mail: feldenres@aol.com
Provides information regarding books, tapes, and materials related to the Feldenkrais Method.

Feldenkrais Recordings
467 Cahill Lane
Santa Rosa, CA 95401
Tel: (800) 722-7349 or (707) 577-8282
Another source of tapes.

Further Reading:

Feldenkrais, Moshe. *Body and Mature Behavior: A Study of Anxiety, Sex, Gravitation , and Learning.* Capitola, CA: International Universe Press, 1970.

——. *Elusive Obvious.* Capitola, CA: META Publications, 1985.

——. *The Master Moves.* Capitola, CA: META Publications, 1985.

——. *Awareness Through Movement: Easy-to-Do Health Exercises to Improve Your Posture, Vision, Imagination, and Personal Awareness.* San Francisco: Harper, 1991.

——. *The Potent Self: A Guide to Spontaneity.* San Francisco: Harper, 1992.

HANNA SOMATIC EDUCATION®

Hanna Somatic Education® is a method in which people learn how to relax chronically tensed muscles and to regain control of various muscle

Each individual, Feldenkrais believed, possesses an inner body wisdom that when allowed will choose the most comfortable and efficient movement patterns for itself. As the individual develops greater awareness of movement patterns and feels the ease and comfort of new choices, a stronger self-image is formed, which directs new, healthy modes of thinking, feeling, and acting.

groups and movement patterns. It seeks to change the body by working with a person's "soma," or internal first-person view of him- or herself. A soma includes a person's internal feelings, movements, and intentions. Hanna Somatic Education seeks to bring all these internal aspects to conscious awareness and combine them with scientific knowledge of how muscles work, thereby helping patients to reeducate their bodies to move freely and without pain.

The History of Hanna Somatic Education®

Hanna Somatic Education (HSE), also called Hanna Somatics, was developed by Thomas Hanna. A philosopher and former chair of the Philosophy Department at the University of Florida, Hanna wrote about the philosophy of the body in his book *Bodies in Revolt: A Primer in Somatic Thinking*. Hanna first coined the term "somatics" in 1976 in order to describe a kind of training that addresses the unification of mind and body. Hanna began with the concept of the "soma," which is the body experienced from within. *Soma* is the Greek word for "body." Historically, somatology referred to the field that eventually divided into anatomy and physiology. This division separated the study of the structure of the body from the study of its functions.

From Hanna's perspective, there was no division between body and mind. He used "soma" to describe a first-person view of the body in which a person is fully aware of his or her own internal feelings, behaviors, and intentions. This first-person perspective is an integral part of Hanna Somatic Education.

In the early 1970s, Hanna met Moshe Feldenkrais, an Israeli physicist and body educator, whose Feldenkrais Method was compatible with Hanna's somatic philosophy. Hanna created the first Feldenkrais training program in the United States, under the sponsorship of the Humanistic Psychology Institute (now the Saybrook Institute), where

Hanna was a director. He continued his study with Feldenkrais for many years at the Novato Institute for Somatic Research and Training, an institution that he founded in 1975.

As he practiced the Feldenkrais Method, Hanna observed characteristic postural difficulties in people of all ages and walks of life. He also noticed that certain techniques were extremely effective in helping clients regain control of the muscles that were holding them in these postures and restricting their movements. These techniques became known as Hanna Somatic Education.

The Basic Principles of Hanna Somatic Education®

Hanna Somatic educators believe that people stand in characteristic postures because chronically contracted muscles hold them there. When muscles are balanced in their tonicity—front, back, and sides—people stand up against gravity in a comfortable, upright posture. When the muscles are more contracted on one side or another, people are pulled in that direction.

Muscles become contracted because the nervous system sends messages, instructing them to shorten their muscle fibers. When this message is sent continually the muscle becomes chronically contracted. The message to contract has become a habitual pattern that the person doesn't control consciously.

In his work with clients, Thomas Hanna identified three reflexes: the red light reflex, green light reflex, and trauma reflex. The red light reflex is also referred to as the startle response or the escape response.

The green light reflex refers to the postural reflex that begins at around six months of age, when an infant first contracts the back extensor muscles. Also called the Landau reflex, it includes the arched back, extended neck, arms, and legs. It enables the infant to sit up, then stand in preparation for walking. It is the activation of our antigravity muscles.

219

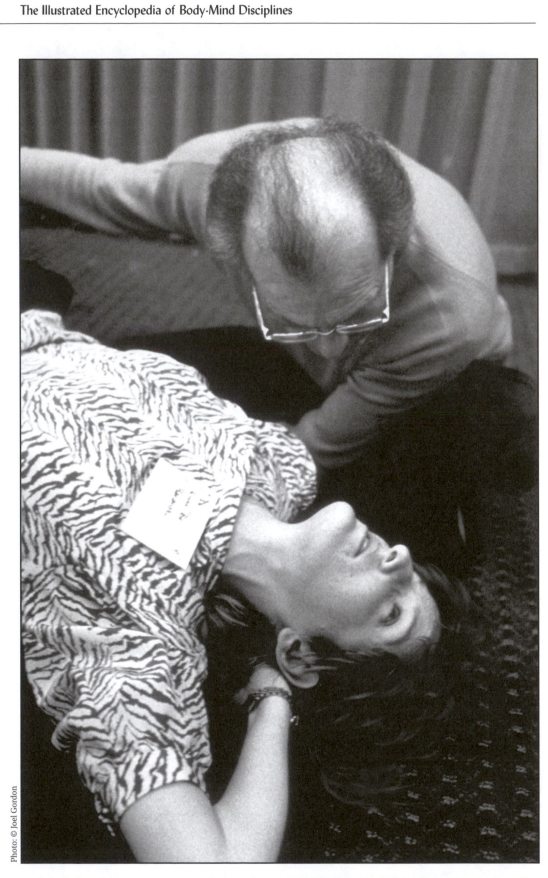

Photo: © Joel Gordon

Philosopher Thomas Hanna uses techniques he developed to help people gain a greater awareness of their own physical sensations.

Unfortunately, some adults remain in this posture out of habit.

The startle reflex is a set of changes that happen rapidly when there is a sudden change in environmental stimulation. This might be a loud noise nearby, or someone saying "Boo!" The reflex includes a set of responses such as eyes widening, muscles contracting, respiration stopping, etc. It takes a while to release these responses and return to normal. With repeated triggering of the startle reflex there will be some chronic muscle holdings. The muscular holdings contribute to a posture in which the person is bent forward, knees bent and pulled together, arms bent, with the head forward. The muscles on the opposite side of the body also become contracted, which may become painful.

The trauma reflex includes motor contractions, which surround any physical or severe emotional trauma—accident, surgery, long-term stress, etc. The trauma reflex posture may result in the person being tilted to one side, or the trunk being tilted to one side, while the head tilts to the opposite side. There may be various rotations: head, shoulders, or pelvis rotated to one side or the other. The rotations may be slight, or very noticeable.

Hanna put forth the concept of sensory-motor amnesia (SMA) to describe the tendency of humans to forget certain movements or ways of relating to muscles or muscle groups, leaving them chronically contracted. This occurs when muscles are contracted from being constantly subjected to different kinds of stress responses or injuries over an extended period of time. Hanna believes the contraction is the result of ongoing brain-stem-level impulses sent to the motor units, causing contractions of muscle fibers.

How to Practice Hanna Somatics

There are two approaches to HSE: hands-on table lessons, guided by the Hanna Somatic educator, and Somatic Exercises™, developed by Thomas Hanna, done by the individual. In the hands-on HSE lessons, a typical session is one-on-one and lasts fifty minutes to one hour. The person is dressed and positioned on a low table. The practitioner guides the person to perform certain movements, evaluating and emphasizing movements according to the person's needs. People can learn the exercises immediately. It is estimated that people average only three visits with a Hanna Somatic educator before they can become comfortable and able to move freely.

In the second approach, individuals do the Somatic Exercises™ on their own. These basic maintenance exercises, also called the "cat stretch," were developed by Thomas Hanna and are done once or twice daily. They take ten minutes to perform. There are many more specific exercises for specific purposes. In fact, these are not really considered exercises, but are reminders to the brain about how to efficiently use the muscles of the body. They are done slowly and gently. There are few repetitions.

Benefits and Cautions

HSE provides significant postural improvements. It is especially effective with conditions that are characterized by chronic muscle contractions. HSE is recommended for the following conditions: accident trauma, whiplash, long-term stress, repeated use stress, difficulties in moving, back pain, and headaches.

Great care needs to be taken with patients suffering from osteoporosis, or with the many conditions that would be aggravated by movement.

—*Eleanor Criswell Hanna, Ed.D.*

Resources:

Novato Institute for Somatic Research and Training
1516 Grant Ave., Suite 212
Novato, CA 94945
Tel: (415) 892-0617
Fax: (415) 892-4388

Provides certification training programs to qualified students. It also conducts individual sessions and workshops.

The Somatics Society
1516 Grant Ave., Suite 212
Novato, CA 94945
Tel: (415) 892-0617
Organization for somatic educators and bodyworkers. Provides information on the practice of somatics, and publishes newsletters as well as Somatics: Magazine-Journal of the Bodily Arts and Sciences. *This membership organization is run by Novato Institute for Somatic Research and Training, also at the same address.*

Further Reading:

Criswell, Eleanor. *An Introduction to Somatic Yoga.* Novato, CA: Freeperson Press, 1987.

Hanna, Thomas. *Bodies in Revolt: A Primer in Somatic Thinking.* Novato, CA: Freeperson Press, 1985.

——. *The Body of Life: Creating New Pathways for Sensory Awareness and Fluid Movement.* Rochester, VT: Healing Arts Press, 1993.

——. *Somatics: Reawakening the Mind's Control of Movement, Flexibility, and Health.* Reading, MA: Addison-Wesley, 1988.

HELLERWORK

Hellerwork combines hands-on bodywork movement education and dialogue to release the accumulated stress and trauma that cause people to become rigid in their bodies, in their movements, and in their thinking. Hellerwork allows the client to experience the inseparability of body, mind, and spirit by releasing the aches and pains stored in a type of connective tissue called fascia, thereby freeing up movement patterns, as well as mental patterns, that waste energy. Its techniques, developed from those of Rolfing, differ in that Hellerwork emphasizes movement education over hands-on bodywork; Hellerwork aims to teach its clients how to live without pain.

History of Hellerwork

Joseph Heller, the founder of Hellerwork, was born in Poland in 1940 and received his early education in Paris. He emigrated to the United States at the age of sixteen, settling in Los Angeles. In 1962 he began working as an aerospace engineer for NASA.

In 1972, in the midst of an intense involvement with humanistic psychology, Joseph Heller gave up engineering and trained with Dr. Ida Rolf in order to learn her method of structural integration (techniques to rid the body of habitual patterns of storing stress) for the body called Rolfing. In 1973 he became a Structural Patterner after studying with Judith Aston, the creator of the discipline known as Aston-Patterning®. In the mid-1970s, while maintaining a very successful Rolfing practice, Heller received advanced training from Dr. Rolf and from Dr. Brugh Joy, a noted physician, author, and innovator in the field of preventive medicine and the use of energy as a

The Novato Institute

The Novato Institute of Somatic Education and Training is the only place to find training in Hanna Somatics. It is a certified training program that began in 1990. The Institute also provides seminars, books, audiotapes, and videotapes through Somatics Educational Resources. Practitioners can also join the Somatics Society, an organization for bodywork professionals.

means of healing. In 1976 Heller became the first president of the Rolf Institute.

As a result of his unique combination of expertise and training in structural integration, movement education, and body energy awareness, Mr. Heller began to synthesize a new form of bodywork that emphasized movement reeducation. In 1978, he left the Rolf Institute and moved to the San Francisco Bay Area, where he founded Hellerwork and began training certified practitioners.

The Principles of Hellerwork

Although Hellerwork is effective for temporary pain or tension relief, practitioners recognize that pain and tension are usually the result of an overall pattern of imbalance occurring in the body. Rather than treating the pain or tension "symptom," Hellerwork focuses on rebalancing the entire body, returning it to a more aligned, relaxed, and youthful state. To fully understand how Hellerwork works, one must learn about connective tissue and gravity.

According to Heller, any tissue in the body that has a connecting function is considered to be connective tissue. The form of connective tissue that Hellerwork primarily affects is called fascia. Fascia is a plasticlike tissue that wraps all muscles and all of the individual fibers and bundles of fibers that make up muscles as well. Fascia comes together at the end of the muscle and becomes the tendon, which attaches the muscle to the bone. The fascial system of our body can be seen as one multilayered body stocking, with fascial sheaths wrapping the muscles and organs, throughout the body. Because of this, stress in any one area of the body has an effect on every other part of the body.

In its optimal condition, fascia is a loose, moist tissue and in a balanced body, the fascial body stocking stays loose and mobile, facilitating movement. However, under continual stress or lack of movement, fascia becomes rigid and layers of fascia begin to glue to one another, causing the "knots" people experience in their backs or necks. The sheaths of fascia stick in a systematic way, based on our habitual patterns of holding and movement. Holding patterns are often created by emotional memories stored in the tissue of the body; movement patterns are often a result of genetic predisposition or unconsciously learned behaviors from parents and primary caregivers. Although people associate tension and stiffness with their muscles, it is actually the connective tissue around the muscles that accumulates most of this stress.

In Hellerwork, the practitioner uses concentrated deep tissue bodywork on fascial areas in order to release and alleviate tensions. Only then can the body attain its optimum alignment. Also, by eliminating stress and pain, Hellerwork practitioners believe the body should be able to rid itself of repressed mental memories and physical and emotional traumas that function as an obstacle to good physical and mental health.

Hellerwork in Practice

During a session a practitioner interacts with a client in three major ways: working with his or her soft tissues while the client rests on a table; leading him or her through movement experiences; and discussing the relationship between body sensations, emotions, and thought.

At the start of the first session, the practitioner takes a health history and establishes with the client the goals for the series. The client then undresses to his or her underclothing and has "before" pictures taken as the practitioner observes the client's body for structural imbalance and restrictions in movement. The client then lies down on a bodywork table and the practitioner proceeds to work with his or her hands on the rigid parts of the client's soft tissues. Through pressure, movement, and stretching, the practitioner restores fluidity to those tissues and rearranges the parts so that they fit better in their alignment with gravity. When the structural work is done the practitioner works with the client in establishing a new movement pattern that supports the new alignment. During the session, the practitioner talks with the client, highlighting the more common attitudes and emotions associated with the areas of the body that have been worked with in that session. As the client becomes aware of these emotions he or she has the opportunity to become more responsive to them, so he or she is less likely to limit self-expression. When the client has integrated the changes in his or her structure with new movement patterns and attitudes the series is complete.

The Benefits and Risks of Hellerwork

The reported benefits of Hellerwork include increased flexibility and adaptability, increased energy levels, and a sense of wholeness and well-being. Although not a treatment for any specific condition, Hellerwork is said to reduce and even eliminate musculoskeletal pain from trauma and stress.

Hellerwork is particularly effective as first aid after trauma to the musculoskeletal tissues. It is not a treatment for any disease, conditions of organs, or symptoms of the nervous system. Use of Hellerwork is not advisable when pressure on the soft tissues cannot be tolerated.

All certified Hellerwork practitioners have completed the training program offered by Hellerwork International, LLC.

In addition to being trained to deliver the Hellerwork series, they have received extensive training in anatomy, movement, psychology, and energy systems.

—Sandy Sullivan
for Hellerwork International

Resources:

Hellerwork International, LLC
406 Berry Street
Mount Shasta, CA 96067
Phone: (916) 926-2500 and (800) 392-3900
Fax: (916) 926-6839
e-mail: Hellerwork@aol.com
Web site: www.hellerwork.com
Offers a list of Hellerwork practitioners. Also provides information about the discipline, as well as training opportunities.

Further Reading:

Heller, Joseph, and William Henkin. *Bodywise: Regaining Your Natural Flexibility and Vitality for Maximum Well-being.* Oakland, CT: Wingbow Press, 1986.

IDEOKINESIS

Ideokinesis is a method of movement therapy that utilizes the capacity of the nervous system to correct awkward or

---

The Role of Verbal Communication in Hellerwork

In Hellerwork, practitioners use verbal dialogue with their clients to discuss the relationship between their client's body sensations, emotions, and thinking.

During the bodywork session, the practitioner highlights the more common attitudes and emotions associated with the affected area of the body. As the client becomes aware of these emotions, they become easier to recognize and deal with, resulting in a discernible change in movement and mental outlook. When the client has integrated the changes in his or her structure with new movement patterns and attitudes, the session is complete.

inefficient movement. The term *ideokinesis* derives from two Greek words, *ideo,* meaning "idea," and *kinesis,* meaning "movement." Ideokinesis views the neurological system as the messenger of ideas or patterns of movement that stimulate and organize muscular and skeletal activity. Through anatomy lessons, exercises, and guided imagery, ideokinesis imparts healthy patterns of movement to the nerves and ultimately to the whole muscular and skeletal structure of the body. Either on its own or combined with other movement training, ideokinesis can aid in overcoming physical impairment caused by illness or injury. It is also considered a means of learning patterns of movement that enhance coordination, reduce tension, and promote a general sense of well-being.

The History of Ideokinesis

Ideokinesis is an outgrowth of techniques Mabel Elsworth Todd discovered when, as a teenager in upstate New York, she struggled to cure herself after suffering a back injury. Once she had completely recovered, Todd developed her techniques into a form of movement therapy that she practiced first in Boston, then in New York City. By the late 1920s she was attracting a steady stream of patients to her private clinic and lecturing on her method at Columbia University and the New School for Social Research. Todd's books, *The Thinking Body* (1937) and *The Hidden You* (1953), record the substance of her teachings and remain essential to the study of ideokinesis. But Todd's method might have been forgotten without the efforts of a former student, Lulu Sweigard, and a former patient, Barbara Clark. They introduced her method into the curriculum of New York University and the Juilliard School of Dance, ensuring that her legacy would be passed on to students in the 1950s and 1960s. *Human Movement Potential*, published shortly after Sweigard's death in 1974, is an important updating of Todd's original practice and gave it the name ideokinesis. While

ideokinesis is not well known to the general public and has no national professional organization or certification procedure, it is studied and used by a network of private practitioners throughout the United States. Many practitioners combine it with dance, Rolfing, or physical therapy.

The Theory of Ideokinesis

Ideokinesis is based on the idea that movement is an event in which each of three systems of the organism—neurological, muscular, and skeletal—plays a specific and integrated role. The event starts when the neurological system acts as a messenger and transmits impulses from the brain to the muscular system. The muscular system, in turn, acts as a motor, responding to the impulses. It moves the third component in the event, the skeletal system or framework.

The particular focus of ideokinesis is the subcortical level of nervous activity. Todd described the delicate subcortical nerves as "the hidden you," since it is through these nerves that ideas and images about the totality of the body are realized. If thoughts about the body are habitually faulty or weak, then the subcortical nerves will transmit debilitating messages to the rest of the body and movement will be impaired. To improve movement, ideokinesis accordingly concentrates not on increasing flexibility or muscular strength, though these often occur, but on changing the neurological system's coding of movement. This is accomplished through exercises and guided imagery, which modify both conscious and unconscious thought about body movements and positions.

Experiencing Ideokinesis

A class in ideokinesis generally opens with a discussion of anatomy, physiology, and body mechanics, which furnishes some of the mental images used in the positions and movements to follow. Beginning-level work often centers upon the constructive rest position, a recumbent position in which the arms are folded softly over the body and the legs are flexed at the knees and kept together. As the constructive rest position is assumed, the participant is instructed to conceive of her or his body as an empty suit of clothes. The ideokinesis teacher then uses suggestive language to evoke a process of gentle pressing that simultaneously removes wrinkles from the imagined suit of clothes and tension from the real body of the participant.

In a comparable fashion, work on sitting, standing, walking, and other basic movements makes use of exercises, mental images, and suggestive language. Participants attempt to perform various movement patterns while calling to mind the biomechanical and metaphorical images the teacher has introduced in the class. Participants work in pairs, with one participant executing the movement, while the other touches her or him lightly to clarify the initiation point and pathway of the movement.

By contrast, the experience of ideokinesis done on a one-to-one basis will vary from person to person, depending on the specific methods of the practitioner and the needs of the client. Instruction in the biomechanics of movement might be omitted and attention given over to diagnosis of difficulties and the establishment of a regimen of remedial exercises.

The Benefits of Ideokinesis

When practiced consistently, ideokinesis can help restore range of motion and improve the integration of sensory and motor skills. Further, it is credited with producing or restoring homeostasis, a condition in which all the systems and subsystems of the organism function harmoniously. In a state of homeostasis, the individual experiences enhanced freedom of movement, release from tension and fatigue, increased vitality, and a sense of well-being that often leads to the discovery of unexpected inner potential.

—*Andre Bernard*

Further Reading:

Matt, Pamela. *A Kinesthetic Legacy: The Life and Works of Barbara Clark.* Tempe, AZ: CMT Press, 1993.

Sweigard, Lulu. *Human Movement Potential: Its Ideokinetic Facilitation.* Lanham, MD: University Press of America, 1988.

Todd, Mabel E. *The Thinking Body: A Study of Balancing Forces of Dynamic Man.* Pennington, NJ: A Dance Horizons Book, 1968.

KINETIC AWARENESS

Kinetic awareness is a discipline that aims to increase knowledge of the human body on both physical and emotional levels. It aims to improve the individual's mental image of his or her body while also revealing ways that physical tension affects health, attitude, and emotional well-being. Practitioners of kinetic awareness believe that through the careful exploration of the body's responses to concentrated physical pressure, people can gain a heightened sensitivity to posture and movement, both in daily life and in specialized activities such as sports, dance, and martial arts.

How Kinetic Awareness Developed

Kinetic awareness was developed by dancer/choreographer Elaine Summers in the 1960s. Her dance career was interrupted at an early age when she began to experience symptoms of osteoarthritis, a potentially crippling disease of the joints. Doctors told her that within five years she would be unable to walk. Eventually, through her own determination, she was able to resume her dance career. During the period of her recovery, she studied with Carola Speads, whose system of physical reeducation evolved from the work of Elsa Gindler, a bodywork innovator. Summers's method of bodywork grew out of these studies and her own search for treatment of her physical condition, and upon experiencing positive results, she began to teach it to others.

Rubber Balls and Kinetic Awareness

Through experimentation, Summers developed an extensive system of techniques to increase physical awareness and release muscular tension. A special feature of this method is the use of rubber balls of various sizes to highlight body parts in isolation.

When an individual rests his or her body on a ball, the ball provides a focal point of attention; the individual naturally concentrates on the muscles and body part directly above the ball, where pressure on the body is greatest. It both supports and stretches the body. Muscular tension dissipates because of the pressure of the ball and the intentional movement of the body as the individual slowly shifts his or her position over the ball.

As an individual moves, the ball tests the elasticity and responsiveness of the muscles and joints. The intensity of the pressure created by the ball is a direct result of the size and firmness or softness of the ball and, therefore, can be controlled. People often feel a pleasurable ease and warmth in the part of the body where the ball has been and an alert quietness in the mind from the focused attention and overall relaxation that occurs from this.

As practitioners work, they release the unnecessary tension that causes many individual aches and pains. The work helps to prevent future injuries by revealing the body's warning signs. Practitioners also see how the mind and emotions manifest themselves in the body. For example, anger, sadness, or joy can each create a particular physical response in the body. Similarly, how people feel physically can create a certain mood, which then affects behavior. Through kinetic awareness individuals discover that they have choices about

how they move, and that it is possible to let go of habits and images of the body that restrict them. Moving with awareness is a profound way to reconnect the mind and the body.

Practicing Kinetic Awareness

Kinetic awareness can be taught both in classes and private sessions. People will often experience benefits such as relief of pain or greater range of movement after one or two sessions, but kinetic awareness can be practiced on an ongoing basis—many dancers and performers incorporate it into their training.

A typical class begins with an evaluation of body sensations while the participant lies quietly on the floor. Close attention is paid to breathing and slow movement explorations, with or without rubber balls. The individual focuses on one body part at a time, moving slowly through its full range of motion while noting any sensations. A person might become aware, for example, that certain parts of the body are dull and have little sensation, while others are hypersensitive. He or she also begins to discover that tension can exist in very specific, concentrated locations in the body. Practitioners of kinetic awareness assert that each person has preferred ways of moving, and that these favored modes naturally exclude other possibilities for movement. Summers believes that moving every part of the body through its potential range, often and without pain, encourages the body to attain physiological balance.

After the initial warm-up is complete, the teacher will suggest an exercise that enables the students to work at their own pace on the part of the body that is chosen as a focus. Throughout the session, the teacher will invite the students to share their feelings and observations. The process may include some explanation of anatomy to further an understanding of the musculoskeletal system and how it works. After the first phase of kinetic awareness, people can then choose to explore more advanced phases that employ multiple simultaneous movements and a full range of speed. The technique is adaptable; there is ample room for creativity and experimentation.

Benefits of Kinetic Awareness

As people practice kinetic awareness, they gain a deeper understanding of their bodies. They are able to release the unnecessary tension that causes many bodily aches and pains and they can prevent future injuries by becoming familiar with the body's warning signs. Furthermore, advocates of this discipline emphasize that the mind and emotions are expressed in the body. By improving physical condition and relieving stress through kinetic awareness, a person is able to create a feeling of well-being that will affect behavior. Through this practice, then, individuals reportedly discover that they have the capacity to choose how they move and they can enjoy more freedom and self-expression through movement.

—Ellen Saltonstall, J. Robin Powell, Ph.D, and Michelle Berne

Resources:

The Kinetic Awareness Center
1622 Laurel Street
Sarasota, FL 34236
Provides information about kinetic awareness as well as referrals to qualified teachers.

The Kinetic Awareness Center
P.O. Box 1050
Cooper Station

New York, NY 10276
Provides information about kinetic awareness as well as referrals to qualified teachers.

Further Reading:

Saltonstall, Ellen. *Kinetic Awareness: Discovering Your Bodymind.* New York: Kinetic Awareness Center, 1988. (Available through the Kinetic Awareness Center)

MEIR SCHNEIDER SELF-HEALING METHOD

The Meir Schneider self-healing method ("self-healing") combines massage, movement exercise, and other methods, including vision improvement exercises for those who need them, into a comprehensive rehabilitation system. It focuses on establishing communication between the mind and the body, and understanding the needs of the body as it strives to heal itself.

How Self-Healing Developed

Meir Schneider, Ph.D., LMT, was born in Ukraine in 1954. He was blind at birth, with cataracts and other serious vision problems. Shortly after he was born, the family emigrated to Israel. By the time he was six years old, five unsuccessful surgeries had left his lenses shattered, which resulted in admitting less than 1 percent of light in one

---

Alleviating Stress

Kinetic awareness encourages the individual to experience the pleasure of movement for its own sake. Practitioners of kinetic awareness maintain that a strong link exists between a person's mental state and the level of muscular tension in the body. This discipline seeks not only to relieve muscular tension resulting from daily stress and agitated emotional states, but also to achieve a corresponding enhancement of psychological well-being through holistic treatment of the human being.

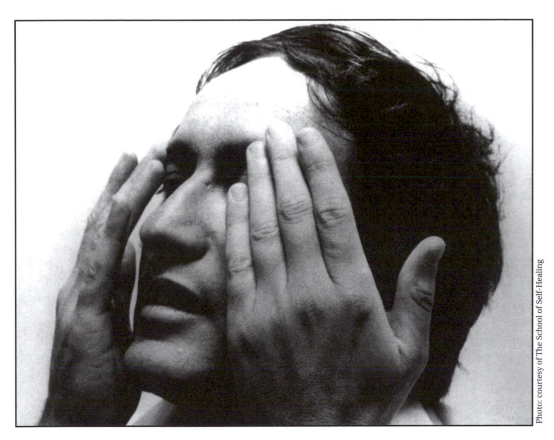

Meir Schneider practices the vision exercises of his self-healing method.

eye and 5 percent in the other. Doctors said that nothing further could be done. Meir was given a certificate of legal blindness and taught to do his schoolwork in Braille. He refused to use a cane or guide dog, and insisted on doing everything a sighted child could do, even riding a bicycle, although he sometimes ran into walls. He was confident that he would gain functional eyesight one day.

At age sixteen, he learned about the Bates method of vision improvement, as well as massage. He began to develop his own theories and insights about movement and the body. He practiced eye exercises, self-massage, and movement exercises up to thirteen hours a day. Worried about false hopes, his family and friends told him he was wasting his time. At first he saw lights and shadows only in a blur, but soon he began to distinguish some of the shapes as win-

dows. Within eighteen months he could read print without glasses. After years of effort, he learned to see well enough to earn an unrestricted driver's license.

With the Bates exercises, he relaxed his eyes, adjusted them to varying levels of light, and trained his brain to use his eyes in different, more effective ways. But he also needed self-massage to improve circulation and relieve the underlying strain of his face and upper body. Movement exercises helped to balance his vision. Through all of this experience, Schneider discovered how deeply the function of any one organ or area of the body is related to that of the whole body.

While still working to gain functional vision, he began to work with clients who experienced chronic pain, multiple sclerosis, and other problems. The massage and movement techniques he had developed from his own experience resulted in improvement in his early clients. He opened his first clinic with two of these clients, a youth with muscular dystrophy and a young woman with polio. His clinic and work gained national attention in Israel. In 1977 he founded the Center for Self-Healing in San Francisco. A few years later, he opened the School for Self-Healing.

Today, Schneider's work with muscular dystrophy is the subject of scientific studies. An internationally known therapist and educator, he is the author of *Self-Healing: My Life and Vision*, and *Meir Schneider's Miracle Eyesight Method*, a recently published vision seminar on tape, and coauthor of *The Handbook of Self-Healing*.

Philosophy of Self-Healing

Schneider believes that the body has a powerful, innate ability to heal itself. Using the body only as a tool to accomplish our everyday goals, most of us lose touch with this ability.

For many people, the body is unexplored territory. Only a fraction of the total capacity of muscles, lungs, and brain are regularly called upon. For example, we overuse about 50 of the body's approximately 600 muscles, and underuse the rest. Stress-related tension is a major cause of this problem. It creates "frozen" areas where muscular tension restricts movement, feeling, and circulation. People respond to stress with shallow breathing, eventually impairing lung and heart function. Chronic stress exacerbates disease. For people with serious health problems, it

aggravates the course of the disease and inhibits the body's natural tendency to repair itself.

Schneider believes that these problems stem from a lack of communication between the body and mind. For many of us, so much of our attention is directed away from ourselves—to other people, work, the constant barrage of external stimulation—that sensations within go unnoticed. In our culture, we tend to listen to our bodies only in times of extreme crisis. By developing an intuitive sense of the body's needs we can overcome serious health problems and increase health and vitality. This is the goal of self-healing therapy.

The School for Self-Healing offers training in the Meir Schneider self-healing method. Level one graduates are eligible in some places for massage therapy certification. Graduates of the full 760-hour program are recognized as self-healing practitioner/educators. Many students enroll in the beginning and intermediate stages of training in order to work with their own or a family member's health problem. Some students are already health care professionals or bodyworkers, while others are newly entering the massage-bodywork field.

Self-Healing Therapy

A self-healing therapy session is usually about one and a half hours long. The client wears underwear or a swimsuit. With the therapist's guidance, the client explores the body-mind link by experiencing a combination of many different

---

What Makes Self-Healing Unusual Among the Bodyworks?

- It combines massage and movement equally.
- It includes vision improvement work.
- Self-healing offers detailed programs, carefully tailored to the needs of the individual at a given time, to nurture specific organs or organ systems that are fragile or damaged.
- It emphasizes client motivation and empowerment. Self-healing is above all an educational process, and the client becomes an active, inventive partner of the therapist.

kinds of movement—massage, self-massage, visualizations of movement, breathing, coordination exercises, and eye exercises when appropriate. The session often begins with a movement that is problematic, difficult, stiff, or uneven. It is repeated at times as a checkpoint to see if there is any improvement. The methods that prove most successful during the session are incorporated into a home exercise program. In this way, deeply ingrained, harmful movement patterns, such as the habit of tensing up in order to move, can be reprogrammed.

For example, a bodybuilding champion came to Schneider with constant pain in her shoulders, neck, and knees, which resulted in diminished performance. "Many bodybuilders have such tight muscles and joints, they can't pull a T-shirt on, and they're in constant pain," she told him. Athletes often exhibit this kind of harmful use of the body, which eventually jeopardizes their performance. He taught her to isolate specific movements, to use only the correct muscles for a specific action without compensating with the others, to stay soft, and to move through a sense of relaxation. Her muscles became longer and fuller, the pain disappeared, and her weight-lifting performance improved.

Benefits of Self-Healing
The Meir Schneider self-healing method has helped athletes and musicians improve their performance. It prevents and alleviates the occupational health hazards of computer work and other detailed eye-hand tasks. It has been successful with breathing, neuromuscular, joint, heart/circulatory, digestive, posture and spine problems, injuries, chronic pain syndromes, poor vision from nearsightedness, farsightedness, astigmatism, lazy eye, a wide variety of eye diseases, and many other health problems.

—*Carol Gallup*

Sensory Awareness

Sensory awareness is a practice in freeing ourselves from conditioned habits, fears, and tensions that keep us from being what we really want to be and doing what we really want to do. The process promotes direct awareness of our sensations: sight, hearing, touch, taste, smell, and especially the subtle kinesthetic sense of body movement. In practicing this kind of awareness, we experience how we relate to ourselves, other people, and the world around us. We begin to be present for what is happening from moment to moment—to be here, now—with greater interest and joy, and more creative responsiveness to things as they are.

The Development of Sensory Awareness
In Germany, at the beginning of the twentieth century, a young woman named Elsa Gindler contracted tuberculosis, for which, at that time, there was no known cure. Her doctor asked, "What have you done to yourself?" and she took this question literally. From that moment on she began giving full attention to how she behaved and what happened inside her body, from the time she awoke in the morning until going to sleep at night. In so doing, her lungs began to function normally and she recovered her health.

Sensory awareness is the name now given to such "restorative observation"—this interested, nonjudgmental attention to the sensations of tension and release felt throughout the body as one moves in response to life's continually changing events. Through such attention, Gindler became aware of natural processes and learned to work with them instead of against them, particularly in regard to breathing and interaction with the pull of gravity, which attracts us to the earth at every moment.

Gindler not only cured herself of TB, but discovered that awareness of what is happening in the "physical" body can

231

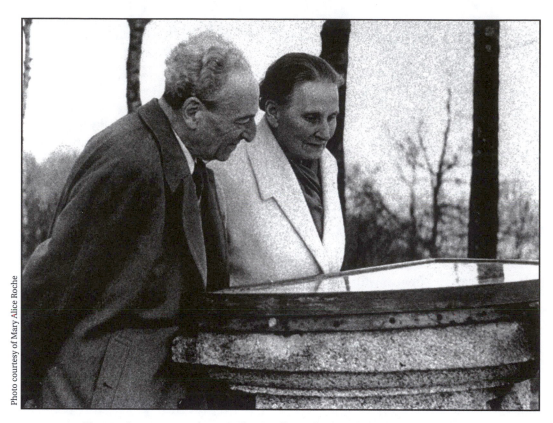

Photo courtesy of Mary Alice Roche

Pioneers in movement therapy, Elsa Gindler and Heinrich Jacoby in Zurich, 1957.

bring about liberation from "mental" anxiety. This practice brought about a state where she was no longer disturbed by her own thoughts and worries. She came to understand that calm in the physical field is equivalent to trust in the psychic field.

At about the same time, a young musician named Heinrich Jacoby was asking himself why some of the singers on the operatic stage had beautiful voices but were blocked musically, and others could master the music, but not move with it. He came to see how "talent" and "lack of talent" were mainly results of conditioning. A person was talented or untalented depending on the imposed ideas of family, teachers, society, culture, rather than on inherent capacities.

His thesis was that every human being born without physical defects has the biological equipment for every natural function, and that these include all possibilities of living, moving, experiencing, and creating. He demonstrated with thousands of people that there is an unrealized human potential for receiving impressions and allowing expression in every mode that can continue to unfold throughout our lives—if we are not blocked by our own limiting mental attitudes.

When these two people came together, they found in each other's discoveries the missing part of their own work. Jacoby was a highly educated "intellectual," while Elsa Gindler had no formal education beyond public school, and taught a bodywork called "gymnastik"—through which she had already recognized that one's attitudes are not just abstract thoughts, but tensions embedded in the physical tissue. When Gindler and Jacoby became colleagues, "mind" and "body" came together. In their classes students might consciously experience a state of balance that was not "physical" or "mental," but both—not only new ways of

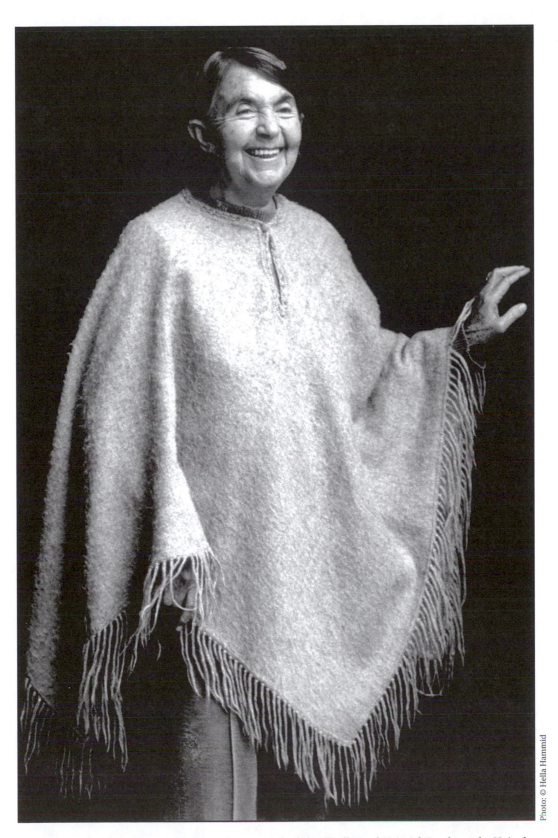

Photo: © Hella Hammid

Charlotte Selver brought the movement therapy work of Elsa Gindler and Heinrich Jacoby to the United States and named it "sensory awareness."

233

moving, but new ways of seeing and hearing, of thinking and relating, of being creative in many ways.

Students of Gindler and Jacoby have carried their work around the world: to Germany, Switzerland, England, Israel, Spain, the United States, Mexico, Canada, and Japan. Sometimes it is the practice as such that is offered, sometimes the practice offers a transforming approach to various professions such as musical performance, dance, child care, or psychotherapy. Dr. Lily Ehrenfried took the work of Gindler and Jacoby to France, where she established a new kind of physical therapy, called *gymnastique holistique*. The AEDE (Association des Eleves de Dr. Ehrenfried et des Practiciens en Gymnastique Holistique) was formed in 1986, and now has practitioners in ten countries in Europe and the Americas.

The Gindler/Jacoby theories and practice were brought to the United States in the 1930s by several of their students, including Else Henscke Durham; Clare Fenichel; Carola Speads (who called the work physical reeducation); and Charlotte Selver. Each offered the practice in her own way.

Selver coined the name "sensory awareness," presenting the first classes in "body awareness" and "nonverbal experience" ever given at the New School for Social Research in New York and Esalen Institute in California. The Charlotte Selver Foundation, now the Sensory Awareness Foundation, was established in 1971 to support her work. The psychologist Erich Fromm studied extensively with Selver and found the work "of great significance for the full unfolding of the personality." Fritz Perls incorporated much of what he learned from her into his gestalt therapy, while Alan Watts, who presented many joint seminars with Selver, called this practice "the living Zen."

Typical Session of Sensory Awareness

Sensory awareness sessions are simply an inquiry into what it feels like to be a living human being—when you are aware of what you are feeling and how you are living. There are no set "exercises." Experiments inspired by the felt needs of the student or students at that moment are outlined by the leader. Afterward, there is reporting as to what a student might have discovered. There are no preconceptions as to what ought to happen or be felt; what is felt is neither "right" nor "wrong"; it just is.

All living is movement, and these experiments are not only large movements, such as walking, running, dancing, stretching, etc., but the most subtle: inhalation and exhalation, the pulsing in a wrist, the vibration of the vocal cords in the throat as a person speaks or sings, the resting of a hand on a cheek, or on a shoulder, the lifting of a partner's arm, or having one's arm lifted. In just noticing how these movements feel as they take place, the habitual tensional patterns that produce inappropriate and painful movements of the body can change.

Sensory awareness is offered privately, in regular group sessions, and in workshops. There are no formal training courses for leaders; leaders and students

This work makes possible a way of being that is full of life, more security, and more courage to dare something new. The wonder is the blessed feeling that comes when I can be more fully, as if each cell in me were happy to exist.

—Ruth Veselko, a longtime Gindler/Jacoby student and Sensory Awareness teacher in Switzerland, speaking of her own experience.

come to a mutual understanding as to when the student is ready to become a leader, usually after many years' practice.

Benefits of Sensory Awareness

As sensory awareness experiments are followed over a period of time, muscles may become more elastic, aches and pains fade, illnesses subside. Fear may be replaced by self-confidence. Movement and thinking may become more spontaneous and creative. There may be less effort and greater joy in relating to others and taking part in private or professional activities. But the fundamental aim is just to wake up—to experience life in every bit of us and be happy to exist at this moment.

It is recommended that one study with an experienced sensory awareness leader, to help you begin to explore this unique practice of making friends with your body, of discovering all of the possibilities that can unfold when you learn to trust in the innate wisdom of the body-mind.

—*Mary Alice Roche*

Resources:

Sensory Awareness Foundation
c/o Sara Gordon
955 Vernal Ave.
Mill Valley, CA 94941
Tel: (707) 794-8496
Distributes various publications concerning the practice of sensory awareness.

Sensory Awareness Leaders Guild
c/o Louise Boedeker
411 West 22nd Street
New York, NY 10011
Tel: (212) 675-5730
Recommends qualified sensory awareness leaders in the United States and abroad.

Further Reading:

Brooks, Charles V. W. *Sensory Awareness: Rediscovery of Experiencing Through the Workshops of Charlotte Selver.* New York: Viking Press, 1974.

SOMA NEUROMUSCULAR INTEGRATION

Soma neuromuscular integration, or "soma bodywork," utilizes ten individual sessions that address particular and progressive soft-tissue manipulation, primarily through working with the fascia, or connective tissue. Developed by Dr. Bill Williams and Dr. Ellen Gregory Williams in 1978, Soma was developed, and continues to be taught, as a way of enabling people to function more optimally by providing greater access to the body-mind. People who inhabit their whole and integrated body-mind frequently experience greater levels of emotional openness, creativity, and self-reliance.

Importance of Body and Mind

Soma neuromuscular integration was developed by Bill M. Williams, Ph.D., and Ellen Gregory Williams, Ph.D. Dr. Bill Williams taught and collaborated with Ida Rolf in the early development of her well-known ten-session work in fascia manipulation. He was a member of the founding board of directors that established the institute teaching Dr. Rolf's methods. Dr. Ellen Williams is a psychologist who after many years of talk therapy realized that there must be an involvement with the body to effect deep and lasting psychological change. In his early years as a Rolfer he continued to be aware of the interaction of the body and the mind and wanted to develop a training program that would more effectively address and work with integrating the whole person. Dr. Williams was one of the first to develop a hands-on training to combine the physiological and psychological approaches to healing.

The Three-Brain Model

Fascia is the tissue that wraps muscles and gives them their shape. Ideally, muscles should be able to move independently

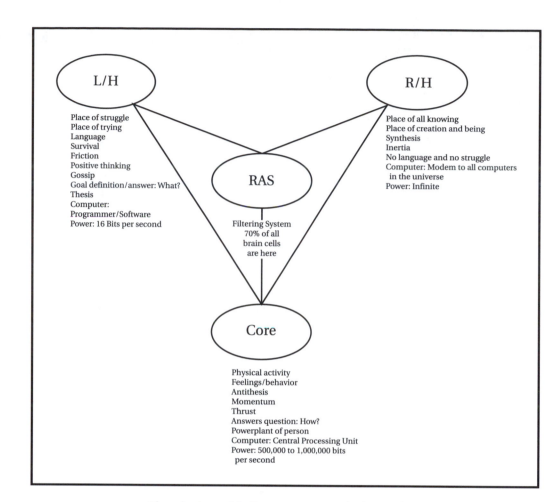

Three-brain model of soma neuromuscular integration.

and slide over each other, but often as a result of age, injury, or physical or emotional stress, the fascia that wraps the individual muscles glues together, causing the fascia and the muscles to lose functional and structural differentiation. Someone who has experienced a serious neck injury may attempt to turn his or her head from side to side, but instead of using only the muscles necessary to accomplish the rotation, the muscles of the neck and shoulders act as one, and turning the head ends up requiring rotation of the entire upper torso. Such gluing is a restriction in movement that is expensive in terms of energy output and general vitality.

By working directly on the fascia, the soma practitioner frees the musculature, allowing it to assume a more effective structural relationship with the fascia. As a result, one stands taller with less effort, and moves with greater ease and comfort. In addition, chronic muscle or joint pain is almost always reduced or eliminated as muscles have the opportunity to lengthen and assume optimal relationships with surrounding fascia.

Neural tissue is embedded within the myofascial system. In the process of freeing restricted and adhered fascia, soma practitioners work directly with the nervous system, sending sensory information to the brain that allows the body new options to organize itself in more comfortable, more energy efficient, more satisfying ways. Practitioners believe that soma bodywork teaches the body to self-correct and continuously reprogram itself to greater levels of ease and freedom.

According to Marcia Nolte, codirector of the SOMA Institute: "Life is change and change is movement, movement in our bodies, our feelings, our thoughts. It is the loss of the ability to move and change our bodies and our thinking that continues over time to diminish our ability to experience life. soma bodywork focuses on accessing more somatic options. Soma therapists are not working toward the evolution of a 'perfect person' by replacing old patterns with new, 'right' ones, but rather toward a less rigid, more authentic individual who responds creatively rather than reacts to his or her environment."

To help accomplish this, soma therapists work with the three-brain model developed by Dr. Williams. The three-brain model is a way of understanding human consciousness and the activity of the nervous system. It is based in part on neuropsychiatric research, which has clearly outlined specific differences between the roles and functions of the left and right sides of the brain. In simplified terms, the left half of the brain is more logical and the right side is more creative. The third "brain" in the model is the corebrain, which consists of nerve plexi located in the abdomen. According to Dr. Williams, it is the source of bodily energy and the means by which the left and right hemispheres translate cognition into activity.

Soma therapists believe that being stuck or dominant in any one "brain" prevents optimal functioning. They endeavor to educate people as to how to integrate all three "brains." The structural organization resulting from the soma bodywork, the integrative exercises, and somatic education are all designed to improve access to the three "brains."

Ten Sessions

There are ten sessions in soma bodywork treatment. These sessions last for approximately ninety minutes to two hours and progress layer by layer, working progressively deeper. The practitioner and client work together to slowly release and rebalance layers of tissue until reaching the deepest layers of "the core."

Unresolved feelings can surface in the rebalancing process. Past trauma that may have been understood intellectually will continue to remain buried in restricted tissues until it is addressed, released, and repatterned. The repatterning part of the work is accomplished through journaling with special goals, the three-brain model of body-mind functioning, a notebook of integrative movement, and individual somatic learning.

Results

The results of soma bodywork are not limited to the relief of symptoms, although relief occurs consistently. The results are believed to include increased levels of energy and performance, fewer stress-related symptoms, increased flexibility, increased alignment and freedom of movement, heightened awareness emotionally and physically, greater self-reliance, and creativity.

—*Karen Bolesky and Marcia W. Nolte*

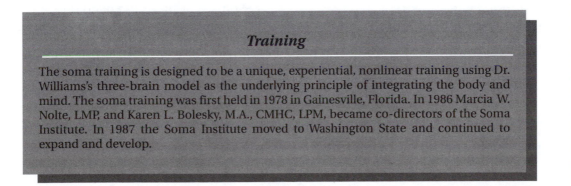

Training

The soma training is designed to be a unique, experiential, nonlinear training using Dr. Williams's three-brain model as the underlying principle of integrating the body and mind. The soma training was first held in 1978 in Gainesville, Florida. In 1986 Marcia W. Nolte, LMP, and Karen L. Bolesky, M.A., CMHC, LPM, became co-directors of the Soma Institute. In 1987 the Soma Institute moved to Washington State and continued to expand and develop.

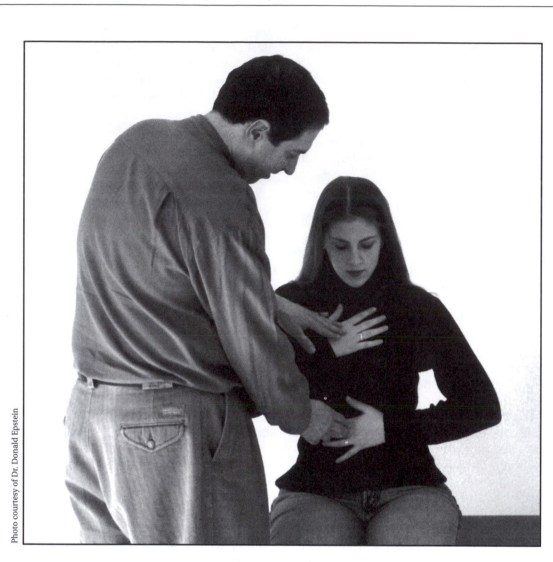

Photo courtesy of Dr. Donald Epstein

Dr. Donald Epstein uses the techniques of touch and breath awareness, which form the basis of somato respiratory integration.

Resource:

Soma Institute
730 Klink
Buckley, WA 98321
Tel: (360) 829-1025
Fax: (360) 829-2805
Web: www.soma-institute.com

Provides the professional licensing program and the certification program in soma neuromuscular integration and somassage. Trainings are held in Washington state. The Soma Institute is licensed by the Washington Workforce Training and Education Coordinating Board, and the Washington State Board of Massage. It also lists soma bodywork practitioners.

SOMATO RESPIRATORY INTEGRATION

Somato respiratory integration (SRI) is a system of breathing and touch that is used to allow a person to heal himself or herself. While it is not used to remedy a specific ailment, SRI invites participants to access the body's inner rhythms and experience the present moment more fully. The body's rhythms are charted in a twelve-stage process, through which a person experiencing SRI will progress.

Over nearly two decades Dr. Donald Epstein developed network chiropractic and network spinal analysis. He noticed specific patterns of breath, movement, and self-touch that spontaneously occurred in his clients after receiving network care. Eventually he categorized these expressions into twelve stages of consciousness, each with its own pattern of breath, touch, and movement. The stages are suffering, polarities and rhythms, being stuck in a single perspective, reclaiming power, merging with an illusion, preparing for resolution, resolution, readiness in emptiness, light beyond form, ascent, descent, and community.

Most of the exercises are done while lying down or seated. At the start of an SRI session, participants are instructed to breathe gently while using their hand to feel the rise and fall of their chest and abdomen. The breathing patterns may involve various combinations of nose and mouth breathing. This exercise is used to transfer a peaceful rhythm to the person's hand, equipping it to heal other regions of the body. The individual then places his or her hands on various areas of the body to allow them to move in alignment with the rhythms. The exercises are used to find the most peaceful areas of the body and spread these areas of peace to other regions. They are a tool used to help an individual pay attention to him- or herself in a meaningful way.

A practitioner intends to educate the client in each of the twelve possible rhythms of healing. An entire SRI session may involve connecting with up to four rhythms. The time it takes to transfer a rhythm will vary with a person's experience. This technique is valued for being simple and effortless. The body becomes increasingly able to dissipate stored tension or energy. The benefits of SRI will occur progressively over the twelve distinct stages of the healing process. With each session, the natural movement of the body overtakes the thinking mind.

SRI does not attempt to force any particular outcome or catharsis. The intent is to acknowledge and accept the body's rhythms without changing them. By observing the way a person moves, touches, and breathes, SRI is used to increase a person's self-awareness and respect for his or her own healing process.

The SRI exercises are best learned under the guidance of a trained SRI facilitator. SRI is not intended as a replacement for any form of therapy, nor as a treatment for specific health conditions. It is ultimately intended as a self-care system that may be used in conjunction with other healing modalities.

—Donald Epstein

Resources:

Innate Intelligence Inc.
444 N. Main Street
Longmont, CO 80501
Tel: (303) 678-8086
Provides information about SRI workshops and a list of those who have taken the SRI programs.

Further Reading:

Epstein, Donald, and Nathaniel Altman. *The Twelve Stages of Healing.* Novato, CA: New World Library, 1994.

TRAGER PSYCHOPHYSICAL INTEGRATION

Trager psychophysical integration is a type of bodywork that uses the human ability to feel pleasure and other sensations as the basis for developing and maintaining a healthy body. According to Trager theory, a healthy body is both the container for and a reflection of a healthy mind and spirit.

Practicing the Trager approach can result in relief from pain and greater freedom of motion. It can also assist in correcting long-standing patterns of posture and movement that cause discomfort, unhappiness, and unfulfilled life potential.

History of the Trager Approach

Trager psychophysical integration was developed by Milton Trager, M.D. As a young man Trager was an aspiring boxer. At the gym, the trainers and boxers used bodywork to alleviate muscular pain after rough workouts. One day Trager gave his trainer a rubdown and discovered that he had a gift for bodywork. Shortly thereafter Trager quit boxing and began to practice his own intuitive form of bodywork on family, friends, and clients in his Miami neighborhood. He experienced success in cases of sciatica, polio, and many other conditions from which people had found no relief through conventional medicine.

After eight years of private informal practice, Trager sought out more formal training and certification. At age forty-one, Trager entered the Universite Autonoma de Guadalajara in Mexico, where he studied medicine. While there, he impressed the doctors, professors, and Catholic nuns with his work with a four-year-old polio victim. After working with her for just forty minutes, the girl, who had been paralyzed from the waist down for two years, could move her foot in four directions. The demonstration caused the university to organize a clinic for Trager, where he continued to treat polio victims throughout his years of study.

In 1959, Trager opened a private practice in general medicine and physical rehabilitation in Waikiki, Hawaii. In 1974, while visiting Los Angeles, he worked on a patient with muscular dystrophy. At the patient's request Dr. Trager agreed to try to teach his approach to the patient's regular therapist. Trager's attempts to teach his approach in the past had been unsuccessful. This time he first had the therapist place his hands over Trager's own hands as he worked. Then he had the therapist place his hands on the patient while Trager worked on top of them. Finally, he let the therapist work alone. Trager knew he was successful when the patient exclaimed, "That's it, Doctor, he's got it! It almost feels like you are doing it!"

In 1973 Trager gave the first public demonstrations of his approach at the Esalen Institute in California. There he met Betty Fuller and found that he could teach her in the same fashion that he had taught the therapist. Fuller immediately recognized the significance of Trager's work and persuaded him to let her form an organization that would allow others to study it. The Trager Institute was founded in 1980 with Fuller as director.

By 1977 Trager had closed his private practice in Hawaii to devote all of his time to his growing number of students. At present there are more than 900 students throughout the world, more than 1,000 certified practitioners, and fifteeen certified instructors.

The Principles of the Trager Approach

Trager believes that human beings are the sum total of all the experiences of their lives. These experiences are ingrained in both the body and the mind. Changes in reflex responses, tissue condition, and behavior are possible, he believes, because of the deep neurological associations between sensory stimulations, emotional feelings, attitudes, and concepts, as well as the body's motor response to all of them. He believes that clients should come to him ready to learn more about their bodies and minds rather than simply to receive treatment.

Trager's method of manipulating the body is actually a form of movement reeducation. The Trager practitioner is not concerned with moving particular muscles or joints. Instead, he or she uses motion in muscles and joints to produce pleasurable feelings. These

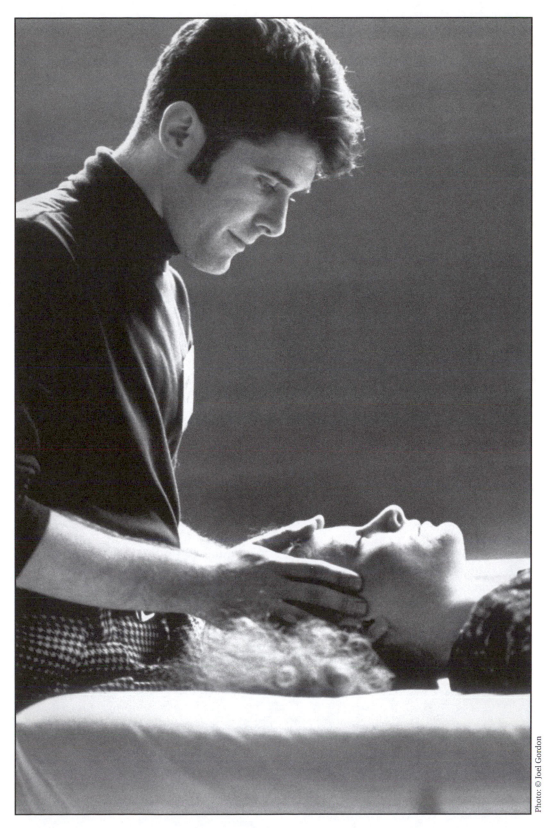

A Trager practitioner, in a relaxed state of consciousness called "hook-up," transmits pleasurable sensations to a client.

enter the central nervous system and begin to trigger tissue changes by means of the many motor-sensory feedback loops between the mind and the muscles. The Trager practitioner does not change the condition of tissue with his or her hands. He or she uses the hands to remind the nervous system how it can feel. This feeling elicits tissue response within the client to achieve this relief and pleasure again. Over the course of many sessions a client learns how to move and hold one's body in a healthier, more beneficial manner.

A Typical Session

A Trager psychophysical integration session takes from one to one and a half hours. No oils or lotions are used. The client wears a bathing suit or underclothing and lies on a well-padded table in a warm, comfortable environment. The practitioner gently and rhythmically moves the body of the client, first as a whole and then by moving individual limbs and parts, in such a way that the client feels the sensation of free, effortless, and graceful movement.

In order to facilitate a successful bodywork session the practitioner enters a relaxed state of consciousness known as "hook-up," in which he or she physically remembers pleasurable sensations. The practitioner transmits these pleasurable sensations through his or her hands directly to the client's body tissue, encouraging the tissue to release into a lighter and freer physical state. When the Trager practitioner encounters stiffened limbs or hardened muscles, his or her response is to apply gentle pressure to release tight, painful tissue and restore it to a deeply relaxed physical state. After getting up from the table, the client is given some instruction in the use of mentastics, a system of simple, effortless movement sequences developed by Trager to maintain and enhance the feeling of balance, freedom, and flexibility that was instilled by the table work. Clients can also take classes in the exercise of mentastics. These are run in a workshop format.

Benefits and Cautions

For most clients, the effects of a Trager session appear to penetrate below the level of conscious awareness and continue to produce results long after the session itself. Benefits include the disappearance of specific symptoms, such as discomfort or pain; heightened levels of energy and vitality; better posture and carriage with less effort; greater joint mobility; a deep relaxation of the body and mind; and a new ease in daily activities.

Although the Trager session involves gentle and light movement and bodywork, it is not advisable for those suffering from joint, bone, and disk disorders; complicated or high-risk pregnancies; broken bones, or blood clots.

—*Nancy Allison, CMA, with Deane Juhan*

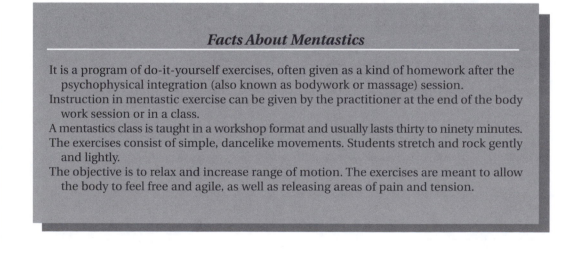

Facts About Mentastics

It is a program of do-it-yourself exercises, often given as a kind of homework after the psychophysical integration (also known as bodywork or massage) session.

Instruction in mentastic exercise can be given by the practitioner at the end of the body work session or in a class.

A mentastics class is taught in a workshop format and usually lasts thirty to ninety minutes.

The exercises consist of simple, dancelike movements. Students stretch and rock gently and lightly.

The objective is to relax and increase range of motion. The exercises are meant to allow the body to feel free and agile, as well as releasing areas of pain and tension.

Resources:

Trager Institute
21 Locust Ave.
Mill Valley, CA 94941-2806
Tel: (415) 388-2688
Fax: (415) 388-2710
e-mail: TragerD@trager.com
Manages the certification program in Trager psychophysical integration and mentastics movement education. Training is conducted throughout North America and Europe. The Trager Institute is accredited by the California Nursing Continuing Education Board and the Florida State Massage Board.

Further Reading:

Trager, Milton, and Cathy Guadagno. *Trager Mentastics: Movement as a Way to Agelessness.* Barrytown, NY: Station Hill Press, 1987.

Part X: Somatic Practices

Brain Gym® • Contact Improvisation • Continuum • Eurythmy •
Gurdjieff Movements • Pilates Method of Body Conditioning® • ROM Dance •
Skinner Releasing Technique • Spatial Dynamics℠ • T'ai Chi Ch'üan

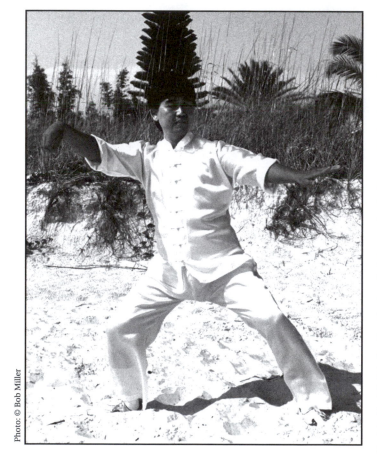

Photo: © Bob Miller

Many people regularly practice t'ai chi ch'üan to stay fit and healthy.

Somatic practices are movement practices that develop one's mental, emotional, and spiritual experience of life by awakening greater awareness of the sensations of his or her physical body as it moves through space. The term somatics was coined by the American philosopher Thomas Hanna (1928–1990) in the 1970s. Deriving it from *soma*, the Greek word for "body," Hanna coined the word somatics to describe "the field of study of the human being as experienced by him or herself from the inside." Hanna's definition includes many disciplines described in other sections of this encyclopedia. However, this section focuses on disciplines that were devised not for relief from a particular ailment or pain, but for those seeking to enhance one's understanding and awareness of what it means to be fully alive in a human body.

History

Throughout history, various cultures have used movement to impart mental, emotional, or spiritual lessons. T'ai chi ch'üan, one of the oldest extant methods, was developed in China between the years 2205 BCE and 1100 CE, although its sources can be found in the even more ancient practices of qigong. Called "great dances" by

Emperor Yü, one of its earliest developers, t'ai chi's sequence of movements was developed collectively by many generations of philosophers, healers, and artists. They were all influenced by Taoism, an ancient Chinese religion that encourages a keen observation of the patterns of movement and change in nature as a means to help human beings understand the physical, mental, and emotional changes that occur during the course of human existence.

Many ancient Western educational and spiritual traditions also developed movement practices. Most of these, including those believed to have been developed by the Greek philosopher and father of geometry Pythagoras and those developed by Jewish and Christian esoteric sects, have been lost to us. They were often practiced in secret and generally frowned upon by the dominant sects of the Judeo-Christian tradition, which condemned the body and its sensations.

For hundreds of years most Western culture, including educational methods and spiritual practices, maintained a separation of spirit and flesh, mind and body. In the latter part of the nineteenth century, however, some philosophers began to reexamine the possibility of using physical exercises to promote healthy mental and emotional functioning. One of the best-known explorers of this period was the Armenian philosopher George Gurdjieff (1866–1949), whose "movements for educating the whole person" were inspired by "sacred dances" he observed in a remote part of Central Asia.

As the twentieth century dawned, the concept of learning mental, emotional, and spiritual lessons through body movements began to echo in many quarters. In 1919 the Austrian philosopher Rudolph Steiner (1861–1925) opened the Waldorf Schools to teach eurythmy, his movement practice to promote spiritual growth based on sound vibrations. Working from a different perspective, the German physical culturist Joseph Pilates (1880–1965) developed contrology, now known as the Pilates Method of Body Conditioning®, to free people from the stress and mechanization of living in the industrialized world. Pilates' sequence of exercises borrows heavily from the physical postures and concepts of the practice of hatha yoga.

In recent times, the concept of enhancing one's experience of life through movement practices has been embraced by innovators in many other professions. Educational theorists Paul and Gail Dennison developed Brain Gym™ as a corollary to contemporary educational practices. Dancers/choreographers Steve Paxton, Emilie Conrad-Da'oud, and Joan Skinner developed contact improvisation, continuum, and Skinner release technique, respectively, from their own creative explorations of movement. Occupational therapists, such as Diane Harlowe—one of the originators of ROM dance—and clinical psychologists, such as Jaimen McMillan—the originator of Spatial Dynamics℠—have created new movement sequences that also have become popular in many contexts outside their original healing work.

Theories of Somatic Practices

The primary theoretical construct that ties these practices together was first elucidated by the ancient cultures of China, India, and the Middle East and has been given voice in our own time by physicists studying the physical laws governing the universe. This ancient construct holds that the entire universe is in constant motion. As parts of the universe, humans are subject to the same laws of movement. By learning to experience how those laws of movement are reflected in our own bodies, we improve our physical condition. We also develop an intuitive understanding of how these physical principles affect our everyday experience. These physical laws become metaphors for ways of thinking, feeling, and living.

Somatic practices help participants focus on the messages they receive from their bodies and become more aware of their physical sensations in the present moment. Each method begins by teaching a person a physical skill. In some practices, such as t'ai chi ch'üan, Pilates Method, or Spatial Dynamics, the movement patterns are extremely specific and must be precisely replicated. In others, such as contact improvisation, continuum, or Skinner release technique, the form of the movement is spontaneously created by exploring a particular concept of movement. Whether the form is set, like an ancient spatial architecture, or improvised, like a free jazz tune, the process used develops one's sensitivity to subtle changes in the body and its relation to its spatial environment. By developing heightened physical sensitivity, a person can experience freer, more graceful, original, or daring movements, creating a sense of pleasure, accomplishment, or calm.

Experiencing a Somatic Practice

Somatic practices are taught in just about every part of the world today. They may be experienced in public and private schools, recreation and growth centers, at business seminars, or in private studios. Classes are generally taught in groups, although private instruction is sometimes available. Classes may be geared for any age level or special needs group. In addition to conditioning the physical body and offering a pleasurable social interaction, these practices seem to imprint themselves on both the body and the imagination of the mover, empowering and freeing him or her to face the challenges of life. In addition, many participants claim that these practices have expanded their sense of connection to the rest of the universe and awareness of what it means to be a human being.

—*Nancy Allison, CMA*

Resources:

International Somatic Movement Education and
    Therapy Association
148 West 23rd Street, 1H
New York, NY 10011
Tel: (212) 229-7666

The Somatics Society
1516 Grant Avenue, Suite 212
Novato, CA 94945
Tel: (415) 892-0617
Fax: (415) 892-4388
*Organization offering seminars and information
on many somatic practices. Publishes the bi-annu-
al magazine-journal* Somatics.

Further Reading:

Arnheim, Rudolf. *Visual Thinking.* Berkeley: University of California Press, 1969.

Gardner, Howard. *Frames of Mind: The Theory of Multiple Intelligences.* New York: Basic Books, 1985.

Hall, Edward T. *The Hidden Dimension.* New York: Doubleday & Co., 1966.

Schneider, Michael S. *A Beginner's Guide to Constructing the Universe.* New York: Harper-Collins, 1994.

Brain Gym®

Brain Gym®* is a system of exercises that joins physical and mental development in ways designed to improve the person's ability to learn and perform in all areas of endeavor. The training focuses on linked brain and motor skills but also includes exercises for the release of stress, now considered a major factor in children and adults with learning differences. Practice in Brain Gym has been shown to accelerate progress at school for students of all ages and skill levels, and to enhance success at work and in recreational pursuits.

Coping with Challenging Situations

Brain Gym was developed by Paul E. Dennison, Ph.D., in the late 1960s. The director of several learning clinics in the Los Angeles area, Dennison was discouraged by inconsistent results in some of his patients. He researched techniques and information from early childhood developmental theory, brain research, developmental optometry, applied kinesiology, language acquisition theory, dance and movement therapy, and his own field of learning theory to formulate a way to improve the skills of his patients. Dennison coined the term "Brain Gym" to describe the movement activities he developed, which were simple enough for anyone, of any age, to do, while effective enough that anyone could benefit.

After the initial success of Brain Gym, Dennison collaborated with his wife, Gail, in exploring its potential as a self-help tool of broad application in business, sports, and the arts. In 1987 they established a research-and-information center on body-mind development, the Educational Kinesiology Foundation, that oversees the training of Brain Gym instructors and coordinates the international network of Foundation faculty and Brain Gym instructors.

In 1991, Brain Gym was recognized by the National Learning Foundation (NLF) as one of twelve "successful learning innovations." Established in response to the White House Task Force on Innovative Learning's 1989 Action Plan, the NLF's mission is to make the most effective innovations in education available nationwide.

Whole Brain Learning

Brain Gym is based on theories about the connection of mind and body in the formation of dynamic, balanced intelligence. The human brain has two hemispheres, each in control of one half of the body and a distinct type of mental function. The left hemisphere is in charge of the body's right side and carries out analytic processes, while the right hemisphere activates the left side and works with visual and spatial perception. Though the right "gestalt" hemisphere can absorb large amounts of sensory information simultaneously, it cannot easily express the material without the participation of the left "analytic" hemisphere. According to the Dennisons, modern educational systems are themselves imbalanced since they emphasize left-brain, logic-oriented skills at the expense of the comprehension and creativity of whole-brain learning.

Stress impedes whole-brain learning by stimulating the "fight-or-flight" reaction in which there are profound physical changes. These changes include elevated pulse and blood pressure, an increased breathing rate, slowed digestion, and unfocused vision—all normal, healthy responses to threat, and useful to mobilize energy to escape from or overcome the threat. However, these responses can make learning difficult at best and, if prolonged, can lead to illness. Using movement to activate the parts of the brain where logical, rational thinking takes place, Brain Gym helps the brain to recover from the fight-or-flight response, evaluate the nature of the threat, and respond appropriately. As the brain responds, the overall stress level drops, and competence increases. In the case of children, this is crucial to their entire process of growth and change since stress disturbs the organism at every level of its relationship to the world.

Brain Gym® Exercises

There are several ways to use Brain Gym. A series of individual sessions with a certified instructor usually gets the quickest results. Each sixty- to ninety-minute session is focused on a specific goal, and starts with PACE (positive, active, clear, and energetic), a series of steps that prepare the participant for the work ahead.

Then the instructor and the student go through a process called a "balance." Together they identify where the brain is working smoothly, and where it's responding less efficiently. The instructor guides the student through basic Brain Gym or in-depth edu-k movements, to help the brain make those connections more effectively. Whole-body activities, exercises to activate eye-hand coordination, movements for fine motor coordination, and others may be used, depending on each individual's needs.

By the end of the balance, the student notices positive changes in attitude, posture, and skills. The student is assigned exercises to do daily at home. These exercises, called "homeplay," support and stabilize the cumulative benefits of the balance. Parents are encouraged to do exercises at home with their children, and often the whole family will do Brain Gym together.

Benefits of Brain Gym®

Today, Brain Gym is used in thousands of schools in the United States, Canada, Europe, Australia, New Zealand, Africa, and Russia. Improvements are reported in all areas of academic skills, including self-esteem, memory, recall, test-taking, listening and attention, technical and creative writing, reading speed and comprehension, oral reading and self-expression. People with learning difficulties such as dyslexia, ADD, and ADHD report improved focus, comprehension, and physical coordination with Brain Gym. Reports indicate, students get more out of other methods when Brain Gym is added.

—*Lark Carroll*

* Brain Gym® is a registered trademark of the Educational Kinesiology Foundation.

Resources:

The Educational Kinesiology Foundation
P.O. Box 3396
Ventura, CA 93006-3396
Tel: (800) 356-2109
Web site: www.braingym.com
Lists Brain Gym instructors in your area, provides copies of the newsletters Brain Gym Journal *and* Edu-K Update, *and offers schedules of courses.*

Further Reading:

Dennison, Gail E., and Paul E.Dennison, Ph.D. *Brain Gym.* Ventura, CA: Edu-Kinesthetics, Inc., 1986.

——. *Brain Gym: Teacher's Edition*, Revised edition. Ventura, CA: Edu-Kinesthetics, Inc., 1994.

Brain Gym's Popularity

In 1991 the White House Task Force on Innovative Learning acclaimed Brain Gym as one of twelve "successful learning innovations" because of its effectiveness in improving basic math, reading, and writing skills. Its reputation is now international, and schools in countries such as New Zealand have incorporated Brain Gym into their curricula.

———. *Edu-K for Kids.* Ventura, CA: Edu-Kinesthetics, Inc., 1987.

———. *Personalized Whole Brain Integration.* Ventura, CA: Edu-Kinesthetics, Inc., 1985.

Dennison, Gail E., Paul E. Dennison, Ph.D., and Jerry V. Teplitz, J.D., Ph.D. *Brain Gym for Business.* Ventura, CA: Edu-Kinesthetics, Inc., 1995.

Hannaford, Carla, Ph.D. *Smart Moves. Why Learning Is Not All in Your Head.* Arlington, VA: Great Ocean Publishers, 1995.

CONTACT IMPROVISATION

Contact improvisation is a form of dance that explores the relationship of mind and body during the experience of interactive touch and improvised movement. While it is generally performed in group classes and jam sessions, and involves ensemble exercises, training focuses on the skills and the attitudes required to create a duet without cues from a choreographed scenario or speech. In fact music is often not used in contact improvisation. The process starts by tuning the partners' capacity to "listen" and respond to touch and leads to dancing that ranges freely from gentle gestures to acrobatic movements. In a typical dance, the partners lean, roll, and fall on *and* with each other; they may also lift or invert the other. At any level of expertise, the dancing builds a momentum that encourages trust, risk-taking, and physical dialogue from participants. Contact improvisation continues to be best known as a component of professional dance, but awareness of its psychological and physical benefits has won it growing popularity as an "art sport" for amateurs. During the past few years, it has also been approached as a mode of mind/body healing and as an adjunct to the martial arts of Asia.

The Development of Contact Improvisation

Although contact improvisation is now included in many dancers' repertory of techniques, it originated in the 1960s amid a wave of experiments that challenged the traditions governing the conception and presentation of dance. Stylized movement, mythic narrative, and stage spectacle were jettisoned in an effort, led first by the Merce Cunningham and then the Judson Church Group, to find ways to connect dance to the realities of contemporary life. Judson Church productions featured movement taken from work, sports, and the martial arts and often investigated ordinary activity, such as sweeping a floor. What was eventually called contact improvisation first appeared in 1972 in "Magnesium," a piece presented by Steve Paxton, a choreographer and dancer who had been a member of both the Cunningham Company and the Judson Church Group. The dancers of "Magnesium" did not attempt to "perform" anything; they instead reacted to one another, improvising their movements and going with the flow of the experience. Later in 1972, Paxton presented a performance evolved from "Magnesium." It retained the use of a group of improvising dancers but focused on the interaction of mixed- and same-sex partners and became the prototype for his subsequent work with contact improvisation.

Assisted by teachers such as Nancy Stark Smith and Daniel Lepkoff, Paxton started to offer workshops and performances in contact improvisation. By the late 1970s, it had its own publication, the *Contact Newsletter*, later renamed the *Contact Quarterly*, and was becoming a major force in the development of postmodern dance. Dance companies that based their work on contact improvisation were mushrooming in the United States, and by the early 1980s, dancers in cultural centers throughout the world, especially Amsterdam, Berlin, and London, were adapting its principles.

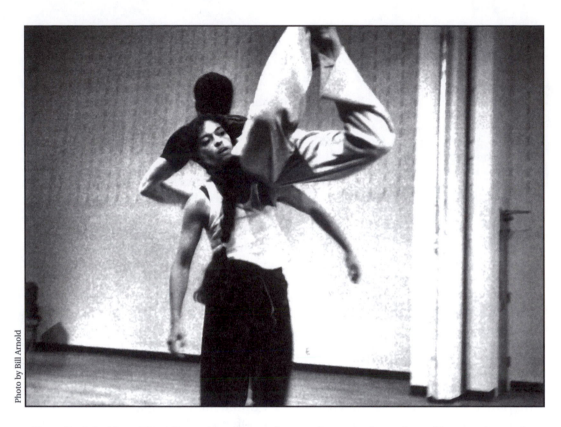

Photo by Bill Arnold

Nancy Stark Smith and Steve Paxton, developers of contact improvisation, a dance-like somatic practice.

Contact improvisation entered the world of body-mind therapy through an outpouring of popular support. It had been attracting a huge amateur following during the 1970s and 1980s and gradually made its way into the curricula of many colleges and universities. In this context of self-discovery and liberal arts study, contact improvisation began to be viewed as a technique accessible to anyone interested in enhancing their understanding of body-mind communication. For some, contact improvisation became a complement to the practice of t'ai chi, aikido, or yoga. For others, it offered a means of helping children, senior citizens, and people with disabilities. Today, three organizations, Touchdown, DanceAbility, and Mobility Junction, are at the forefront of the work being done to incorporate contact improvisation into therapy programs for people with special needs.

The Principles of Contact Improvisation

Despite the diversity of its sources and improvised structures, contact improvisation has a remarkably consistent look and feel, whether done by professional or amateur dancers. This is because, like a conversation, it has a few ground rules that everyone understands and follows as they meet and exchange responses. Trust is a top priority. The dancers need to release tension and uncertainty and meet one another in an open, relaxed way. Otherwise they will not be able to establish the connection that is essential to the process of reciprocal improvisation. Trust and physical listening are key factors in determining the actions of the dancers. They drop concern for the look of the body in order to concentrate on the flow of energy between them and their partner. The outcome is a collaborative process described as "a cross between jitterbugging, wrestling, and making love." The dancers focus on the physical sensations of touching, leaning, supporting, and falling with one another. Awkwardness matters only if it is a symptom of one dancer's lack of focus and withdrawal from the spontaneous release into the here-and-now of physical experience. The emphasis on being present in the moment links contact improvisation to the martial arts, yoga, and meditation. All these disciplines encourage the individual to let go of blocks that prevent him from apprehending the energy that constantly courses between mind and body.

Experiencing Contact Improvisation

Students work with one another, learning to establish connection through light physical touch and to move together in a shared kinesphere. A kinesphere may be pictured as a bubble of space in which the body moves. It is usually envisioned as the 360 degrees of space encircling an individual, but in contact improvisation the kinesphere is the joint creation of dancers who become adept at falling and rolling together, sliding off each other, spiraling around, and leaning into each other. They learn to find "tables" or body surfaces on one partner that can support the balanced weight of the other.

The structure of a class in contact improvisation depends on the teacher's particular interests and on the needs and abilities of individual students. Beginning-level classes concentrate on the basic skills for performing duet and group improvisation. Exercises in touch increase the skin's ability to register information about the speed and angle of movement. Other exercises help the body to release and become receptive. Students learn to roll and slide on the floor and on each other with ease; to use the body's surfaces for support; to flow with the momentum of movement; to reverse and invert the body's orientation; and to circle and spiral in space.

More complex duet and group improvisation is the focus of classes at the intermediate and advanced levels. Mastery of an exercise known as "flying" is often the last skill to be taught. The dancers vault in the air, are caught by their partners, and perch momentarily over the head of their partner. Gender equality is valued at this as at all levels of training: men lift women and vice versa.

A portion of each class is generally reserved for free-form dancing by students. The action is likely to begin in a "round robin." Some members of the group improvise while the others form a circle around them. As the dancing proceeds, the organization of the "round robin" becomes increasingly fluid. People join and leave the dancing at will, improvise with various partners, or dance alone.

The Risks and Benefits of Contact Improvisation

Though injuries are rare in contact improvisation, it is a strenuous activity and many participants take the precaution of wearing kneepads. It is also advisable to review one's personal boundaries before taking up contact improvisation. Those with a history of trauma or abuse may find it disturbing.

Advocates regard contact improvisation as a unique blend of sport, art, and meditation and credit it with numerous health benefits. It can release tension, promote an overall sense of well-being and ease, boost vitality, and aid concentration. Further, as a non-sexual form of intimacy, it affords a safe way to sort through volatile issues of gender, trust, bonding, control, and spontaneity in human relationships. Some proponents would add that contact improvisation is most effective and complete when experienced as a metaphor for the movement and change pervading all aspects of late twentieth-century life.

—*Paul Langland*

251

Resources:

Contact Collaborations
c/o Forti Studio
537 Broadway
New York, NY 10012
Provides information about contact improvisation training and performance; maintains a video archive of contact improvisation.

Contact Quarterly
P.O. Box 603
Northampton, MA 01061
Tel: (413) 586-1181
A journal with articles on contact improvisation and compiles an international directory of contact improvisers.

Movement Research
296 Elizabeth Street
New York, NY 10012
Tel: (212) 477-6635
Provides information about contact improvisation classes.

Further Reading:

Novack, Cynthia J. *Sharing the Dance: Contact Improvisation and American Culture.* Madison, WI: University of Wisconsin Press, 1990.

CONTINUUM

Continuum, a movement program developed by Emilie Conrad-Da'oud in 1967, encourages participants to resonate with the motions and rhythms of our primordial origins, which are subtle, undulating movements pulsing in the fluids of our bodies. One of the benefits of this practice is to facilitate the release of mental and physical illness from the body and promote health through engagement on a biological level.

Origins of Continuum
Continuum springs from the work of one woman, Emilie Conrad-Da'oud, who was born in New York City in 1934. Conrad-Da'oud is a classically trained dancer who spent five years as a choreographer in Haiti in the late 1950s. Upon her return to the United States in 1960, Conrad-Da'oud remained fascinated with the throbbing drum rhythms of Haitian music and dance. She wondered if the richness of Haitian dance might draw from roots deeper than culture. She wondered whether its power might stem from a biological source.

Guided by all that she had absorbed from the richness of the sacred dances of Haiti, Conrad-Da'oud spent seven years deconstructing their movements and exploring their origins. Inspired by Damballah, the snake deity from the vodou religion of Haiti, Conrad-Da'oud gained insight into the powerful origins of these movements. As a serpent with its belly to the earth, Damballah brought the undulating movements of the water to land, and it was these motions that Conrad-Da'oud recognized in Haitian sacred dances as a link between humankind's water-based origins and our current, land-based lives.

From 1974 to 1979, Conrad Da'oud's work was researched by Dr. Valerie Hunt, professor of kinesiology at UCLA. Hunt's findings questioned conventional notions of movement education at the time. She found that, through a practice such as continuum, we can access our own cellular world, or effect changes in our body on a cellular level, and encourage our body's capacity to innovate when faced with injury or illness.

Many movement education programs deal with the body as an object while continuum presents it as a process. In other words, continuum explores the body on a fluid and cellular level, believing the body is not bounded by form; there is a constant exchange in our fluids and cells with those of the environment, and we are in continual participation with the planetary process.

These ideas have influenced the fields of dance, physical therapy, deep tissue therapy, as well as disciplines such as chiropractic, physical fitness, and somatics. People from many different disciplines in the alternative health community explore continuum and apply to their own practices the idea of the human being as a fluid, innovative, boundless being, with movement inherent to our very selves.

Theory of Continuum

The continuum program represents Conrad-Da'oud's distillation of Damballah's wavelike motions with our own human biology. A human's first environment, in the uterus, is liquid. According to Conrad-Da'oud, our fluid origin is inseparable from our surrounding environment. In other words, the fluids of the biosphere resonate with the fluid of our bodies and we are in concert with our world. For these reasons, continuum holds that human beings are primarily aquatic and become terrestrial.

Conrad-Da'oud also sees human beings as "biomorphic," which means that we include all life-forms. We are all part of a larger process, along with other animals, plants, and Earth itself. Conrad-Da'oud emphasizes that the human body emerges from the matings of earlier life, from protozoa to mammals, the vestiges of which lie within us, along with the vastness of biological intelligence.

Continuum encourages participants to explore themselves as biomorphic beings and to establish a mental and physical rapport with the various life-forms within them. Participants allow their primordial movements—which curve, arc, and spiral—to emerge. Through rapport with our biological heritage, Conrad-Da'oud has found that our complex fluidity can provide an environment for creativity and innovation to occur. In relation to "healing," the suggestion is made that innovation can create neural pathways that can bypass trauma, allowing life to move on in new and surprising ways.

The Experience and Health Benefits of Continuum

Conrad-Da'oud's work involves a great deal of attention to the movement of breath. All movement begins with inhaling and exhaling. By invoking a softening of the breath, participants of continuum disrupt habitual patterns and encourage an increased mobility of breath to access greater flexibility and adaptability. This new dexterity of breath invigorates nerve fibers and connective tissues that have become entrenched in the old patterns. Ultimately, these breathing exercises increase our capacity to receive cellular nourishment and bring about a healing environment to areas that have become barren and atrophied.

Physical and emotional trauma and genetic deformities sometimes leave the body with limited functionality. Among the paralyzed, for example, the traditional neural pathways have been injured. By breathing in a manner that creates a wavelike motion, we can cause micro-movements to spread into dormant areas, often returning function to areas that traditional medicine cannot affect.

Continuum, more than anything else, provides a context for questioning and comprehending not just physical movement but all aspects of our functioning. Our whole thinking-feeling-moving-electrochemical-electromagnetic organism participating within its biological and cultural environment can be lived as one unbroken movement. Participants come to understand that our responsibilities, the significance and meanings we give our world, can be seen as one process of flowing movement.

—Compiled in consultation with
Emilie Conrad-Da'oud

Resources:

Continuum Studio
1629 18th Street 7
Santa Monica, CA 90404
Tel: (310) 453-4402
Fax: (310) 453-8775
Offers workshops in Continuum.

EURYTHMY

Eurythmy is a movement art that translates verbal and musical sounds into movement of the human body. According to eurythmy, there are three most basic ways in which life expresses itself. They are movement, form, and language. By integrating these elemental expressions of life and creating a harmonious expression of them, eurythmy is believed to reach the spiritual nature behind all living things, giving this spiritual nature a clear voice and a visible reality.

The Origin of Eurythmy

Eurythmy was conceived in 1912 by Rudolf Steiner, the Austrian-born founder of the spiritual movement known as Anthroposophy. *Eurythmy* is a Greek term meaning "harmonious rhythm" and was chosen because Steiner saw rhythm as the very basis and center of life. Around the time that he began to consider the notion of eurythmy, Steiner founded the Anthroposophical Society, a movement intended to help further his teachings, particularly his belief in the existence of a spiritual realm that can be perceived by people with highly developed mental faculties.

A philosopher and visionary, Steiner asserted that all human beings—with proper training and preparation—have the potential to participate in the spiritual world. To this end, he devised a system of education called the Waldorf School movement, which uses such disciplines as eurythmy to teach individuals from the earliest age about their inner spirituality and their relationship to the world around them. Eurythmy also can be performed on stages before audiences or employed as a therapy for treating various types of illness. There are currently more than thirty eurythmy training centers located throughout the world.

Language and Music as a Basis for Movement

In eurythmy the human voice and language are often used as the basis for movement. Human sound can be thought of as carrying all of life within it. The name of a thing, a person, or an experience can be seen as more than just a separate description. The sounds chosen to represent something can be seen as a reenactment of the unique spiritual and physical qualities of the thing in question, as holding the essential qualities of the thing itself. And so when eurythmy is performed, the gestures are not symbols, they are expressions of the essence of the thing itself.

The human voice is a remarkable instrument, capable of transforming our inner experiences into another medium—sound. When the sounds of language and song are intoned, they set into motion unique yet invisible waves or gestures through the air. In eurythmy these gestures are artistically expressed to reveal the outer forms belonging to each consonant or vowel, each musical tone or interval.

The Philosophy of Eurythmy

For Steiner, eurythmy was not a physical illustration or interpretation of language and music, but instead a true expression of sound through the body. Claiming to see a shifting field of energy around each human being, Steiner identified a system of body movements that correspond to the shapes of the energy field as it responds to each spoken word and musical sound. To an uninformed member of the audience, eurythmy may seem to be a mix of mime, dance, and sign language performed to music, singing, or spoken word. Steiner, however, declared that eurythmic movements are equivalent to sound, not artistic representations of it. To him, eurythmy is one means of assisting humankind in returning to an earlier state in which people were more aware of their inner being and the invisible processes of the world. In the *Introduction to Eurythmy,*

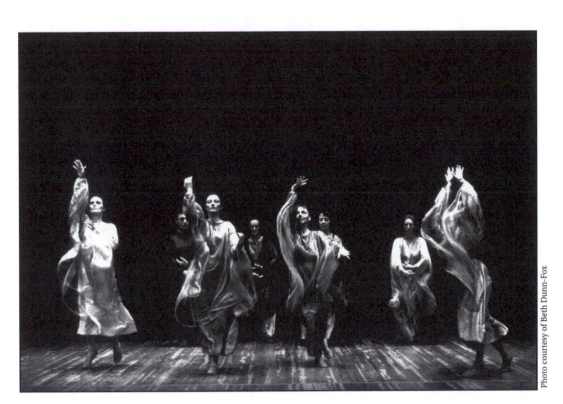

The techniques of eurythmy can be used to create concert dance.

Steiner stated: "The seeds of movement are manifest in the human larynx and its neighboring organs when someone speaks . . . or when he produces musical sounds. If one had some artificial device by which one could see at such a moment how the air mass is stirred to rhythmic vibration by the incipient movements of the larynx and its neighboring organs, he would realize . . . how the entire man is revealed through it."

Eurythmy in Practice

In studying eurythmy, a person learns about the different qualities found in the sounds of language and tones of music. Eurythmy classes begin with movement exercises that help students better understand and be more comfortable with space, with people around them, and with their own movements. Subsequently, one is taught specific movements or gestures that correspond to each letter of the alphabet. Initially,

movements are acted out in silence, and later they are performed in collaboration with live music or spoken words. In a speech eurythmy class, students examine the elements of language Steiner felt appeared in poetry, drama, and fiction. In a tone eurythmy class, they study the gestures Steiner believed were inherent in music. Performance of eurythmy on a stage can incorporate colorful costumes and dramatic lighting, which heighten the mood created by the actors and musicians.

Benefits of Eurythmy

Students who have studied eurythmy at Waldorf schools reportedly benefit from improved coordination, agility, and flexibility, and a greater sense of physical well-being; for these reasons, eurythmy is also commonly used as therapy. Group practice of eurythmy creates a strong sense of teamwork, as individuals jointly overcome their reluctance to use physical expression in public. Furthermore, since eurythmy is taught as a means to explore the psyche, this very personal, revealing experience can have the effect of bonding those who undergo the process together. As well as these reasons for practicing eurythmy, Steiner insisted that the most important benefit is mental: decreased dependence on the world of the senses and increased perception of the spiritual world.

—*Beth Dunn-Fox*

Resources:

Anthroposophic Press
RR 4 Box 94 A-1
Hudson, NY 2534
Tel: (518) 851-2054
Fax: (518) 851-2047
Publishes many Rudolf Steiner texts, including several on eurythmy. A catalog is available upon request.

Eurythmy Association of North America
13726 23rd Avenue NE
Seattle, WA 98125
Tel: (206) 361-6113

Eurythmy Spring Valley
285 Hungry Hollow Road
Chestnut Ridge, NY 0977
Tel: (914) 352-5020
Fax: (914) 352-5071
e-mail: bdeury@aol.com
Provides a professional training program accredited by the Association of Eurythmy in Dornach, Switzerland. Weekly courses and summer workshops are also offered for those interested in experiencing eurythmy for refreshment and self-development.

Waldorf Schools in North America Director of Schools
Web site: www.io.com/user/karisch/
waldir.html
Waldorf schools, many of which offer eurythmy classes for children, teens, and adults, are located throughout the United States and Canada.

Further Reading:

Steiner, Rudolf. *Curative Eurythmy*. Hudson, NY: Anthroposophic Press, 1984.

——. *Eurythmy as Visible Speech*. Hudson, NY: Anthroposophic Press, 1984.

——. *An Introduction to Eurythmy: Talks Given Before Sixteen Eurythmy Performances*. Hudson, NY: Anthroposophic Press, 1983.

——. *A Lecture on Eurythmy*. London: Rudolf Steiner Press, 1977.

GURDJIEFF MOVEMENTS

The Gurdjieff movements were developed by the Armenian teacher George Ivanovitch Gurdjieff as the way for his pupils to experience in movement the reality of his teaching. Practice of the Gurdjieff movements has meaning only when undertaken in the context of an entire program of activities and studies of the system of Gurdjieff's ideas. The aim of the movements is to bring together the mind, body, and feelings through the performance of different kinds of exercises, rhythmic sequences, series of postures, and dances.

George Ivanovitch Gurdjieff

George Ivanovitch Gurdjieff was born in 1866 in Alexandropol, now known as Gumri, in what is now Armenia. He was raised and educated in Russian Armenia at a time and place in which there was a confluence of new technologies and scientific ideas of the West with the traditions, thought, and religions of the East.

In his autobiographical account, *Meetings with Remarkable Men* (published posthumously in 1963), he writes of his father, a well-known ashokh, or bard, who was part of an oral tradition

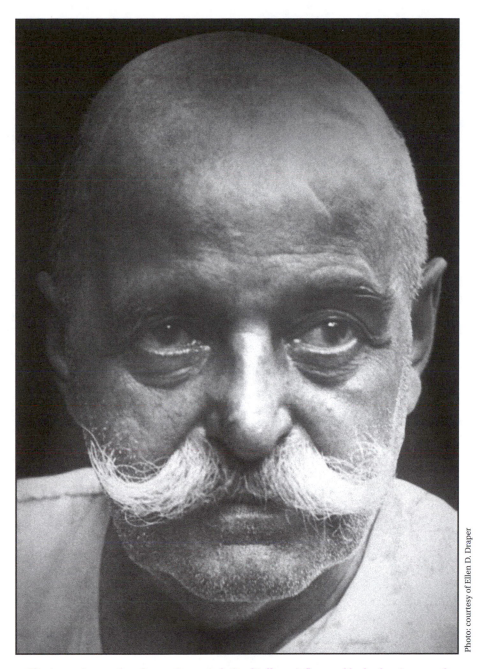

The Armenian teacher George Ivanovitch Gurdjieff was influenced by both science and religion.

stretching back to the distant past. The legends that he heard from his father left a mark on his whole life. His tutors, men of science and religion, trained him for both the priesthood and medicine, and he pursued his studies with burning interest. In *Meetings with Remarkable Men*, Gurdjieff describes several close escapes from death as well as encounters with "magic" and other manifestations of realities beyond the explanations of science and logic. As he came of age in the midst of these unfathomable mysteries and inexplicable events, Gurdjieff felt dissatisfied with the answers of contemporary knowledge and began his search for other sources of wisdom. He and fellow "seekers of truth"—young people with questions similar to his own, including engineers, doctors, archaeologists, and musicians—journeyed for several years through central Asia and northern Africa to find the answers to their questions about the meaning of life.

Eventually they found a school in a remote, nearly inaccessible monastery, whose exact location remains a mystery. It was here that Gurdjieff first witnessed sacred dances.

In the early 1900s, Gurdjieff came to Moscow with a teaching that attracted groups of artists and intellectuals, including P. D. Ouspensky (1878–1947), one of his best-known disciples. As the Russian revolution drew near, Gurdjieff and a small group of followers moved to Tiflis (now Tbilisi, Georgia) and established the Institute for the Harmonious Development of Man. It was here that he first taught "sacred gymnastics"—now known as the Movements. He was joined at this time by the composer Thomas de Hartmann and his wife, and by the Russian painter Alexandre de Salzmann and his wife, Jeanne, a teacher of Dalcroze eurythmics, a study of the relationship between music and movement. When World War I made it impossible for him to continue his work there, Gurdjieff and his pupils continued their journey to Essentuki, Russia, in 1917, to Istanbul, Turkey, in 1920, and finally to France. In 1922, he reestablished the Institute for the Harmonious Development of Man at the Chateau du Prieuré at Fontainebleau, near Paris. During the 1920s and 1930s, Gurdjieff further developed many of the central methods and practices of his teaching, including the movements. His work began to attract people throughout Europe, and in 1924 he visited America for the first time.

During the years between 1924 and 1935, Gurdjieff reduced the work of the institute, putting most of his energy and attention on writing. After 1935, assisted by Jeanne de Salzmann, he expanded the work of the institute in France and visited the United States three more times, enlarging his work there. He died in Paris on October 29, 1949.

For forty years after Gurdjieff's death, his primary pupil, Jeanne de Salzmann, guided the ongoing efforts of Gurdjieff Foundation groups throughout the world. She oversaw the publication of his writings, and between 1950 and 1984, she produced a series of documentary films of the movements as an archive of the Gurdjieff teaching. Today, movements classes are part of a whole program of activities conducted at the Gurdjieff Foundations in Paris, London, New York, Caracas, and other major cities. The Gurdjieff work remains an oral tradition, passed from teacher to pupil in a living chain of transmission.

At the heart of Gurdjieff's teaching is the perspective that human beings are a vital link in a universal process. Unfortunately, they are "asleep" to their unique cosmic place and to the full potential of their individual essential natures. Each person is like someone who lives in the smallest room of his or her house, never suspecting there are other rooms, filled with treasure.

According to Gurdjieff's teaching, what is needed in order to discover each person's own hidden treasure is a new kind of attention that comes from the physical and emotional sides of one's nature as well as from the mind. Gurdjieff was a merciless critic of the usual kind of education, which he said only "stuffs" the mind with unrelated information and opinions. He constantly told his pupils that they should verify for themselves everything he taught and accept nothing until they had personally experienced its truth.

The Movements

With the aim of an education for the whole human being, Gurdjieff introduced the study of ideas, group meetings, practical physical work, and the movements. Participation in the movements is one of the primary means through which students are able to experience the power that mechanical habits such as posture, tension, facial expression, etc., have over their inner states. The practice of experiencing one's actual way of being, or *self-study*, according to Gurdjieff, is the beginning of *self-knowledge* and inner freedom. Practice of the movements offers the opportunity for such study and the foretaste of such a liberating knowledge.

The task of the dancers is to learn to participate with the whole of themselves. What is seen is the movement itself, as if the series of postures were the outer image of an inner and more subtle energy. Understood in this way, one realizes that the aim of the movements is not to create a psychic state of some kind, but to develop a specific attention leading to an immediate and practical experience of the inner structure of the human being and of the cosmological order to which humanity belongs.

Movements classes are composed of students working together in a group, with more experienced pupils directing and guiding the course of each class. There are exercises of different qualities, including movements of forceful dynamism and quiet prayer, men's and women's dances, and exercises that demonstrate the cyclic movements of mathematical laws. Each dance or exercise is composed of sequences of fixed postures executed in specific rhythms and tempos in which a demand is made to stretch the attention beyond its usual limits. Practicing these exercises, one finds it possible to truly inhabit the body; from there, one may then open to the transformative power that a better quality of attention can bring.

The music used to accompany the sacred dances comes from various sources. Gurdjieff had a keen sensitivity to and memory for the music he had heard since his early childhood and during his travels in Asia. Between 1919 and 1924, he began to write music for the sacred dances in close collaboration with the composer Thomas de Hartmann. Later, de Hartmann and others expanded this literature, and pianists accompanying today's movements classes play these earlier compositions as well as improvise music based on similar scales and harmonies. The task of the pianist, like the pupils working in the class, is to seek to understand the meaning of each exercise as it is being practiced.

A New Potential

The study of the Gurdjieff movements, when undertaken in conjunction with the study of his system of ideas, offers the means for inner discovery and development. Through this practice, the mind and the feelings are able to combine with the movements of the body to express the potential of the whole human being.

—*The Gurdjieff Foundation of New York*

The Sacred Dances

During his youth, Gurdjieff traveled to regions of Central Asia in search of answers to the questions that tormented him. In remote monasteries, he first witnessed certain sacred dances that made a lasting impression on him. This is dramatized in Peter Brook's film, *Meetings with Remarkable Men*, when the young Gurdjieff asks, "What is the meaning of these movements?" An older pupil answers, "They tell us of two qualities of energy moving without interruption through the body. As long as the dancer can keep in balance these two energies, he has a force that nothing else can give. . ."

Further Reading:

Gurdjieff, G. I. *Beelzebub's Tales to His Grandson.* Aurora, OR: Two Rivers Press, 1993. (A facsimile of the original 1950 edition published by Harcourt Brace and reissued by E. P. Dutton in 1964.)

———. *Beelzebub's Tales to His Grandson.* New York and London: Viking Arkana, 1992. (A revised translation of the original.)

———. *Meetings with Remarkable Men.* New York: E. P. Dutton, 1963; New York and London: Arkana, 1985.

———. *Life Is Real Only Then, When "I Am."* New York: E. P. Dutton, 1978; New York and London: Viking Arkana, 1991.

———. *Views from the Real World: Early Talks in Moscow, Essentuki, Tiflis, Berlin, London, Paris, New York and Chicago as Recollected by His Pupils.* New York: E. P. Dutton, 1973; London: Viking Arkana, 1984.

Ouspensky, P. D. *In Search of the Miraculous: Fragments of an Unknown Teaching.* New York: Harcourt Brace and World, 1949.

———. *The Psychology of Man's Possible Evolution.* New York: Knopf, 1954.

*The film *Meetings with Remarkable Men,* created by Jeanne de Salzmann and Peter Brook, is available on videocassette through Corinth Video.

PILATES METHOD OF BODY CONDITIONING®

The Pilates Method of Body Conditioning®* consists of a series of exercises designed to develop a complete and balanced individual by strengthening and stretching the body while fully engaging the mind. Founded more than seventy years ago by Joseph Pilates, this method has been quite popular among dancers and professional athletes. While the exercises may appear to be just physical, there is a conscious aspect that is essential. Students use concentration and mental focus to control body alignment and breathing and to perform exercises with grace and control. The exercises are intended to create a graceful efficiency in one's everyday movements. Many practitioners also report a direct "mental rejuvenation" as a result of performing these exercises.

The History of the Pilates Method of Body Conditioning®

Joseph H. Pilates was born in Germany in 1880. He was a frail and sickly child suffering from rickets and asthma. Determined to be strong and healthy, Pilates worked extremely hard at bodybuilding, and by the time he was fourteen years old, he had become so physically fit that he was able to pose for anatomical charts. He then went on to become a boxer, diver, skier, and gymnast.

In 1912 Pilates moved to England, where he continued his boxing training and taught self-defense classes. During World War I he was interned with other German nationals on the Isle of Man. While there he began devising his personal exercise methods and started designing special equipment to help with the exercises. He also helped rehabilitate injured internees and encouraged others to practice his technique in order to stay healthy.

In 1923 Pilates left England for America, and on the way he met and married a woman whose own ideas about exercise fused with and encouraged his. Together they founded the first Pilates studio in New York City.

For many years the Pilates Method was extremely popular among dancers and professional performers in New York City, while it remained virtually unknown elsewhere. Dancers embrace the method for its ability to fine-tune the body, giving the dancer great strength and energy while maintaining long, lean muscles with tremendous flexibility. In

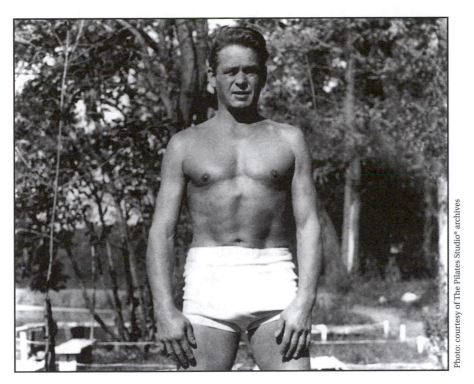

Photo: courtesy of The Pilates Studio® archives

Physical culturist Joseph H. Pilates, founder of the Pilates Method of Body Conditioning®

more recent years this system's popularity has grown to encompass people of all ages and all stages of fitness. Today, such medical professionals as physical therapists and chiropractors are recommending and adopting Pilates as a means of rehabilitation and preventative medicine, and certified studios now can be found throughout the world.

Pilates' Philosophy of Body/Mind Development

Joseph Pilates believed that fitness required more than just physical education. He believed in the development of the whole person—body, mind, and spirit. Pilates referred to his unique system of exercise as the "art of contrology." In his book *Return to Life*, he states, "Contrology develops the body uniformly, corrects wrong postures, restores physical vitality, invigorates the mind, and elevates the spirit." Pilates felt that with improved physical functioning, one's endurance improves, allowing more time and energy for what

he called "playing," spending quality time with family and friends, enjoying a movie or a play, or reading a book. Pilates believed that having increased energy for such activities would undoubtedly have a positive effect on one's mind and spirit.

Control, Centering, Precision, Flowing Movement

These are the key principles of the Pilates Method. Throughout a session, one concentrates on all of these aspects. To be effective the movements have to be performed correctly, according to precise standards. For this reason, concentration is considered as important as the physical movements. The mind focuses on controlling all aspects of the movement: maintaining body alignment, doing exercises exactly as indicated by the instructor, using graceful, flowing movements, and keeping the breath flowing. An essential element of the Pilates Method is the concept of the body's "center," referred to as the "powerhouse of the anatomy." This circular "belt" around the body encompasses the lower back and abdominals; an immediate benefit one feels as a result of practicing Pilates is strength in the abdominal muscles and relief of chronic lower back discomfort.

The Pilates® Studio and Classes

Today these studios often look strange yet elegant with equipment, mats, and various apparatus, all built to Joseph Pilates' specifications. While there are several machines used, the main piece of equipment is known as the universal reformer. It looks similar to the frame of a single bed with a sliding carriage attached to four springs. After adjusting the number of springs to regulate the resistance, the student pushes or pulls against a metal bar or straps. The exercises are done sitting, lying down, kneeling, and standing. Emphasis is not on maximum resistance but on the student's ability to work with and control the springs. The springs help with a stretching and contracting action in the muscles.

Individuals may begin practicing Pilates at any level of fitness. The exercises are learned slowly, and strength is built gradually. Students are encouraged to progress at their own rate. Once fundamental exercises have been mastered, new and more challenging ones are introduced, each in a very particular order, thus building up a repertoire of exercises. There are hundreds of various exercises and, depending on the individual's progress, as many of these will be taught as deemed necessary by the instructor.

At the initial session, the client's physical history is discussed, a certified instructor takes the student through the initial series of exercises from beginning to end. An experienced certified instructor will be able to assess a person's particular strengths and weaknesses quickly and gauge what exercises are to be included in, or omitted from, the personal routine. From the beginning, basic principles are taught, including how to engage lower abdominal muscles, how to roll through the spinal column evenly and smoothly and how to maintain correct body posture and alignment.

While there is a specific sequence to the system, lessons are customized to suit the individual, with special problems taken into account. Each person does a complete series of exercises on specialized equipment and on a flat cushioned mat; in Pilates, the apparatus work and mat work are of equal importance. Within each exercise, repetitions are kept to a minimum, focusing on quality rather than quantity. This allows for a very high level of concentration and precise, careful movements and insures that muscles are never worked to exhaustion. The instructor often sets the rhythm, keeping the workout dynamic and energetic, yet always gentle and never hurried. One rarely hears music or chatting because students are encouraged to concentrate fully on the exercises and on their breathing. Many studios offer small group classes with rarely more than four students per instructor. Once a student has learned to perform the basic exercises correctly and confidently he or she can choose to supplement studio time with work done at home on a cushioned mat. Students can generally expect results after approximately ten consistent lessons, although some react more quickly.

The Pilates Method always considers the body as a whole rather than separate body parts. Every exercise will engage the entire body while paying particular attention to one main muscle group. At the end of each session the whole body is stretched and strengthened equally. Although a person's heart rate may increase, the Pilates Method is complementary to rather than a replacement for aerobic exercise.

Benefits of The Pilates Method®

Depending on the individual, benefits of using Pilates exercises may include improved posture, longer, leaner muscles, improved all-over strength (especially in the abdominal region), greater flexibility, general ease of movement, relief of chronic aches, more energy and endurance, and a higher level of concentration and focus in all aspects of one's life. A added benefit is that students invariably leave a Pilates studio feeling invigorated.

—Leah Chaback,
certified instructor and teacher trainer

*Pilates® and the Pilates Method of Body Conditioning® are registered trademarks.

Resources:

The Movement Center
39 Broadway
Kingston, NY 12401
Tel: (914) 331-0986
A certified, fully equipped Pilates studio that offers private, semiprivate, and group lessons.

The Pilates Studio
2121 Broadway
New York, NY 10023
Tel: (800) 4-PILATES
e-mail: mrpilates@aol.com
Web site: www.pilates-studio.com
A certified, fully equipped Pilates studio.

Further Reading:

Friedman, Philip, and Gail Eisen. *The Pilates Method of Physical and Method Conditioning* New York: Warner Books, 1981.

Pilates, Joseph, and William John Miller. *Return to Life Through Contrology.* Boston: Christopher Publishing House, 1960.

ROM DANCE

ROM dance is an exercise and relaxation program created for people with chronic pain and other physical limitations. ROM is the acronym used in physical therapy to describe the range of motion as flexibility of joints. These exercises, recommended by doctors and therapists, are combined with the basic principles of t'ai chi ch'üan, an ancient Chinese exercise practiced for health and longevity. T'ai chi ch'üan trains the participant to be calm while alert, both strong and flexible, and to relax in the midst of activity. These elements are applied to ROM dancing, teaching the participant to move gently and slowly in order to maintain the ability to move in spite of pain. It also allows the participant to develop sensitivity to subtle changes in the body that may eventually reduce pain and limitations. Through regular practice, this slow, fluid exercise is purported to enhance mental focus, body awareness, and imagination.

The History of ROM Dance
ROM dance was created in 1981 by Diane Harlowe, M.S., an occupational therapist and researcher, and Tricia Yu, M.A., a t'ai chi instructor and health educator, at St. Mary's Hospital in Madison, Wisconsin. Patients had complained that their exercises were boring and monotonous. Harlowe and Yu designed this unique routine of stretches and movements, which take about seven minutes to complete, to encourage their patients to keep moving everyday.

The program had the following objectives: assisting and inspiring the participants in following any medical recommendations for involvement in daily exercise/rest routines; increasing frequency, enjoyment and perceived benefit of involvement in daily exercise and rest; enhancing the ability to cope with stress and pain through use of relaxation techniques; improving body awareness; and promoting a general sense of well-being.

Originally designed as an eight-week community health education program, it is now taught by physical and occupational therapists, nurses, dance and recreation therapists, and t'ai chi ch'üan instructors in hospitals, senior centers, nursing homes, outpatient clinics, patients' homes, and rehabilitation clinics.

The Principles of ROM Dance

The seven major ROM dance principles are adapted from the ancient body-mind principles of t'ai chi ch'üan. *Attention to the present* awakens all the senses of the ROM dance practitioner as he or she is guided to look, listen, smell, or feel all the physical sensations coming to and from the body-mind. *Diaphragmatic breathing* and *postural alignment* help relax and nourish the body and mind. As a result, the respiratory and musculoskeletal systems function more fully and easily. *Moving more slowly than normal* enhances *awareness of movement* sensation and builds strength as well as sensitivity in the body and the mind. Avoiding unnecessary tension or force creates *relaxed movement* which encourages healthy functioning of the circulatory and nervous systems. Exercising the imagination by reciting poetic images from nature while doing the ROM dance seems to evoke soothing, nurturing, healing feelings of warmth and a sense of personal involvement and well-being.

ROM Dance in Practice

ROM dance, which takes about seven minutes to complete, can be performed both sitting and standing. It incorporates movement in all ranges for the large joints, and includes a special exercise routine for the small joints of the hands.

The program includes instruction in both exercise and relaxation. It is designed to be practiced as a daily routine to help maintain flexibility. The relaxation and pain management training provides participants with strategies for relaxing both during periods of rest and when dealing with stress or pain in the middle of daily activities.

The Benefits and Risks of the ROM Dance Program

The program can help people with a variety of disabilities maintain a range of motion and cope with stress and pain. It can also be used as the warm-up and cool-down phases of more extensive exercise programs.

ROM dance is based on movements usually recommended for rheumatoid arthritis. It has also been successfully used in the following areas: fibromyalgia; hand therapy; psychiatry; geriatrics; oncology (cancer); Parkinson's disease; stress management; pain management; lupus; and the practice of neurology.

Those interested in learning and practicing ROM dance should be advised that it is not a substitute for medically recommended exercise therapy unless approved or modified by a physician or therapist. Also, the following risks should be noted: people with severe neck problems or hip replacements should check with their doctors before attempting the movements; dancers should avoid straining or forcing any movements and should personally modify them when necessary; and those using this dance program should always apply proper body mechanics when standing and sitting.

Because the movements of ROM dance are gentle and take only a few minutes a day to perform, nearly everyone—including individuals in wheelchairs—can do them. The program may improve flexibility and mobility while promoting a general sense of relaxation in a safe, slow, and gentle manner.

—Patricia Yu, M.A.

Resources:

The ROM Dance Network
P.O. Box 3332
Madison, WI 53704-0332
Tel: (608) 242-9133
Fax: (608) 242-9140
Links practitioners and professionals, disseminates information and instructional materials, and organizes seminars and training workshops. Provides the ROM Dance Multimedia Instructional

An Example of the Guided Imagery Used in ROM Dance Sessions

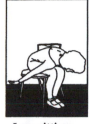

I am sitting—
at a quiet beach—

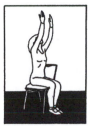

I scoop the warm water over my head
covering me with a warm waterfall—

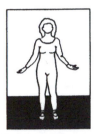

I gather the sun's warmth
over my shoulders and
it feels good—

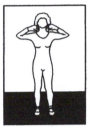

Someone comes to my beach who will be my friend—
we know that somehow in some way—
we will be together.

Kit, which is available to both professionals and individuals for personal home practice. It includes videos for both standing and wheelchair exercise, guided relaxation and music audiotapes, as well as a text for instructors.

SKINNER RELEASING TECHNIQUE

The Skinner releasing technique (SRT) is a movement discipline used to alleviate physical pain and tension. Based on the philosophy that all human beings have the potential to move with natural grace, SRT taps into intrinsic, primal coordination and the experience of movement at a deep kinesthetic level by using movement along with poetry, music, and imagery. It encourages people to understand how their bodies move and to visualize how their bodies can function without discomfort.

The Development of the Skinner Releasing Technique

Joan Skinner was dancing in the companies of Martha Graham and Merce Cunningham during the late forties and early fifties. Between her ballet class in the morning and her modern class in the afternoon she began to explore dance technique in her apartment in Greenwich Village, New York. She found an old banister that she used for a barre and set up mirrors so that she could see herself at the 3/4 angle from the front and back simultaneously. She kept a notebook in which she posed questions about the techniques she was learning in her dance classes. Teachers at that time used the terms "pull up—grip—hold on," and she wondered how one could breathe as nature intended while gripping and holding. Then she suffered a back injury that would not heal, and she was advised to consult an instructor who specialized in the Alexander technique—one of only three such instructors in the country at that time. The Alexander technique made sense to Joan because it did not compress the body with gripping but opened and extended it in a multidirectional way. It facilitated natural breathing, and it took the pressure off the injury so that it could heal.

After leaving New York, Joan spent three years working alone to develop what is now known as SRT. She began by applying the Alexander principles to ballet barre movements. In searching for that multidirectional balance, the barre exercises broke down to where she spent time balancing on one leg—without gripping and holding the balance. In the beginning this meant wobbling and losing balance and then getting back on the leg. The work then became kinesthetic—that is, she began perceiving movement at a subtle level of the muscular sensation.

When she went to the University of Illinois in 1966 to teach a traditional modern dance class, she introduced some of her new knowledge and techniques to her students. She used images and metaphors for kinesthetic experiences she wanted her students to have. They responded powerfully to the imagery and would drop the structure of the class to stay with an image. Joan realized that something important was happening to them, so she allowed the class to become less structured, a concept that formed the foundation of the Skinner releasing technique.

SRT in Practice

A typical class in the Skinner releasing technique includes three parts: tactile studies; floor work with guided imagery; and movement studies for the group, guided by the instructor. Music and sounds are interwoven throughout the session. The SRT pedagogy progresses from introductory work through ongoing levels to the advanced.

The tactile studies in SRT help students experience kinesthetically the releasing of fixed tension patterns in the shoulders, back, or legs. Almost everyone has acquired patterns of tension, sometimes hidden, in the body during the process of growing up under numerous stresses. Trained dancers often find these tension patterns in the body *underneath* their training. The tensions are blocks—distortions of the alignment of the natural body. Releasing these blocks allows for realignment of the body. This makes it possible to move with greater flexibility, range, speed, and strength.

A unique aspect of SRT is its integration of technique with creative process through the use of imagery. For example, if an instructor wants to focus a class on the concept of "autonomy of the limbs" he or she might begin with a tactile study focusing on the hip joint. The instructor guides student partners to gain a physical experience of more freedom of movement at the hip by instructing one partner to rotate and extend his or her partner's leg while the partner is passive, relinquishing control of his or her leg. Eventually the active partner is instructed to let go of the leg, allowing the passive partner to continue the movements alone. Later in the class, the same concept is developed through the use of a metaphor, a poetic image given by the teacher that stimulates an improvised exploration. To begin this creative process, students lie on the floor while the teacher, using a procedure similar to relaxation technique, verbally guides students into a state just under conscious control. This state is free of anxieties, and sensory perception is sharpened. In this state, one can be physically transformed by a mental image. Propelled by the image, students begin to move up from the floor, to improvise from the image of freeing the legs, and eventually to dance as the concept of "autonomy of the limbs" plays through the body-mind.

How SRT Works

The objectives of the technique are similar to traditional dance techniques:

optimal alignment, flexibility, strength, coordination, balance, speed, clarity of articulation, and control of nuance. But the means are distinctly different, in that the nature or essence of a movement finds its own form, fostering creativity.

The Skinner release technique deals with the universals within all dance forms. The individual discovers how she or he can move with the essences of basic body movements, such as turning or spinning, rather than a specific stylized form of the movement. Gradually, SRT practitioners are encouraged to improvise in more complex and challenging ways with the movement, at the same time they are focusing on a principle, such as—*no one segment of the body compresses against any other segment.* Thus the practitioners develop maximum technical freedom without being constricted within a specific dance style and ideally can adapt to any form.

Some professional dancers use SRT as a practice to enhance their study of a specific dance technique. Some practice SRT as their only dance technique. Many declare that their technical progress speeds up and their growth as artists deepens with these SRT experiences. Nonprofessional dancers who study SRT are frequently artists in other media: musicians, painters, and poets, as well as doctors, psychologists, physicists, and pregnant women. SRT's organic, holistic approach to body-mind integration becomes part of a way of life. The technique gives the individual an understanding of the uniqueness of his or her own body and the way in which a movement flows through it.

Benefits of SRT

As it is the primary objective of the discipline to maximize the movement potential of all its practitioners, it can be useful to people of all ages. The use of guided imagery allows individuals to explore important issues and encourages people to get in touch with their creative and expressive selves. Individuals who experience the Skinner release technique report reduced levels of stress, relief of chronic pain, improved alignment, increased flexibilty and strength, as well as increased energy and vitality.

—*Joan Skinner*

Resources:

The New York Public Library for the Performing Arts
Dance Collection
c/o Lincoln Center Plaza
New York, NY 10023-7498
Tel: (212) 870-1657
Provides information about SRT.

Skinner Releasing
Emily Herb, Administrator
University of Washington Dance Program
Box 351150
Seattle, WA 98195-1150
Tel: (206) 233-8803
Fax: (206) 726-0616
e-mail: ejherb@aa.net
Manages workshops and seminars on the practice of SRT. Offers listings of certified teachers of SRT worldwide.

Further Reading:

Books:
Knaster, Mirka. *Discovering the Body's Wisdom.* New York: Bantam Books, 1996.

Journals:
Davidson, Robert. "Transformations: Concerning Music and Dance in Releasing." *Quarterly Dance Journal*, Winter. 1985.

Skinner, Joan, Bridget Davis, Sally Metcalf, and Kris Wheeler. "Notes on the Skinner Releasing Technique." *Quarterly Dance Journal*, Fall 1979.

Skura, Stephanie. "Releasing Dance Interview with Joan Skinner." *Quarterly Dance Journal*, Fall 1990.

Spatial Dynamics[SM]

Spatial Dynamics[SM] is a discipline that concerns itself with the human being's movement and interaction with space through spatially oriented movement activities. Focus on how the body moves through space is used as a catalyst for developing awareness of the potential of the body. It is a core premise of Spatial Dynamics that this awareness influences psychological, emotional, intellectual, and spiritual development.

How Spatial Dynamics[SM] Developed

In the mid-1970s a young clinical psychology student named Jaimen McMillan was struck by the disconcerting similarity in the postures and movement patterns of patients suffering from similar complaints. In the case of autistic children, for example, where it could be determined that they had never been exposed to others with the same disorder, their movement repertoires were so similar as to appear almost rehearsed. It was clear that a particular condition affected the movement patterns of the patient. McMillan wondered if one could possibly work in the opposite direction. If, indeed, the disorder had a negative effect on a patient's movement patterns, could practicing more wholesome movement patterns have a positive effect on the person's disorder? McMillan's initial attempts in this direction yielded encouraging results.

It became clear to him that in order to use spatial movement therapeutically in an appropriate and scientific way, one's own movements had to be worthy of imitation, one had to develop new concepts of space and new ways of perceiving movement, one had to know which effects a given movement elicited, and one had to work from a holistic movement picture of the *balanced* individual.

Attracted by the artistry and uprightness of the discipline of fencing, McMillan began his movement research through extensive training with the saber and attained "fleeting moments of mastery." In comparing his experiences with those of others who had achieved success in their fields, he considered a common factor largely overlooked in the study of sport, physical education, therapy, and movement in general: the concept of *enlivened space.*

His inclination to experience and understand *enlivened space* led him to begin rigorous training in various disciplines, including two ancient martial arts and yoga, which incorporated Eastern philosophies that allowed him to develop mental power and experience the effects of *concentrated space.* He also studied water, sound, sculpture, projective geometry, and eurythmy, which helped him learn about fluidity of movement and the processes of change through movement.

McMillan was also influenced by the work of such revolutionary twentieth-century thinkers as Albert Einstein and anthropologist Edward T. Hall, in particular their concepts of time and space. From Rudolf Steiner came the concepts of the evolution of space, and the connections between the human soul and the dimensions of space. These concepts contributed to the development of Spatial Dynamics.

McMillan worked, traveled, and studied in Europe for the next ten years. He went on to receive diplomas in physiotherapy, massage, movement therapy, and Bothmer gymnastics. He continued to collect and develop suitable movement activities that aid the processes of growth, health, and integration. This body of exercises has come to be known as Spatial Dynamics.

Philosophy of Spatial Dynamics[SM]

In Spatial Dynamics, space is perceived as a vibrant medium and movement as a dynamic force that is at our disposal to span distances psychologically as well as physically. The concept of space is further differentiated to designate an ever-widening range of possibilities for self-knowledge and interaction with others. Working first from the "body-space" in Spatial Dynamics exercises, practitioners can explore moving through the "personal," or surrounding space; the "interpersonal," or meeting and exchange space; to the "public," or social space; and finally to the "supra-personal," or macrocosmic space.

Out of the totality of spatial work, many exercises and games that aid in balance, orientation, and spatial differentiation have been developed and brought together. Many of the exercises are taught in slow motion so that one can learn to follow, distinguish, and control the quality of the movement. At no time, even when performed more rapidly, are they done automatically. Great emphasis is placed on the individual's need for awareness and freedom. The exercises incorporate a developmental sequence that spans the years of movement development, corresponding to the unique spatial need of any given age and stage of development. For young children, they have the quality of playful imagination and joyfulness, whereas for adults they bring calm and enable one not merely to change but to choose one's own habits.

Perhaps the most distinctive characteristic of Spatial Dynamics is the conscious interplay between the opposing forces of gravity and levity. The earth represents a force that pulls everything toward one point, which is called *gravity*. For Spatial Dynamics practitioners, the sun represents a force that draws and lifts toward the periphery, toward infinity. This force is called *levity*. A third force, *rhythm*, is born out of the interaction between these two.

The concept of enlivened space has educational, artistic, and athletic applications. A movement artist can learn to create consciously by bringing the three above-mentioned forces (gravity, levity, rhythm) into play through deliberate differentiation. An observer perceives an athlete or dancer who orchestrates these forces successfully as graceful. An actor may employ these techniques to transcend his or her own personality and represent the forces called for in whatever role is being played. A child who has a learning block may move to the next step in the learning process if the correct movement experiences that are missing in his or her development are given.

Practicing Spatial Dynamics^SM

One of the goals of Spatial Dynamics is to enable people to experience, and effectively enliven and employ, their spheres of activity in daily life. As a discipline it can be practiced alone, even subtly during the course of the day, pursued one-on-one with a teacher, or carried out in larger groups. Another important aspect of Spatial Dynamics is its unique approach to posture as a spatial process rather than as a set position or "pose." The social aspect of the exercises is visible in group work, in which the extensions of each individual's movements create weavings of geometrical patterns with others.

The Role of Bothmer Gymnastics in Spatial Dynamics^SM

The Bothmer exercises are spatial gems, developed to augment the Waldorf School curriculum for grades three through twelve. (The Waldorf School was a special institution set up by Rudolf Steiner in 1919.)

Spatial Dynamics makes use of the Bothmer exercises and in addition has expanded the range of its spatially oriented movement activities to touch the whole spectrum of life, from a unique approach to childbirth preparation all the way to working with the elderly, including preparation for death and dying.

Benefits of Spatial Dynamics℠

McMillan and Spatial Dynamics graduates have made an impact on the field of psychosomatic illness, most notably with eating-related disorders such as anorexia and bulimia, with space-related phobias such as claustrophobia and agoraphobia, and with problems involving nervousness, lack of awareness, and lack of "presence." Movement therapists, physical therapists, chiropractors, and orthopedic doctors have implemented Spatial Dynamics principles successfully in the area of physical medicine.

—*Jaimen McMillan*

Resources:

Spatial Dynamics Institute
423 Route 71
Hillsdale, NY 12529
Tel/Fax: (518) 325-7096
Provides in-service training programs in the discipline of Spatial Dynamics. Annual public conferences are also held at varying locations around the country.

Further Reading:

Hall, Edward T. *The Hidden Dimension*. New York: Anchor Books, 1969.

McMillan, Jaimen. *Posture: Giving Yourself Space*. Hudson, NY: Lindisfarne Press, 1998.

Schwenk, Theodor. *Sensitive Chaos*. Ann Arbor, MI: Rudolf Steiner Press, 1972.

Steiner, Rudolf. *Man: Hieroglyph of the Universe*. Translated by G. and M. Adams. Ann Arbor, MI: Rudolf Steiner Press, 1972.

Whicher, Olive. *Sunspace*. Ann Arbor, MI: Rudolf Steiner Press, 1989.

T'AI CHI CH'ÜAN

T'ai chi ch'üan is an ancient Chinese exercise art, a system of activating the body for the simultaneous development of physical, emotional, and mental well-being. Composed of a slow, continuous series of circular movements, it is said to develop balance, stamina, and grace. It is one of the oldest exercise arts, going back to about 2205 BCE, but it wasn't fully established as a body-mind technique for increasing the span of a healthy life until 1100 CE. From the Chinese viewpoint a healthy life includes emotional stability and a high degree of mental efficiency as well as physical stamina.

A Long History

For centuries, many civilizations have devised systems to improve health and reduce occurrences of disease and illness. Believed to be one of the earliest systems of this nature, the "great dances" were devised by the Chinese emperor Yü in 2205 BCE. He maintained that these exercises, if done daily, would stimulate the body's natural circulatory process, combat disease, and keep the mind alert by tending to the activity of the stipulated patterns and rhythms. It was also believed that performing these organized and structured movements awakened "positive and agreeable feelings" in the practitioner, thereby calming the emotions as well.

As centuries passed, the exercises became more intricate than those of the previous century until, as history has it, the twelfth century, when Chang San-Feng profoundly extended the range of self-understanding physically and spiritually. He created the uniquely structured form of t'ai chi ch'üan as a set of movements that build upon one another, movements that are interconnected and require the full concentration of the practitioner.

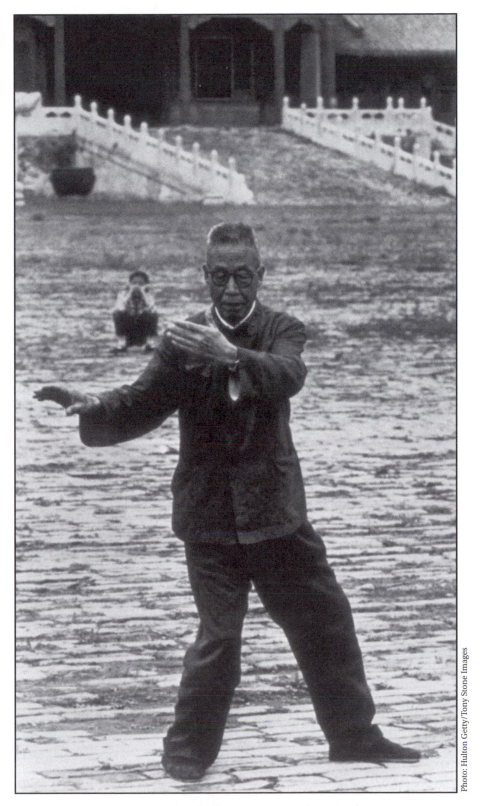

Photo: Hulton Getty/Tony Stone Images

A Chinese man practices t'ai chi ch'üan in the Forbidden City, Beijing, China.

Connected and Flowing Exercise

T'ai chi ch'üan is never to be practiced, as Chinese t'ai chi masters say, automatically, as for example the way one can recite the alphabet with the thoughts wandering elsewhere. It is a complex composition of multiple themes. The varied patterns pass from one part of the body to another so that no part is overworked and the mind stays interested. The mind directs the action and participates in it.

T'ai chi ch'üan is a long exercise, continuous for twenty-five minutes. This basic length of time is an essential ingredient. According to experts, it is just long enough to overcome resistance and laziness; to develop physical strength, patience, and persistence; to give every part of the body varied exercise, but not long enough to fatigue the body or the mind.

The way of moving in t'ai chi ch'üan looks soft, continuous, light, and fluid, giving the appearance of effortlessness. Yet in order to do it the body must be firm, stable, and strong. The mind must be alert and active. The movements of t'ai chi ch'üan are circular, made in curves, arcs, and spirals. According to t'ai-chi masters, moving in circles conserves energy, creates security, and lessens nervousness.

During the process of action, muscles are never tensed to their maximum ability. The amount of effort-tension used depends entirely upon the demands of the position or movement itself. For instance, it requires more energy to stand on one leg than on two. The muscles naturally behave differently in each case. Force is never added to a movement; one tries to use exactly as much force as is necessary to perform the movement. As Chinese t'ai chi masters say, "Use one pound to lift one pound." The approach of t'ai chi ch'üan is to balance force with necessity, which awakens the practitioner to the proper use of strength and helps him or her find a harmonious relationship with the natural force of gravity.

Balance is an essential aspect in the practice of t'ai chi ch'üan. Through the control of every nuance, muscles and joints are strengthened. Proper posture and lightness of movement are inevitable results of good body balance. Balance on the physical level also contributes to mental and emotional stability.

T'ai chi ch'üan is connected and flowing. Each unit, each moment of movement, is joined to the next without a visible break. Calmness and lightness are evoked by such fluidity. There is no cessation of movement throughout the entire twenty-five-minute exercise. Stamina and endurance grow as one develops the ability to sustain an even continuity.

It is a slow exercise. The breathing is meant to stay natural, the heartbeat steady. The tempo of the movement is related to a healthy heart rate. Slowness develops patience, poise, and power. But that is not to say that t'ai-chi is without changes in dynamics. Changes of delicate force and strength, stillness and activity are in constant alternation throughout the form. The variation in dynamic flow produces flexibility, pliability, and resilience.

Yin and Yang

The symbol for t'ai chi ch'üan is a circle divided by a flowing line that represents the movement of a wave. Filling the circumference of the circle are two curved shapes of equal size, one white, representing yin, and one black, representing yang. There is a small dot of the opposite color in each shape, showing the sympathetic character of each to the other. The dynamic flow within the symbol represents movement and the continuity of the life force.

The Chinese masters recognized and worked with the mind's desire for diversity. The form was designed to engage what the Chinese believe to be the two vital energies of life, which they call yin and yang. Yin represents all things receptive and quiet. Yang represents all things assertive and active. The many ways in which yin and yang are contrasted within the form add to the development of good coordination and heightened perception as well as memory. With the mind satisfied and the body exercised, a sense of total relaxation and well-being results.

A Lifelong Practice

T'ai chi ch'üan is generally taught in small group classes, but some teachers also offer private lessons. It is usually taught indoors in studios with wooden floors. In temperate climates it is often taught and practiced out of doors, where students can breathe freely and fully and perhaps more easily feel themselves in harmony with their natural surroundings. Loose comfortable clothing is worn. Students may be barefoot, in socks, or in soft Chinese slippers, depending on the surface of the floor. Music is never used when teaching the discipline, as it distracts students from the awareness of the dynamic rhythms within the form.

T'ai chi ch'üan can be practiced in every phase of life: as a child, adult, and senior citizen. While beginners are generally separated from advanced practitioners in classes, it is always possible for experienced practitioners to learn something new by starting at the beginning once again, or for beginners to learn by feeling the flow of movement of an experienced practitioner.

Reasons to Practice T'ai Chi Ch'üan

Many people believe the practice of this discipline can be a calming preparation for any task. Many people report that by doing even some of the form, their mind focuses away from their anxious self, and emotional and psychological problems seem to evaporate. Other people report that t'ai chi has helped them become more mentally and physically proficient and limber. With quickened physical reflexes comes an easier acceptance of new ideas and a quickened capacity to discard old habits. Emotionally, self-consciousness is diminished and self-assurance awakened. Many practitioners assert that practicing the form has helped them develop patience, awareness, and endurance.

—Sophia Delza

Resources:

T'ai Chi Chüan/Shaolin Chuan Association (TCC/SCA)
33W624 Roosevelt Road
P.O. Box 430
Geneva, IL 60134
Tel: (708) 232-0029
Conducts demonstrations, seminars, lectures, and certification program for members. Publishes annual booklet on the practice of martial arts.

T'ai Chi Foundation, Inc.
5 East 17th Street
New York, NY 10003
Tel: (212) 645-7010
Founded in 1979, this is an educational organization that strives to make the practice of t'ai chi ch'üan more accessible to Western society through promoting international conferences. In addition, it operates a resource center that provides information about this discipline.

Further Reading:

Delza, Sophia. *T'ai Chi Ch'üan: Body and Mind in Harmony.* Rev. ed. New York: State University of New York Press, 1985.

Emerson, Margaret. *Breathing Underwater: The Inner Life of T'ai Chi Ch'üan.* Berkeley, CA: North Atlantic Books, 1993.

Hooten, Claire. *T'ai Chi for Beginners: 10 Minutes to Health and Fitness.* New York: Berkley Publishing Group, 1996.

PART XI: MARTIAL ARTS

Aikido • Capoeira • Ju Jutsu • Judo • Karate • Kendo • Kung Fu Wu Su • Taekwondo

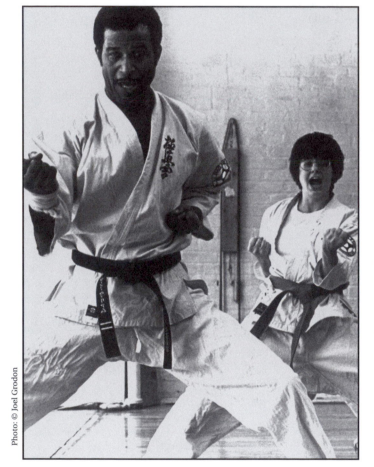

Photo: © Joel Grodon

Martial arts integrate body and mind in athletic practices of self-defense.

Martial arts are forms of combat that advocate the integration of mind and body as the basis for the study and practice of physical forms of self-defense. Although many different styles of martial arts have evolved over time, many of those practiced today are similar in their belief that the highly charged, dynamic quality of a physical confrontation is a powerful metaphor for life. Today martial arts are practiced the world over by people who enjoy the vigorous physical conditioning they demand, as well as the inner path of psychological and spiritual transformation and growth they offer. A list of martial arts and countries where they developed appears in the table that accompanies this entry.

Three Theories

It has been suggested that hunting skills comprised the early forms of combat for primitive man. As these techniques were used, their degree of sophistication generally increased. However, the origins of the martial arts remain speculative and open to controversy among writers, historians, and researchers. Three general theories exist to explain how martial arts developed throughout time.

One theory holds that ancient fighting techniques of the Greeks and Romans spread into Asia following the routes of commerce and trade. Indeed, some combative elements can be found in literary writings and sculptures of Greece and Rome. However, the complexity of specific Asian martial arts techniques appear to be lacking in literary descriptions or sculptured poses uncovered thus far in archaeological investigations.

A second theory maintains that martial arts could be traced to either China or India. A common myth credits Bodhidharma, a prince of India and founder of Buddhism in China, with teaching specific exercises to monks at the Shaolin Temple that later evolved into formal combative techniques. Under close scrutiny, this theory contradicts historical fact, and has lost favor with experts and historians.

The third theory argues that similar techniques of several martial arts that differed coincidentally evolved in parallel form in widely separate regions of the world. Unique characteristics of these similar techniques later evolved as a function of certain conditions, such as social structure and physical demographics. As examples, slaves from Africa who were brought to Brazil initially developed capoeira techniques in chains and restraints, which limited the development of hand strikes while emphasizing kicking movements from a handstand position. In China, individuals who were taller developed systems that emphasized kicking (northern region) while individuals of shorter stature resorted to systems that stressed close-range hand movements (southern region). In the Philippines, Chinese merchants from the Fukien province taught kuntao to the royal families of people of Mindanao as a token of their friendship and good faith. The "hard" style that evolved here reflected the more external, combative focus of the Filipino martial arts in general.

Central to the problem of documentation is the fact that martial arts were often shrouded in a veil of secrecy. The older teachers did not reveal their knowledge readily. Secret teachings were not passed on to the student until after many years of training and dedication to the art and teaching alike. If no suitable successor to the tradition could be found, the art often died with the master. Information was also often transmitted orally (as opposed to any documentation in written form), leading to further gaps in any traceable history.

Today, the martial arts of Asia have emerged as a significant component of American culture. It is difficult to find an individual who does not have some sense of familiarity with or recognition of these ancient disciplines when reference is made to them. Following World War II, a number of servicemen who had been exposed to these esoteric practices endeavored to pass on their teachings to other Americans. Fueled by developments in media presentations, the growth of interest in martial arts—seldom even mentioned forty years ago—has been quite phenomenal. Depiction of martial arts in films, television, and popular magazines is now commonplace.

The Basic Principles of Martial Arts

The physical foundations of the martial arts as a whole have roots in self-defense movements that make use of punches, hand strikes, blocks, kicking, jumping, grappling, rolling techniques, chokes, joint manipulations, locks, and throws. Aside from empty-hand techniques, many systems of martial arts make use of weapons, which might include a staff, stick, blade, or projectile instrument. Martial arts disciplines that stress these combative components are often labeled "external."

Other martial arts disciplines emphasize an esoteric component in their teachings that has been described as "internal" in nature. These practices and exercises include specific types of breathing techniques, performance of unique rituals, use of special hand-body configurations, chanting or recitation of specific combinations of letters or words, cultivation and manipulation of "internal energy," and sitting, standing, and movement meditation exercises. These more esoteric practices are taught for improving physical performance, enhancement of health, and psychological and spiritual development. Practice of traditional, regimented, prearranged forms often serves to unify both external and internal aspects of martial arts.

Each of the different systems of martial arts has defining characteristics that identify the nature of the art. For example, t'ai chi ch'üan is a Chinese art that consists of smooth, flowing, gentle movements with no hesitation observed between various postures and rounded, curling gestures that involve kicks, strikes, and evasive actions. Originating in Africa, capoeira is now practiced widely in Brazil and is characterized by a dancelike, acrobatic movement style accompanied by music and song and takes on the form of a game being played as a performance. Another example is aikido, which is a contemporary Japanese art of self-defense based upon principles of non-resistance to and harmony with one's opponent that makes use of circular movements to gain control of an attacker's momentum, thus neutralizing aggressive actions.

Learning Martial Arts

While each discipline of martial arts is unique, some general principles underlie the pursuit and study of all the disciplines. Instructions are often given in a group setting, with classes being taught anywhere from three to seven days a week for one, two, or even more hours per session. An instructor or set of instructors will lead the class and often insist upon the display of proper behavior, attitudes, moral conduct, and discipline throughout the class. Training can be demanding physically and mentally and requires dedication and perseverance to progress through a defined ranking system.

Benefits and Risks of Martial Arts

Millions of people worldwide study martial arts disciplines. They report many positive effects, including the following: an increase in mental clarity and means of achieving self-discipline; maximum physical fitness; general well-being through proper breathing techniques; an outlet for aggression; increased personal power through internal energy development exercises; and increased self-confidence from the knowledge of valuable self-defense techniques.

People with severe physical limitations may have difficulty participating in the more vigorous "external" forms of martial arts. Choosing which martial art to study should entail some knowledge of the physical techniques involved, the mental, emotional, and spiritual goals stressed, and exposure to the teaching style of a particular instructor. The degree to which the philosophical aspects of a practice are emphasized will depend upon the individual teacher, but the physical self-defense aspect of these disciplines remains the defining feature that distinguishes them from other body-mind disciplines.

—*Michael Maliszewski, Ph.D.*

Further Reading:

Books:

Draeger, Donn F., and Robert W. Smith. *Comprehensive Asian Fighting Arts.* Tokyo: Kodansha International, 1969.

Maliszewski, M. *Spiritual Dimensions of the Martial Arts.* Tokyo: Charles E. Tuttle, 1996.

Journals:

The Black Book: The Quarterly Martial Arts Supplies Guide and Master's Desk Reference. Erica Talorico, editor. Bellmawr, NJ: Marketing Tools, Inc. (204 Harding Ave., Bellmawr, NJ 08031)

Journal of Asian Martial Arts. Michael DeMarco, editor. Erie, PA: Via Media Publishing Company. (821 W. 24th St., Erie, PA 16502)

COUNTRY	MARTIAL ART
India	kalarippayattu, thang-ta
China	t'ai chi ch'üan, wing chun, pa kua, Hung-gar
Korea	taekwondo, hapkido, tang soo do, hwarang-do
Japan	kendo, aikido, ju jutsu, judo, karate
Okinawa Islands	Goju-ryu, Shito-ryu, Uechi-ryu, Shorinji-ryu
Indonesia	pencak silat, kuntao
Philippines	arnis, escrima
Thailand	muay Thai, krabi-krabong
Africa, then Brazil	capoeira, ju jutsu
USA	jeet kune do, talahib-marga

AIKIDO

Aikido is a Japanese martial art. The word *aikido* means the path to the coordination of body, mind, and spirit. It is a defensive system of continuous, circular movements meant to counter the attack of an armed or unarmed opponent. Continued practice in aikido allows you to effectively anticipate and successfully defend yourself with minimum effort against an attack.

History of Aikido
The founder of aikido, Morehei Ueshiba (1883–1969), also known as O Sensei, or "great teacher," was influenced by two things—religion and martial arts. In Tokyo in 1902, O Sensei studied kendo (Japanese sword technique), and jujutsu, the traditional art of hand-to-hand and small weapons combat. Ueshiba would continue these studies all his life, earning several certificates in various schools. He also studied sojutsu, or spear fighting, sumo wrestling, and kokodan judo.

Ueshiba studied extensively with Onisaburo Deguchi, founder of Omoto-Kyo, a religion based on the traditional Shinto religion. After his father's death, Ueshiba went to live in Deguchi's organic farming community near Kyoto. There he studied spiritual works that later influenced his philosophy of martial arts. In 1920 Ueshiba opened his first martial arts school, Ueshiba Academy. By 1922 his teachings evolved into a discipline he called aiki-bujutsu, known generally as Ueshiba-ryu Aiki-bujutsu. Later, the art became known as aikido, the way of harmony, reflecting O Sensei's concern with the peaceful resolution of conflict.

In the thirties and forties, the practice of aikido spread throughout Japan and was recognized by the state as a martial art. During the Second World War, Ueshiba retreated to the country to build a shrine to aikido. After the war, aikido's focus on conflict resolution allowed for its practice during the American occupation. In 1961 the first practice hall opened outside of Japan in Honolulu, Hawaii. Ueshiba died in 1969.

Concepts and Principles
The central concept of aikido is the peaceful resolution of conflict. To this end, O Sensei envisioned it as training for the spirit and mind, as well as the body. All techniques in aikido are defense techniques and guide the aggressor's attack to its conclusion, resulting in the aggressor's downfall. These techniques are meant to show the aggressor the error of his or her judgment and end the attack. The defender, called *nagi*, protects himself and his attacker, known as *uke*, with these techniques. Rank is given according to knowledge of technique and ability to perform basic movements. Ranking tests are given, but they are not competitive.

On a physical level, the focus and direction of ki, or vital life energy, is very important in practice; ki is developed through breathing exercises. The pelvis, center of ki, is the origin of all movement in aikido. From the pelvis, ki is channeled through the arms and legs, and eventually to the hands. This process is called extension, another important principle of aikido. The embodiment of these concepts produces flowing, circular movement that is the trademark of aikido.

Aikido Practice
All aikido practice takes place in a dojo, a room with mats on the floor and a shrine to O Sensei at one end. For practice all students wear a *gi*, a heavy white cotton suit, a kimono jacket, pants, and belt. Students in the lower ranks, known as the five kyus, wear white belts. Advanced students in the higher ranks, or dans, wear black belts. Senior students in the dojo are often given permission to wear black wide-legged pants called hakama. All advanced students wear hakama.

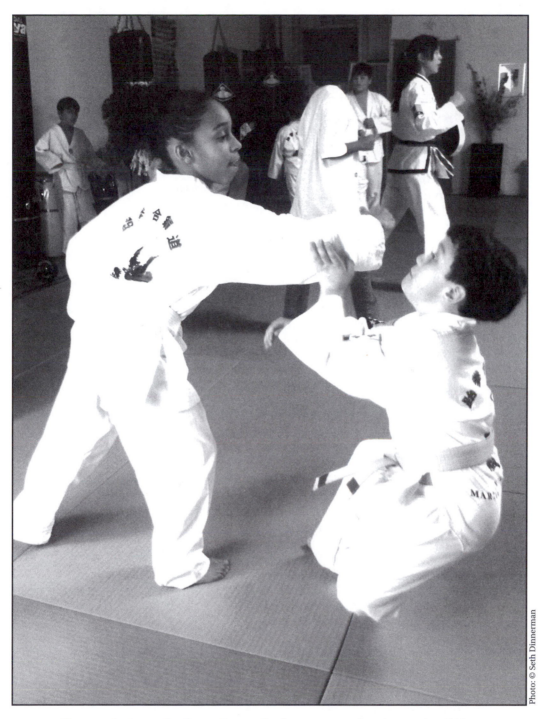

Photo: © Seth Dinnerman

Young students practice the continuous circular movements that characterize aikido.

Etiquette is important in aikido. Class begins and ends with a set sequence of quiet bowing to the shrine, to the teacher, and at the end of class, to fellow students. Students are expected to bow to the shrine on entering and leaving the mat. Bowing is a gesture of respect rather than worship.

After opening the class, the instructor, also called Sensei, leads the class in a warm-up. Then the instructor demonstrates a technique with a senior student. In the course of most classes, a few techniques will be practiced. Often each student will take a partner and work on the technique. Both students in each pair practice being the attacker who takes the fall, and in turn play the defender. By changing roles, students learn to cooperate with each other. They are expected to adapt their practice to their partners. Injuring your partner is considered bad form in most dojos, since injury takes a student out of class. Aikido classes often are silent, which fosters students' concentration on the technique; concentration is important since all aikido techniques can injure the attacker.

The attacker's falls in aikido are called ukemi; these movements, like other aikido defensive techniques, are circular and flowing. Ukemi maneuvers are just as important as defense movements, called nagi. For example, the forward roll in aikido begins from standing, and flows from the leading arm, across the back, down to the leg, and back to standing. This roll should always be flowing, without any jarring movement.

An Ideal Martial Art

Because of its psychological and physical benefits, aikido is an ideal martial art for life. Practice builds strength, coordination, and flexibility. As students advance, the tempo of practice accelerates, bringing aerobic benefits. On an intellectual level, many students find mental focus and clarity through their practice. The benefits of aikido have taken O Sensei's students all over the world to open dojos. Today, O Sensei's son, Kisshomaru Ueshiba, heads aikido schools worldwide.

—Clio Pavlantos, M.A., CMA, Second Kyu USAF, in collaboration with Marvin Bookman, Third Dan USAF.

Resources:

United States Aikido Federation, Eastern Region
142 West 18th Street
New York, NY 10011
Web site: www.usaikifed.org
Eastern United States division of the international organization founded by O Sensei and now headed by his son, Doshu Kisshomaru Ueshiba. The USAF provides lists of affiliated dojos in America and abroad. Publishes the Federation News, *a newsletter promoting aikido.*

CAPOEIRA

Capoeira is an ancient martial art that has its roots in African culture but developed fully and attained an immense popularity in Brazil. Like other martial arts, capoeira strives to integrate mental as well as physical strength in order to perform combat maneuvers with dexterity, skill, and grace. Yet capoeira differs from other martial arts in that rhythmic music, including singing, clapping, and the playing of instruments, is integral to the unique spirit and practice of the discipline.

African Origins
Although there are many theories about

The Role of Etiquette

Etiquette is very important in aikido. All students are expected to bow to the shrine of O Sensei when they enter or leave the dojo and at the beginning and end of class. This is a sign of respect rather than worship. Class begins and ends with a set protocol of meditation, bowing to the shrine, to the teacher, and, at the end of class, to fellow students.

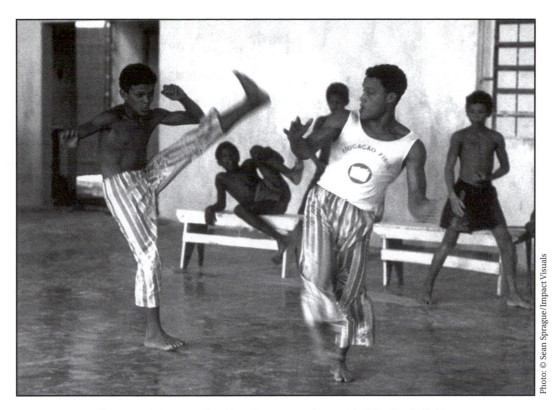

Boys practicing capoeira, Alagados community center, Salvador de Bahia.

Photo: © Sean Sprague/Impact Visuals

the origin of capoeira, most scholars agree it can be traced back to certain hand-to-hand combat forms and dances of central Africa. Two African dances are most often credited with being the origin of capoeira: sanga and n'golo. Both dances exhibit characteristics that are integral to the practice of capoeira today. Sanga was an ancient war dance, also known as a sword dance, in which warfare and dance movements were inextricably linked. The dance element is significant because the ability to leap, twist, roll, and dodge the arrows and blows of opponents is one of the most important skills of capoeira. N'golo was an acrobatic dance used as competition between the young males of the Mucope people in Angola.

Capoeira traveled with the Atlantic slave trade to Brazil. Among themselves, slaves trained in capoeira as a form of physical resistance, stressing the fighting aspects of the discipline. When the slave owners were present, the dance aspects of capoeira were emphasized. Slave owners outlawed capoeira and made the practice punishable by death. Well into the twentieth century, capoeira was an outlaw art, performed secretly by slaves or by thieves and criminals. Roving bands of capoieristas (those that practice capoeira) were employed as thugs and enforcers by businessmen and would attack taverns and police, further advancing the negative image of the discipline.

It was through the efforts of two modern masters, Manoel dos Reis Machado (known as Mestre Bimba) and Vincente Ferreira Pastinha (known as Mestre Pastinha) that capoeira eventually became an acceptable part of Brazilian life. Mestra Bimba is known as the great innovator. He invented the style called capoeira regional, which emphasizes the offensive, fighting aspects of the martial art. Known as the great traditionalist, Mestre Pastinha was a proponent of the style called capoeira angola, which aims to maintain the ritualistic, defensive, aesthetic, and philosophical aspects of the discipline.

Today many styles of capoeira are practiced throughout Europe, the United States, and South America. It is taught in private academies and in many universities. The Capoeira Foundation in New York City promotes the study, research, and performance of the art.

Six Principles of Capoeira

Capoeira is based on the African cultural values from which it arose. The religious traditions and rituals of central Africa form the basic philosophical underpinnings of the practice of the art.

In *Karate/Kung-Fu Illustrated*, August 1988, scholar Alejandro Frigerio identified six characteristics of modern capoeira angola:

- Complementation is the importance of playing with, not against, the opponent. It is similar to a "cutting session" in jazz, in which the musicians try to outplay each other with the ultimate goal of creating beautiful music. Through complementation the most creative interaction possible is achieved.
- Malicia is the art of being evasive or deceptive. One aspect of malicia is to look vulnerable until the opponent attacks, then gracefully defend and/or counterattack. In other words one should play closed (or controlled), while appearing open (undisciplined or vulnerable).

- It is not enough merely to defeat the opponent; one must prove superior skill by displaying it with style or beautiful movement. This style and grace are as important as the victory.
- Both slow and fast movements are important to capoeira angola. Most movements are slow and deliberate—they teach control and precision, which then enable practitioners to perform the movements very quickly and effectively and to improvise new moves.
- Capoeira angola is a sophisticated discipline with subtle rules and rites. If a player displays ignorance of these unwritten rules, he or she is considered an inferior player, uneducated in the proper, traditional way. Secret personal and religious rituals called mandingas protect a player from harm.
- Finally, unlike other martial arts, the jogo, or play of capoeira, is performed for others. The viewers should be entertained by the skill, deception, and humor of the play. The practitioners of this discipline should always be aware of the effect their display has on those attending and develop their play accordingly.

Performance

The play of capoeira takes place in what is known as a roda, which is a circle formed by the players and onlookers. Included in the circle is the bateria, which is an ensemble of musicians and singers.

Music is one of the most important elements of the art of capoeira. Different

Lack of Hand Techniques in Capoeira

There is little use of offensive hand techniques in capoeira. Some scholars have attributed this to the belief that slaves had to fight with their hands immobilized by chains and therefore developed advanced foot and leg techniques. Other commentators contend that it is more likely that the absence of hand techniques is based on an old central African proverb that says, "Hands are to build, feet are to destroy."

songs and rhythms inspire the players to more intense levels of performance and function to calm them down if the dance becomes too heated. The order of songs is part of the ritual aspect of capoeira.

The berimbau, a musical bow with one string, is considered "the soul of capoeira." Attached to the bow is a hollowed-out gourd that acts as a resonator box. Tones are produced when the bowstring is struck by a thin flexible stick (baqueta). A small rattle (caxixi) is also held in the hand that holds the baqueta. Each instrument has a prescribed position in the circle.

The ritualized practice of capoeira begins when two players enter the circle and kneel at the foot of the berimbau. One player sings a ladainha, a ritual song of commencement. If his opponent doesn't respond with a song of his own, the first begins another song, acorrido, a song for going out to play. The song is then passed on to one of the musicians as the jogo-de-capoeira (play of capoeira) begins.

Capoeira is characterized by dynamic movements such as cartwheels, handstands, circling kicks, and acrobatics. Performers use agility, guile, and superior technique to maneuver the other into a defenseless position, rendering him or her open to a blow, kick, or sweep. Only one's hands, head, and feet are allowed to touch the floor. Disqualification occurs when a player is knocked down.

Improvisation is greatly admired. It allows the capoeirista to create openings and keep the action of the performance innovative and fluid. Also prized are evasive techniques and implied strikes, especially when one fighter has been maneuvered into an indefensible position.

Why Practice Capoeira?

Capoeira aims to teach its practitioners how to face harsh experiences while remaining flexible and receptive, how to respond to violence with evasion and grace, how to use the trials and tribulations of life to develop physical strength, spiritual strength, and wisdom in thought and action. It is an ancestral wisdom that aims to create balanced and productive bodies, minds, and lives.

Resources:

The Capoeira Foundation
104 Franklin Street
New York, NY 10013
Tel: (212) 274-9737
e-mail: dancebrazl@aol.com
Provides information on capoeira, including information on instructors.

Further Reading:

Almeida, Bira. *Capoeira: A Brazilian Art Form.* 2nd ed. Richmond, CA: North Atlantic Books, 1986.

Dimock, Anne. "Capoeira Angola." In *Black People and Their Culture: Selected Writing from the African Diaspora.* ed. by Linn Shapiro. Washington, DC: Smithsonian Institution, 1976.

Kubick, Gerhard. "Capoeira Angola." In *Angolan Traits in Black Music, Games and Dances of Brazil: A Study of African Cultural Extensions Overseas.* Lisboa: Junta de Investigacoes Cientifica do Ultramar, Centro de Estudos de Antropologia Cultural, 1976.

Lewis, John Lowell. *Ring of Liberation: Deceptive Discourse in Brazilian Capoeira.* Chicago: University of Chicago Press, 1992.

Ju Jutsu

Ju jutsu is a type of fighting that involves grappling, throwing, and limb twisting. Although variously spelled as jiu jitsu, ju jitsu, or even ju jutso, the name refers to the yielding principle of the art, which refers to the ability to submit to an opponent's direction of attack while attempting to control it. The Japanese character *ju* has several meanings: soft, pliable, submissive, adaptable, yielding, and harmonious. The character *jutsu* means skill or technique. Yet the common translation of ju jutsu as the "gentle art" is somewhat misleading. Many ju jutsu techniques can be very forceful and damaging to the opponent. Sometimes great strength is needed to ensure the defeat of an opponent, though expert technique can make it appear to be effortless. Perhaps it is the fact that ju jutsu is an art that adapts to the opponent and the situation, using leverage, balance, and the minimum amount of effort necessary to gain an advantage over the aggressor, that has earned it the name the "gentle art." In ju jutsu, the mind is used to evaluate the opponent's weaknesses and anticipate the next move, while the body controls the opponent's balance and positioning.

The History of Ju Jutsu

Ju jutsu is considered the forerunner of the popular martial arts judo and aikido. It dates back a thousand years, being known as tai-jutsu, yawara, and hakuda during the course of its development into what is recognized today as ju jutsu. Grappling and throwing arts have long existed in Japan, and there are a number of legends about the emergence of ju jutsu. According to one popular story, ju jutsu originated with a Japanese physician named Akiyama. He traveled to China to study medicine and, while there, learned an art known as hakuda, which consisted of kicking, striking, seizing, and grappling.

Upon his return to Japan, Akiyama began to teach hakuda. According to the legend, he had few techniques, so his students grew bored and left him. Angered, Akiyama went to meditate at the Tenjin Shrine. During a snowstorm on his journey, he saw a pine tree broken beneath the weight of snow. Nearby

there was a slim willow tree bending under the snow, its branches so pliable that the snow slipped from them, leaving the tree unbroken. Akiyama later meditated at the shrine and is said to have come upon 303 different martial art techniques that applied the principle he had seen demonstrated by the willow. He opened a new school in which flexibility and suppleness were all important, naming it Yoshin-Ryu, or Willow Tree School.

The 1500s are considered a turning point for ju jutsu. During this time of the art's greatest popularity, there were more than 700 schools sharing few standard techniques. No method existed that could be considered a complete and independent system of unarmed fighting.

Many sources regard the Takenouchi Ryu, founded in 1532 by Takenouchi Hisamaro, as the core ju jutsu ryu (school) from which all "empty-handed" (meaning without weapons) ju jutsu sprang. Ju jutsu had traditionally been taught in conjunction with, and as a complement to, archery, swordsmanship, and other forms of armed fighting. Takenouchi Ryu, also known as Kogusoku, parted with weapon-oriented training, establishing a pure method of unarmed ju jutsu.

Modern Ju Jutsu

It is doubtful that the "empty-handed" ju jutsu practiced today bears much resemblance to the ancient art from feudal Japan. Although Takenouchi established a formal system of unarmed combat, ju jutsu still continued to flourish mainly as a part of the samurai training.

In the mid–seventeenth century, changes in ju jutsu began to emerge. Increasingly, ju jutsu systems started to develop independently from weapons training.

In the nineteenth century, schools opened to teach people other than samurai who were interested in studying the martial arts. The new schools of ju jutsu lacked the real combat training of the older schools, and many methods became theoretical as the need for practical application disappeared. This kind of ju jutsu came to be the most well known, and eventually spread to the West. A few old schools still exist, practicing their dangerous art according to tradition. Over the years, ju jutsu, like karate, judo, and many other arts, developed as a form of sporting and good-natured competition. Because of this, lethal techniques were further removed from the training programs.

Since the 1970s, when the martial arts benefited from tremendous growth due to the Bruce Lee cinema phenomenon, many offshoots from the traditional styles have sprung up, and with the help of no-holds-barred contests, ju jutsu and grappling arts are enjoying renewed popularity.

Ju Jutsu Training

Ju jutsu does not require any particular clothing to be effective, unlike the high kicking arts that require loose clothes for proper execution. The student is expected to wear traditional clothing, not for effectiveness, but out of respect for the history of ju jutsu.

Many of the training procedures date back to the early days of ju jutsu, when this discipline was still part of the samurai's training. For example, ju jutsu is practiced mostly with the partners facing each other. This custom originates from the battlefields of the old samurai. Sometimes a samurai would stand facing the enemy before his soldiers and scream out a challenge, his name, his ryu (school), or even a favorite technique. A samurai from the enemy camp would come forward and accept the challenge. Such a duel could determine the outcome of the whole battle.

While ju jutsu is often identified as pure grappling that incorporates arm locks, joint manipulation, throws, and breakfalls, the art also includes devastating kicks and punches. Training in ju jutsu progresses from the learning of basic techniques to the practice of choreographed or prearranged series of fight moves, to freestyle or improvisational practice.

The many techniques of ju jutsu include *atemi waza* (striking techniques), *tachi waza* and *nage waza* (standing and throwing techniques), and *ne waza* and *katame waza* (lying and grappling techniques). Just as in other martial arts, ju jutsu training includes prearranged fight patterns or choreography called *jigo waza* (defense techniques). *Jigo waza* is a methodical way to learn how to apply the basic techniques. Randori, or free sparring, is a means of learning one's strengths and weaknesses because it tests the student's fluency with spontaneous moves and responses. In randori, students avoid causing injury but may use any techniques at their disposal.

As the name implies, ju jutsu is not a contest of muscular strength. Excellent balance, leverage, and speed are needed to get the most out of the technique. Throws, holds, and locks are carried out in a manner that, if not handled with care, could be devastating to the opponent. Calling for an awareness of anatomy, ju jutsu focuses on the vital points on the body and the effective use of force on the joints and limbs. Nevertheless, competitors are taught to stop short of harming each other. Modern ju jutsu is designed to render an opponent helpless without causing injury.

The Nature of Ju Jutsu

Because ju jutsu originated in Japan, there are similarities in etiquette and terminology with martial arts such as karate and judo. The training takes place in a dojo, or training hall. As in karate, the philosophy of ju jutsu is based on Zen Buddhism. According to this philosophy, the dojo is considered more than a place to practice. The vigorous training that occurs there helps practitioners to understand themselves.

Through competition and practice, students develop confidence and learn about commitment, determination, discipline, and conquest of fear. The lessons learned in the dojo help the student to deal with conflicts and stresses that occur outside the dojo. In this way, ju jutsu training is a source of self-enlightenment.

The mental aspect of ju jutsu complements the physical aspect. The philosophy of ju jutsu stresses the power of ki (also known as chi), or inner spirit and energy. According to this thinking, each time attackers commit themselves to a movement, they are also committing their ki. Skilled students of ju jutsu can control this energy by applying the principle of yielding, which means using opponents' attacks and movement against themselves: if the opponent pulls, the defender pushes; if the opponent pushes, the defender pulls.

It is believed that by controlling the opponent's ki one can also control his mind, and therefore his whole being. Because this art is potentially destructive and must be used responsibly, ju jutsu, like other martial arts, places strong emphasis on character and self-control. Students must be patient and tolerant, with the ability to resist confrontations if deemed unnecessary. By studying ju jutsu, students learn not only to control their opponents but, more important, about self-control, commitment, discipline, and rising to challenges.

—Stefan Nikander

Resources:

American Judo and Jujitsu Federation (AJJF)
c/o Central Office Administrator
P.O. Box 993312
Redding, CA 96099-3312
e-mail: ajjfdanzan@aol.com
Web site: www.ajjf.org
Founded in 1958, this is a nonprofit corporation that promotes the DanZan Ryu system of ju jutsu.

American Jujitsu Institute (AJI)
c/o 1779 Koi Koi Street
Wahiawa, HI 96786
Tel: (808) 621-6274

Fax: (808) 622-2179 (call first to set up fax)
e-mail: pra0005@pixi.com
Web site: www.pixi.com/~pra0005/aji.html
Founded in 1939, AJI is the oldest martial arts organization in the United States. It sponsors tournaments and offers instruction, testing and certification, and seminars and clinics.

World Martial Arts Association
P.O. Box 1568
Santa Barbara, CA 93102
Tel: (805) 569-1389
Fax: (805) 569-0267
Promotes and teaches martial arts such as ju jutsu, judo, aikido, and karate.

Further Reading:

Ferrie, Eddie. *Ju Jitsu: Classical and Modern.* Wiltshire: Crowood Press, 1990.

Nakae, Kiyose, and Charles Yeager. *Jiu Jitsu Complete.* Secaucus, NJ: Carol Publishing Group, 1995.

Palumbo, Dennis G. *The Essence of Hakkoryo Jujutsu.* Boulder, CO: Paladin Press, 1995.

Uphoff, Joseph A., Jr. *Jujitsu: The Art of Precision.* Colorado Springs, CO: Arjuna Library Press, 1993.

JUDO

Judo is a modern Japanese martial art that has its roots in the ancient martial art of ju jutsu. It integrates mental as well as physical strength in order to perform a series of combat maneuvers and movements with dexterity, skill, and grace. Like other martial arts, this discipline places a strong emphasis on spiritual balance, serenity, as well as mental and physical fitness as an approach to life. It is characterized by techniques that are used to upset the balance of an opponent, eventually neutralizing him or her. Today judo is often thought of as an aggressive, competitive sport, but in its original form it was nonviolent and basically defensive.

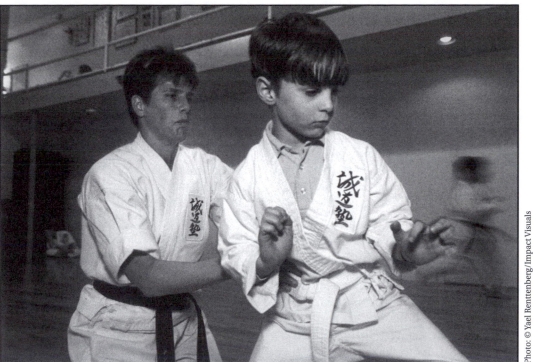

A young student learns judo, the Japanese martial art primarily consisting of movements using bare hands.

Origins of Judo

The story of judo begins with Terada Kanemon, a warrior who in the eighteenth century developed a specific art of combat using only bare hands, from the many techniques of ju jutsu. He called this martial art judo, which means "way of gentleness."

The modern art of judo, however, is attributed primarily to the work of Kano Jigoro. Born in 1860, he grew up as a member of a wealthy family in Kobe, Japan. He was very dedicated to the study of ju jutsu. Even though the discipline had a long and respected tradition as a martial art, at that time ju jutsu was used by bandits and thieves and had a very negative reputation.

Kano Jigoro explored ways to bring together the techniques he had learned studying with different master teachers. He wanted to create a "sporting discipline" that would educate and train young people in a time of peace. He revived the name judo to describe his new "martial sport."

In 1882 he opened his own school (dojo) in Tokyo. His method was very popular, and by 1889 he had 600 students. In that same year he gave a demonstration of judo in Marseilles, France; the popularity of judo spread, and the first dojo outside of Japan was established in Paris under the directorship of Jean-Joseph Renaud and Guy de Montgrillard.

Between 1902 and 1912 Kano Jigoro was sent on official missions by the Japanese government to teach the principles and techniques of judo throughout China and Europe. Soon there were dojos throughout Japan, China, and Europe. In 1922 Kano Jigoro established another school in Japan called the Kodokan. It became the official international center for all the dojos.

Although Kano Jigoro did not believe that public competition was an appropriate aim of the study of judo, some students enjoyed competing with each other. Public competitions were held between European, Chinese, and Japanese dojos until the outbreak of World War II.

After the war, international judo competitions resumed. Weight categories, such as those used in boxing, were established. This step gradually led to an ideological split between those who began to see judo more and more as a competitive sport and those who remained dedicated to Kano Jigoro's view of judo as a personal art of training the mind and body. Today Judo is one of the most widespread sports in the world, but very few dojos teach the spirit of gentleness that was at the heart of Kano Jigoro's technique.

The Fundamental Principles of Judo

Kano Jigoro believed that his art of unarmed self-defense was a means to teach a philosophy or art of daily living. A serene, disciplined mind, working in conjunction with controlled body actions, was used to bring down an opponent and, applied in a larger sense, to live life in peace and well-being. Control of body and mind results from a supple body, perfect balance, constant alertness, emotional detachment, and proper breathing techniques.

The techniques of judo are practiced with a partner and require quick shifts of body and mind. The fundamental movements derived from ju jutsu are designed to neutralize the opponent, but the overall aim of the technique, according to Kano Jigoro, is to "understand and demonstrate the living laws of movement." The movements involve the body, arms, and legs. They are taught carefully and repeated many times in the course of training.

Today the principal movements of judo also include kumi-kata, which is the action of gripping an opponent; nage-waza, a series of throws; katame-no-kata, which are techniques of control; osaekomi-waza, classified as the action of immobilizing an opponent on the ground; shime-waz, which are strangulation techniques; and finally kansetsu-waz, which are techniques of bending and locking the joints.

Once the fundamental movements are learned, the partners practice training in a freestyle combat called randori. In this quick dancelike practice, Uke, the one who submits, is thrown to the mat and immobilized by Tori, the one who throws. Suppleness of body, perfect balance, serenity, and alertness are all tested and developed here.

Learning Judo

Judo is taught on large rectangular tatami mats. Traditionally the mats were made of straw, but today they are often made of pressed foam. Students are barefoot and wear a special uniform called a judogi. It is made of thick white or unbleached cotton. It consists of large, baggy trousers called *zubon*, a wide-fitting jacket with wide sleeves that come halfway down the forearm called a sode, and a belt called an obi.

Judo training is organized in stages. When a student passes a particular stage he or she is allowed to wear the colored belt associated with that stage. A white belt represents a beginner, a black belt the most advanced practitioner.

Even though today judo is more often a test of strength between the two opponents, the underlying principles of the spirit of the founder and of all martial

Principle Movements of Judo	*Corresponding Japanese Name*
bending & locking of the joints	Kansetsu-waz
control techniques	Katame-no-kata
strangulation	Shime-waz
throws	Nage-waza
immobilizations on the ground	Osaekomi-waza

arts are still at the core of this body-mind discipline.

Benefits of Judo

Judo is one of the more popular martial arts disciplines, and many people worldwide have reported a variety of benefits. These include a significant improvement in physical fitness; sharpened mental clarity and emotional balance; increased self-discipline; and the self-confidence from the knowledge of valuable self-defense techniques.

—*Nancy Allison*

Resources:

American Judo and Jujitsu Federation (AJJF)
c/o Central Office Administrator
P.O. Box 993312
Redding, CA 96099-3312
e-mail: ajjfdanzan@aol.com
Web site: www.ajjf.org
Founded in 1958, this organization promotes the teaching of ju jutsu and judo in the United States.

International Judo Federation (IJF)
21st Floor, Doosan Bldg.
101-1 Ulchiro 1ka, Choongku
Seoul, Korea
Tel: (82 1 2) 759-6936
Fax: (82 1 2) 754-1075
e-mail: yspark@ijf.org
Web site: www.ijf.org
World's governing body of judo. Provides information about competitive judo, including international and Olympic events.

World Martial Arts Association
P.O. Box 1568
Santa Barbara, CA 93102
Tel: (805) 569-1389
Fax: (805) 569-0267
Founded in 1979, this group promotes and teaches several martial arts, including ju jutsu, judo, aikido, and karate.

Further Reading:

Caffary, Brian. *The Judo Handbook: From Beginner to Black Belt.* New York: Galley Books, 1989.

Frederic, Louis. *A Dictionary of the Martial Arts.* Translated and edited by Paul Crompton. Boston: Charles E. Tuttle Company, 1995.

Tegner, Bruce. *Judo: Beginner to Black Belt.* Ventura, CA: Thor Publishing, 1991.

KARATE

Karate originated as a method of hand-to-hand combat, but today is also practiced as a sport and a form of self-discipline. The name *karate* is formed from the Japanese characters "kara," meaning empty, and "te," meaning hand, and is therefore often translated as "empty hand." Karate students, known as karateka, learn highly effective weaponless ("empty hand") techniques of attack and defense using their arms and legs. The philosophy of karate is based on Zen Buddhism, which places great value on inner calm, clear thinking, self-knowledge, and a heightened awareness of one's relationship to others and the world. Therefore, karate not only is a form of physical training and self-defense but is also used to develop spiritual and mental well-being.

Okinawa, the Birthplace of Karate

Karate developed in Asia over the course of several centuries. Its roots lie in the different forms of unarmed combat that arose among peasants who sought to protect themselves from neighboring invaders. Buddhist monks of the Shaolin Monastery in the Hunan province of China also refined a method of fighting to protect themselves against troops and robbers. At the Shaolin Monastery, the Zen Buddhist monk Bodhidharma equipped his disciples with the strength and discipline to approach enlightenment by instructing them to practice fighting moves. The teachings of Zen Buddhism became the basis for the mental and spiritual training that is essential to the martial arts.

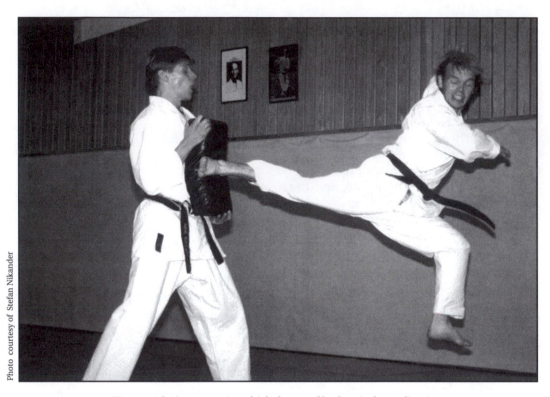

Photo courtesy of Stefan Nikander

Karate techniques require a high degree of body-mind coordination.

The island of Okinawa, located almost midway between Japan and China, became a place that allowed traders, soldiers, travelers, and local inhabitants to exchange goods, ideas, and fighting techniques. It was here in the seventeenth century that several martial arts styles arose, collectively known as Okinawa-te ("Okinawan hand"). In the early twentieth century, the various styles of Okinawa-te were unified under the name of karate by Funakoshi Gichin, who is considered the founder of modern karate. Funakoshi promoted his sport by traveling through Japan staging tournaments and demonstrations, and karate gained in popularity. The karate practiced at this time was used as a form of violent combat. Because of this, karate-do was established as an alternative to the lethal version of karate. The suffix *do* means "way" and conveys the sense that the new approach was intended for spiritual and physical development, not war. In karate-do, blows are never completed but, instead, stop just short of impact; in karate-do competitions, karateka are evaluated on their form and the quality of their execution of prescribed moves.

By 1930 every major university in Japan had a karate club. With the outbreak of World War II, karate was taught to the Imperial Japanese Army. When Japan surrendered in 1945, General Douglas MacArthur placed a ban on all martial arts training, greatly hindering the spread of karate. In 1948, one year after the United States occupation forces lifted the ban on karate instruction, Funakoshi started to rebuild the sport. He gave a demonstration at a U.S. air base, and the impressed American commanders gave permission for instruction to take place on their military bases. Funakoshi himself toured the U.S. air bases giving demonstrations. It was this effort that saved karate, and introduced the way of the empty hand to the West. Karate was officially introduced to the United States in 1953.

Two years later, the Japanese Karate Association was formed, and by 1957 karate had reached Europe. Millions of people currently practice karate, and the sport is known throughout the world.

The Styles

Karate is not a single unified system—in fact, hundreds of styles of karate exist. Many of these styles originated in the years after karate's first introduction in Japan. Some were advanced by Okinawan masters following in Funakoshi's footsteps, while others were outgrowths from Funakoshi's karate school. However, all of the other styles are outgrowths of five major branches: shotokan, wado ryu, goju ryu, shito ryu, and kyokushinkai. Each style has its own strengths, techniques, and applications. By comparing different styles, individuals seeking to study karate may find the school most suited to their ability and temperament.

The Nature of Karate

Karate is practiced in a dojo, or training hall. According to the philosophy of karate, the dojo is not just a place to practice fighting techniques. It is also where karateka learn to become emotionally sound and mentally disciplined. Perfecting the technique requires a long and demanding training schedule. Through triumphs and failures, karateka must remain committed to the study of karate and be willing to work hard.

In karate, as in all the martial arts, etiquette is an important part of training and practice. Karateka bow before entering the training area of the dojo as a sign of respect for their training community. Before they practice fighting, the students bow to each other. At the beginning and end of every training session, they line up and bow to the sensei, or master. When karateka bow, they are not only showing respect but also learning to display an inner calm and power that emanates an aura of inner strength and invulnerability. Practitioners of karate believe that confidence, character, dignity, and self-awareness are as important as physical technique.

The student's uniform is called a karate gi. A belt called an obi is worn by all karateka and marks the level they have reached in their training. The belts vary in color, with each color corresponding to a specific level of progress. When belts were first introduced, students started with a light color and dyed them darker shades each time they passed the examination and advanced to the next level. If the karateka studied long enough and made significant progress, the belt eventually became black.

Karate Training: Sport, Physical Exercise, Self-Defense, and a Way of Life

Karate employs the whole body and is used to gain and maintain physical fitness. While karate techniques stress relaxation, muscular effort is needed to accelerate the arms and legs. Physical training exercises are performed to improve stamina, power, and flexibility.

Karate moves include kicking, striking, and blocking with the arms and legs. The practitioner attempts to focus as much force as possible at the point and moment of impact. Blows are made to the opponent with the forearm, elbow, knee, heel, and the ball of the foot. All are toughened by practice blows against padded surfaces or pine boards. Tameshiwara, or "power breaking," is one of the most spectacular and well known of karate training techniques. This involves breaking pine boards up to several inches thick with the bare hand or foot. But like all the techniques of karate, Tameshiwara is a personal measure of concentration and self-confidence as much as a test of physical strength.

Proficiency in karate comes through drills and repetition of techniques. Extensive repetition requires patience, stamina, and discipline. The philosophy of karate is based on Zen Buddhism, which promotes these qualities and aims to bring the mind and body into harmony. A person training to perfect the basic teachings of karate develops resilience, respect, and the knowledge of self-sacrifice.

Semi-sparring introduces the beginner to an actual fighting situation. Under controlled conditions, students face each other, one as the attacker, the other as the defender. Moves are pre-arranged and may look somewhat stiff in their execution. In contrast, real fighting is fast and unpredictable. The free-form movement that occurs in real fighting is difficult to teach, so the movements are broken down into their simple components. As students progress, new techniques are learned and added to the repertoire of movements that they have mastered. In the beginning, defensive blocking and counterattacking are performed as separate movements, but as students advance, the lapse in time between the two should gradually disappear until the block and counter flow fluidly.

The karate kata, or form, is a series of carefully arranged offensive and defensive moves performed against imaginary opponents. Only one person performs the kata at a time, and thus no contact is involved; in tournaments, panels of judges evaluate the execution of the kata. To an outsider, the kata appears to be a confusing sequence of movements and may resemble a dance more than a fight. Nevertheless, it is a fundamental element of karate. Besides teaching the student the basic fighting movements, the kata helps the student to bring his or her body under the control of the mind and will. At an advanced level, the kata training includes very quick strikes and reactions. Those who have mastered kata seem to be able to anticipate their opponents' movements.

In the hands of a well-trained individual, karate can be the most lethal of martial arts. To some, it is an exciting form of competition, while others enjoy it as a form of physical fitness training. But to Funakoshi Gichin, and to thousands of serious teachers and students of karate throughout the world, it is a powerful vehicle of discipline and self-knowledge.

—*Stefan Nikander*

Resources:

American Amateur Karate Federation
1930 Wilshire Boulevard, Suite 1208
Los Angeles, CA 90057
Tel: (213) 483-8261
Fax: (213) 483-4060
A national governing body for karate. The federation promotes karate with the intention of improving the physical and mental health of the public through the practice of karate.

U.S.A. Karate Federation
1300 Kenmore Boulevard
Akron, OH 44314
Tel: (216) 753-3114
Fax: (216) 753-6967
A national governing body for karate. The federation certifies instructors, conducts classes, and organizes competitions.

Further Reading:

Aiello, Jerry L. *Warrior Within: A Guide to Applying Your Warrior Spirit.* Berkley, MI: Aiello Group, 1992.

Aigla, Jorge H. *Karate-Do and Zen: An Inquiry.* Santa Fe, NM: Do Press, 1994.

Funakoshi, Gichin. *Karate-Do: My Way of Life.* New York: Harper and Row, 1975.

Hassell, Randall G. *The Karate Spirit.* St. Louis, MO: Focus Publications, 1995.

Johnson, Nathan. *Zen Shaolin Karate: The Complete Practice, Philosophy, and History.* Boston: Charles E. Tuttle, 1993.

Nakamura, Tadashi. *Karate: Technique and Spirit.* Boston: Charles E. Tuttle, 1986.

Nicol, C. W. *Moving Zen: Karate as a Way to Gentleness.* New York: William Morrow, 1982.

KENDO

Kendo is the Japanese martial art of swordsmanship. The name literally means "the way of the sword." It is considered the oldest of the Japanese martial arts and is based on rigorous physical and mental training and self-discipline. Essential to the practice of kendo is the knowledge and anticipation of the opponent's thoughts in order not only to defend oneself from the attack of others, but to better understand oneself and others in daily life.

History of Kendo

Kendo has a long and respected tradition in Japan, with techniques as old as swordsmanship itself. They were first used by the bushi, or warrior class, that developed in the northern provinces of Japan in their fights against the Ainu tribes. Throughout Japanese history the techniques have been called ken-jutsu, heiho, toho, gekken, hyoho, to-jutsu, tachi-uchi and hyodo. These techniques were passed on from father to son and from teacher to student through oral tradition.

The samurai, an elite class of bushi, started training in these techniques in the tenth century. It is estimated that from the start of this training until 1876 more than 600 different schools of swordsmanship flourished throughout Japan. In 1876 the first Meiji emperor forbade the samurai to carry swords due to the many fights and political intrigues between the samurai and noble class.

The exact origin of modern kendo is credited to a variety of sources. According to Louis Frederic in his *Dictionary of the Martial Arts*, Sakakibara Kenkichi, an expert of the Jikishin kage school of swordsmanship, improved upon a technique using the shinai, or bamboo sword. He gave demonstrations of his new technique throughout Japan in 1873. Sakakibara's desire was to revive the art of Japanese swordsmanship without its violent applications. The name *kendo* was given to the new

peaceful discipline by the Abe-ryu, or school headed by the Abe family. Modern kendo, or Japan kendo style, was a collaboration by the six leading kenjutsu schools at the end of the feudal era in 1876.

The first academy of kendo was founded in Tokyo in 1909. Both men and women were taught, and the new martial art gained a large following throughout Japan. The study was primarily confined to Japan until 1955, when it was introduced on an organized scale to France and the United States. In 1970 the first international tournament was held in Japan.

Since that time kendo has gained a high reputation internationally and is practiced throughout the world. Kendo is practiced in thirty-seven countries today, and there are thirty-four member countries of the International Kendo Federation. The federation sponsors an international competition every three years.

The Basic Principles of Kendo

The goal of kendo is to overcome the opponent by overcoming the self. This involves tremendous self-discipline and intense mental concentration, often in the face of great physical pain. Unlike tai chi ch'üan or aikido, which admonishes the practitioner to "go with" the opponent, the philosophy of kendo is that it is a battle to the death and only the strongest will remain alive when the fight is over.

To dominate the opponent the kendoka (someone who practices kendo) must unite his or her ki with the ki of the universe. According to Japanese belief, ki is the vital life energy flowing through all things and all people. Kendo philosophy states that the power of ki can be channeled and directed through concentration.

This ability to channel the ki is first realized through the kendo stance, in which the kendoka absorbs the ki from the earth by pulling it up through the soles of the feet into the legs, torso, and eventually the top of the head. The

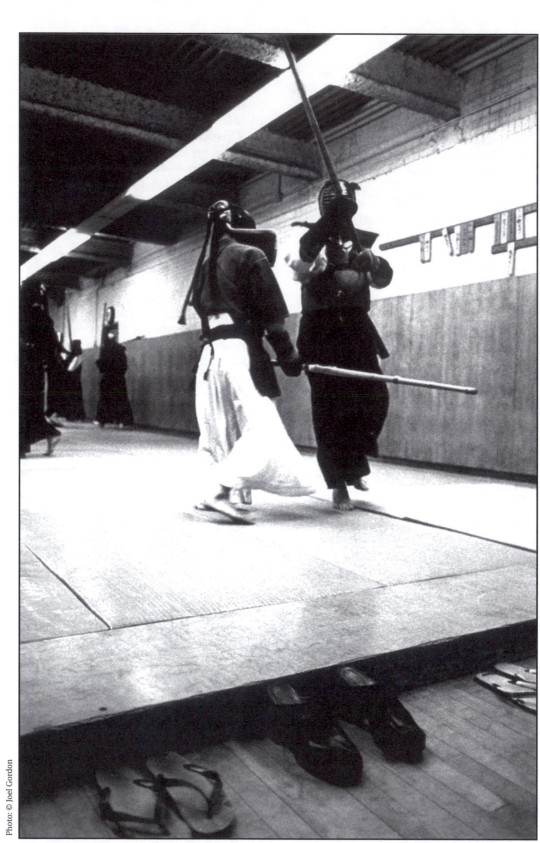

Photo: © Joel Gordon

Masks, shinai (swords), and costumes reveal the ancient roots of kendo, the Japanese art of swordsmanship.

spine must remain straight in order to avoid impeding the flow of ki. The effect of a bent spine on the flow of ki can be compared to the effect of pinching or bending a garden hose on the flow of water. As the water is dammed up in the hose, so it will be with the flow of ki in the body if the spine is broken or bent.

Even more fundamental than the stance is the flow of breath, which is slow and deep. It is pulled through the nose into the tanden, or hara, which is located about three inches below the navel, midway between the navel and the spine. The tanden is considered the physical and psychological center of the human being. It is here that individual ki and universal ki unite to form a powerful fighting energy. At the moment that a blow is struck, the attacker releases a powerful sound called ki-ai which is the concentration and focus of ki toward the kendoka's goal.

The focus of the eyes is another way in which the kendoka seeks to dominate his or her opponent. The kendoka must "see through" his or her opponent, penetrating to the mind with his or her eyes. This allows the kendoka to predict his or her opponent's next move. At the same time the kendoka must "see as far away as possible." By seeing "far away" the opponent becomes like a person seen against a mountain—a small insignificant dot that cannot stop the kendoka from achieving his or her goal.

Mental energy is paramount to the training in kendo. Only through mental concentration can total control and power be achieved. Yet the kendoka's mind must be like that of a baby, soft and focused. In this way the kendoka can stay totally concentrated in the moment and be prepared for any attack.

Typical Session of Kendo

A typical kendo class is a rigorous, ritualized workout, which usually lasts for two hours. The dojo (training hall) is a large open room with a wooden floor. At one end of the room is the joza, or altar. Each class begins and ends with a bow to the joza as a sign of respect, specifically to the sensei, or master teacher, but metaphorically to all ancestors and all knowledge that have gone before.

Students wear the armor and traditional dress of samurai warriors. Navy blue hakama, or wide skirt-like pants, and gi, or jacket, are worn. In the feudal era, only samurai were entitled to wear the hakama, a symbolically pleated garment. Each of the five front pleats represents a virtue from the bushido, or samurai code of honor. The first pleat stands for humility, the second for justice, the third for courtesy, the fourth for knowledge, and the fifth for trust. The two back pleats represent yin and yang, the two opposite cosmic energy principles that unite symbolically in one straight line down the back of the hakama.

A taiko drum on the joza is beaten to signify the beginning of class. After the initial bow, students generally form a circle to perform basic calisthenics warm-up exercises. Then suriashi (footwork exercises) are practiced walking the length of the dojo. The exercises progress from slow to fast and from simple to complex, beginning with the basic kendo sliding step, by which the foot never leaves the ground, to complex patterns involving multiple changes of direction and thrusts of the shinai.

The class proceeds to waza, or techniques. Waza include instructions in how to hold the shinai and how to attack. Beginning with a single target, the training advances to multiple targets, all of which must be quickly and precisely hit during the length of one long exhale.

In more advanced classes the teacher will eventually signal that it is time to put on the steel grilled head masks called *men*. At that point students line up, in order of their ranked ability, with the highest ranking students nearest the joza. They sit in zazen, a traditional kneeling posture in which the mind, breath, and body are brought to a state of calm readiness. Gloves and mask rest in front; the shinai is placed to the left of the body. The sensei puts on a protective head scarf and mask, and then upon verbal cue all the students do the same.

Now in full armor the keiko, or practice, begins with a bow to the joza, the sensei, and the opponent. Beginning with specific thrusts, advancing to series of thrusts, the keiko eventually progresses to full contact, where kendokas practice a series of fights, each lasting about three minutes. The keiko continues until the taiko drum is beaten once again.

The students return to their line of rank and repeat in exact reverse order the ritual movements that began the keiko—bowing, removing the *men* and head scarf, and finally kneeling again in za-zen for a brief period of meditation. Classes often conclude with the sensei giving a "teaching" on the spirit of kendo.

Benefits of Practicing Kendo

Because of its psychological and physical benefits, kendo is one of the most popular martial arts in Japan. Practice builds strength, coordination, and flexibility. On an intellectual level, many students are able to sharpen their mental focus and clarity through practice. Through the rigorous training and self-discipline of kendo, kendoka learn first to master themselves, and through that how to master all opponents and adverse situations. The physical, mental, and emotional knowledge gained through the study of kendo can be applied to all endeavors in life. Many of the political and industrial leaders of modern Japan study kendo.

—Nancy Allison, CMA, with Daniel T. Ebihara and Bruce Robertson-Smith

Resources:

Canadian Kendo Association
205 Riviera Drive
Markham, ON L3R 5J8
Canada
Tel: (416) 445-1481
Fax: (416) 445-0519
Provides information on kendo in Canada.

Eastern Kendo Federation
c/o Mozart H. Ishizuka
445 Fifth Avenue, Suite 21E
New York, NY 10016

Scoring in Kendo Competition

Precision, speed, and coordination are the qualities admired in a kendo attack. Bruce Robertson Smith, a first-degree black-belt student, explains that scoring a point in kendo is not as clear-cut as scoring a point in soccer or basketball. Three judges, standing in a triangular formation around the contest area, must all agree that the kendoka has earned the point.

Earning a point involves many things. First of all, the kendoka must strike the exact target that he or she calls out at the instant of the attack. Kendo recognizes nine target spots on the body: the right, left, and middle of the forehead; right and left forearms; the right, left, and center of the torso; and the center of the throat. Only the point or upper third of the shinai can effectively be used to strike a target area. The movement of the attack must be aesthetically pleasing, much like the criteria for earning points in competitive gymnastics. Finally, the energy expressed through the ki-ai must be full and strong. These criteria, known as kikentai-no-ichi, literally translated, mean "life force-sword-body-one."

Tel: (212) 679-1230
Fax: (212) 679-1236
Offers information about dojos in the New York area.

Great Lakes Kendo Federation
c/o Dr. Tsuyoshi Inishita
2423 Fenwick Road
University Heights, OH 44118
Tel: (216) 321-1187
Disseminates information about kendo in the Midwest.

Pacific Northwest Kendo Federation
616 SW 135th Street
Seattle, WA 98146
Tel: (206) 246-2239
Provides information on kendo in the Northwest.

South East Kendo Federation
2830 Carolyn Drive
Smyrna, GA 30080
Tel: (404) 434-7166
Furnishes regional information on kendo practitioners.

Southwest Kendo Federation
c/o Charles Riddle
12101 Randy Lane
Burleson, TX 76208
Offers resources to those practicing kendo in the American Southwest.

Further Reading:

Kiyota, Minoru. *Kendo: Its Philosophy, History, and Means to Personal Growth.* New York: Columbia University Press, 1995.

Sasamori, Junzo. *This Is Kendo: The Art of Japanese Fencing.* Rutland, VT: Charles E. Tuttle, 1964.

KUNG FU WU SU

Kung fu wu su refers to a multitude of Chinese martial arts and gymnastic movements, and encompasses nearly 400 disparate styles. For instance, it includes combative styles such as hung gar and more defensive styles such as t'ai chi ch'üan, and even includes acrobatic exercises. Advanced practice of kung fu requires almost life-long study combined with knowledge of Chinese culture, customs, and history.

History of Kung Fu Wu Su

Some forms of kung fu wu su date back approximately 5,000 years. The form that is the basis of most forms practiced today is said to have been perfected by Taoist monks, who practiced it to protect themselves from bandits and brigands in ancient China. The system itself is so potent that China's first great monarch, Huang Ti, known as the Yellow Emperor, had it systematically taught to his troops to improve their fighting ability. Kung fu, as we know it today, flourished in both northern and southern China, but throughout the years evolved in different ways. Generally speaking, southern styles emphasize hand techniques, while northern styles emphasize leg techniques.

The term *kung fu wu su* has a direct translation from its Chinese characters, and a philosophical meaning derived from that translation as well. *Kung* means "discipline technique"; *fu* means "person"; *wu* means "martial art"; and *su* means "technique" or "skill." But the word as a whole encompasses much more. The philosophical idea of kung fu is to develop three distinct but necessary characteristics: *dar* (character); tse (mental ability); and tee (physical ability). The aim is to live a positive and harmonious life.

The concept of self-defense is as old as humanity. But the first definitive martial arts systems evolved in China, and it is assumed that the Chinese had already cataloged and codified a basic system of self-defense as early as 4,500 years ago, which they called kung fu or wu su. In time, Taoist monks began to experiment with various divergent styles, beginning with five animal styles:

the crane, tiger, snake, dragon, and monkey. The second great transformation in the system came from India, when a traveling Buddhist monk, Bodhidarma, introduced advanced breathing techniques and meditative exercises, which were incorporated into kung fu about 550 years ago. This reinforced what came to be known as the Shaolin style, named after the temple where it was taught. Bodhidarma was enshrined by his Chinese name, dor-mor, for adding to and strengthening an already established system.

China's history has been tumultuous, and conflict and warfare eventually disrupted the tranquillity of the Shaolin Temple. The Shaolin Temple era ended with the Ming Dynasty (1368–1644 CE), when the reigning emperors began to regard the two Shaolin temples, one in southern China, the other in the north, as a threat to their authority. They effectively embarked on a campaign that led to the destruction of both temples. With the demise of their temples, Shaolin monks scattered throughout Asia, teaching kung fu wherever they went.

The Varied Styles of Kung Fu

The differing styles of kung fu evolved through need or observation. For example, besides the animal styles, which are based on observation of animal movements, there are also styles based on natural phenomena, such as moving shadow. Other styles are based on distinct physical features like white eyebrow, a state or condition such as drunken monk, or even a physical substance, such as green jade.

There are twenty-five groupings in kung fu that identify the various styles. These groupings include everything from an astrological classification, like chee sin, or seven stars style, to insects, like tong lon, or praying mantis style. All these groupings can be classified into four general categories:

- The first classification is based on appearance. Some may emphasize the "hard" way with strong, devastating blows and movements. Others may emphasize the "soft" way, where the opponent's strength may be used against him, but is just as effective in subduing an adversary. For example, gin kong is considered a hard style because of its aggressive nature, and t'ai chi is a soft style because of its emphasis on defensive movements. Some disciplines, such as northern Shaolin style, may be a combination of both.
- The second classification is based on geography. Pa kua, a style that emphasizes distinct stepping movements, comes from north central China. Jow gar and hung dar, styles that emphasize strong hand techniques, come from southern China.
- The next classification is based on the character of the style. T'ai chi, with its emphasis on inner force and evasive maneuvers, is considered an internal discipline. An example of a discipline that is external in nature is hung gar, because of its preference for force and rapid attack movements. A combination of both can be found in the northern Shaolin style.
- The final classification is based on the purpose of the style. It may be the grabbing, grappling style of chin-na fa, or a weapon style like the steel sword or kong chien. The terminology used to define each style often reflects its content.

Most styles of kung fu employ punching and kicking techniques, but others use grappling and throwing techniques, and/or ground fighting. Most utilize a variety of weapons, both long and short, such as the long or sleeve staff, small-bladed weapons, straight sword or machete, long-bladed weapons such as the spear or trident, and throwing weapons such as stars or spikes. Nearly all the styles incorporate meditation, breathing techniques, and body conditioning. The end result is a vigorous combination of external and internal methods, designed to promote knowledge of self-defense and enhance general

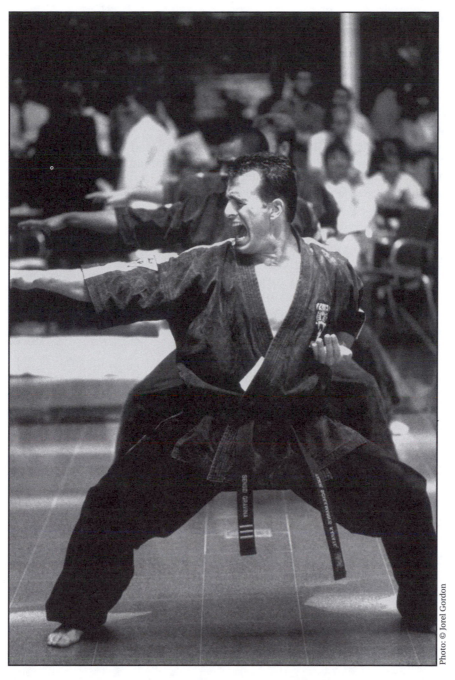

Photo: © Jorel Gordon

The chinese martial art of kung fu consists of nearly 400 different styles.

health. The overall makeup is derived from philosophical and theoretical concepts from Taoist and Buddhist teachings, designed to keep both the body and mind agile and resilient.

Kung fu embodies more than just physical aspects. Ancient masters in China considered it a way of life, not just a sport or pastime. In its true essence, it is an ethical discipline that permeates every aspect of life. Since kung fu is more than a martial arts technique, it can be achieved by any disciplined person. If one does a task well, and acts in a correct and moral manner, he or she is said to have kung fu. The purpose of kung fu practice is to create not a fighting machine, but a complete individual—one who aspires to continual growth as a total person and who contributes to the well-being of the community.

When choosing a style to practice, consider your own needs and desires as an individual. There are kung fu schools or temples that will emphasize one style or manner of practice. Others may offer a combination of styles. Eventually, you will gravitate toward the method that is best suited to your nature.

The Instruction of Kung Fu Wu Su

The study of kung fu wu su in all its diverse forms can take a lifetime. The basic course in martial arts practice can take up to five years to complete. High-level studies will take longer. The length of the training depends on how much the individual student wants from the study and how much time and effort he or she gives to the training. The basic applications include body conditioning to calisthenics to basic self-defense techniques. The training is all-inclusive. It can also be extensive in other areas if the student is given a grounding in philosophy, concentration, kung fu medicines, breathing, meditation, and diet. Not many temples or schools will offer such a varied and extensive program of study.

Benefits of Kung Fu

People study kung fu for many reasons. Some seek a measure of self-protection. Others are drawn by its refined, elegant movements. Some are enthralled by the sheer power generated by its defensive and offensive techniques. And some are enticed by the arcane self-healing practices rooted in the system, such as the enhancement of chi, or life force, the positive energy within all of us. Some individuals seek to develop this chi to its highest level, to channel this energy to protect and heal themselves and others from illness. Kung fu is a system that seeks a dynamic flow between mind and body. In the beginning, it may test one's commitment to learning and mastering the different movements and their applications.

—*Oswald Rivera*

Resources:

Chinese Kung-Fu Wu-Su Association
28 West 27th Street, 8th floor
New York, NY 10001
Tel: (212) 725-0535
Provides information on different martial arts disciplines.

T'ai Chi Ch'üan/Shaolin Chuan Association (TCC/SCA)
33W624 Roosevelt Road

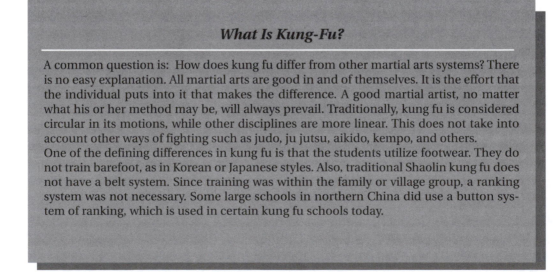

What Is Kung-Fu?

A common question is: How does kung fu differ from other martial arts systems? There is no easy explanation. All martial arts are good in and of themselves. It is the effort that the individual puts into it that makes the difference. A good martial artist, no matter what his or her method may be, will always prevail. Traditionally, kung fu is considered circular in its motions, while other disciplines are more linear. This does not take into account other ways of fighting such as judo, ju jutsu, aikido, kempo, and others.
One of the defining differences in kung fu is that the students utilize footwear. They do not train barefoot, as in Korean or Japanese styles. Also, traditional Shaolin kung fu does not have a belt system. Since training was within the family or village group, a ranking system was not necessary. Some large schools in northern China did use a button system of ranking, which is used in certain kung fu schools today.

P.O. Box 430
Geneva, IL 60134
Tel: (708) 232-0029
Founded in 1987, this organization promotes and offers instruction in t'ai chi ch'üan and Shaolin chuan kung fu. Conducts demonstrations, seminars, lectures, and certification programs for members, and publishes a bimonthly newsletter.

World Martial Arts Association (WMAA)
P.O. Box 1568
Santa Barbara, CA 93102
Tel: (805) 569-1389
Fax: (805) 569-0267
Promotes many kung fu wu su disciplines and instructs practitioners on the technical aspects of these disciplines.

Further Reading:

Mitchell, David. *Shaolin Temple Kung-Fu.* London: Stanley Paul, 1990.

Parulski, George R. *The Secrets of Kung-Fu: A Complete Guide to the Fundamentals of Shaolin Kung-Fu and the Principles of Inner Power.* Chicago: Contemporary Books, 1984.

Wong, Kiew Kit. *The Art of Shaolin Kung-Fu: The Secrets of Kung-Fu for Self-Defense, Health, and Enlightenment.* Rockport, MA: Element, 1996.

TAEKWONDO

Taekwondo is one of the most popular martial arts in the world. Its offensive and defensive movements are uniform for all of those that practice the discipline, which makes it easy to set standards of accomplishment and skill. It is also used by many people as an effective system of self-defense. People of all ages and walks of life have taken up this contemporary Korean martial art to improve their stamina, physical fitness, and mental acuity, and to learn to defend against attack. The practice of taekwondo has a rich heritage, and its practitioners adhere to strict ethical and moral guidelines.

History of Taekwondo

The contemporary art and modern sport of taekwondo can be traced to tae kyon, a discipline characterized by its emphasis on kicking techniques. Some experts believe that tae kyon was an offshoot of su bak, the martial art said to have been practiced more than 1000 years ago by Hwarang warriors in Korea. The Hwarang (which means "flowering youth") were a national group of outstanding youths handpicked for training in swordsmanship and archery. The chosen youths were guided by a code of ethics, known as the Code of Hwarang, prescribed by the eminent Buddhist monk Wongwang. The Code of Hwarang dictated that followers would loyally serve the king, be obedient to their parents, be honorable to friends, never retreat in battle, and kill justly.

In peacetime, there was little use for the practice of tae kyon to the common man. At the time of the Silla dynasty (688–935 BCE), Korea became a highly centralized Buddhist state. The fine arts flourished, and the practice of martial arts was suppressed because of their offensive, warlike capabilities.

The contemporary art of taekwondo was founded by General Choi Hong Hi in 1946. Choi came from a military family; he studied tae kyon as a child and karate while forced to serve in the Japanese army. Originally, taekwondo was nothing more than transplanted Japanese karate with a bit of tae kyon. In fact, the term taekwondo (*tae* meaning "foot," *kwon* meaning "fist," *do* meaning "art" or "the way") was adopted by the Korean Taekwondo Federation as the Korean translation of karate (*kara* meaning empty, *te* meaning hand). Today, however, the World Taekwondo Federation is the undisputed governing body, sanctioning all taekwondo competitions and certifying all belt rank

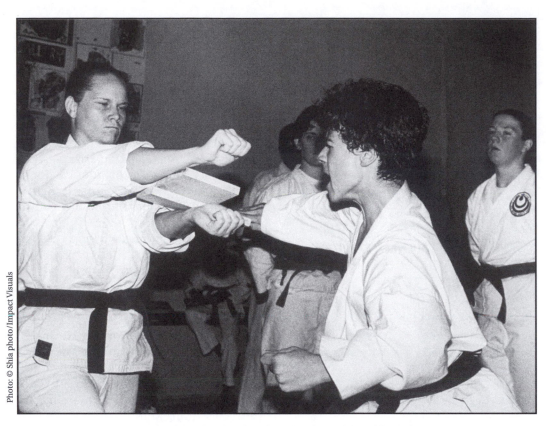

A taekwondo student breaks a board with hand for a blue belt test.

promotions at the black-belt level and above. In addition, the body and movement structure of the contemporary, karatelike taekwondo has been modified into a modern sport form within the past ten years. Notable changes include a higher fighting stance, faster footwork, a new set of pre-arranged patterns, and an emphasis on sport competition and its rules rather than self-defense applications.

The Basic Principles of Taekwondo

While the physical movements of taekwondo are simple, dedicated practice is necessary for them to become natural and spontaneous. As a result, the practitioner develops discipline and perseverance, as progress is sometimes slow. The mental discipline, self-confidence, and self-control gained through prolonged practice bring taekwondo practitioners the utmost determination and stability of both mind and body.

As a sport, taekwondo's uniform technique sets a standard for all practitioners. As a martial art, the basic techniques of taekwondo serve as a powerful system of self-defense skills. In competition, taekwondo techniques are evaluated on the practitioner's ability to perform them individually in the air, in series as self-defense techniques with an opponent, and in application through sparring.

Taekwondo Class

Taekwondo is taught in a dojang (training hall), which is usually a simple room with a wooden floor. In the more traditional taekwondo dojang, one will find a makiwara (striking post), used to develop focus and power in striking. In the modern, sport-oriented dojang, however, this is replaced with a heavy punching bag, and various types of padding, such as chest, head, and foot protectors, and padded punching gloves are used.

At the beginning of each class, students line up in rows. The sabumnim (master) will then yell out a few commands, and students will bow to him, to the senior student, and the flags of Korea and the country where the training hall is located. Then the students will stand for a few minutes in meditation. During meditation, students are asked to clear their minds of thoughts and to relax as well as prepare for serious practice. Once these preparations have concluded, physical training begins.

Classes in taekwondo generally last one hour or ninety minutes. The first fifteen minutes are spent stretching the legs and hips. Students spend the next fifteen minutes practicing sets of basic blocking, striking, and kicking techniques in the air. This is followed by a fifteen-minute practice of predetermined offensive and defensive movements known as hyung or poomse. The next fifteen minutes are generally spent on the practice of basic self-defense techniques, including defenses against the straight punch, wrist grabs, and holds of various types. The next ten minutes are used for the practice of sparring, which allows students to use their skills against an opponent in a controlled environment. This is where many students feel they benefit the most from training in that they are able to see firsthand how their skills have improved. The final five minutes of class are spent in meditation to calm the mind, shed the fighting mentality, and ease back into daily activities.

The conclusion of class finds students reciting the Code of Hwarang, bowing to their master, the senior student, and the flags once again. Practitioners then take a few minutes to sweep the dojang floor and clean any mirrors that may be present. The bowing and cleaning are humbling mechanisms. They instill in the student a sense of respect for one's elders and seniors, the training hall, and one's surroundings. It is hoped that this will carry over into the practitioner's daily life.

Benefits of Practicing Taekwondo

As taekwondo practitioners refine their physical abilities, they improve in many seemingly unrelated areas. A relaxed state of mind, improved patience, sharpened concentration, and numerous other benefits accompany new self-defense skills. Above all, taekwondo students embrace the philosophical and ethical beliefs that define the discipline, beliefs that function to guide the student in his or her daily life.

Since its Olympic debut in 1988, taekwondo's popularity has spread at a remarkable rate across the world. Profiency in basic taekwondo techniques takes only a few years. While the earning of a black belt takes roughly three or four years, it is typically thought to be just the beginning of a lifelong journey toward self-actualization.

—*Mark Wiley*

Resources:

International Taekwondo Association
P. O. Box 281
Grand Blanc, MI 48439
Tel: (810) 232-6482
Promotes the practice of taekwondo in the United States.

Korean Ki Do Federation HQ
Seoul, Kang Nam Gu, Non Hyun Dong
122-2 Nam Yang Bldg. 300
Korea
Tel: (02) 540-2156-7
Provides information for international organizations and associations.

United States Taekwondo Association
220 East 86th Street
New York, NY 10028
Tel: (212) 772-8918
Disseminates information about taekwondo in the United States.

United Taekwondo International
4707 48 Street, 2nd floor
Camrose, Alberta T4V 1L2
Canada

Tel: (403) 672-3500
Offers information about the practice of taekwondo in Canada.

Further Reading:

Books:

Cho, S. Henry. *Taekwondo: Secrets of Korean Karate.* Rutland, VT: Charles E. Tuttle Co., 1992.

Corcoran, Jon, and Emil Farkas. *The Original Martial Arts Encyclopedia.* Los Angeles: Pro Action Publishing, 1993.

Draeger, Donn F., and Robert W. Smith. *Comprehensive Asian Fighting Arts.* Tokyo: Kodansha International, 1980.

Haines, Bruce. *Karate's History and Traditions.* Revised edition. Rutland, VT: Charles E. Tuttle Co., 1995.

Park, Y. H., and Jeff Leibowitz. *Fighting Back: Taekwondo for Women.* East Meadow, NY: Y.H. Park Publications, 1993.

Shaw, Scott. *Hapkido: Korean Art of Self-Defense.* Rutland, VT: Charles E. Tuttle Co., 1996.

Journals:

Young, Robert W. "The History and Development of Tae Kyon." *Journal of Asian Martial Arts* 2, 2 (1993): 44–69.

PART XII: YOGA

Integral Yoga • Iyengar Yoga • Kripalu Yoga

Yoga is an ancient Hindu method of body-mind integration used to achieve spiritual enlightenment. Literally translated from Sanskrit, the language of the Hindu spiritual texts, yoga means "union." This union refers to the joining of the individual human spirit with the motivating spirit of the universe. Over thousands of years many methods of reaching this desired spiritual union evolved. These methods include such activities as the study of metaphysics and philosophy, meditation, the development and cleansing of the physical body, and living a life of service and devotion. As practiced in the United States today, most yoga classes focus on hatha yoga, the method of developing spiritual enlightenment through physical mastery of the body. Hatha yoga practice includes stretching, flexing, and balancing the body in many different positions, internal cleansing techniques, and breathing exercises. In many yoga classes, such as those offered in health clubs or recreation centers, the physical aspects of hatha yoga are often more emphasized than the spiritual. With or without the spiritual goal, the many forms of yoga now practiced offer a means of gaining and maintaining physical, emotional, and mental health and well-being.

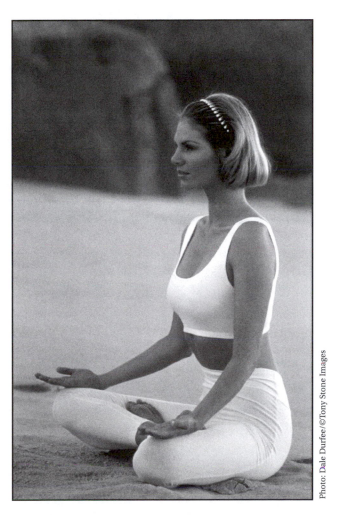

Photo: Dale Durfee/©Tony Stone Images

Yoga is practiced to center and calm the body and mind.

The History of Yoga

Archaeologists and yoga scholars believe that images found on ceramics during excavations in India's Indus River basin are of yoga asanas, or postures, and show that the practices of yoga flourished in India as far back as 3000 BCE. Sometime between the fifth and second centuries BCE the Indian philosopher Patanjali gathered many of the basic techniques and concepts of raja, or kingly yoga, into a book called the *Yoga Sutras*. The most common forms of yoga practiced in the West today are derived from the concepts and practices that Patanjali recorded.

Yoga was incorporated into the Buddhist religious tradition by Buddhism's founder, Prince Siddhartha Gautama. The young Indian prince was well versed in the theories and practices of yoga when he left his home in search of the cause of human suffering. The solutions he found form the philosophical basis of Buddhism. Followers of Gautama, also called the Buddha, or the "enlightened one," lived peacefully in India until around the third century BCE, when the political climate became less tolerant of non-Hindus. It was at this time that the monks and disciples of Buddhism began to migrate in large numbers across the Asian continent.

Over time the Buddhist monks became a vital part of the cultural fabric of their adopted countries, and the yoga-based practices they brought with them were integrated into the native religions of China, Japan, and other Asian countries. In each country distinctive variations of the original Indian yogic practices developed. In his three-volume work, *The Complete Yoga Book*, James Hewitt states that ancient yogic techniques traveled in similar ways as far east as Siberia, mixing with Inuit shamanic practices and as far west as the Middle East, where they were incorporated into Islamic Sufi practices. Both Hewitt and the scholar Mircea Eliade believe that Indian yogic practices also influenced the mystic sects of Christianity.

The philosophy and practices of yoga have slowly infiltrated Western culture throughout the twentieth century. With the British colonial expansion into India, knowledge of the physical, psychological, and metaphysical practices of yoga increased. The World Parliament of Religions, held in Chicago in 1893, brought many yoga teachers to America for the first time. In 1911 the American writer William James described in his classic study of the psychology of religious experience, *On Vital Reserves*, the considerable benefits one European friend received through the practice of yoga. By the 1930s Indian practitioners of yoga, such as Paramhansa Yogananda, were lecturing in England and in the United States. By 1946 Paramhansa's book *Autobiography of a Yogi*, describing the concepts and meditative practices of yoga, was available throughout the English-speaking world.

In the 1950s and 1960s yoga practices become more popular throughout the United States, with many books published on the subject and many yoga schools established. In 1970 Swami Rama, founder of the Himalayan Institute in Pennsylvania, was the subject of research at the Menninger Foundation in Topeka, Kansas. According to journalist Linda Johnsen, writing in *Yoga Journal International*, he shocked researchers by "his abilities to stop his heartbeat for extended periods of time and to remain fully lucid while his brain registered the delta waves normally associated with sleep" ("Hatha Traditions: How to Find a Class That's Right for You," *Yoga International's Guide to Yoga Teachers and Classes*, 1996). It was this research that first drew the attention of much of the mainstream Western scientific community to the link between human consciousness and physical functioning.

Today many Westerners practice yoga on a variety of levels—from full body-mind-spirit union to the maintenance of physical well-being. Many types of yoga classes are available in most major cities and even in smaller towns. There are a multitude of training programs where yoga practitioners, from beginner to advanced, can develop their practice.

The Spiritual Goal of Yoga

To understand the practice of yoga it is helpful to understand something about its spiritual goal. The spiritual goal of yoga is closely connected with the Hindu philosophical view concerning the relationship between spirit and matter. According to that view, the spirit animating the universe and the spirit animating every individual human being are one and the same. Every single thing on this planet, from the simplest blade of grass to the most complex human being, is, according to the Hindu view, a materialized form of this same spirit.

The desire motivating this spirit, as Mircea Eliade describes in his widely respected book *Yoga: Immortality and Freedom*, is simply "to be known." So this spirit incarnates and reincarnates into more and more complex forms of matter according to a moral code known as the law of karma. When the spirit reaches human form it has the ability through many disciplined practices to realize its true nature as part and parcel of the whole. This is a long and varied process involving many changes of human consciousness or awareness. *Samadhi* is the Sanskrit word that describes the blissful state of human consciousness attained when the individual human spirit experiences itself once again as part of the universal cosmic spirit.

The Nine Systems of Yoga

Reaching samadhi requires great discipline and much dedication. Over thousands of years many different systems of yoga practices evolved to suit the needs and personalities of different people. The different systems often share so many concepts and techniques that it is difficult to find one classification method upon which all yoga scholars, and certainly all yoga teachers, would agree. However, the following represents the nine generally recognized paths toward the goal of samadhi.

- **Raja yoga**, also known as royal, kingly, classical, ashtanga, or eight-limbed yoga, is the path of mental mastery. Mental mastery here refers to the basic yogic belief that the disciplined focus of mental energy is the necessary basis for spiritual awareness. Raja yoga recognizes that this energy cannot be tapped unless the body is strong, healthy, relaxed, and balanced. Students of raja yoga work through the first seven limbs, or stages, which cover physical stretching, strengthening, toning and cleansing exercises, breathing exercises, ethical and philosophical inquiry, and meditation practices to reach samadhi, which is considered the eighth limb.
- **Hatha yoga**, the path of bodily mastery, is the best-known and most practiced form of yoga in the West. Perhaps because of its focus on the body itself, the benefits of hatha yoga may be felt most easily without having to accept the spiritual component.

For this reason many scholars believe that the practices of hatha yoga are merely a preparation for raja yoga. Hatha yoga practices include asanas, or postures in which one balances, stretches, and strengthens the body; kriyas, or methods of cleansing the internal body; and pranayama, or special breathing exercises. Together these constitute a thorough method of hygiene that cleanses and tones the internal organs and glands and the musculo-skeletal, respiratory, digestive, and nervous systems.

- **Mantra yoga** is the practice of influencing consciousness through repetition of certain syllables or phrases known as mantras. The word or phrase is considered to be a mystical distillation of the cosmic energy of the universe. It can be repeated aloud or silently in the mind. In Western scientific terms, spoken mantras may be understood as sound vibrations affecting one's emotions, similar to the way music often does. Transcendental Meditation, which was brought to the West by Marahishi Mahesh Yogi, is a form of mantra yoga.

- **Yantra yoga** uses visual images as the focal point for concentration in order to affect consciousness in the same way that mantra yoga uses sound. Yantra images may be sculptures or paintings of deities or teachers, but more often they are mandalas—symbolic, geometric images of the relationship between the individual and the universal energy. Traditional mandalas are ornate paintings incorporating many Hindu or Buddhist deities in a sort of map of the spiritual universe, but simple abstract images are also common in the West today.

- **Kundalini or laya yoga** is a method of yoga in which cosmic energy is imaged as a sleeping serpent coiled three and a half times around the base of the spine. In this image the mouth of the kundalini, or serpent, is grasping the sushumna, a narrow nerve channel through the spine. Difficult asanas, strenuous pranayama, mantras, yantras, muscular contractions or locks called bandhas, and concentrated meditative practices are all used to encourage the kundalini to climb up the sushumna through the seven chakras, or spiritual centers, that correspond to physical places along the length of the spine. As the kundalini passes through each center it purifies the channel and awakens specific physical and psychic powers. While the traditional practices of kundalini yoga are often considered dangerous, the imagery associated with the chakra system is frequently used in other systems of yoga and has affected the development of many Western body-mind disciplines as well.

- **Jhana yoga,** the path of spiritual knowledge and wisdom, emphasizes philosophical inquiry and meditation to reach spiritual enlightenment. For instance, students are encouraged to reflect on the nature of the world, reality, and the meaning of life, and their true selves. This is the path of intellectual pursuit and does not involve the body directly. A follower of jhana yoga would be comparable to Albert Einstein. Einstein was not a yoga practitioner, but the way he focused his intellect to inquire deeply into the nature of the universe had the disciplined and dedicated quality of a yogic meditation. Interestingly Einstein's ground-breaking theories about the relationship of energy and matter began a shift in Western physics that continues to move ever closer to the Hindu philosophical view of the universe.

- **Bhakti yoga** is the path of love and devotion. It emphasizes living a life that demonstrates one's pure and selfless love of the divine. The Hindu god Krishna is often a focus for this form of yoga in India. The rites of this path include singing songs and dancing dances of devotion. Members of the Krishna Consciousness Movement are among the devotees of this path. While it has traditionally been one of the most popular paths for the people of India, Westerners are generally less comfortable with its practices.
- **Karma yoga**, the path of selfless action and service, might be exemplified by Mahatma Gandhi or Mother Teresa. Even though Mother Teresa practiced Catholicism, the way in which her devotion to her religion led her to serve humanity is similar to the way in which a follower of karma yoga is taught to dedicate all of his or her actions to the good of others.
- **Tantric yoga** as a general term can refer to any method of yoga using physiological techniques such as hatha or kundalini yoga, but is more specifically used to describe the path of union through harnessing sexual energies. In tantric yoga sexual union is seen as a way to spiritual illumination. Its practices include asanas, pranayama, mantras, and yantras employed in preparation of and during sex, which is performed as a ritual uniting of the male and female aspects of the one universal energy. (The Hindu spiritual texts have many names for these aspects, which are represented in Hindu art as gods and goddesses in the act of sexual embrace, but they are more familiar to Westerners through their Chinese names of yin and yang.) Because tantric yoga is an ecstatic path that embraces the earthy aspects of life, it has often been abused as a spiritual path, but the goal of tantric yoga, like the goal of all yogas, is spiritual union, and when practiced in earnest requires the same discipline and dedication.

The Yoga Experience in the West

Most yoga practiced in the West today primarily combines elements of hatha, mantra, and raja yoga. Because of the enormous overlap of the elements of various yogic systems, jhana, karma, kundalini and/or yantra yoga may also be combined in contemporary practices. Classes are generally taught in groups, but individual lessons are also available. They are generally taught indoors, but some ashrams, or teaching centers, offer classes outdoors, where the energy of the sun and fresh air can enhance the pleasure and effectiveness of the exercises. Often the room will have an altar where flowers, incense, candles, or a mandala or a photo of the founder of the school will rest. Students and teacher generally wear comfortable cotton clothing, which allows for the flow of air to the skin.

Yoga classes may be extremely vigorous and fast-paced or very gentle and slow-moving, depending on the tradition of the school and teacher. Many yoga classes will begin with the chanting of a mantra. The Hindu sacred syllable *oM* is often used. The purpose of chanting is to utilize the power of sound vibrations to focus and influence consciousness.

Classes generally proceed to a series of asanas. Hundreds of asanas and many different techniques concerning the approach to and sequence of them have been developed by different gurus, or teachers. But whether the class is vigorous or gentle,

309

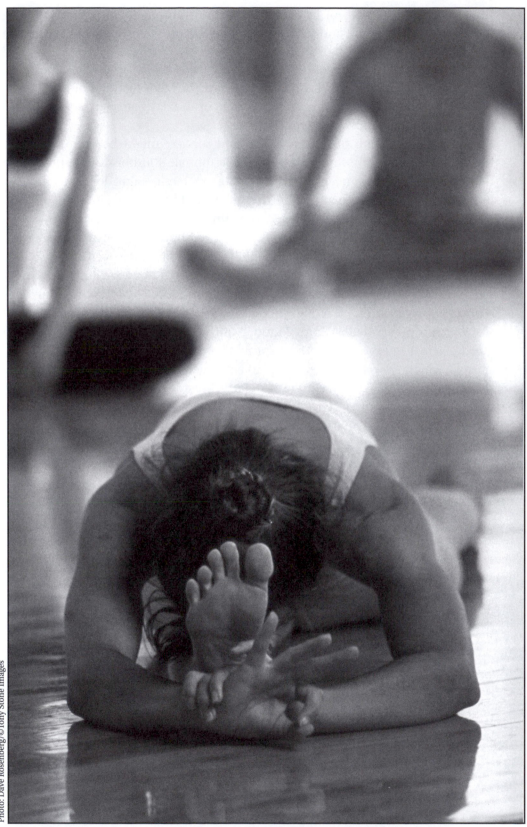

Yoga practices, such as this forward bending pose, develop physical and mental concentration.

students will be urged to focus their attention on the initiation, sequencing, and quality of movement as they enter, hold, and leave each pose. Each pose has a specific purpose and name. For example the cobra pose, named for the characteristic pose of the animal, is a backward lengthening and bending of the spine performed while lying on the stomach. It's used to develop flexibility in the spine, strength in the abdomen, and an openness in the personality and spirit. Focusing on the flow of breath while in the pose calms the nervous system and mind, gently preparing the body and mind for deeper meditation.

The asana portion of the class is generally followed by a series of pranayama, or breath-control exercises. Through pranayama, yoga students aim to create steady flowing movement of prana, or life force, through the system. As the breathing becomes deeper, more controlled, and rhythmical, the mind becomes calm and focused.

With a cleansed and strengthened body and a calm and focused mind, the student is better prepared to begin meditation. The meditation portion of the class is designed to create a heightened sense of peace and awareness and to focus, empty, and control the mind. It is through the practice of meditation, after many years of long and disciplined study, that yogis believe the state of samadhi may be reached.

Benefits

With or without the goal of samadhi, the benefits of yoga can be numerous. Many practitioners attribute health, vitality, and peace of mind to the practice of yoga. Western scientific studies have shown it to be effective in strengthening muscles and bones, improving circulation and respiration, reducing blood pressure and heart rate, relieving stress and physical pain, sharpening intellectual functioning and motor skills, and aiding in relief from physical and emotional addictions.

With the plethora of classes and approaches available, it is important to take the time to find a well-trained teacher, in a style and class of yoga that is compatible with the goals and temperament of the student. Once found, the potential benefits of yoga seem to be limited only by the dedication of the student.

—Nancy Allison, CMA
with consultation by Lillo (Leela) Way

Yoga Therapy

Yoga therapy is an emerging field of physical therapy most often practiced on a one-on-one basis. Yoga therapy is not a complete method as are the nine ancient systems, but uses the therapeutic properties of yoga breathing, posturing, and meditative techniques to aid the healing process. Yoga therapy functions much like a visit to a doctor or a therapist, at which certain exercises are prescribed to treat particular symptoms, and verbal dialogue between the therapist and client addressing the body-mind nature of the ailment may ensue.

Resources:

Himalayan International Institute of Yoga, Science
    and Philosophy
78 Fifth Avenue
New York, NY 10011
Tel: (212) 243-5995
*Offers courses and lectures on all aspects of yoga
practice and workshops for yoga teachers. The
school is dedicated to helping individuals develop
physically, mentally, and spiritually.*

The International Association of Yoga Therapists
109 Hillside Avenue
Mill Valley, CA 94941
Tel: (415) 381-0876

International Sivananda Yoga Vedanta Centres
    Worldwide
Sivananda Ashram Yoga Camp
8th Avenue
Val Morin, Quebec
Canada
Tel: (819) 322-3226
Fax: (819) 322-5876

Yoga Journal
2054 University Avenue
Berkeley, CA 94704.
Tel: (510) 841-9200

Further Reading:

Arua, Pandit U., et al. *Yoga Sutras of Patanjali
    with the Exposition of Yvasa: A Translation and
    Commentary.* Vol. 1. Honesdale, PA: Himalayan
    Publishers, 1986.

Eliade, Mircea. *Yoga: Immortality and Freedom.*
    New York: Pantheon Books, Bollingen Series
    LVI, 1958.

Hewitt, James. *The Complete Yoga Book.*
    New York: Schocken Books, 1977.

Satchidananda, Yogiraj Sriswami. *Integral Yoga
    Hatha.* New York: Holt, Rinehart and Winston,
    1970.

Vishnudevananda, Swami. *The Complete Illustrat-
    ed Book of Yoga.* New York: Harmony Books,
    1980.

INTEGRAL YOGA

Integral yoga is a modern approach to the ancient body-mind discipline of yoga. Its practice combines six ancient methods of yoga to help individuals discover inner peace and happiness. The methods it combines are hatha yoga, which uses body postures (asanas), breath control (pranayama), and relaxation techniques; karma yoga, which teaches the selfless service of oneself for the good of others; raja yoga, which stresses concentration and meditation on ethical perfection; japa, or mantra, yoga, which uses the repetition of sounds to help focus the mind in meditation; bhakti yoga, which stresses love and devotion to God or the Divine Being; and jhana yoga, which encourages self-inquiry and the investigation of the meaning of life and the nature of knowledge and reality.

Guiding Principles of Integral Yoga

The goal of integral yoga is to help people achieve what practitioners believe is the birthright of every individual—that is, to realize the spiritual unity behind all the diversity of life and to live harmoniously as members of one universal family. This goal is achieved by maintaining a well-balanced life with a body of optimum health and strength, the senses under total control; a clear, calm, well-disciplined mind; a sharp intellect; a will that is strong and yet pliable; a heart full of unconditional love and compassion; an ego as pure as crystal; and a life filled with supreme peace and joy. Integral yoga strongly encourages such principles as truth, nonviolence, and universal brotherhood.

The Development of Integral Yoga

In the early part of the twentieth century Swami Sivananda Saraswati (1887–1963) of Rishikesh, India, developed an approach to yoga that integrated several of the ancient methods of yoga. Several of his disciples spread this approach to yoga around the world. One of them, Swami Satchidananda, founded Integral Yoga International (originally the Integral Yoga Institute) in the United States in 1966.

For the past forty years Swami Satchidananda has promoted world peace through ecumenism—the recognition that, intrinsically, all religions embrace the same ultimate truth and belief in one God, which may be worshiped variously through many names and forms. He frequently conducts Light of Truth Universal Services, where clergy of all faiths worship together, each according to his or her own tradition.

Integral Yoga International now has more than forty Integral Yoga Institutes (IYIs) and Integral Yoga Centers (IYCs) throughout the United States and abroad. The headquarters of Integral Yoga International is Satchidananda Ashram–Yogaville, located in Buckingham, Virginia. The center encompasses almost 1,000 acres of woodland and fields. Here, people of all faiths and backgrounds come together to study and practice the principles of integral yoga.

The focal point of Satchidananda Ashram–Yogaville is the Light of Truth Universal Shrine (LOTUS), which embodies Swami Satchidananda's teachings and his efforts to foster world peace and religious harmony. Inside the shrine each major faith is represented by an altar, on which rests a carved inscription from the scripture of that particular faith. Other known faiths and those that may one day develop, but which are still unknown to us, are also represented by illuminated arches. The theme of LOTUS is "Truth Is One, Paths Are Many," and this aphorism may also be extended to integral yoga. Integral yoga is a system that synthesizes the various yogic approaches with one goal in mind: to help the individual experience physical, mental, and spiritual harmony.

—*Rev. Kumari de Sachy, Ed.D*

Resources:

Satchidananda Ashram–Yogaville
Route 1, Box 1720
Buckingham, VA 23921
Tel: (804) 969-3121
Fax: (804) 969-1303

Headquarters for Integral Yoga International that provides teacher training courses, silent retreats, and classes and workshops in hatha yoga, meditation, yoga philosophy, vegetarian diet, and other various branches of yoga. These are offered regularly, year-round. Guests are welcome to visit the ashram.

IYENGAR YOGA

Iyengar yoga is a specific approach to the ancient body-mind discipline of yoga. It was developed in the 1940s by B. K. S. Iyengar. Iyengar's approach to yoga incorporates all of the methods of classical or eight-limbed yoga. Yoga begins with the study of universal and individual ethical values. This is followed by the physical practice of stretching, strengthening, toning, and cleansing the body through postures. After a time breathing exercises are introduced. This foundation leads to the various stages of meditation. Iyengar Yoga is unique in its specific approach to asana, or body postures, and pranayama, or breathing practices.

The History of Iyengar Yoga

B. K. S. Iyengar was born on December 14, 1918, in Karnataka, in southern India. At the age of sixteen Iyengar moved to Mysore to live with his uncle, Shree T. Krishnamacharya, who had founded a yoga school. Iyengar's early experiences with yoga postures were tremendously painful and made him aware of his own stiffness. Through perseverance Iyengar found he was able to do more and more, achieving a remarkable skill in his own practice. Soon he was performing demonstrations and teaching at his uncle's school. In 1943 he married a woman named Ramamani, who inspired him to develop his unique approach to the practices of asana and pranayama.

After his marriage Iyengar moved to Pune, in the state of Maharastra. There he established his own yoga school, which is currently operating as Ramamani Iyengar Memorial Yoga Institute, in memory of his beloved wife, who passed away in 1973. Iyengar's renown as an accomplished yogi began to spread in India and in the West. His first of many visits to the United States was to Ann Arbor, Michigan, in 1974.

The first U.S. teacher-training center for the Iyengar method was formed in San Francisco, California, in 1976 following a visit by B. K. S. Iyengar to Berkeley, California. The center was run by his students at that time. Presently there are schools teaching his approach worldwide. Teacher training includes classes in anatomy, physiology, kinesiology, yoga philosophy, and student/teacher relationships as well as asana and pranayama. Iyengar is called guruji by his students, which is an Indian term of affection for a beloved teacher. He has written five books on yoga. He continues to teach in India, the United States, and throughout the world today.

Unique Aspects of Iyengar Yoga

Iyengar yoga relies on standing asanas more than do other styles of yoga. Students first learn to balance in the field of gravity and develop a richer contact with the Earth through the feet. Iyengar believes that active development of the posture inherent to human beings—that of standing on two legs—enhances the understanding of other types of poses. Experience gained in the practice of standing poses is used in all other types of asanas—seated, twisted, inverted, and back bending.

Another unique aspect of Iyengar yoga is the use of props such as chairs, weights, benches, mats, belts, and blankets, which help stretch and strengthen the body. Iyengar yoga teachers accommodate students with special needs through the effective use of props. In his teaching, Iyengar saw that students new to yoga tend to struggle at a muscular level, which creates a disturbance in the breath. He found that a prop used for support can alleviate muscular effort, thus helping the student achieve a freedom of breath. This encourages quieting of the mind and senses, bringing the student to a state of meditation in the asana.

A Summary of B. K. S. Iyengar's Approach to Yoga

In Iyengar yoga, the asana practice can be quite rigorous. Yoga asanas sometimes resemble typical Western exercises or stretches. Thus, according to Iyengar, a change is required in the typical Western mind-set, a movement away from a mechanical, purely physical practice toward an integrated, mindful approach. Yoga describes the body as consisting of five layers: anatomical, physiological, psychological, intellectual, and bliss. Iyengar stresses that yoga develops all five layers, not just the physiological layer.

—*Janet MacLeod*

Kripalu Yoga

Kripalu Yoga is a modern approach to the ancient body-mind discipline of yoga. It was developed by Amrit Desai, a yoga practitioner inspired by Kripalvananda, an Indian master of kundalini yoga. The kripalu approach to yoga combines asanas, or postures, which involve folding, stretching, bending, and balancing the body in a variety of positions; pranayama, or breath control; and meditation. Kripalu

Yoga is meant to give practitioners peace of mind, and good health, and to develop spiritual awareness so that their inner divinity which, according to Hindu and yogic tradition, is inherently present in everyone, can manifest itself.

Kripalu yoga is taught in three specific stages. The first stage is called "willful practice." The purpose of this stage is for practitioners to learn to perform the postures correctly; to learn to take deep, full breaths; to coordinate their breaths with the movements; and to pay close attention to body alignment.

When students have mastered this first stage they move on to the second, called "will and surrender." In this stage, postures are performed with the concentration focused fully on the body and the physical sensations that are being experienced. In this second stage practitioners hold the postures longer than in the first stage. Holding the postures longer provides a physical challenge that allows practitioners to face their own physical and mental resistances. Devakanya G. Parnell, the director of resident yoga education at the Kripalu Center in Lenox, Massachusetts, has described it this way: "When you come to your toleration point during prolonged holding, you encounter your self-perceived limitations and learn how to consciously transcend them" ("Hatha Traditions: How to Find a Class That's Right for You," by Linda Johnson in *Yoga International's Guide to Yoga Teachers and Classes, Yoga International,* 1996). This aspect of kripalu yoga is meant to help students with similar experiences in everyday life. It helps build confidence and self-reliance.

The third and final stage is reached when practitioners perform postures in a spontaneous flowing pattern, following their bodies' intuition and desires. This is known as Meditation in Motion™. In this, the hallmark of kripalu yoga practice, it is believed that the practitioner is able to sustain a tangible relationship with his or her own divine nature. At this level practitioners have truly released all of the obstructions that keep them from recognizing their essential divine nature.

In addition to its spiritual goals, regular practice of kripalu yoga has a variety of health benefits. It can reduce stress, increase flexibility, and enhance one's sense of well-being. Practitioners consider this a method for uncovering physical, emotional, and mental tensions, allowing for insight into these problems and for relaxation.

Resources:

Kripalu Center
P.O. Box 793
Lenox, MA 01240-0793
Tel: (413) 448-3152
Toll-free: (800) 741-SELF
A spiritual retreat center that offers workshops in yoga, meditation, and holistic health. Weekend, weeklong, and monthlong programs are available.

PART XIII: MEDITATION

Relaxation Response • Transcendental Meditation

Meditation, the art of turning one's attention inward in order to achieve more lucid consciousness, is a technique of character development most closely associated with Asian cultures. Since the 1960s, meditation has been more widely practiced in the West. Westerners are meditating to relieve stress, to assist in the healing of physical disorders, to increase athletic performance, to learn how to improve their concentration, and to enhance their experiences in psychotherapy. Meditation is also used in the practice of yoga and the martial arts, and as a form of inward personal discipline that many pursue as lifetime spiritual practice. As an imported product from Asian cultures, its study and practice has also led Westerners to a greater appreciation of their own contemplative traditions.

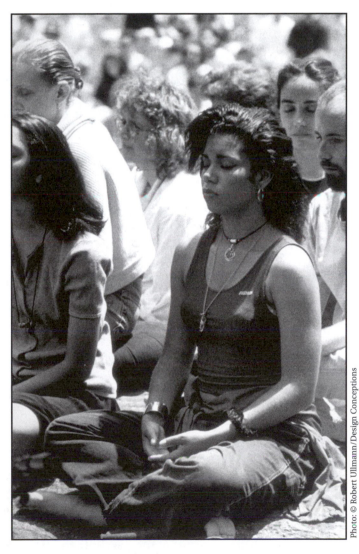

Photo: © Robert Ullmann/Design Conceptions

Meditation is a quiet, inward-turning experience.

The History of Meditation in the West

Meditation has been practiced in the East by Asian and Indian cultures for thousands of years and has been known by Western travelers to Asian countries for centuries.

Meditation was also an integral part of European Renaissance culture and occult Christianity, which helped spread the practice to the West. This was particularly true among the mystical religious schools, such as the Rosicrucians.

In the New World, German mystical communities settled in the original thirteen colonies, especially in Pennsylvania, where persecuted religious groups could come practice freely in an atmosphere of tolerance. Some of these groups practiced ascetic forms of meditation informed by Eastern religion and philosophy.

By the mid-nineteenth century, New England transcendentalists, such as Ralph Waldo Emerson and Henry David Thoreau, had read the few Eastern scriptures in circulation at the time and integrated ideas about meditation and yoga into their own literary and philosophical meditations. The transcendentalists used a walking form of meditation they called sauntering. They also practiced looking within one's self, or quiet contemplation, while immersed in nature.

By the last quarter of the nineteenth century such international movements as the Theosophical Society, which was first founded in the United States in 1875 and then reestablished in India in 1878, were disseminating information about Eastern contemplative practices to a public eager for the exotic as well as for alternative sources of spiritual discipline.

Asian Meditative Techniques Are Formally Introduced to the West

Formal training in Asian meditative techniques did not come to the United States until 1893, when the first wave of Asian teachers spoke to American audiences at the World Parliament of Religions, held in Chicago. In the aftermath of the Parliament, Swami Vivekananda of the Ramakrishna Vedanta order in India began teaching meditation to New Englanders who were attending Miss Sarah Farmer's Greenacre School of Comparative Religions in Portsmouth, New Hampshire.

Americans heard a firsthand account of Buddhist forms of meditation when Anagarika Dharmapala lectured at Harvard University, at Mrs. Ole Bull's Cambridge Conferences on Comparative Religions in 1904, and when the Zen abbot Soyen Shaku gave teachings across the United States in 1906. Asian teachings on meditation were spread in the 1920s and 1930s by spiritual leaders and visionaries such as Paramhansa Yogananda, Gurdjieff, and Jidhu Krishnamurti. European and American writers such as Aldous Huxley and Gerald Heard popularized the meditative tradition of Hindu Vedanta in southern California during World War II. Swami Akhilananda taught Vedantic meditation in Boston during the same period.

Zen meditation became particularly popular in the 1950s among members of the "Beatnik generation," like poet Gary Snyder. Writers such as J. D. Salinger and psychotherapists such as Karen Horney became followers of the lay Zen teacher, Daisetz T. Suzuki, who by then was lecturing in New York. Zen meditation was further popularized through the writings of the psychotherapist and ex-Episcopalian priest, Alan Watts during this same period. Public espousal of the Zen way by such intellectuals helped shift meditation into a position where it could be detached from questions of faith and approached as a countermeasure to materialism and stress. This view of meditation became a principal focus of the counterculture movement of the 1960s, when thousands of young people took up Asian spiritual practices in an effort to liberate their minds from the strictures of the established society.

Since that time there have been two major developments regarding meditation as a practice and as a subject of scientific research: First, a uniquely American spiritual tradition of meditation now distinct from Asian sources has evolved; and second, the practice of meditation in various forms is making its way into the health care system and into scientific laboratories, where rigorous investigation is now being carried on by a new generation of younger scientists who are also meditation practitioners.

Understanding the Forms of Meditation Practiced in the West

One way to understand the many different forms of meditation now flourishing in American culture is to ask from what tradition a particular form of practice comes. This is because there is no application of any kind of technique without some kind of philosophy to explain what is happening to consciousness as a result of the practice.

For example, Transcendental Meditation represents the tradition of Vedantic Hinduism according to the teachings of the Indian guru Maharishi Mahesh Yogi. Here, in the Hindu tradition of Vedanta, the practice of meditation is understood in terms of self-realization, particularly as the experience of awakened consciousness, where one is said to realize that the subjective self and the Absolute Self of the universe (Atman), or pure consciousness (chit) are one and the same.

The different branches of Buddhist meditation strive for a completely different state of consciousness. Theravada Buddhist meditation seeks *nibanna* (nirvana), a "burning out of the flame of sense desire," while Mahayana Buddhist meditation strives to reach emptiness (sunyata). Both forms of Buddhism believe that there is no such thing as an underlying permanent self, which means that the experience of enlightened consciousness in meditation is quite different from that of Hindu Vedanta.

Two other significant forms of meditation, and ones that have direct clinical application in medicine today, are Herbert Benson's relaxation response program at the Harvard Medical School/Mind-Body Medical Institute and the Stress Reduction Clinic at the University of Massachusetts Medical Center, run by Jon Kabat-Zinn. Both programs, well organized and intended to be educational, have been franchised out to schools, prisons, hospitals, and other therapeutic programs.

Benson's program began with an intensive study of Transcendental Meditation and then shifted to the study of meditation practiced by monks of Tibetan Buddhism, which is a combination of Hindu Tantra, Indian Mahayana Buddhism, and the native religion of Tibet, called Bon. Benson now teaches a generic form of meditation he calls the "relaxation response." In Jon Kabat-Zinn's program, patients referred to the stress-reduction clinic are trained in Vipassana (or mindfulness meditation), which comes from Southeast Asia; specifically, it is the Theravada tradition of Burmese Buddhism. At the same time, many meditators in the West practice Zen sitting, the Japanese form of Mahayana Buddhism, which originally came through China and Korea from India.

A Few Aspects of Meditation

While there is no really typical meditation session, Benson believes he has isolated the generic first steps common to all meditative and contemplative practice: a quiet environment, a relaxed position, and focus on the slow repetition of a sound or word. To this he has recently added readings from the inspirational texts of a practitioner's religious tradition.

A normal meditative session might last twenty minutes and be practiced once or twice a day. The subject usually sits comfortably in pleasant, quiet surroundings, preferably in a room with lowered illumination. The session might begin with a moment of deep relaxed breathing. The meditation task that follows might be to contemplate an object, such as looking into a candle flame, meanwhile paying attention to the cycle of one's breath. The task might be to keep the mind clear of attachment to any thoughts. It might be to just witness what goes by in the field of consciousness without thought or judgment.

The inability of a subject to succeed in the task at first should be no cause for alarm. Concentration merely means returning to the task without judgment. Each time the mind wanders, free of guilt or recrimination, one simply returns the mind to its original focus. Eventually, the surface of the mind becomes quieter and quieter, until sustained concentration becomes possible. Reentry into normal waking reality should be gradual, and as relaxed as in the beginning. A typical session might then end with some gentle stretching.

Potential Benefits of Meditation

Physiologically, it is believed that relaxed forms of meditation lead to a decrease in heart rate, a decrease in blood pressure, an increase in breathing volume, but a decrease in number of breaths taken per minute (typically sixteen in-breaths and out-breaths in the normal waking state; four in the meditative condition), increased alpha waves as recorded on an electroencephalogram, and synchronization of measured brain waves between the cerebral hemispheres.

Benson believes that meditation activates the parasympathetic nervous system, which quiets the nerves. Practice twice daily for twenty minutes produces a thermostatic effect, allowing the stressed nervous system—normally in a state of fluctuation—to have a standard by which to adjust itself. Studies have shown that when the practice finally takes effect, hypertensive medication can be cut in half, cramping in mild to moderate premenstrual syndrome can be modulated, standard light therapy for psoriasis can have an accelerated effect, and so on.

There are many other forms of meditation than quiet sitting, however. Each form has its own pattern of physiological effects, sometimes quieting, sometimes arousing the nervous system. There is walking meditation, for instance, in which the subject perambulates slowly around, remaining exquisitely mindful of each step. There is continuous but slow movement meditation in traditional sequences, as in Chinese qigong and t'ai chi ch'üan. There is meditation associated with rapid breathing, as in certain forms of kundalini yoga. In general, different types of philosophical teachings usually lead to radically different patterns of physiological response, making generalizations about meditation as a generic practice very difficult.

In most cases, it is not the kind of meditation one does that counts, but rather the similarity of outcomes among different kinds of techniques that leads to moral and aesthetic improvement, an enhanced sense of well-being, and enriched relationships. These are the criteria against which successful practice, either under an advanced teacher or by oneself, should be measured.

— *Eugene Taylor, Ph.D., and Marilyn Schlitz, Ph.D.*

Further Reading:

Books:

Benson, Herbert, and Miriam Z. Klipper. *The Relaxation Response*. New York: Avon Books, 1976.

Epstein, Mark. *Thoughts Without a Thinker: Psychotherapy from a Buddhist Perspective*. New York: Basic Books, 1995.

Kabat-Zinn, Jon. *Wherever You Go, There You Are: Mindfulness Meditation in Everyday Life*. New York: Hyperion, 1994.

Murphy, Michael, and Steven Donovan. *The Physical and Psychological Effects of Meditation: A Review of Contemporary Research with a Comprehensive Bibliography*. 2nd edition. Edited with an Introduction by Eugene Taylor. Sausalito: Institute of Noetic Sciences, 1996.

Prabhavananda, Swami, and Frederick Manchester, eds. *The Upanishads, Breath of the Eternal: The Principal Texts*. New York: New American Library, 1957.

Suzuki, Daisetz Teitaro. *An Introduction to Zen Buddhism*. Edited by Christmas Humphreys, with a foreword by C. G. Jung. London: Rider, 1983.

Taimni, I. K. *The Science of Yoga: The Yoga-Sutras of the Patanjali*. 4th Quest Book ed. Wheaton, IL: Theosophical Publishing House, 1975.

Journals:

Tricycle, a magazine of Buddhism in America, which began publication in 1991.

RELAXATION RESPONSE

The relaxation response is a body-mind process that is characterized by significant physical changes, such as lower blood pressure, a decreased heart rate, and increased body temperature as well as a general sense of intense calm. Dr. Herbert Benson, through an examination of the psychological and physiological aspects of meditation, found that the relaxation response can be brought about by the use of meditation, yoga, repetitive exercises, hypnosis, prayer, and other forms of stress management.

The Development of the Relaxation Technique

In the late 1960s, Herbert Benson, M.D., a Harvard cardiologist, began to study the physical effects of meditation. Later he traveled to India to study Tibetan monks who meditate every day. Dr. Benson was one of the first scientists to study advanced meditators using Western scientific methods. He measured some of the physical changes, such as blood pressure and body temperature, that occurred as the monks meditated. He found that while the monks were in a meditative state their body processes slowed. He documented the fact that meditation was associated with lowered blood pressure and heart rate and an increase in body temperature, all of which are associated with calmness. He labeled these meditation-induced physical changes in the body the relaxation response.

The Relaxation Response

Studies prove that if people could relax the body they could potentially prevent some of the harmful effects of psychological stress. Hundreds of scientific studies have shown that there are negative effects from psychological stress; these effects are mental or intellectual, behavioral and physical. Psychological stress can make it harder to think effectively and behave appropriately and can also cause physical changes associated with the development of medical illness.

The relaxation response is the opposite of the stress response, or what has been termed the fight-or-flight response. When most animals in the wild are faced with life-threatening situations, their bodies respond with a predictable arousal pattern that prepares them to either fight a threat or run away from danger. In humans, this response prepares the body for vigorous muscular activity by stimulating the sympathetic nervous system to increase heart rate, blood pressure, and muscle tension. The fight-or-flight response was necessary for the survival of humans when confronted by wild beasts. Today, the same response is stimulated to varying degrees when we are faced with everyday stresses, most often threats to our ego, such as taking tests or being late.

The work of Dr. Benson suggested an important symmetrical relationship between the fight-or-flight response and the relaxation response. Whereas repeated or prolonged elicitation of the fight-or-flight response has been associated with medical illness related to stress and arousal, repeated or prolonged elicitation of the relaxation response has been associated with the prevention of stress-related disease.

Through his examination of the psychological and physiological components of meditation on Tibetan monks, Dr. Benson theorized that the positive effects of meditation could be acquired without the belief in Eastern religions or altered states. The most important thing was that patients learn to generate the calming effects associated with the relaxation response. The way in which an individual learned to generate the effect was unimportant. He then set out to devise a general strategy that would bring about the desired response. He found that the relaxation response would occur using many different disciplines including yoga, repetitive exercise, hypnosis, and other forms of stress management. Dr. Benson and his colleagues concluded that only two specific steps were necessary to produce the relaxation response: the first is attentional focus on a single repetitive word, sound, prayer, phrase, image, or physical activity; the second is to passively return to a specific focus when distractions occur.

How to Elicit the Relaxation Response

In a typical training session the client enters the therapist's office and is instructed to sit in a comfortable chair. The therapist then begins giving the following guidance in a quiet voice:

1. Sit quietly in a comfortable position and close your eyes.
2. Deeply relax all your muscles, beginning at your feet and progressing up to your face. Keep them deeply relaxed.
3. Breathe through your nose. Become aware of your breathing. As you breathe out, say the word "one" silently to yourself. For example breathe in . . . out, one; in . . . out, one; etc. Continue for twenty minutes. You may open your eyes to check the time, but do not use an alarm. When you finish, sit quietly for several minutes at first with closed eyes and later with opened eyes.
4. Do not worry about whether you are successful in achieving a deep level of relaxation. Maintain a passive attitude and permit relaxation to occur at its own pace. Expect other thoughts. When distracting thoughts occur, ignore them and continue repeating "one." With practice, the response should come with little effort. Practice the technique once or twice daily, but not within two hours after any meal, since the digestive processes seem to interfere with the subjective changes.

Benefits of the Relaxation Response

The relaxation response has been associated with improvements in many medical conditions, including hypertension, cardiac arrhythmia, chronic pain, insomnia, side effects of cancer therapy, side effects of AIDS therapy, infertility, as well as preparation for surgery and X ray procedures.

—Richard Friedman, Ph.D., Patricia Myers, Herbert Benson, M.D.

Resources:

Mind/Body Medical Institute
Beth Israel Deaconess Medical Center
Harvard Medical School
110 Francis Street
Boston, MA 02215
Tel: (617) 632-9530
Provides a well-respected treatment program that teaches how to elicit the relaxation response.

Meditation and the Relaxation Response Technique

Meditation and its potential role in health is often misunderstood because of its association with mystical Eastern traditions. While Eastern cultures accept the concept that regular meditational practice can result in positive psychological benefits, they also believe that it can result in an altered state of consciousness or a change in the perception of reality. Because meditation is so heavily associated with altered states, the Western medical community has been slow to acknowledge that the practice of meditation could be used by patients to produce positive healthful effects.

Further Reading:

Benson, Herbert. *The Relaxation Response.* Richmond, VA: Outlet Books, Inc., 1993.

——. *Timeless Healing.* New York: Fireside, 1996.

Benson, Herbert, and William Proctor. *Beyond the Relaxation Response.* New York: Putnam/Berkley, Inc., 1984.

TRANSCENDENTAL MEDITATION

Transcendental Meditation (TM), is a simple technique that is used to help individuals access their inner creativity and wisdom while also improving their physical health. According to TM theory, which is based on the ancient Vedic tradition of yoga, certain meditation techniques can quiet the mind, allowing the body to enter a state of deep relaxation. Veda, meaning "knowledge," is a science of life and consciousness that is rooted in ancient India. TM was introduced in 1957 by Maharishi Mahesh Yogi. He has since traveled the world, promoting and teaching TM. As a result, more than 5 million people from different countries, religions, and educational backgrounds have learned the TM technique.

The Life of Maharishi Mahesh Yogi

Maharishi Mahesh Yogi was born in 1918 in India. "Maharishi," meaning "great sage," is a title of honor. Maharishi graduated in 1941 with a degree in physics from Allahabad University in India. Shortly after his graduation, he met Swami Brahamananda Saraswati, a renowned spiritual leader in India, and asked to study with him. Maharishi was accepted and became his disciple for more than thirteen years.

After Swami Brahamananda Saraswati died in 1953, Maharishi spent two years in seclusion in the Himalayan Mountains, where he developed the system of Transcendental Meditation. In 1957, at the eighty-seventh birthday celebration of his teacher, he announced his plan to spread TM around the world. To accomplish this, in 1959 he founded the Spiritual Regeneration Movement. His reputation greatly increased in the early 1960s, when his teachings gained the interest of the musical group the Beatles and other celebrities from the West. Subsequently, TM became more popular in the United States. Maharishi toured the United States in 1967 and delivered lectures at several prominent universities. By the 1970s, TM had spread to more than 100 countries.

Currently, people participate in Maharishi's teachings to different extents. There are many students who follow Maharishi's versions of various branches of Vedic science, including systems of medicine, architecture, and prediction. For them, Maharishi's teachings influence various aspects of one's lifestyle. His teachings have also inspired a political movement, organized in sixty countries as the Natural Law Party. At the same time, there are many other people who study only the meditation technique without changing their lifestyles or political beliefs. They attend classes where the TM technique is taught and use the skill to help achieve their own personal physical, emotional, and spiritual goals.

Principles of Transcendental Meditation

According to Maharishi, consciousness is not merely a function of the human nervous system; it is actually a field in nature, just like gravity or electromagnetism. This field pervades the physical universe and is the source of the creativity and intelligence in nature, as well as in an individual's life. Although this model of consciousness is derived from the Vedic tradition of ancient India, some have noted its similarities with a contemporary Western scientific theory concerning all matter and energy in the

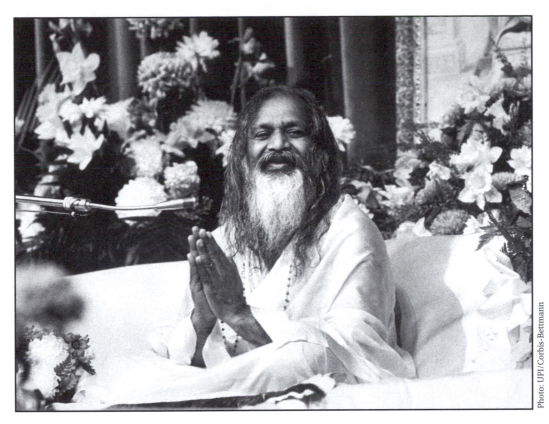

Photo: UPI/Corbis-Bettmann

Maharishi Mahesh Yogi, founder of Transcendental Meditation.

universe known as the unified field of natural law.

Vedic science claims that the human brain and nervous system can function as instruments capable of directly experiencing the unbounded field of consciousness. TM practitioners believe that when a person is in a quiet, settled state the mind will naturally move toward experiencing this field. TM is a technique to transcend the superficial, active level of the mind, allowing it to experience this latent and unlimited source of energy, creativity, and intelligence.

Coming from India, where meditation techniques abound, Maharishi was frequently asked if all meditation techniques—and therefore all benefits of meditation—are the same. He asserted that there are profound differences between practices. Most meditation techniques, Maharishi said, involve concentration or control of the mind.

He advocated a departure from these methods. To Maharishi, control of the mind actually stops the process of transcending normal consciousness. Instead, meditation should be completely natural and effortless, requiring no concentration or control of the mind. Meditation should simply allow the mind to follow its own natural tendency toward the expanded field of consciousness, a field of bliss and inner happiness.

Experiencing Transcendental Meditation

Even though the process of Transcendental Meditation is designed to be simple and effortless, properly learning the techniques is very precise. Learning to meditate in the Vedic tradition has always involved personal instruction from an expert or guru. Therefore, TM practitioners believe that those who are interested in meditating should learn from a qualified teacher.

TM is practiced for fifteen to twenty minutes twice a day. A person begins meditation by sitting in a comfortable position with the eyes closed. Then, mantras—meaningless syllables or phrases—are silently repeated. Proponents of TM believe that meditation quiets the mind, which helps the body enter a unique state of relaxation, deeper than ordinary rest with eyes closed. As a person begins to relax his or her mind, he or she begins to experience finer levels of thought. Ultimately, a person transcends the finest level of thought and experiences the source of thought, the field of pure consciousness.

Benefits of Transcendental Meditation

There has been a significant effort among advocates of TM to integrate traditional teachings with Western science. Since the mid-1970s hundreds of research studies have been conducted that confirm that TM can yield both psychological and physical benefits. It has been found to reduce stress, anxiety, and depression, and increase creativity, happiness, and self-esteem. It has also been used to increase one's energy, improve memory, and reduce insomnia and high blood pressure.

Some students use the TM technique to improve memory and quicken their ability to solve problems. People have also used these benefits of TM to become more productive at their jobs. It has also been used as a part of programs designed to help people recover from drug or alcohol addiction. In each of these cases, the TM technique is used as a practical skill to help a person in his or her daily life

—Compiled in consultation with Robert Roth

Resources:

Maharishi University of Management
1000 North 4th Street
Fairfield, IA 52557
Tel: (515) 472-7000
Web site: www.miu.edu
An accredited university, offering standard academic disciplines in addition to Transcendental Meditation.

Maharishi Vedic University
1401 Ocean Avenue
Asbury Park, NJ 07712
Tel: (908) 774-9446
Offers a program of instruction in the Vedic sciences.

Transcendental Meditation Program
Tel: (888) LEARN TM
Web site: www.tm.org

Further Reading:

Denniston, Denise. *The TM Book: How to Enjoy the Rest of Your Life.* Fairfield, IA: Fairfield Press, 1986 .

Roth, Robert. *Transcendental Meditation.* New York: Primus, 1987.

Yogi, Maharishi Mahesh. *Science of Being and Art of Living.* London: SRM Publications, 1967.

A seven-step course in Transcendental Meditation is offered by hundreds of Maharishi Vedic universities and schools throughout the world. The course consists of two lectures about the principles of TM and four days of instruction in meditation—about two hours each day. After the course is completed, additional personal instruction is also available.

PART XIV: PSYCHO-PHYSICAL EVALUATION FRAMEWORKS

Enneagram • Kestenberg Movement Profile • Laban Movement Analysis •
Movement Pattern Analysis

Psycho-physical evalua-
tion frameworks are orga-
nized theoretical structures
and notation systems that
correlate body movement
with psychological attri-
butes and patterns. These
frameworks see the process
of movement as a complex
and multifaceted affair.
Each method combines, in
its own way, an objective
approach to observing and
recording the subtle aspects
of movement with an appreciation for the subjective
elements of the experience
of moving. Because each
method aims to create a
comprehensive model of all
the possible combinations
of movement elements,
these frameworks can be
applied to many athletic
and aesthetic activities,
therapeutic modalities, and
educational programs for
diagnostic as well as prescriptive purposes.

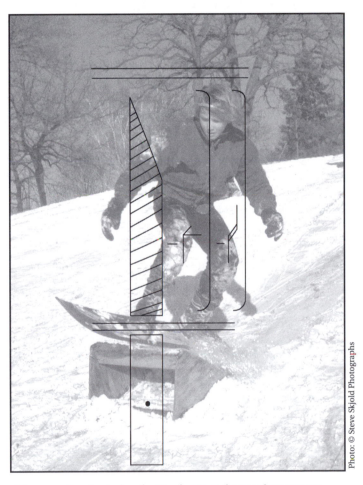

Photo: © Steve Skjold Photographs

Many psycho-physical evaluation frameworks use abstract notation to record observed movement. Pictured above is motif writing used in Laban movement analysis.

The majority of psycho-physical evaluation frameworks in use today and included
here are inspired by the work of Rudolph Laban (1879–1958), an Austro-Hungarian
movement theorist. The methods included in this section are distinguished by their
founders' efforts to collect first all the variations of movement they could observe
before developing theoretical frameworks linking physical movements to psychological

characteristics. They recorded these observations by means of various abstract symbol systems that generally developed right along with their theoretical concepts. From data collected, the various frameworks were then formulated. In this way a comprehensive map of the possible range of movement patterns and their relationship to patterns of emotional life was created.

What These Frameworks Have in Common

The frameworks described in this section are linked by several basic concepts. First and foremost is the belief that physical movement is reflective of inner psychological patterns, preferences, and coping mechanisms. While some frameworks like the Enneagram model focus more on behavioral actions, the Laban-based models, including Laban movement analysis, Kestenberg movement profile, and movement pattern analysis, base their observations specifically on the qualitative changes in movements through space over a period of time.

These frameworks are also linked by their belief that people have preferred movement repertories that are unique and special to them. Health, growth, and understanding are often facilitated by experiencing behavioral actions, movement qualities, combinations, and patterns outside this preferred movement repertory. In this way these frameworks are related to the ancient and contemporary holistic body-mind disciplines that see physical, emotional, and spiritual health in terms of balance and harmony.

Using the Frameworks to Help You

The modes of practice of these particular disciplines are extremely varied. In fact, a client doesn't so much "practice" them as make use of the information and new insights they provide. In some cases it is possible to visit a practitioner of one of these disciplines for a personal assessment. For example, you can go to an enneagram seminar and discover where you fit in that method's map of the gestalt of human consciousness. Or you can learn about your own decision-making process by having your movement pattern analyzed by a certified movement pattern analyst.

But it is more likely that if you were to go to a dance teacher, sports coach, or a massage or movement therapist, he or she might be working with one of these psychophysical evaluation frameworks. The teacher, coach, or therapist is the "practitioner" of this discipline. The framework provides a model within which to assess your condition, understand the whole physical and psychological dynamic of your situation, and plan a step-by-step program to help relieve your pain, improve your performance, or assist you in reaching your goals.

—Nancy Allison, CMA

Further Reading:

Fouts, Roger, and Stephen Tukel Mills. *Next of Kin: What Chimpanzees Have Taught Me About Who We Are*. New York: William Morrow and Company, Inc., 1997.

Moore, Carol-Lynne, and Kaoru Yamamoto. *Beyond Words: Movement Observation and Analysis*. New York: Gordon and Breach, 1994.

North, Marion. *Personality Assessment Through Movement*. London: Macdonald and Evans, 1972.

ENNEAGRAM

Enneagram is a model of human personality that provides nine personal strategies, or ways of being in the world, called types. In Greek *ennea* means "nine" and *gram* means "graph" or "model." The system provides a framework, language, and conceptual vocabulary for understanding people and behavior. In offering personality descriptions that account for differences between people, the model greatly enhances people's ability to understand themselves and to appreciate that others approach the same situation from different perspectives. When used well, the enneagram system opens up new possibilities for people in management, leadership, teaching, learning, and personal growth.

Nine-Pointed Star

Many ancient sacred traditions such as esoteric Christianity, Sufism, and Judaism describe variants of the enneagram model. This implies an old, common source for the current model. There are other strands that lead into the modern-day enneagram. For instance, the Platonic tradition from ancient Greece, in which the philosopher Plato describes nine perfect essential states of being and a tenth state called unity, is a philosophy that resonates with the enneagram as well.

In this century George Ivanovitch Gurdjieff (1872–1949), the spiritual philosopher and teacher, brought a nine-pointed star diagram to the West, purportedly from Sufi sources. Gurdjieff used the star, and the internal-flow pattern that unites the points in a specific way, in his private teaching work. According to Gurdjieff theory, by using the star he was able to describe the changing attitudes and perceptions that occur when people feel either secure or stressed. Gurdjieff painted a huge enneagram on the floor of the Institute for the Harmonious Development of Man, the name of his school where students practiced movements aimed at developing personal awareness.

Oscar Ichazo, a European born in the early 1930s and a noted contemporary enneagram author who claimed to have learned the system from Sufi masters in Afghanistan, added the next development to the enneagram system. He named the central focus of each of the types after Christianity's seven capital sins—anger, pride, envy, avarice, gluttony, lust, sloth—and added two more, deceit and fear. This frame of reference has become widespread, but it does not imply that it is a system of Christian psychology.

In 1972 the first teacher of the enneagram in the United States, a Chilean psychiatrist named Claudio Naranjo, a student of Oscar Ichazo, taught the system to a group of psychologists, psychiatrists, and students in Berkeley, California. This group painstakingly aligned the central features of the enneagram types with the *Diagnostic Survey Manual,* a canon in the psychological community used by all American and Canadian clinicians for diagnostic purposes. While the *DSM* describes pathologies (deviations from normal psychological functioning), the enneagram describes in general terms the broadly correlating characteristics of normal and high-functioning people. For example, in enneagram theory point six represents constant fear and vigilance; enneagram practitioners believe that this corresponds with the psychological term *paranoid*. In a like manner, every point on the enneagram correlates to a contemporary psychological pathology.

Naranjo's other contribution was to explore the enneagram using panels of the types; in this method groups of people of the same personality type work together to explore the intricacies of the inner structure of their thought and behavior patterns. These early panels provided the empirical proof for the key distinguishing characteristics of the types.

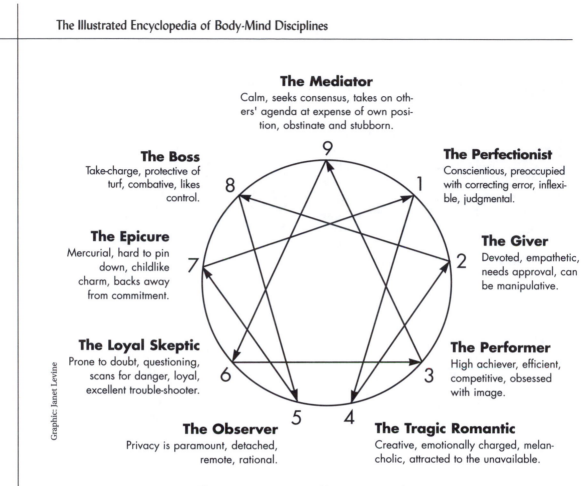

The Mediator
Calm, seeks consensus, takes on others' agenda at expense of own position, obstinate and stubborn.

The Boss
Take-charge, protective of turf, combative, likes control.

The Perfectionist
Conscientious, preoccupied with correcting error, inflexible, judgmental.

The Epicure
Mercurial, hard to pin down, childlike charm, backs away from commitment.

The Giver
Devoted, empathetic, needs approval, can be manipulative.

The Loyal Skeptic
Prone to doubt, questioning, scans for danger, loyal, excellent trouble-shooter.

The Performer
High achiever, efficient, competitive, obsessed with image.

The Observer
Privacy is paramount, detached, remote, rational.

The Tragic Romantic
Creative, emotionally charged, melancholic, attracted to the unavailable.

Graphic: Janet Levine

The enneagram system of human personalities.

The first books on enneagram theory were published in the United States in the mid-1980s. Today research on the correlation between the enneagram model and Western psychological theory is being conducted at Loyola University in Chicago, the Center for Integral Studies in San Francisco, and less formally in many other seminaries and graduate schools.

What Is Type?

People have to survive in the world and need to exhibit traits and characteristics that will enable them to make their way and form relationships. Personality is about defense mechanisms, characteristic habits of thought, emotions that underpin thoughts, interpersonal aptitudes and abilities, and a way of handling the body to manage energy. While all people have access to all these areas, in many instances one area predominates and people fall broadly into physical,

mental, and emotional types. The enneagram recognizes these distinctions too, and the diagram is organized in triads that are made up of these distinct energies—the emotional triad (points 2,3,4), the mental triad (points 5,6,7), and the instinctual/body triad (points 8,9,1).

In traditional psychology, personality type has been identified through pathology, or deviations in personality makeup. Many psychologists and psychiatrists believe that if people can understand how their personality disintegrated, they can be helped to reintegrate themselves. Psychotherapists are trained to find how the personality defense mechanisms have broken down, rather than to concentrate on what is working.

The enneagram system provides a new way to understand ourselves. The model offers a format for normal and high-functioning people to examine what their reactive or habitual behavior patterns conceal. Enneagram theory pinpoints nine patterns of avoidance: error, emotional needs, failure, ordinariness, connection, deviance (being different), pain, vulnerability, and conflict. Our sense of self is manufactured largely out of one of these avoidances in our emotional experience. When we face up to, process, and integrate those aspects of ourselves we have been denying, the self can emerge as a whole, and the grace of compassion for self and others becomes possible.

The system offers the choice for proactive, rather than reactive, behavior and the opportunity to cease going on "automatic" without realizing what one is doing. Knowledge of enneagram type (e-type) frees people to expand the way they think about themselves, to find compassion for themselves and others, to manage emotional energy with more skill, and to end habitual behavior.

Finding Your Type

The key to using the enneagram system is recognizing one's type. To do this a group of interested people will typically see a videotape or listen to an audiotape describing the nine types. There are obvious dangers and consequences of mistyping and stereotyping. As people (especially youths) become more knowledgeable about their own personality, they need to be honest and objective about their own defining characteristics. If after this process they are still unsure of their enneagram type,

a one-to-one interview is available to help those interested in this model to identify their type.

Enneagram consultants do not tell people their type. While multiple-choice tests are sometimes used to help determine type, enneagram consultants believe that knowledge of type is useful only if it is part of a process of self-recognition and self-discovery. The forty-five minute individual interview is designed to unobtrusively elicit patterns of thought and emotion, deeply held inner motivations, and habits. The questions asked in the interview and the manner of asking them have been developed from thousands of interviews conducted by the Center for Enneagram Studies in Berkeley, California. Through this process the enneagram system brings many people revelatory understanding of their individual beliefs, values, and ideas. Finding one's e-type is only the initial step; learning how to work with one's strategy, and to grow in understanding, compassion, and acceptance of oneself and others is the journey. To this end, the body-mind methods of the many sacred traditions, such as heightened self-knowledge, breathing practices, meditation, and developing a sense of groundedness, are all helpful.

Benefits and Inherent Risks

People who use the enneagram system have reported that it enriches and facilitates interactions between people and offers opportunities for more thoughtful, effective, and honest relationships.

Enneagram Study Today

There are currently many enneagram centers and hundreds of enneagram teachers throughout the United States and the world. In 1994 the First International Enneagram Conference was cosponsored by and held at Stanford University in Palo Alto, California. In 1996 the First National Enneagram Institute for Educators was cosponsored by and held at the Milton Academy in Milton, Massachusetts, which is becoming a laboratory for enneagram applications in education, particularly learning and teaching styles.

Business managers, educators, and students feel that the system helps them develop a sense of their motivations and the patterns behind their thoughts and actions.

However, there are dangers inherent in the system. Stereotyping, or not seeing the individual in the type, is a distinct danger. A shallow understanding of the system on the part of the practitioner, whether teacher or student, ignores the facets that account for individual differences. Perhaps the gravest danger in the system lies in people prematurely mistyping themselves and others.

—Janet Levine

Resources:

The International Enneagram Association
849 Independence Avenue, #B
Mountain View, CA 94043
Tel: (415) 903-8300
Fax: (415) 967-0995
Offers a full listing of enneagram centers and teachers both in the United States and internationally.

The National Educators Institute for Enneagram Studies
Program Director: Janet Levine
Milton Academy
170 Centre Street
Milton, MA 02186
Tel/Fax: (617) 696-9410
e-mail: Jlevinegrp@aol.com
Web site: www.enneagram-edge.com
Provides information about training in the enneagram system for the educational sector.

Further Reading:

Books:

Naranjo, Claudio. *Enneatype Structures.* Nevada City, CA: Gateways, 1990.

Palmer, Helen. *The Enneagram.* San Francisco: Harper San Francisco, 1988.

——. *The Enneagram in Love and Work.* San Francisco: Harper San Francisco, 1994.

Riso, Don Richard. *Personality Types: Using the Enneagram for Self-Discovery.* New York: Houghton-Mifflin, 1987.

Rohr, Richard, and Andreas Ebert. *Discovering the Enneagram.* New York: Crossroad, 1992.

Journals:

The Enneagram Monthly. Troy, NY.

KESTENBERG MOVEMENT PROFILE

The Kestenberg movement profile (KMP) is a method of psychological assessment based on observations of patterns of movement. While observers have long recognized that bodily movement styles often reflect various aspects of personality and feelings, a framework was needed to unravel the mind-body connections in a systematic fashion. Such a framework was developed in the 1960s by Dr. Judith S. Kestenberg and the Sands Point Movement Study Group, consisting of Drs. Hershey Marcus, Jay Berlowe, Esther Robin, Arnhilte Buelte, and Martha Soodak. A new generation of students such as Susan Loman, Mark Sossin, and Penny Lewis continue to develop the approach in the 1990s. The KMP provides a methodology and theory for observing and interpreting body movement patterns and has been used effectively for evaluation as well as prescriptive purposes by psychologists, anthropologists, and dance/movement therapists.

The Sands Point Movement Study Group

Kestenberg first observed the close integration of body and mind in Vienna in the 1930s while studying patients with neurological brain damage. Later, as a child psychiatrist in New York, she speculated about ways in which psychological disturbances might be expressed in body movement. In 1953 she began what was to be a twenty-year longitudinal study of the movement patterns of three newborns. Unfamiliar with any system of movement notation, she recorded the babies' movements by moving her pen in accordance with their motions. Her pen traced rhythmic and semi-rhythmic lines across the paper, creating tracings that looked like electrocardiogram graphs. However, it was not yet clear to her how this data could be interpreted.

In 1960, the Sands Point Movement Study Group—four psychiatrists, a movement specialist, and a dance therapist—eager to learn together and cross disciplinary lines, gathered to study movement in a more systematic way. They were led to the work of the movement specialist Rudolf Laban, who had emphasized that movement patterns are closely associated with styles of thinking and feeling. For example, Laban pointed out that people who "tackle" decisions tend to prefer strong, quick, direct movements; those who slowly ponder decisions tend to prefer light, sustained, and indirect movement patterns. He created a system of notation that allowed an observer to record, categorize, and interpret movement in relation to the mover's inner intention.

The Sands Point group studied Laban's system and adapted it to serve their interest in child development and psychological evaluations. In particular, they elaborated on Laban's observation that changes of muscle tension may reflect inner feelings and needs. They found that in children, just as Laban had theorized, bound muscle tension often reflected states of anxiety or caution, and that relaxed or free-flowing movements were associated with feeling at ease. How could they study this phenomenon more carefully?

Warren Lamb, one of Laban's students, suggested that Kestenberg's tracings of the babies' movements documented changes in muscle tension and offered a way to study changes of tension flow. Equipped with this methodology, the Sands Point Movement Study Group discovered particular patterns of muscle-tension changes characteristic of children's basic everyday functioning, such as eating, crawling, or jumping. Throughout development these rhythmic patterns serve not only such bodily functions, but also other psychological needs.

For example, sucking rhythms used for nursing also serve self-soothing functions and thus are important throughout the life span. Particular rhythmic patterns typically become prominent during the early phases of development, from birth to age six, paralleling and reinforcing the process of maturation; as an example, short stop-and-go rhythms common in the two-and-a-half-year-old function to help bladder control and also encourage energetic activity and competitiveness. A slow, swaying rhythm, common in three-year-olds, supports and encourages nurturing behavior and creativity.

From 1972 to 1990 additional observations were gathered at the Center for Children and Parents, a private institution in Roslyn, New York, founded by Kestenberg. These were used to refine and verify the Kestenberg movement profile and its interpretive scheme. As confidence in the profile grew, it became the basis for the evaluation of movement preferences, developmental achievement, cognitive (thinking) abilities, self feelings, and social skills.

The Kestenberg Movement Profile and Personality Types

While individuals exhibit all ten biologically based rhythmic patterns identified in the Kestenberg movement profile, they generally favor two or three rhythmic patterns, infusing them into many of their activities. For example, some people eat with a "jumping" rhythm, gulping their food, while others "drift" along, finishing long after everyone else. Severe deficiency of one pattern may undermine the development of certain qualities, such as assertiveness or the ability to relax. By tracing someone's "rhythms of tension flow," as these patterns are called in the Kestenberg movement profile, one can begin to create a profile of the subject's preferred ways of meeting personal needs.

In addition to tension-flow patterns, over sixty-three specific movement qualities have also been studied and used to create a detailed and comprehensive movement profile for the psychological assessment of individuals. Combinations of these qualities reflect the individual's style of coping with the environment, self-image, use of psychological defenses, learning styles, cognitive thinking patterns, and ways of relating to others. Laban had theorized, and Kestenberg's research confirmed, that in order to collect accurate, useful observations of movement patterns it is necessary to observe more than one movement quality at a time. Observing movement from this frame of reference creates a complex palette of data from which to draw psychological implications.

The richness of the material leads the observer to the discovery of multiple interconnections between mind and body. One movement quality often underlies cognitive processes and social modes of relating. For example, an individual who favors "spreading" movements over "enclosing" motions also generally prefers to explore widely in an environment and take in many diverse perspectives. Such a person also tends to feel comfortable relating to quite a number of different people. One who prefers enclosing movements generally favors focused investigations and explorations, more singular perspectives, and also tends to be more comfortable relating to others on a one-to-one basis. Of course, most people have access to both patterns of movement and both modes of thinking and relating, but demonstrate distinct styles and preferences in specific contexts.

Applications of the KMP

The Kestenberg movement profile can be used in natural, real-world settings as well as more controlled therapeutic ones. Adults engaging in a conversation or children engaged in free play can be profiled. It has also been used successfully in different cultural settings.

As a preventive measure, the Kestenberg movement profile's model of childhood development suggests age-appropriate activities for children and remedial movement patterns where deficiencies are found. The profile also aids in the treatment of problems in interpersonal relations. For example, by comparing profiles of family members, the therapist can study the areas of harmony and clash between individuals. The therapist can then analyze how certain movement patterns inhibit and mislead communication. Individuals can be made aware of the movement-level basis of their clashes and learn to build on their areas of harmony, find more compatible movement patterns, or at least understand their clashes on a more comfortable movement level.

Parents can learn to attune to their infants, use affined movement patterns, and develop a body-level mode of communication. The process of becoming attuned with others can begin quite early. Kestenberg taught pregnant women to trace the tension flow rhythms of fetal movements. This facilitated getting to know and *relating* to the baby *before birth,* and *bonding* with it *after birth.*

The Kestenberg movement profile also serves as a guide for dance/movement therapists who utilize movement as a form of treatment. Psychologists, physical therapists, and physicians who also examine the language of the body have found the KMP effective as part of the diagnostic process and in the determination of appropriate avenues of therapy.

—*Janet Kestenberg Amighi and Susan Loman*

Resources:

Allegheny University of the Health Sciences
1505 Reay, Mail Drop 905
Bellet Bldg., 10th Floor
Philadelphia, PA 19102
Tel: (215) 246-5020
Offers a program in the KMP.

Antioch New England Graduate School
Keene, NH 03431
Tel: (603) 357-3122
Provides a training program in the Kestenberg movement profile.

The Laban-Bartenieff Institute for Movement
  Studies
11 East 4th Street
New York, NY 10003
Tel: (212) 477-4299
Teaches the Kestenberg movement profile to qualified individuals.

Further Reading:

Books:

Kestenberg, J. S. *Children and Parents: Psychoanalytic Studies in Development.* New York: Jason Aronson, 1975.

Kestsenberg, J. S., and M. Sossin. *The Role of Movement Patterns in Development II.* New York: The Dance Notation Bureau Press, 1979.

Kestenberg, J. S., J. Amighi, S. Loman, P. Lewis, and M. Sossin. *The Meaning of Movement: Developmental, Multicultural and Clinical Perspectives as Seen Through the Kestenberg Movement Profile.* New York: Gordon and Breach, 1998.

Lewis, P., and S. Loman, *The Kestenberg Movement Profile: Its Past, Present Applications and Future Directions.* Keene, NH: Antioch New England Graduate School, 1990.

Journals:

Loman, S., and H. Merman. "The KMP: A Tool for Dance/Movement Therapy." *American Journal of Dance Therapy* 18, No. 1 (1996): 29–52.

LABAN MOVEMENT ANALYSIS

Laban movement analysis (LMA) is a system that provides a comprehensive language to describe, interpret, and study movement. Central to LMA is the idea that movement is an outward expression of inner intentions and that movement is a combination of the physical, emotional, and mental attributes of human behavior. LMA allows for the analysis and synthesis of the physical and psychological processes of moving. As such, the language of LMA is applicable to many fields of body-mind study.

The History of Laban Movement Analysis

Rudolf Laban, artist, scientist, and philosopher, was born in 1879, in what was then Bratislava in the Austro-Hungarian Empire. He spent much of his life in France, Switzerland, and Germany until, in 1936, artistic conflicts with the National Socialist Party (the Nazi Party) led him to relocate in England, where he lived until his death in 1958.

From 1913 to 1917 in Ascona, Switzerland, he began developing an abstract-symbol system that notated movement. Originally this system provided the impermanent art of dance with a means for documentation and historical preservation. But Laban's broad range of interests coupled with his scientific approach to the study of movement led him to develop a system of notating all types of movement.

Between 1920 and 1936 Laban was most active in Berlin. He established two dance companies, Tanzbuhne Laban and Kammertanzbuhne Laban. Laban's system of notation was published in 1928 as *Kinetography Laban*, which became known as *Labanotation* in the United States. Laban established dance schools throughout Germany and gained a reputation for his prolific work in developing movement choirs, orchestrating large groups of laypeople in movement displays of pageantry and community.

His life work continued in England from 1936 to 1958. His book *Modern Educational Dance*, published in 1948, became the basis for a curriculum in movement education in public schools. He also began teacher-training programs in movement with recognition from the Department of Education and Science.

Laban's legacy continues through his writings, his notation system, and through his groundbreaking investigation into nonverbal expression and the creative unconscious sources of movement expression. Several of Laban's students, including Irmgard Bartenieff, Warren Lamb, Judith Kestenberg, and Anne Hutchinson Guest, have continued his work and expanded its range of application to a variety of fields. Lamb, for instance, applied the theories to the corporate sector to help professionals understand their own and others' decision-making processes. And Kestenberg works with children in a body/movement-conscious psychotherapy.

The Ingredients of Movement

To facilitate a fundamental understanding of all human movement, the Laban movement analysis system articulates and differentiates the ingredients of movement expression. These ingredients combine in infinitely varying ways to become the work actions, human behaviors, and dance styles of cultures throughout the world. Although movement is a constantly changing state, these ingredients continuously emerge as observable points of emphasis in movement patterns. LMA places these movement ingredients into four major categories: body, effort, space, and shape.

Body This category focuses on how movements are executed physically. It looks at specific body parts and relationships between body parts, identifies how movements are initiated, and describes simultaneous or sequential phrasing of movement. The body category also distinguishes between postural and gestural movements and examines the rhythms created as one goes from being still to moving and vice versa.

Effort This category covers qualitative changes in the energy of movement. It addresses movement in terms of weight, space, time, and flow. Fluctuations of weight occur between light or strong, space is direct or indirect, time is quick or sustained, and flow is free or bound. These eight effort elements combine in a multitude of configurations that Laban described as "states" and "drives." These "states" and "drives" appear as moments of significant change and yield the endless rhythmic variation evident in human movement. For example, the language may serve to compare and contrast the percussive, strong, quick accent of a tap dancer's movement and the delicate, light, sustained, free promenade of a ballet dancer.

Space This category examines the way the body moves through the space around it and addresses issues of proximity, direction, pathway, location, and relationship. The LMA framework identifies a personal kinesphere as a bubble of space that travels with an individual through the general space. Proximity refers to the relative distances between people or between a person and an object. Appropriate proximity varies from culture to culture and is an important aspect of social behavior. To further delineate three-dimensional space, Laban imagined a human being standing inside various geometric forms or crystals such as a sphere, cube, octahedron (an eight-sided crystal), icosahedron (a twenty-sided crystal), or dodecahedron (a twelve-sided crystal). The vertices, edges, and facets of this crystalline architecture suggest possible pathways through space.

Shape In shape description, Laban movement analysts observe the forms the body makes and the process of shape change as one moves between forms. It provides a vocabulary for identifying design elements that appear in the arrangement of body parts in relationship to one another. In addition to familiar descriptions of shape such as curved, angular, symmetric, or asymmetric, shape is viewed as a dynamic process, the outward shape change revealing a variety of inner attitudes. The change in body shape that occurs when an individual is actively engaging or responding to the outer environment, as in building a sand castle, appears very different from a change in the body shape that results from a deep sigh or other internally motivated action. This framework provides a way to describe the plasticity of the body, the forms it reveals, and the way in which its form constantly changes.

Any movement event is a complex layering of many movement elements. Variables of body, effort, shape, and space are all occurring simultaneously. The Laban framework provides differentiated concepts within each category. The vocabulary that results from this conceptual understanding of movement enables observers to identify the most important characteristics of a movement event and to describe how these characteristics change through time.

LMA in Practice

LMA provides a means of moving from description of movement to interpretation and creating plans for change or improvement in movement expression. In athletics, performance arts, martial arts, and fitness training, LMA is used to break an action down into its separate elements and then to determine which elements are most important in performing the action most efficiently, effectively, and/or expressively. From this assessment it is possible to move actively toward developing and refining the specific movements that contribute to virtuosity within any physical skill. In the same way LMA can also serve as a diagnostic tool in injury rehabilitation and in maximizing movement patterns

for health and efficiency. Since LMA recognizes that movement can express inner intentions and psychological motivations, the system also provides concrete tools for deciphering the non-verbal language of movement expression as viewed within the fields of psychology, sociology, and anthropology. As a conceptual framework, it provides movement educators with a concrete language for the clarification of somatic goals and an assessment of progress. As a system that provides specific links between mental, physical, and emotional realms of human functioning, its range of potential application extends to any inquiry concerned with the intersection of body and mind experience.

—Ed Groff, M.F.A., CMA

Resources

The Laban-Bartenieff Institute of Movement
    Studies
11 East 4th Street
New York, NY 10003-6902
Tel: (212) 477-4299
An institute providing comprehensive training in LMA that offers a certificate program.

The Dance Notation Bureau
33 West 21st Street
New York, NY 10001
Tel: (212) 807-7899
An institute providing certificate training in Labanotation.

Motos Humanus
P.O. Box 11036
Denver, CO 80211
Tel: (303) 421-2023
An organization serving the needs of Laban-based movement professionals through publications, conferences, advanced training seminars, and professional consultation.

Laban Centre for Movement and Dance
University of London Goldsmith's College
London SE 14 6NW
England

Tel: 01-692-4070
A school offering undergraduate, postgraduate, and special courses in Laban studies.

The Language of Dance Center
17 Holland Park
London W1135D
England
A school offering comprehensive training in Labanotation.

Further Reading:

Bartenieff, Irmgard, and Dori Lewis. *Body Movement: Coping with the Environment.* Revised edition. New York: Gordon Breach Science Publishers, Inc., 1980.

Dunlop, Valerie P. *Modern Educational Dance.* Revised edition. Boston: Plays Inc. Publishers, 1990.

Guest, Ann Hutchinson. *Your Move: A New Approach to the Study of Movement and Dance.* Revised edition. New York: Gordon and Breach Science Publishers, Inc., 1990.

Laban, Rudolf. *A Life for Dance.* New York: Theatre Arts Books, 1975.

Laban, Rudolf. *The Mastery of Movement.* Revised by Lisa Ullman. Boston: Plays Inc. Publishers, 1975.

North, Marion. *Personality Assessment Through Movement.* London: Macdonald and Evans, 1972.

MOVEMENT PATTERN ANALYSIS

Movement pattern analysis focuses on the relationship between mind and body in the structure and coding of movement. Though it can be applied to a broad range of activities, it is generally used in executive training programs to improve individual skills in decision making, communication, and group interaction. There is no prescribed regimen of exercise in movement pattern analysis. It assesses habitual structures of behavior in order to provide information that will help in the choice and attainment of life goals.

The History of Movement Pattern Analysis

Movement pattern analysis has its roots in the system of movement analysis first developed in the early twentieth century by Rudolf Laban, an Austro-Hungarian artist, scientist, and philosopher. The rise of Hitler forced Laban to flee to Great Britain where, from 1941 to 1946, he and F. C. Lawrence, a management consultant, conducted a study of industrial production tasks. Their findings contradicted the mechanistic principles of time/motion study, which governed thought about efficient factory production at that time.

Laban and Lawrence approached factory work as if it were a form of dance, paying particular attention to the characteristic mental attitude needed to perform each individual movement of the task. They argued that this dynamic patterning, which Laban called effort phrasing, should be the basis for determining a worker's suitability to a job. Struck by the repetitive nature of factory work, they also encouraged workers to make motions that, strictly speaking, were inefficient but lent a satisfying rhythm to their tasks. Workers at factories who adopted the Laban Lawrence industrial rhythm, also called Laban personal effort assessment, increased their output, suffered less stress, and felt more complete as human beings.

At the end of World War II, Warren Lamb joined Laban's group and began to explore ways of applying effort assessment to managerial work. He observed the behavior of managers in their offices and devised a system for correlating effort phrasing with the decision-making skills required for a number of managerial activities. First marketed in the 1960s as action profiling, Lamb's method had an enormous impact on the corporate community, particularly in

Great Britain. Action Profiling gave companies a new, effective means for allocating responsibility and building successful management teams. In 1992 disagreements over the Laban heritage forced Lamb to leave his first organization, Action Profilers International, and rename his method movement pattern analysis.

The Theory of Movement Pattern Analysis

Lamb's method is based on the belief that movement is a direct, faithful register of a person's inner intention, whether conscious or unconscious. The nature of the intention is evaluated through study of a particular type of movement, which Lamb named integrated movement. These movements, which seem to appear when a person is most fully revealing of his or her inner intentions, are distinguished by the fact that they flow throughout the entire body, moving from the core outward, or from the extremities inward.

Information for assessment of the decision-making process is derived from extended observation of integrated movements. The shape these movements take in space, rising or falling, spreading or enclosing, retreating or advancing, is noted and correlated with qualities of effort. According to Lamb, who follows Laban on this principle, effort is manifested in four qualities: flow, weight, space, and time. Each of these four attributes of movement is indicative of a specific inner attitude of the mover. For example, flow, or the quality of ongoingness of the movement, is indicative of an inner attitude of progression. A controlled movement reflects a sense of caution, whereas a free-flowing movement indicates an inner attitude of abandon. By attending to the relationship between effort and shape in integrated movement, it is possible to determine "where" a person is in the decision-making process. A picture of her or his entire decision-making process can be produced with data drawn from prolonged study. The profile is as distinctive and indelible as a fingerprint.

Experiencing Movement Pattern Analysis

Movement pattern analysis is conducted like a job interview or an ordinary conversation. The client remains fully clothed and in some instances may not be aware of the precise purpose of the meeting. The movement pattern analyst asks questions concerning the client's job or life. As the conversation proceeds, the analyst assesses the client's integrated movements and records the data on coding sheets formulated by Lamb. The results are then discussed with the client and possibly with the client's employer.

When a group such as a management team is evaluated, movement pattern analysis is done in two stages. In the first stage the members of the group are approached on an individual basis and given information about their decision-making habits. In the second stage the group is studied as an entity with its own characteristic mode of behavior. This second analysis of group movement pattern is used by the group leader and the group as a whole to determine tactics for achieving smoother, more productive teamwork.

The Benefits of Movement Pattern Analysis

A profile of one's decision-making process can be an important means of self-empowerment. It allows decision making to be understood as a pattern of behavior with strengths and weaknesses that can be examined and changed.

—*Warren Lamb*

Resources:

Motus Humanus
Carol-Lynne Moore, Director
P.O. Box 11036
Denver, CO 80211
Organizes workshops and conferences in movement pattern analysis and supervises the training of movement pattern analysts.

Further Reading:

Laban, Rudolf, and F. C. Lawrence. *Effort.* London: Macdonald & Evans, 1947.

Laban, Rudolf. *The Language of Movement.* Lisa Ullman, ed. Boston: Plays, Inc., 1974.

Lamb, Warren. *Posture and Gesture.* London: Duckworth, 1965.

——. *Management Behavior.* London: Duckworth, 1969.

Lamb, Warren, and Elizabeth Watson. *Body Code: The Meaning in Movement.* Princeton, NJ: Princeton Book Company, 1987.

Moore, Carol-Lynne. *Executives in Action: A Guide to Balanced Decision-Making in Management.* 4th ed. London: Pitman, 1992.

Ramsden, Pamela. *Top Team Planning: A Study of the Power of Individual Motivation in Management.* London: Associated Business Programmes, 1973.

PART XV: EXPRESSIVE AND CREATIVE ARTS THERAPIES

Art Therapy • Authentic Movement • Dance Therapy • Drama Therapy • Halprin Life/Art Process • Journal Therapy • Multi-Modal Expressive Arts Therapy • Music Therapy * Poetry Therapy • Sandplay Therapy

Expressive and creative arts therapies are methods that use one or several of the fine arts as a means to effect changes in physical, mental, or emotional functioning. Music, painting and sculpture, dancing, mimicry, and story-telling were all used by early humans to try to create order in a seemingly chaotic universe. By giving aesthetic form to their fears, hopes, and dreams, our ancestors found many ways to cope with the mysterious and sometimes terrifying forces that control the universe. Expressive and creative arts therapies are grounded in this same notion, using the evocative, organizing power of aesthetic expression to help people of all ages face challenges of healing and growing—challenges that can be as difficult in this day and age as they were for our primal ancestors.

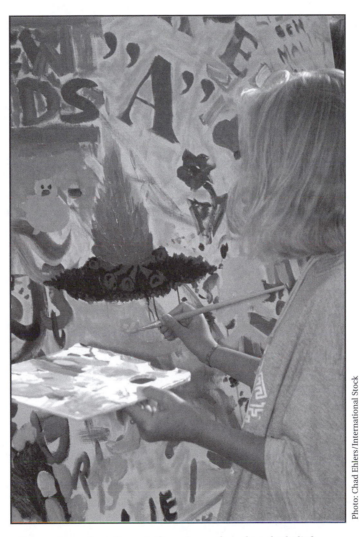

Photo: Chad Ehlers/International Stock

Expressive and creative arts therapies are based on the belief that a person's creativity reveals his or her inner life.

Learning Life Skills Through the Arts

Although the use of the fine arts for therapeutic purposes is comparatively new in Western medicine, the healing and educational power of the arts has been intuitively

341

recognized around the world from the beginnings of human history. For ancient primal cultures and their contemporary relatives, the indigenous peoples of North and South America, Africa, Polynesia, Australia, and Asia, the arts are an intrinsic part of life. In these cultures children develop gross and fine motor skills along with a strong sense of identity as they learn to weave baskets or make pottery, clothing, or hunting equipment in the traditional patterns of their culture.

In these cultures religious celebrations mark the seasons of the year and important events in life, such as birth, reaching adolescence, marriage, and death. These celebrations are often communal events in which participants might prepare traditional costumes, masks, and musical instruments and take part in ritualized singing, dancing, and theatrical presentations. These activities develop physical and intellectual skills in the participants while serving on a deeper level to guide their emotional and spiritual development.

In the highly developed ancient cultures of China, India, and Egypt the arts were an integral part of political, educational, religious, and health practices. These cultures believed that the universe was perfectly ordered by divine forces. They believed that achieving power, success, happiness, and health was a result of learning how these divine forces operate in the universe and working harmoniously with them. One way this could be accomplished was through aesthetic expression. Sound, motion, and light—the elemental materials of music, dance, and visual and performance art—were believed to follow divine cosmological laws. Artists and philosophers, who also functioned as teachers and healers in these cultures, worked to discover aesthetic theories for the arts so that artistic expressions would reflect the divine order of the universe and help people experience a sense of harmony with it. The teachers applied these laws to various artistic disciplines such as music (including chanting), calligraphy, dance, and theatrical performances.

The Changing Role of the Arts

Aesthetic modes of healing, praying, and learning continued unbroken for nearly 5,000 years in the East. As Western culture evolved, the arts began to be separated from these basic human activities. Ironically, the philosophy of Plato (c. 428–348 BCE), known for its promotion of aesthetic beauty, is partially responsible for this change. He believed humans could create a more perfect order in the universe and put forth the idea that human behavior was created from three basic sources: desire, emotion, and knowledge. In Plato's hierarchical philosophy reason and intellect, located in the head, were a more valuable pilot for the soul than the emotions located in the heart, or desires located in the loins or pelvis. From this point of view the physical embodiment of divine laws through art grew to be less valuable than intellectual and theoretical discussions of those laws.

As Western culture passed through the decline of Greece and the rise and fall of Rome, the arts continued to lose their primacy as a means of praying, teaching, and healing. In the Dark Ages that followed, the arts remained connected to religious activities within the Judeo-Christian tradition, but they were no longer valued as a primary method of communicating spiritual knowledge or healing. That tradition denigrated the physical body and all sensory modes of expression and glorified the human mind and intellectual thought as the one true path to spiritual salvation. The arts were treated as crafts in need of direction and control and became a mere adornment to the pursuit of spiritual excellence. Then, during the Renaissance, the arts began to fall prey to the secularized demands of commerce, where they have by and large remained to this day.

However, at the dawn of the twentieth century a confluence of forces in art, politics, and health care served to partially reestablish the role of the arts as a tool for healing in the West. In the first decades of the century Sigmund Freud (1856–1939) and his colleagues, notably Carl Jung (1875–1961), began to explore the connections between physical health and the workings of the human mind and emotions. Freud's theories of the unconscious and its role in the development and behavior of human beings became the basis of an entirely new mode of treatment in Western scientific medicine. Both psychoanalysis, as Freud termed his approach, and analytical psychology, as Jung described his approach, relied on the revelation of personal unconscious imagery to effect a cure. This unconscious imagery is still an important tool for many expressive and creative arts therapists.

At about the same time Western artists such as Pablo Picasso (1881–1973), Arnold Schoenberg (1874–1951), Isadora Duncan (1877–1927), Rainer Maria Rilke (1875–1926), and Konstantin Stanislavsky (1863–1938) were becoming disillusioned with traditional art forms, which they felt were outmoded and had lost their ability to inspire. They began creating modern art forms full of vibrant abstract images reflecting personal perceptions. By the time World War II rocked the Western world in 1939 there was a large body of artists in Europe and the United States exploring the power of the arts to capture, reflect, and organize unconscious content. Many of these artists intuitively recognized the therapeutic value of their own artistic activities, and they explored its potential in private teaching situations. Open-minded doctors, aware of the therapeutic successes of some of these artists, invited them into the hospitals, which were strained by the large number of people suffering from physical and emotional trauma as a result of the war. Predominantly dancers and visual artists, but also musicians, writers, and theater artists, entered the hospital setting, and the new modalities of music, dance, art, poetry, and drama therapy were born.

After 1945 the nascent expressive arts therapies were introduced into other institutional settings such as schools, prisons, and senior citizen homes. Experiential exploration and theoretical development continued throughout the 1950s with more and more creative artists developing unique practices and approaches to healing and changing through the arts. With the social upheaval of the 1960s and its demand for more meaningful forms of living, the creative and expressive arts were enlisted once again in growth centers across the country. For example, at the Esalen Institute in California and the Omega Institute in New York, the arts became a means by which ever greater numbers of people sought to expand their understanding of themselves and their role in the universe.

Today each of the expressive arts therapies (music, dance, visual art, poetry, and drama) is represented by a national organization that sets standards for the training of therapists and offers a forum for the many technical and philosophical issues confronting the field. In addition, an ever-growing number of related creative arts practices serve individuals in their efforts to heal and grow physically, mentally, emotionally, and spiritually.

The Process of Creation as Exercise for the Brain

All the expressive arts therapies and creative arts practices share the belief that creating a work of art is in and of itself therapeutic. The process, not the end product, is the most important part of the work. For instance, creative dance sessions can extend the range of movement and develop the physical coordination of people with cerebral palsy, muscular dystrophy, or polio. Painting and sculpting can develop hand-eye coordination in the physically healthy as well as the physically challenged. Music classes that focus on the use of the voice can help people with asthma discover a new relationship to their lungs and the process of breathing.

Contemporary research into the nature of the brain suggests how the practice of creative arts brings about these seemingly miraculous improvements. Researchers have discovered that the right side of the brain controls the left side of the body and is also responsible for imaginative, nonlinear thought. The left side of the brain, which controls the right side of the body, is also the location of all logical, rational, analytic, and verbal skills. Creative arts use both imaginative and analytical skills calling on both sides of the brain, developing brain cells and nerve connections that drugs and specific repetitive physical exercises simply cannot awaken.

Creating Art to Improve Social and Emotional Skills

Social and emotional skills are also explored through the process of making art. Creating a work of art independently requires developing an ability to turn one's attention alternately inward toward the creative impulse and outward toward the form that is being created, and to develop a dialogue between the two. The communication skills developed in this process are similar to those needed for healthy, satisfying interpersonal relationships. In a like manner, creating a group dance, musical composition, or visual art installation can serve as a laboratory for the development of group social skills.

Whether the participant is creating alone or in a group, the form of the work being created always serves as the reference point for the developing physical or emotional skills. It is a basic tenet of all expressive arts therapies and creative arts practices that the form of a work of art reflects the inner feelings of the creator or creators. Whether the feelings are conscious or unconscious, expressive and creative arts practitioners believe we can perceive, describe, and share those feelings more effectively by giving them expression in an aesthetic form and then reflecting on that form and our process in creating it. Both the form itself and the process of creating it become metaphors for how we live our life.

Reflecting on the Work

The process of reflecting on the work of art will vary depending on the orientation of the therapist, counselor, or group leader. Therapists who adhere to the Freudian therapeutic model will observe and discuss the content of the work of art, interpreting it symbolically in relation to seven psychosexual stages of development of the child in relation to its parents. Therapists with a Jungian orientation will compare the content to characters and themes from world mythology, sensing in them the unfolding of an individual human consciousness in relation to "the collective unconscious," a sort of world library of human experience. Followers of transpersonal or humanist psychology, founded by Abraham Maslow and Carl Rogers respectively, will probably not engage in the process of interpretation at all, trusting entirely in the ability of the individual or the group to direct their own psycho-spiritual healing through the process of making art.

Experiencing Expressive Arts Therapies and Creative Arts Practices

While the formalized use of expressive arts therapies began in institutional settings and remains an important part of healing and education in hospitals, prisons, shelters, and schools, it is also possible to explore these practices, individually or in a group, in private counseling or growth centers throughout the United States today. No special talent is required, simply an enjoyment of an art form and a desire to explore and grow. Many creative arts leaders advertise workshops in magazines and newspapers. Expressive arts therapists practicing privately can be located through their national organizations.

Each therapist or group leader will have his or her own approach to working with individuals, groups, and the specific art form. Some therapists or group leaders will focus on spontaneous creation, or improvisation, as the major activity of a session or workshop. For others the main activity may be the practice of specific movements, or playing or listening to particular pieces of music, or reading particular poems. Here the emphasis is not so much on the ability of art to capture and reflect unconscious content but on the power of a previously created form or the experience of a particular element of artistic technique to effect a desired change in the body and mind of the practitioner. Many therapists or group leaders will combine both approaches in their creative arts sessions.

In group work the role of observer can be as important as the role of creator. Participants often observe group members in the act of creating, or view others' completed works of art. Just as the ancients recognized the value of creating art, active observing has long been recognized for its cathartic and therapeutic effects on our mind and body, too. Responding verbally to a work of art can also help us learn to understand our emotions and their effects on others. And by sharing our responses with the creator we complete a loop of communication, allowing the creator to learn how others experience his or her creation/emotional expression.

A Method with Physical, Mental, and Emotional Benefits

Whether approached in group or individual modes, expressive art therapies and creative arts practices offer great possibilities for developing a deeper understanding and appreciation of our physical, mental, and emotional coping strategies and learning new living and communication skills. With an open heart, willing mind, and dedication to the process, the arts offer an unlimited opportunity to explore and share the unfolding of our essential humanity.

—*Nancy Allison, CMA*

Resources:

Expressive Arts Program
California Institute of Integral Studies
9 Peter Yorke Way
San Francisco, CA 94109
Tel: (415) 674-5500
*Offers a master's degree in counseling psychology
with a specialization in expressive arts therapy.*

Expressive Therapies Program
Lesley College
29 Everett Street
Cambridge, MA 02138
Tel: (617) 349-8425
*Offers a comprehensive graduate program in
multi-modal expressive arts therapy.*

International Expressive Arts Therapy Association
P.O. Box 64126
San Francisco, CA 94164
Tel: (415) 522-8959
*A professional organization dedicated to multi-
modal expressive arts therapy.*

Further Reading:

Arnheim, Rudolf. *Towards a Psychology of Art.*
Berkeley: University of California Press, 1966.

Berger, John. *Ways of Seeing.* Magnolia, MA: Peter
Smith, 1977.

Dewey, John. *Art as Experience.* New York: Peri-
gree Books, 1959.

McNiff, Shaun. *The Arts in Psychotherapy.* Springfield, IL: Charles C. Thomas Pub. Ltd., 1981.

ART THERAPY

Art therapy is a method used to help people release inner thoughts and emotions by making visual art. The process of creative expression, through forms of visual art such as drawing, painting, sculpture, or collage, is thought to aid a person's healing and recovery. Therapists may work with a person to decipher symbolic representations of his or her feelings, thoughts, or perceptions. This form of therapy may appeal to people who otherwise find it difficult to express or understand a problem or emotion. Art is used as an intuitive, physical method of manifesting hidden feelings and overcoming difficult problems.

The Origins of Art Therapy

Although the field of art therapy formally emerged in this century, the use of visual images to express inner emotions and master external events extends as far back as prehistory. Masks, ritual pottery, carefully designed costumes, and musical instruments were all created as outer expressions of powerful spiritual beliefs and were used in rituals. The use of art in so many rituals suggests two healing aspects of art: its potential to achieve or restore psychological equilibrium and its ability to alleviate or contain feelings of trauma, fear, anxiety, and psychological threat to the self and the community.

In the late 1800s and early 1900s, a growing number of European psychologists were becoming interested in studying visual art made by patients with mental illnesses. In 1912, psychiatrists Emil Kraeplin and Eugen Bleuler were among the earliest therapists to try to diagnose psychopathologies by interpreting their patients' drawings. Later, Sigmund Freud reported that patients of his who were unable to describe their dreams in words would frequently say that they could draw the images from their dreams. This observation encouraged the belief that artistic expression could reveal the inner world of the human psyche.

Psychologist Carl Jung's work also influenced the development of art therapy. Jung was particularly interested in the psychological meanings and uses of art expressions, including his own drawings and those of his patients. Unlike Freud, who never asked his patients to draw their dream images, Jung often encouraged his patients to draw. "To paint what we see before us," he said, "is a different art from painting what we see within." Jung believed that there was an important connection between the images that people made and their inner thoughts. Jung studied art created around the world and noted recurring and seemingly universal symbols he called archetypes. These archetypes are cultural images that represent basic elements of unconscious thought and human development. Jung's theory of archetypes became a foundation for understanding how symbolic imagery reveals meaning in artworks, and is still used by many therapists today.

In the 1940s, art therapy became a profession in the United States largely due to the work of Margaret Naumburg. She founded the Walden School in 1915, where she used students' artworks in psychological counseling. She agreed with the predominant psychological viewpoint that art expression is a way to manifest unconscious imagery. In Naumburg's view, art could provide the client a form of spontaneous expression and communication. She considered these images a form of symbolic speech.

Through the 1950s and 1960s Edith Kramer, an artist, educator, and pioneer in the field of art therapy, pointed to another important benefit of art making. She was a European artist who moved to the United States, where she began teaching art to children. While other therapists sought to decode patients' artworks, Kramer was interested in the value of the act of art making. She believed that there were therapeutic benefits to the creative process itself.

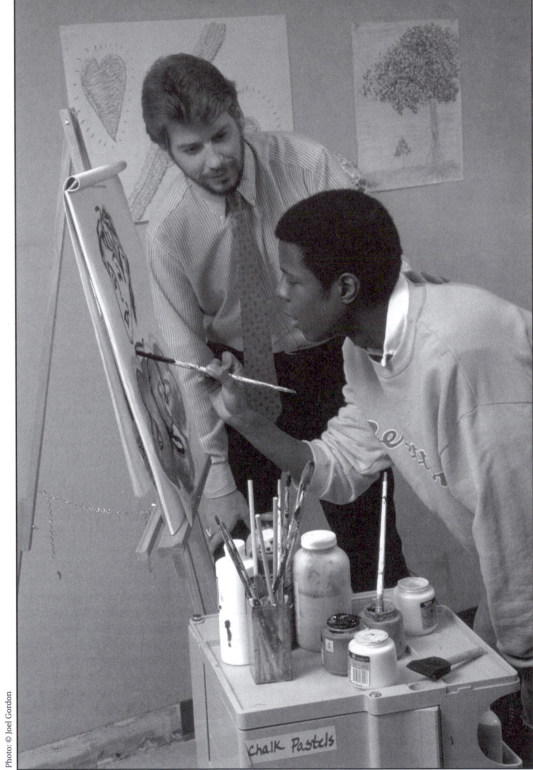

Photo: © Joel Gordon

Art making allows people to release their emotions without verbalizing them.

She stressed creativity, in addition to the communication of visual symbols, as the key to the art therapy process.

How It Works

Art therapy attempts to introduce visual art making as an accessible method of communicating feelings, thoughts, and experiences. This creative process is used to aid a person's healing and recovery. An art therapist will work with his or her patients to help them understand their art expressions. To accomplish this, the therapist and client will review the artworks and discuss possible meanings or emotions expressed in the work. With the help of the art therapist, the patient interprets the images by trying to recognize aspects of his or her self in art expressions. For those clients who cannot verbally articulate the content of their images, such as children, the art therapist may look for repetition of themes over time to provide clues to possible meanings. A therapist will try to understand and clarify the meanings of images while respecting the client as a creative individual capable of contributing to his or her own healing process.

Art as Therapy

An art therapist uses visual art media (such as drawing materials, paints, collage/mixed media, and clay sculpture) and the creative process to help a patient explore issues, interests, concerns, and conflicts through art expression. Art therapists work in a variety of ways and with many different populations. For example, an art therapist in a hospital setting might work individually with psychiatric patients to help them use art to explore emotional conflicts or develop social skills. With a child who has been traumatized by physical abuse, an art therapist might use art activities to help the child explore feelings about the trauma and to reduce feelings of anxiety, fear, or depression. Art therapists often work as part of a treatment team including doctors, nurses, psychologists, social workers, and counselors.

Who Benefits from Art Therapy

An art therapist may work with adults in a psychiatric hospital, an addictions treatment center, a shelter for battered women and their children, a school for the mentally retarded or disabled, a day-care center for the elderly, a rehabilitation hospital, or in a medical facility with physically ill patients. They work with children, adults, families, and groups, and with a variety of patient populations. Some art therapists work as private practitioners, while others are employed by schools, hospitals, clinics, or community agencies.

Art therapy uses art making to enhance communication between therapist and client. The artworks are used as a common language through which clients and therapists can explore feelings, thoughts, and experiences. This makes art therapy a significant contribution to the field of mental health with enhanced promise in the growth of human understanding.

—*Cathy Malchiodi, M.A., ATR, LPAT, LPCC*

Resources

American Art Therapy Association, Inc. (AATA)
1202 Allanson Road
Chicago, IL 60060
Tel: (847) 949–6064
Fax: (847) 566–4580

Art therapists who practice in the United States are trained at the graduate level and receive a master's degree; a strong background in visual art and psychology is generally required to enter a graduate program.

Web site: www.louisville.edu/groups/aata.www
A list of approved training programs, membership information, and resources for books, tapes, and videos is available from the AATA. This organization also publishes Art Therapy: Journal of the American Art Therapy Association.

The Arts in Psychotherapy
Elsevier Science
660 White Plains Road
Tarrytown, NY 10591–5153
e-mail: esuk.usa@elsevier.com
This journal features articles by experts in the creative arts therapies about the therapeutic use of various forms of art. It reports on national and international art therapy conferences and features book reviews.

Further Reading

Case, C., and T. Dalley. *The Handbook of Art Therapy.* London: Tavistock. 1992.

Kramer, E. *Art as Therapy with Children.* Chicago: Magnolia Street Publishers. 1994.

Malchiodi, C. A. *Breaking the Silence: Art Therapy with Children.* New York: Brunner/Mazel, 1997.

McNiff, S. *The Arts in Psychotherapy.* Springfield, IL: Charles C. Thomas, 1981.

Ulman, E., and P. Dachinger, eds. *Art Therapy in Theory and Practice.* Chicago: Magnolia Street Publishers, 1996.

AUTHENTIC MOVEMENT

Authentic movement is a dance-movement process practiced by individuals and groups as a way to learn from the body's own experience, insights, and imagination. It is an outwardly simple but profound process where subjects follow their impulses for movement or stillness in an accepting rather than judgmental way. Rather than consciously choosing what movements to do, they allow their bodies to initiate the movement, thereby making room for the unconscious to participate as well. This process leads to a deepened respect for the body's wisdom and is practiced for diverse purposes such as personal enrichment, spiritual insight, artistic renewal, psychotherapy, or community ritual.

A Different Approach to Movement

Mary Whitehouse, the pioneering dancer, teacher, and dance therapist, began developing this approach to movement in the 1950s and 1960s. She was a modern dancer who had trained with Mary Wigman and Martha Graham. Wigman's emphasis on individual creativity and Whitehouse's interest in the psychological theories of Carl Jung provided a foundation for what is now known as authentic movement.

Whitehouse described "authentic" movement as that which was spontaneous and genuine to that person, rather than learned movement. It arose out of the "self," and occurred when the ego relinquished control over the movement. Throughout her life Mary Whitehouse continued to experiment with this approach to movement, and with various names for it; for example, she called it the "Tao of the body," and "movement in depth."

Janet Adler, a dance therapist well known for her work with autistic children, studied with Whitehouse in 1969–70. She brought her own interest in Freudian psychological theory and a deep interest in shamanism and mysticism. In the late 1970s she began to formalize a set practice and call it authentic movement. She established the Mary Starks Whitehouse Institute in western Massachusetts in 1981, two years after Whitehouse's death, as a place to study and teach this form of movement.

Core Elements of Authentic Movement

The core element of the process shared by most practitioners is the relationship between the mover and the witness. With eyes closed or inwardly focused, the mover responds to his or her inner impulses while the witness watches nonjudgmentally from the sidelines. After a set time of moving, usually without musical accompaniment, there is usually a dialogue between mover and witness. The heart of the process is to honor the expression of the mover's inner experience without judgment.

There are several core values shared by most authentic movement practitioners. The first is that one's body contains wisdom and can be used as a source of insight, healing, and guidance. A second is that the mover's experience during the session—when one spends time in the body, paying attention to how the body moves—is of prime importance. The third is that authority for an individual's experience rests with the individual and not with anyone who moved with that person or an observer.

Authentic movement offers an opportunity for deep rest and recuperation of both body and soul. It cultivates the integration of one's physical, psychological, and spiritual aspects, and it invites the safe inclusion of the full range of healthy human expression—be it playful or somber, solitary or shared. Authentic movement is practiced by people varied in age, physical skill, dance or movement training, and religious belief, and for diverse purposes such as for personal enrichment, spiritual insight, artistic renewal, psychotherapy, or community ritual.

Although the name authentic movement is widely used to identify the process, other names are also used—such as contemplative dance, or the moving imagination. Currently, there is no central organization overseeing practitioners, although steps toward more communication between practitioners is under way.

Experiencing Authentic Movement

During a session, people move in a tremendous variety of ways, from extended periods of complete stillness to vigorous activity. The movement might be minute—even imperceptible—or large and highly stylized. It can be idiosyncratic, mundane, or formal; rhythmic or dancelike or not; familiar or foreign; homely and awkward or graceful and elegant. No movement is inherently unacceptable unless it harms the mover or others. This very broad acceptance of movement possibilities distinguishes this practice from other forms of open improvisation. Unlike most forms of dance, there is no need to please or impress viewers or fellow movers.

In order to establish a safe environment both physically and interpersonally, rules about safety and confidentiality are regularly reinforced and refined. Individuals must be responsible for not hurting themselves or fellow movers (by opening

---

Janet Adler Explains the Dynamics of Authentic Movement

"The witness, especially in the beginning, carries a larger responsibility for consciousness, as she sits to the side of the movement space. She is not 'looking at' the person moving, she is witnessing, listening—bringing a specific quality of attention or presence to—the experience of the mover."

"The mover works with eyes closed in order to expand her experience of listening to the deeper levels of her kinesthetic reality. Her task is to respond to a sensation, to an inner impulse, to energy coming from the personal unconscious, the collective unconscious, or the superconscious. . .The mover and witness usually speak together about the material that has emerged during the movement time, thus bringing formerly unconscious processes into consciousness."

their eyes when necessary, for example, or moving away from unwelcome contact), and are not to share others' experiences outside of the group. These structures and rules allow for significant privacy—both from the outer world and/or from one's fellow movers—considerable intimacy, trust, and an unusually broad freedom in movement possibilities.

Just as important to the authentic movement process is the "sharing after moving" phase that allows the participants to integrate what they have experienced. Depending on the goals of the participants, there might be analytical dialogue in a therapeutic setting, discussion of artistic ideas or images in an artistic working group or rehearsal, personal sharing in a peer group, or no discussion at all in a group practicing for spiritual purposes. This phase might take different forms for people in the same group, or different forms for one person on different days.

In choosing a facilitator one should be conscientious and sensible. Questions about the person's background, training, and goals are appropriate. One should ask for references. It is important to feel intuitively comfortable with the teacher and that the goals for working together are shared.

Benefits

Authentic movement is a contemporary movement practice that provides people from a wide variety of backgrounds and abilities a structure within which they can recuperate their bodies and souls. This process can lead to an enhanced awareness of one's whole self, and provide insights to fundamental issues and questions relevant to one's life.

—*Daphne Lowell*

Resources:

The Authentic Movement Community Directory
Editor: Michael Gardos Reid
2219 Taft Street
NE Minneapolis, MN 55418

Tel: (612) 788–1822
e-mail: 76232.1634@Compuserve.com
Lists practitioners of authentic movement.

Further Reading:

Books:

Pallaro, Patrizia, editor. *Authentic Movement: Essays by Mary Whitehouse, Janet Adler, and Joan Chodorow.* Volume 1. London: Jessica Kingsley Publishers, 1998.

—— *Authentic Movement: Moving the Body, Moving the Self. A Collection of Essays.* Volume 2. London: Jessica Kingsley Publishers, 1999.

Journals:

A Moving Journal: Ongoing Expressions of Authentic Movement. Editors: Annie Geissinger, Joan Webb.

DANCE THERAPY

Dance therapy is founded on the principle that a vital connection exists between personality and the way in which one moves, and that changes in movement behavior can affect the emotional, intellectual, and physical health of an individual. It is used to help people attain healthy, expressive functioning, individually or in group situations. It is especially useful with people for whom verbal therapy is ineffective or overwhelming. While the roots of dance therapy are ancient, it has been recognized as an established form of therapy only since the 1940s.

Dance: An Ancient Form of Self-Expression

The rhythmic movements of dance have appealed to people throughout the ages. Dance is found in nearly every culture and civilization, serving a variety of purposes. In many cultures, dance was and still is used as a cathartic healing tool. Primitive societies used dance in rituals, such as rites of passage and

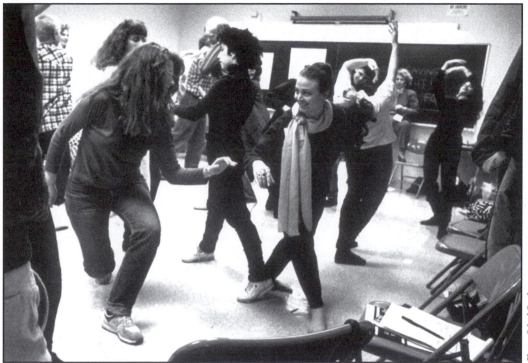

Photo: © Joel Gordon

Mirroring another person's movement, a basic technique used in dance therapy, is often the first step in establishing interpersonal communication.

other religious ceremonies. Dance rituals marked life transitions, helping to integrate individuals with the larger society. Many societies still use dance in similar ways. Experts agree that in early civilizations dancing, religion, music, and medicine were often connected.

Dance Therapy Evolves

In the early part of the twentieth century radical changes in dance movement and expression resulted in what is now called "modern" dance. Up to that time Western theatrical dance had been a highly structured and regimented art form. Modern dance focuses on spontaneity, awareness of natural movement, and more freedom for personal expression. During the first half of the twentieth century there were also new developments in psychiatry that explored nonverbal aspects of psychology and psychopathology. Eugen Bleuler in Switzerland, Jean-Martin Charcot in France, and Henry Maudsley

in England were examining the unique movement behavior of people with mental illness. The field of dance therapy emerged in the 1940s and 1950s amid these innovations in dance and in psychological treatment.

The earliest dance therapists were dancers and dance teachers who were encouraged by psychiatrists to use dance as a method of communicating with withdrawn patients. Marian Chace (1896–1970) is considered an important pioneering force in the establishment of dance therapy in the United States. Chace's dance education included dance from many cultures, dance improvisation, and music theory, and cultivated in Chace an openness to many forms of dance expression. Later, she established her own school in Washington, D.C., where her dance technique, which stressed improvisation and individual expression, gained a reputation for having therapeutic effects.

Communication Through Movement

In 1942, Chace was invited by psychiatrists at St. Elizabeth's Hospital to initiate a dance program for World War II veterans suffering mentally and emotionally from their wartime experiences. Chace was influenced by the ideas of American psychiatrist Harry Stack Sullivan, among others, who stressed that personality is formed through relationships, and that relationships require communication. She believed that schizophrenics and others with mental illness who were isolated in the back wards of psychiatric hospitals could be helped through direct contact and that through movement she could open lines of communication and establish relationships with these patients. Where others had seen only bizarre, random movements, Chace saw a valuable, if distorted, form of communication. Through a technique she called "mirroring" movement, Chace established a connection with an individual by re-creating his or her movement behavior with her own body. Mirroring, as Chace conceptualized, is not an imitation or a mimicry of a patient's movement. Rather the therapist is trying to take on the quality of the patient's movement, to move in tune with the patient in order to better understand what he or she is trying to communicate and to be able to respond in kind. Through this process, Chace discovered that symbols, imagery, and metaphor arose from movement that could be given verbal expression, thus providing a healing catharsis. Chace worked with individuals and groups using dance and movement as a means of communication; she took the expressive and symbolic elements of dance and merged them into a powerful form of therapy.

Other pioneers in the field of dance therapy include Francizka Boas, Liljan Espenak, Blanch Evan, Alma Hawkins, Trudi Schoop, and Mary Whitehouse. All of these early founders of dance therapy were grounded in a modern dance tradition that stressed authentic expression of the self. Each worked independently and developed her own method that studied, interpreted, and supported movement exploration, using the dance therapy session as the "container" of emotional experience. These individuals and others helped develop a broad range of styles and clinical applications with which contemporary dance therapists continue to work today.

In 1966, a group of therapists formed the American Dance Therapy Association (ADTA) in order to set professional standards and establish channels of communication among dance therapists, who were working mostly independently in hospitals and clinics throughout the country. Today, ADTA has more than 1,000 members nationally and internationally. The association publishes the *American Journal of Dance Therapy*, holds an annual conference, and maintains a registry of dance therapists who have met educational and clinical requirements.

The Guiding Principles of Dance Therapy

Dance therapy relies on several theoretical tenets. First and foremost is that dance is an expressive art and as such fulfills the human being's basic need for communication. Believing that each person has a desire to communicate, the dance therapist engages those parts of the person's personality that are expressive, however subtle they may be. Dance therapists believe that the body and mind are in constant reciprocal interaction, therefore changes that occur on the movement level can affect one's total functioning.

Dance therapists also believe that movement reflects personality. Dance therapy utilizes the nonverbal dimension of personality by using the technique of "mirroring," which re-creates the early experiences of the nonverbal mother-infant interaction. The relationship between the therapist and patient is central to the effectiveness of dance therapy. The dance therapist responds to the patient on a body level by mirroring, synchronizing, and interacting with the patient's movement, thus creating a strong therapeutic relationship. This helps explain why dance therapy is particularly effective with patients who are so regressed that verbal therapy is ineffective. Empathy is an important healing agent in dance therapy. By moving with the individual, in similar patterns, the patient feels accepted on an emotional level.

Movement, like dreams and the process of free association, can be symbolic of the underlying unconscious process. Therefore, ideas and feelings that are outside conscious awareness may emerge in movement behavior as symbols. Interpretation of these symbols can help in the process of therapeutic change.

Finally, the act of creating a movement through improvisation is inherently therapeutic since it generates new ways of moving, which generate new experiences of being in the world with other people. Individuals often experience highly charged emotional states during a dance therapy session. The therapist creates a safe and trusting environment in which feelings are explored through dance and words together, working with the individual to assess and interpret his or her movement verbally. Verbal processing helps to connect action, thought, and feeling, enabling the individual to experience greater feelings of personal integration and effectiveness.

Experiencing Dance Therapy

Dance therapy sessions are usually conducted in groups but can also be practiced one on one. Generally, the participants meet in a spacious, empty room where they feel free to move. No special dance clothing is worn. The structure of the session will vary depending on the participants involved and the orientation of the therapist. A session might begin with a warm-up, led by the therapist, and designed to reflect the mood of the patient or group in the moment. The therapist will be trained to pick up subtle movement cues and extend them through the mirroring technique rather than teaching dance steps or choreographed movements. Depending on the orientation of the therapist, he or she will continue to pick up movement and themes from the group based on improvisation or "dance in the moment." The goal of the session is not to perform or to exercise. Instead the therapist creates an environment where any and all movement behavior is valuable. After the development of movement themes and imagery, along with free verbal associations, the session ends with some sort of structured closing.

In 1966, a group of therapists formed the American Dance Therapy Association (ADTA) in order to set professional standards and establish channels of communication among dance therapists who were working mostly in isolation in hospitals and clinics throughout the country. Today, ADTA has over 1,000 members nationally and internationally. The association publishes the *American Journal of Dance Therapy*, holds an annual conference, and maintains a registry of dance therapists who have met educational and clinical requirements. The professional training of a dance therapist takes place on a graduate level. Dance therapists in training study dance/movement therapy theory and practice, psychopathology, human development, observation and research skills, and complete a supervised internship in a clinical setting. The title dance therapist registered (DTR) indicates that the therapist has completed professional education and training as indicated by the ADTA. Academy of Dance Therapists Registered (ADTR) is a title that means qualified to teach, provide supervision to other dance therapists, and practice privately.

Benefits and Risks

The goals of dance therapy include helping people achieve body-level reintegration. It helps individuals improve their communication skills and teaches new ways to interact with others. Dance therapy also provides a safe environment in which to address emotional issues. Dance therapy can help individuals with serious psychological and social difficulties, eating disorders, substance-abuse problems, Alzheimer's disease, and posttraumatic stress disorders. It can also be helpful in dealing with everyday stress and emotional and relationship issues. The elderly, adults, adolescents, children, and infants have all been helped by dance therapy.

—Anne. L Wennerstrad

Resources:

The American Dance Therapy Association
2000 Century Plaza, Suite 108
Columbia, MD 21044
Tel: (410) 997–4040
Fax: (410)997–4048
e-mail: ADTA@aol.com
listserv: adta@list.ab.umd.edu
Founded in 1966, this membership and advocacy group sets dance therapy eligibility standards, holds annual national conferences, provides information about graduate training programs, and publishes the American Journal of Dance Therapy.

Further Reading:

Levy, F. *Dance Movement Therapy: A Healing Art.* Reston, VA: American Alliance for Health, Physical Education, Recreation, and Dance, 1992.

Payne, H. *Dance Movement Therapy: Theory and Practice.* London: Routledge, 1992.

Sandel, S., S. Chaiklin, and A. Lohn, eds. *Foundations of Dance/Movement Therapy: The Life and Work of Marian Chace.* Columbia, MD: The Marian Chace Memorial Fund of the American Dance Therapy Association, 1993.

Stanton-Jones, K. *Dance Movement Therapy in Psychiatry.* London: Routledge, 1992.

DRAMA THERAPY

Drama therapy combines techniques from drama and theater with techniques from psychotherapy in an action-based method that helps people find solutions for social and emotional problems. This creative arts therapy helps people improve their sense of self-worth by discovering their own inner resources and by learning how to function better in groups. In its most well known form, drama therapy uses role play to help participants learn healthier behavior patterns. Drama therapists also use techniques such as improvisation, theater games, concentration exercises, mime, masks, and puppetry, scripted dramatizations, and open-ended scripts to further emotional growth and psychological integration. Drama therapy can offer individuals a vision of something outside the self and beyond a personal, subjective view of the world to expand their universe.

The Origins of Drama Therapy

Drama has been with us since the first cave people came home from a hunt and acted out their daring adventures for an assembled group. Formal theater came much later with dramas that provided moral and ethical lessons for people, as well as comedies to entertain and lighten their burdens. Religious leaders recognized the power of drama as a method of teaching their beliefs to people and added theatrical elements to their rituals. Theater practitioners have long been aware of the therapeutic value of drama.

It took a little longer for the action method of treatment combining psychology, process-drama and theater to be formalized. Although drama therapy has been practiced in Europe, especially in England, for many years, the National Association for Drama Therapy (NADT) was not established in this country until June 1979 at Yale University. The first annual conference was held in July 1980, which makes drama therapy the newest of the creative arts therapies. As of July 1997, there were approximately 300 members of the National Association for Drama Therapy.

How Drama Therapy Helps People

Drama therapy is defined by the National Association for Drama Therapy as "the intentional use of drama/theater process to achieve the therapeutic goals of symptom relief, emotional and physical integration, and personal growth. This creative arts therapy is used to maintain health as well as to treat such dysfunctions as emotional disorders, learning difficulties, geriatric problems, and social maladjustments. Drama therapy, as a primary or an adjunctive modality, is used in evaluation, treatment, and research with individuals, groups, and families."

Put more simply, drama therapy offers practice for living and helps clients discover their own inner resources and promotes their ability to express their feelings. It enhances sensory awareness and helps people learn to use the imagination as a problem-solving tool. It allows clients to play a role different from themselves or to play themselves with a new set of behaviors. For example, many people have difficulty saying no to others. A role play scene could be set up in which the person plays a character who will not give in—who can say no. In effect, he or she rehearses for a real-life situation, practicing in role what he or she wishes to do in reality.

Drama therapy helps people get in touch with their feelings and understand how feelings affect their bodies. For example, when angry, the body can become a tightly coiled spring. Individuals may find it difficult to express anger without violence. Exploration of such emotions and practice in dealing with life situations in a drama therapy session can help a person learn to handle powerful emotions better in real life.

A drama therapy session is a safe place to try out new behaviors or deal with existing situations in a different way without the fear of real consequences. It offers the opportunity to discuss feelings in a judgment-free environment. Perhaps one of its greatest assets is to help clients learn to identify their feelings and verbalize them. Many people think they are the only ones who have a particular problem, but they soon learn that they are not alone. Through sharing and interaction, clients realize their problems are not so different from those of others.

Drama Therapy Techniques

Drama therapists use many different techniques, from full-fledged theater performances to simple sensory-awareness exercises, depending on the person or people with whom they are working. A sensory-awareness exercise may involve simply passing around an unusual piece of fabric and asking, "What does it remind you of?" On the other hand, a theater performance may stimulate the whole audience to become emotionally involved with a problem and to offer alternative solutions. Some theater groups ask members of the audience to come up and play the role the way they think it should be done, involving the audience in solving the situation being examined. Some therapists use clients as the actors in a play, which teaches many levels of cooperation.

Role plays are enacted to give people experience in dealing with difficult situations. Frequently, when a patient is warmed up to an issue, he or she becomes fully involved in the role play and has the same feelings and reactions that occur in the real-life situation. Some comments heard after a good role play are, "Now I know how my mother feels!" Or "I never thought of it that way before." The experience of being in someone else's shoes can be very insightful.

In group drama therapy most therapists structure their sessions similarly with a warm-up first to help the clients feel comfortable and safe. When everyone is ready, the main action, where role play is often used, comes next. Lastly comes the sharing or processing of the session, which is equally if not more important than the action section.

In the processing or sharing part of the session, the players talk about the feelings they had in their role during the scene. If there is an audience, they are encouraged to express their feelings and responses also. Other possibilities are discussed. How else might the scene have gone, or what else could the person say? Everyone is encouraged to make some contribution. The processing discussion is as important as the action, helping people realize that there is always more than one solution to a problem.

Other types of group drama therapy include theater performances dealing with specific problem issues. These are most popular in community and school settings and usually address the kinds of life choices facing students today, e.g., drug and alcohol use, sexual conduct, violence, and problems with parents, teachers, and peers. Other groups present a production that offers information and/or education on a specific subject such as AIDS, drug abuse, illiteracy, dealing with violence, etc. Some performers stay in role to answer questions, and others offer workshops after the performance.

Who Uses Drama Therapy?

Since there are many techniques and variations of drama therapy, it is suitable for all age groups and populations. Most often it is practiced in groups and can be done in a variety of settings. Currently drama therapists are working with every population that can benefit from any of the creative arts therapies, including special education classes, psychiatric patients, persons recovering from substance abuse, trauma victims, dysfunctional families, developmentally and physically disabled persons, prison and correctional facility inmates, anorexic and bulimic patients, AIDS patients, the homeless, the elderly, children, and adolescents. These therapists provide services to individuals, groups, and families in addition to conducting clinical research.

With some groups the drama therapist is brought in to deal with a certain issue or offer training to deal with specific needs of the group. For example, a drama therapist may be contracted to work with a group of managers dealing with sexual harassment. All the exercises, role plays, and explorations will deal with bringing about a greater understanding and sensitivity to that subject.

Choosing a Drama Therapist

When choosing a drama therapist, verify that the person is an RDT, a registered drama therapist. This is the only valid

How to Become a Registered Drama Therapist

RDT, registered drama therapist, is the only valid credential for drama therapists. RDTs are registered through the National Association for Drama Therapy. Standards for registration include expertise in dramatic, theatrical, and performance media; an understanding of psychotherapeutic process with different populations in a variety of settings; integration of the artistic and psychological aspects of drama therapy; and professional expertise in the field of mental health and/or special education. An RDT/BC is board certified to give training in drama therapy.

credential for drama therapists. RDTs are registered through the National Association for Drama Therapy and have met rigorous standards for their credentials. Standards of registration for RDTs include the following: expertise in dramatic, theatrical, and performance media; an understanding of psychotherapeutic process with different populations in a variety of settings; integration of the artistic and psychological aspects of drama therapy; and professional expertise in the field of mental health and/or special education.

—*Patricia Sternberg, RDT/BCT*

Resources:

NADT National Office
15245 Shady Grove Road, Suite 130
Rockville, MD 20850
Tel: (301) 258–9210
The national office keeps an updated list of all RDTs, all registered drama therapists/board certified trainers (RDT/BCTs), and other members of the National Association of Drama Therapy. The RDT Registry is available and may be requested from the national office as well as further information on the organization.

Further Reading:

Bailey, Sally. *Wings to Fly: Bringing Theatre Arts to Students with Special Needs.* Rockville, MD: Woodbine House, 1993.

Emunah, Renee. *Acting for Real: Drama Therapy Process, Technique, and Performance.* New York: Brunner/Mazel, 1994.

Gersie, Alida. *Dramatic Approaches to Brief Therapy.* London: Jessica Kingsley, 1995.

Grainger, Roger. *Drama and Healing: The Roots of Drama Therapy.* London: Jessica Kingsley, 1990.

Landy, Robert. *Drama Therapy: Concepts, Theories and Practices.* Second edition. Springfield, IL: Charles C. Thomas, 1994.

Salas, Jo. *Improvising Real Life: Personal Story in Playback Theatre.* Dubuque, IA: Kendall/Hunt Pub. Co., 1993.

Schatner, Gertrude, and Richard Courtney. *Drama Therapy Vol. I and Vol. II.* New York: Drama Book Specialists, 1981.

Sternberg, Patricia, and Antonina Garcia. *Sociodrama: Who's in Your Shoes?* New York: Praeger Press, 1989.

HALPRIN LIFE/ART PROCESS

The Halprin life/art process is an integrative approach to movement, the expressive and the therapeutic arts. It is used to evoke the creative development and expression of the whole person, and to foster personal, interpersonal, and social transformation. The discipline is based on the belief that dance and the expressive arts, when connected with life concerns, can have a creative and healing role for an individual, the community, and the environment.

One drama therapist explains her work with substance abuse groups: "I begin by saying that drama therapy is an exploration of our strengths. I work with the imagination, helping my patients learn how to use it as a problem-solving tool." She goes on to say, "Oftentimes patients who are invited to attend a drama therapy session will say, 'I'm no actor' or 'I don't know how to act.' My answer to that is, 'It's not acting. It's human behavior and everybody does that.'" The ultimate compliment she hears about the benefits of drama therapy after a session with this population is, "I never knew you could have so much fun without being high!"

The Halprin life/art process was originated by dance pioneer Anna Halprin in the 1950s at the San Francisco Dancer's Workshop Company, a collaborating collective of dancers, musicians, and visual artists. Halprin tried to develop a form of modern dance that could foster the organic and authentic expression of the body, and integrate the emotions and imagination of the dancer. Beginning in the 1960s, Anna Halprin and her company worked with leaders in humanistic psychology, exploring relationships between art and therapy. Upon being diagnosed with cancer in 1972, Halprin devoted her research and teaching to the use of dance as a healing art, working with people challenging cancer, and later challenging AIDS.

Daria Halprin, Anna Halprin's daughter, was an original member of the Dancer's Workshop Company. She developed applications of the Halprin life/art process as a therapeutic and educational model to advance personal transformation. In 1978, Anna and Daria Halprin founded the Tamalpa Institute to teach the Halprin life/art process in training programs, workshops, and classes, all of which incorporate the application of the expressive arts to psychology, education, and health.

The Halprin life/art process addresses three dimensions of human experience: the physical, emotional, and mental. The *physical* is addressed through the study and practice of basic principles of somatic awareness, movement, and dance. The *emotional* is addressed through the study and practice of movement, drawing, and other therapeutic processes. The *mental* is addressed through the study and practice of group facilitation methods, collective creativity, communication skills, creative writing, and the presentation of theory. Each of these three aspects is studied and explored from the point of view of how it interrelates with all the other aspects.

In the Halprin life/art process, expressive art activities follow the model: move/draw/dialogue. This model evokes the physical, emotional, and mental aspects of the individual, often focusing on an identified life theme. For example, working with the theme balance/off balance, a class session might start with an exploration in movement of the physical experience of being in balance and off balance. The student or client would then draw two images inspired by the movement experience, which may be consciously or unconsciously connected with a life experience. The drawings are given titles that serve as a basis for a written piece: prose, poetry, or a dialogue between the two drawings. The theme balance/off balance is then reencountered as the student creates an expressive movement piece, which is consciously connected with the drawings and written script.

According to this discipline, an integrated and healthy life includes and honors creative expression. The Halprin life/art process is interested in how we can live artfully in our world today, and how we can bring the transformative power of art into our daily and community life. Practitioners apply their work as performance artists, teachers, and therapists. As leaders in community settings, they work with people and groups facing life-threatening issues, including cancer, AIDS, eating disorders, physical and sexual abuse, homelessness, addictions, and physical disabilities. Students have applied their work to environmental and cross-cultural issues.

—*Daria Halprin-Khalighi, M.A., CET*

Resources:

Tamalpa Institute
P.O. Box 794
Kentfield, CA 94914
Tel: (415) 457–8555
Fax: (415) 457–7190
e-mail: tamalpa@igc.apc.org
Offers training programs, workshops, and classes in the Halprin life/art process. Upon completion of the Practitioner Training Program, graduates are eligible

to apply for certification as an expressive arts therapist through the National Expressive Arts Association (NETA) and as a movement therapist through the International Somatic Movement Education and Therapy Association (ISMETA). The institute publishes a yearly newsletter, and distributes articles and books representing the Halprin life/art work.

Further Reading:

Halprin, Anna. *Movement Ritual.* Illustrated by Charlene Koonce. Kentfield, CA: Dancer's Workshop/Tamalpa Institute, 1990.

——. *Moving Toward Life: Five Decades of Transformational Dance.* Hanover, NH: Wesleyan University Press, 1995.

Halprin, Daria. *Coming Alive: The Creative Expression Method.* Kentfield, CA: Tamalpa Institute, 1990.

JOURNAL THERAPY

Journal therapy is the act of writing down thoughts and feelings to sort through problems and come to deeper understandings of oneself or the issues in one's life. Unlike traditional diary writing, where daily events and happenings are recorded from an exterior point of view, journal therapy focuses on the writer's internal experiences, reactions, and perceptions. Through this act of literally reading his or her own mind, the writer is able to perceive his or her own problems more clearly and thus feel a relief of emotional and mental tension that has also been shown to improve the immune system functioning of individuals.

The Development of Journal Writing for Well-Being

Although people have written diaries and journals for centuries, the therapeutic potential of reflective writing didn't come into public awareness until the 1960s, when Dr. Ira Progoff, a psychologist in New York City, began offering workshops and classes in the use of what he called the intensive journal method. Dr. Progoff had been using a "psychological notebook" with his therapy clients for several years. His intensive journal is a three-ring notebook with many color-coded sections for different aspects of the writer's psychological healing. The Progoff method of journal keeping quickly became popular, and today the method has been taught to more than 250,000 people through a network of "journal consultants" trained by Dr. Progoff and his staff.

In the late 1970s journal writing for personal growth and emotional wellness was introduced to a wider audience through the publication of three books. Dr. Progoff's *At a Journal Workshop* (1978) detailed his intensive journal process and gave instructions on how to set up an intensive journal for those who could not attend a journal workshop in person. In 1977 a young writer and teacher named Christina Baldwin published her first book, *One to One: Self-Understanding Through Journal Writing,* based on the adult education journal classes she had been teaching. And in 1978 Tristine Rainer published *The New Diary,* a comprehensive guidebook that for many years was the most complete and accessible source of information on how to use a journal for self-discovery and self-exploration.

The Philosophy of Journal Therapy

In the 1980s many public school systems began formally using journals in both English classes and other curricula as well. These journals, often called "dialogue" or "response" journals, offered a way for students to develop independent thinking skills and gave teachers a method for responding directly to students with individual feedback. Although the intention for classroom journals was educational rather than therapeutic, teachers noticed that a simple assignment to reflect on an academic question or problem often revealed important information about the student's emotional life. Students often reported feeling a relief of pressure and tension when they could write down troubling events or confusing thoughts or feelings.

Probably one of the most common reports from people who write journals is that the act of putting thoughts and feelings on paper helps give useful emotional and mental clarity. However, there is scientific evidence that the relief from writing things down is more than just psychological. Dr. James Pennebaker, a researcher in Texas, has conducted studies that show that when people write about emotionally difficult events or feelings for just twenty minutes at a time over three or four days, their immune system functioning increases. Dr. Pennebaker's studies indicate that the release offered by writing has a direct impact on the body's capacity to withstand stress and fight off infection and disease.

After the publication of the Pennebaker studies, the medical and therapeutic communities began taking a closer look at journal writing as a holistic, nonmedicinal method for wellness. In 1985, Kathleen Adams, a psychotherapist in Colorado and the founder/director of the Center for Journal Therapy, began teaching journal workshops designed to give the general public tools that could be used for self-discovery, creative expression and life enhancement. Her "journal toolbox" of writing techniques offers a way to match a specific life issue with a specific writing device to address it. Her first book, *Journal to the Self: 22 Paths to Personal Growth,* was published in 1990. Through a network of certified instructors, the Journal to the Self workshop is available throughout the United States, Canada, and several other countries.

Journal Therapy in Practice

Although there are many psychotherapists who incorporate journal therapy into their sessions by assigning written "homework," there are relatively few who specialize in journal therapy. Therapists who utilize journal writing in a session often begin by asking the client to write a short "check-in" paragraph or two on "what's going on"—how the client is feeling, what he or she wants to work on in the session, and what's happening in his or her life that impacts the therapeutic work at hand. This writing is usually shared with the therapist and an "agenda" for the session is set. The therapist then guides the client through a writing exercise designed to address the therapeutic issues or tasks that the client has brought forward in the check-in or warm-up writing or exercise. The second writing usually takes about ten minutes, and the remainder of the session is spent with the client and therapist talking about the information revealed in the longer writing. The session generally concludes with the therapist offering several suggestions for journal "homework" to be completed between sessions.

Journal therapy is also very effective in groups, and it is common for group members to establish a sense of deep community as writings representing authentic expressions of self are shared.

At present, there is one graduate educational program in poetry therapy at Vermont College of Norwich. This program teaches techniques in journal therapy. Generally, journal therapists first obtain an advanced degree in psychology, counseling, social work, or a related field. They may then enter a credentialing program such as that offered by the National Association for Poetry Therapy, or an independent-study program such as that offered through Kathleen Adams' Center for Journal Therapy or through Dr. Progoff's Dialogue House.

Benefits of Journal Therapy

It is believed that by recording and describing the salient issues in one's life, one can better understand these issues and eventually diagnose problems that stem from them. Journal therapy has been used effectively for grief and loss; coping with life-threatening or chronic illness; recovery from addictions, eating disorders and trauma; repairing troubled marriages and family relationships; increasing communication skills; developing a healthier sense of self-identity; getting a better perspective on life; and clarifying life goals.

—*Kathleen Adams, M.A., LPC*

Resources:

The Center for Journal Therapy
P. O. Box 963
Arvada, CO 80001
Tel: (303) 421-2298
Organization dedicated to the instruction and practice of journal therapy.

The Dialogue House
80 E. 11th Street
New York, NY 10009
Tel: (212) 673-5880
Fax: (212) 673-0582
Provides several intensive workshops that utilize the journal therapy method.

The National Association of Poetry Therapy
P.O. Box 551
Port Washington, NY 11050
Tel: (516) 944-9794
Web site: www.poetrytherapy.org.
Multidisciplinary professional organization for students and practitioners of journal therapy.

Further Reading:

Adams, Kathleen. *Journal to the Self: 22 Paths to Personal Growth.* New York: Warner Books, 1990.

——. *The Way of the Journal: A Journal Therapy Workbook for Healing.* Lutherville, MD: Sidran Press, 1993.

——. *Mightier than the Sword: The Journal as a Path to Men's Self-Discovery.* New York: Warner Books, 1994.

Baldwin, Christina. *One to One: Self-Understanding Through Journal Writing.* New York: Evans & Co., 1977.

——. *Life's Companion: Journal Writing as Spiritual Quest.* New York: Bantam Books, 1990.

Oshinsky, James. *The Discovery Journal.* 2nd ed. Odessa, MD: Psychological Assessment Resources, 1994.

Progoff, Ira. *At a Journal Workshop.* New York: Dialogue House, 1978.

Rainer, Tristine. *The New Diary.* Los Angeles: J. P. Tarcher, 1978.

MULTI-MODAL EXPRESSIVE ARTS THERAPY

Multi-modal expressive arts therapy integrates various forms of arts into a therapeutic relationship to foster awareness, encourage emotional growth, and enhance relationships with others. It promotes healing through the transformative power of both the arts and psychotherapy. By activating the imagination, this therapy enables self-exploration and self-understanding; by working within more than one medium, it amplifies and clarifies self-discoveries; and by expressing these discoveries through images, sound, movement, and words, it expands communication.

The History of Multi-Modal Expressive Arts Therapy

The arts have been brought together to shape and express human experience since the dawn of civilization. Paleolithic cave paintings indicate that early humans used art as a means for passing spiritual, social, and hunting skills from generation to generation. In ancient Greece, dramas incorporating music, dance, and storytelling brought crowds to amphitheaters for a collective experience of the tragic and comedic dimensions of life. Intricate hierarchies of religious and sociopolitical belief were woven into the art and architecture of medieval Europe. Today, many forms of theater, dance, performance art, and multimedia installation art are used in concert to bring people together to participate in cathartic release from life's sorrows and gain a better understanding of individual and communal identity.

While multi-modal expressive arts therapy draws on this entire body of the arts, it is a development of the last half century. After World War II, American veterans' hospitals integrated music, dance, and drama into an alternative method of treatment for veterans struggling to recuperate from the ordeal of battle. In Europe during the 1950s, innovative educators formulated an approach that engaged children in multiple art forms, which they believed would help foster full sensory development. Then, in the 1960s, versatile European and American performance artists began combining various forms of art to convey their messages and touch their audiences.

Changes in education, the fine arts, and medical treatment of trauma opened the way for the gradual emergence of therapy programs that take a holistic approach to both art and healing. By 1969 there was a graduate training program in expressive arts therapy at the University of Louisville in Kentucky. A decade later, expressive arts therapy had become a widely recognized mode of treatment for children and adults with special needs, had its own professional organization, the American Association of Artist-Therapists (later called the National Expressive Therapy Association), and an emergent nascent scholarly literature.

The Theory of Multi-Modal Expressive Arts Therapy

In a doctoral dissertation of 1978, *Intermodal Learning in Education and Therapy*, Paolo Knill postulated that multi-modal

expressive arts therapy is not simply a loose gathering of the arts under the umbrella of therapy, but rather a highly sophisticated way of bringing the imagination into the work of healing. Unlike exclusively verbal therapies, it centers upon the embodiment and transformation of emotions. They are expressed in one medium, then translated into others. As one is led through a series of creative arts experiences, the imagination grows more active, and at the same time emotions are explored, clarified, and transformed, helping people to connect with themselves, with others, and with a greater sense of purpose and meaning in life.

Experiencing Multi-Modal Expressive Arts Therapy

Multi-modal expressive arts therapy is generally experienced as a type of group therapy in a school, nursing home, or some other institutional setting. The length and structure of sessions will vary, based on the specific method of the therapist and the needs of the group or individual participant. Children may have a half-hour session, adult outpatients' sessions may last over an hour, and intensive workshops may go on for several days. The range of structure is no less broad, from sessions with a predetermined format and topic to sessions that encourage spontaneous engagement with the arts and dynamic interaction between participants.

Activity in all but the most loosely structured sessions is usually divided into three phases. A short "warm-up" that helps participants overcome inhibitions and start to tap their imaginations is followed by a longer phase devoted to a series of art activities designed to uncover, explore, and transform the participants' feelings. In the third phase, participants reflect on the sounds, movements, images, or words they have created, as well as the process of forming them.

A multi-modal expressive arts therapy session might begin by having participants stand in a circle and take turns making a movement that expresses their immediate feelings. In the second phase of the session, they might use oil crayons, pastels, or a felt-tipped pen first to transfer that movement onto a large piece of drawing paper, then to elaborate the graphic mark into a picture. Other transformations will probably follow. The therapist might suggest that the participants look at one another's pictures and leave a written response on a nearby piece of paper. Each participant then uses the words and phrases to compose a poem that she or he recites to the group. The sequential unfolding of expression, from physical gesture to recited poem, becomes the basis for a concluding discussion that might consider the interplay of emotion, bodily movement, and verbal expression or the insights gained through group interaction.

The Benefits of Multi-Modal Expressive Arts Therapy

By engaging the imagination, multi-modal expressive arts therapy promotes the creative release of emotions and stimulates the development of self-esteem and a capacity for self-healing. Since it integrates many aspects of personal growth from the sensory to the emotional to the social, multi-modal expressive arts therapy is often used by individuals who are coping with physical or mental disabilities, as well as the effects of aging, loss, and isolation.

Susan Spaniol, Ed.D., ATR
Philip Speiser, Ph.D., CET
Mariagnese Cattaneo, Ph.D., ATR

Resources:

European Foundation for Interdisciplinary Studies (EGIS)
Forchstrasse, 106

CH 8032 Zurich
Switzerland
Fax: 382 33 07
An international professional organization for expressive therapists.

Expressive Arts Program
California Institute of Integral Studies
9 Peter Yorke Way
San Francisco, CA 94109
Tel: (415) 674-5500
Offers a master's degree in counseling psychology with a specialization in expressive arts therapy.

Expressive Therapies Program
Lesley College
29 Everett Street
Cambridge, MA 02138
Tel: (617) 349-8425
Offers a comprehensive graduate program in multi-modal expressive arts therapy.

International Expressive Arts Therapy Association
P.O. Box 64126
San Francisco, CA 94164
Tel: (415) 522-8959
A professional organization dedicated to multi-modal expressive arts therapy.

International School for Interdisciplinary Studies (ISIS)
Forchstrasse, 106
CH 8032 Zurich
Switzerland
Fax: 382 33 09
A training institute in multi-modal expressive arts therapy.

Further Reading:

Books:

Knill, P. J., H. N. Barba, and M. N. Fuchs. *Minstrels of Soul: Intermodal Expressive Therapy.* Toronto: Palmerston Press, 1993.

Levine, S. K. *Poiesis: The Language of Psychology and the Speech of the Soul.* Toronto: Palmerston Press, 1992.

Advanced art-making skills or expensive equipment is not needed to take part in multi-modal expressive arts therapy.

Rogers, N. *The Creative Connection: Expressive Arts as Healing.* Palo Alto, CA: Science & Behavior Books. 1993.

Journals:

Lusebrink, V. "A Systems-Oriented Approach to the Expressive Therapies: The Expressive Therapies Continuum." *The Arts in Psychotherapy* 5 (1991): 395–403.

MUSIC THERAPY

Music therapy is a profession that believes in the therapeutic potential inherent in music. Qualified music therapists use music and/or musical elements such as sound, rhythm, melody, and harmony with individuals or groups to help people improve, change, or better integrate different aspects of their selves. Listening to, moving to, and creating music are used to help resolve emotional, social, familial, cognitive, physiological, and developmental problems. While recognition of the therapeutic powers of music is ancient and widespread, formally, it became a type of therapy in the 1950s.

Connecting the Basic Elements of Music to Human Development

The fundamental elements of music—sound, rhythm, hearing, and movement—and people's prenatal and primary experience with these elements are paramount to music therapists. They consider music's basic elements essential in the development of human beings and deeply rooted in the very beginning of a human life. Research shows that the human fetus can hear at four months of fetal life. A developing fetus hears voices, noises, and the sounds of its own and its mother's heartbeat and digestive system. After birth, a baby continues experiencing rhythm and beat in the sound of its mother's heartbeat and breathing, and in its mother's rocking motions. The baby's very first sign of life at birth, crying, is seen by music therapists as combining the primary elements of music—rhythm, movement, and sound—in the service of self-expression and communication with other people.

Music's Therapeutic Nature

One can find references to the therapeutic powers of music in philosophy, art, and literature throughout the ages. In the Bible, young David, known for his musical talents, is brought to play the lyre before King Saul, in the hope that this would alleviate the King's ill humor (Samuel I, 16, 14–23). Greek mythology ascribed a divine origin to music. In the mythological world, music had magical powers; people believed it could heal sickness and purify the body and the mind. Among the Greeks, music was thought to be an activity related to the pursuit of truth and beauty.

The therapeutic power of music plays an important role in the healing ceremonies of early cultures throughout the world. Healers and shamans use chants, incantations, rhythmic playing of drums and rattles, clapping, and stomping to induce hypnotic or ecstatic states. When in this altered state of consciousness they communicate with the spirit world, which helps them exorcise bad spirits, cure illnesses, and soothe and relax patients.

Everyday experience also points to the psychological effect that music can have on us. Most would agree that even given varying musical tastes, certain types of music create specific moods. A wedding march creates a different mood than does a funeral dirge. Scary movies use ominous music to create suspense. Bands play lively music at sporting events to excite the crowd. A doctor may play quiet easy-listening or classical music in his waiting room to help soothe patients. Mothers sing to and rock their babies in times of distress.

The Development of Music Therapy as a Profession

Music therapy was established as a profession in the United States in the 1950s. Professionals from various disciplines, such as music, education, medicine, and psychology, had been using music while working with various populations and found, through their clinical experience, that music yielded remarkable therapeutic results. In their experience, individuals suffering from severe impairments, be they sensory, motor, mental, or emotional, seemed to show startling improvement when working with music. By 1950, the National Association for Music Therapy (NAMT) was created, and training programs for music therapists were initiated in several colleges and universities. Around this time, methodical research expanded, as well as the formulation of theories, clinical models, and professional publications. In 1998 the American Association of Music Therapy (AAMT) and NAMT merged into one association called the American Music Therapy Association (AMTA).

Today, music therapy is practiced worldwide. It is an extremely varied and flexible profession, found within such disciplines as special education, rehabilitation, psychiatry, psychotherapy, and geriatrics. It is practiced in hospitals, clinics, rehabilitation centers, schools, and private settings.

The Principles of Music Therapy

All models of music therapy encourage an individual to find and express his or her uniqueness through music. Because it focuses on the process of self-discovery and not on the end product, one need not have any musical skills or talent in order to utilize or benefit from music therapy. The music that is produced is not judged as good or bad.

The therapeutic agents of music therapy are dual: on one hand there is music, and on the other, the relationship between client and therapist. Because music is deeply rooted in the early physio-psychological development of an individual, making music touches upon the unconscious in a direct, unmediated way. This enables individuals to connect themselves directly to repressed material, forgotten or masked memories, or to enter into regressive emotional states, which allow further exploration of issues central to the self.

The other therapeutic agent is the relationship between client and therapist. In order for music activity to be therapeutic, it must take place within the framework of a reliable relationship with a therapist, a relationship that is characterized by trust, respect, and a serious commitment to the process. As this relationship becomes more meaningful, so does the musical activity that takes place within its framework.

Some Techniques of Music Therapy

Music therapists use varied techniques and models for their work, which they adapt to their clients' needs and ages as well as the setting of each session (individual vs. group, for example). Nevertheless, all types of music therapy search for the individuality of the client as expressed through music. This search is carried out with active help and support from the therapist.

Many clinical models in music therapy use instrumental or vocal improvisation. Because of its spontaneous and expressive qualities, musical improvisation is a particularly potent method of shedding light on aspects of the self that are many times obscured or blocked by one's conscious thinking or behavior. Music therapists are trained to understand improvised music as a unique personal language. In music therapy, both client and therapist set out to explore and reveal the form and meaning of this special language.

For an adult client with emotional problems, a session might begin with a verbal discussion of a current issue. Then, client and therapist find a way to investigate issues through sound in various

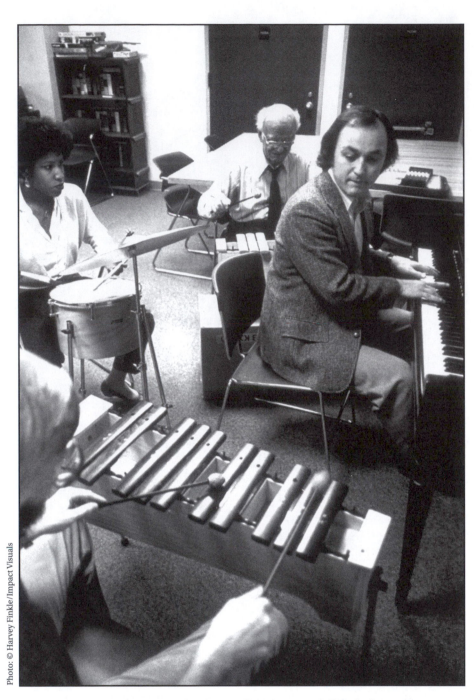

Photo: © Harvey Finkle/Impact Visuals

Musical improvisation requires listening to oneself and others.

ways. For example, one might choose to play an instrument, sing, or write words to a song. This musical experience occurs in the "here and now" but later becomes material for discussion and the development of better self-under-standing.

Another type of music therapy uses recorded music as a stimulus for exploring the self. Clients are induced to a state of relaxation through breathing and suggestive imagery. Music carefully selected by the therapist is played, and the client is invited to explore images, sensations, memories, and visions prompted by the music. Sometimes the client achieves an altered state of consciousness, which is usually extremely positive and relaxing and can lead to self-discovery. After the listening experience, the client is brought out of the relaxed state and is invited to discuss the experience with the therapist. In some models the client is invited to choose preferred selections and listen, move, or paint to that music.

Music is also used in family and group therapy. Special techniques have been developed to utilize music's inherent social character. One outstanding feature of the art of music is the possibility to produce and perceive several sounds simultaneously as with orchestras, ensembles, and choirs. Although something of this sort takes place in all of the performing arts, its effect is most dramatic in music. For example: members of a family in therapy may be asked to choose a musical instrument and then improvise a performance. The "music of the family" proves to be enormously indicative in showing who is "in harmony" with whom in the family, who gets the role of making "disturbing noises" or "clashing sounds," who picks a very loud instrument that prevents everybody else from being heard, or who gives up playing their favorite instrument because someone else demanded it. Group or family musical improvisations often reveal hidden agendas, tensions and dilemmas, self-defeating communication patterns, and other problems. These problems are sometimes easier to perceive, express, and deal with when manifested in music.

The Benefits of Music Therapy

Music therapy is suitable for individuals of all ages, even young babies. Music therapy is used to help autistic children acquire communication skills. It has been shown to improve the skills of individuals with learning disabilities, and to help people deal with emotional, social, and familial problems. Music therapy is utilized in individual, family, and group settings, as well as with couples. It has

been used by therapists to help people recovering from accidents, including individuals recovering from cerebro-vascular accidents and major surgery.

—Adva Frank-Schwebel

Resources:

American Association for Music Therapy (AAMT)
P.O. Box 27177
Philadelphia, PA 19118
Tel: (215) 265-4006
Association for professional music therapists that publishes the journal Music Therapy *and also holds conferences. It also determines credentials for certified music therapists (CMTs).*

National Association of Music Therapy (NAMT)
8455 Colesville Road, Suite 930
Silver Spring, MD 20910
Tel: (301) 589-3300
Association of professional music therapists that provides registered music therapist (RMT) credentials. It also publishes the Journal of Music Therapy *and holds music therapy conferences.*

Further Reading:

Books:

Bonny, H., and L. Savary. *Music and Your Mind: Listening with a New Consciousness.* New York: Harper and Row, 1973.

Bruscia, K. E. *Improvisational Models of Music Therapy.* Springfield, IL: C. Thomas Charles, 1987.

Feder, S., R. L. Karmel and G. H. Pollock, eds. *Psychoanalytic Exploration in Music.* Madison, CT: International Universities Press, 1990.

Maranto, Cheryl Dielo, ed. *Perspectives on Music Therapy Education and Training.* Philadelphia, PA: Temple University, 1987.

Nordoff, Paul, and Clive Robbins. *Creative Music Therapy.* New York: John Day Co., 1977.

Priestley, Mary. *Music Therapy in Action.* St. Louis: MMB Music, 1985.

Sekeles, Charles. *Music, Motion and Emotion: The Developmental-Integrative Model in Music Therapy.* St. Louis: MMB Music, 1996.

Verney, T., and G. Kelly. *The Secret Life of the Unborn Child.* London: Sphere Books, 1981.

Journals:
Noy, P. "The Psychodynamic Meaning of Music–Part II." *Journal of Music Therapy,* 4 (1): 7–23.

POETRY THERAPY

Poetry therapy involves reading, writing, reciting, and/or creating poetry as well as other language arts to cope with emotions related to psychological, physical, and social problems. Poetry therapy uses the imaginative and emotional qualities of all types of literature and is therefore not limited to the specific genre of poetry— metaphor, poetry reading, journal writing, song lyrics, storytelling, and prose writing may be used. It should be noted that bibliotherapy, the use of reading to help individuals, has an extensive history and is now considered a part of poetry therapy. For all practical purposes, the terms are now synonymous. Many professionals such as social workers, psychologists, nurses, physicians, counselors, and special education teachers use poetry therapy as a tool in their work. Other professionals have received advanced training in poetry therapy methods and developed it as their primary method of practice.

Poetry: An Ancient Form of Therapy

The notion of poetry as therapeutic has ancient roots. For ages poetry has been a method through which people have pondered the human condition and expressed their sorrows, joys, and epiphanies. The ancient Greeks made Apollo the god of both poetry and healing. In the early eighteenth century psychiatrists started using the various expressive arts in order to soothe patients' anguish and as a medium to encourage dialogue and social interaction. The general population has also used poetry and literature as a form of catharsis. For example, one might be cheered by a limerick, or be comforted by an eloquent expression of grief that a person feels speaks to his or her own emotions. Robert Haven Schauffler wrote a prescriptive book called *The Poetry Cure: A Pocket Medicine Chest of Verse,* which was published in 1925. The book contains numerous poems that are categorized for use with specific life problems.

The formal development of poetry therapy as a discipline begins with Jack J. Leedy, a psychiatrist, who in 1969 founded the Association for Poetry Therapy (APT) in New York. In 1973, Arthur Lerner, a psychologist and poet, founded the Poetry Therapy Institute in California. In 1981, APT became formally incorporated as the National Association for Poetry Therapy (NAPT). The NAPT sponsors annual conventions and has helped set standards and procedures for certification and registration of poetry therapists.

Human Experience Captured in Symbols and Images

Language and feelings are central to both poetry and therapy. Similar to other arts therapies such as music and dance, poetry therapy concerns itself with symbolism, verbal and nonverbal expression, rhythm, order, and balance. Psychotherapy, for example, often addresses an individual's interpretation of certain past events and/or fears about the present and future. Poetry has the capacity to capture similar human experiences through symbols and images. Also, the rhythm of certain poems can affect the reader's mood. Some poems might be used for a calming effect, while others might be used to energize clients.

Poetry therapy provides a vehicle for individuals to express what might be

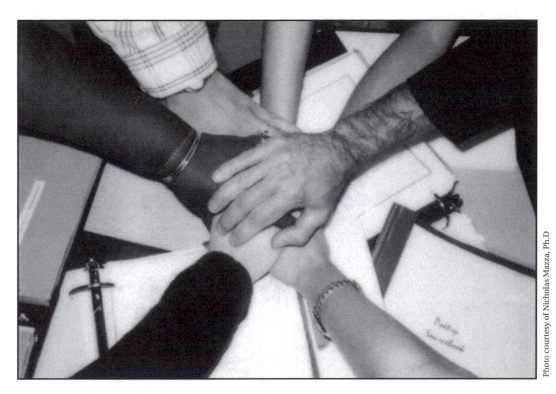

Sharing emotions through poetry can help people break through feelings of isolation.

difficult to express under ordinary circumstances. By talking about a poem, one can relate personal material. Often an emotional identification can be made with a poem that reflects a person's thoughts or feelings on a particular matter. The poem can also help the person to feel that he or she is not alone. Writing a poem (or letter, story, or journal entry) can be empowering by providing a sense of order and control to an individual. The act of writing integrates one's thinking, feeling, and behaving. The sharing of reactions to poetry or the sharing of one's own work also has the potential to build interpersonal relationships and communication skills.

The Techniques of Poetry Therapy

There are a variety of techniques that can be used depending upon the professional's education and training. For example, a social worker might use a poem to validate a feeling or promote insight with a depressed individual in a therapy session. In this situation the poetry is part of the therapy. A poet might start a writing program in a runaway shelter. In this case, the purpose might be educational or life enriching rather than therapeutic; however, the therapeutic aspects of writing are recognized. Following are a number of ways in which poetry is used to help people:

- *Introduce an existing poem to an individual, group, or family and invite reactions.* The theme of the poem should relate to the issues of the individual or group. If a person is having a hard time making an important decision, then a poem such as Robert Frost's "The Road Not Taken" could be connected to the struggle of the individual. A discussion of possible "roads" that the person might take could follow.
- *Collaborative poems.* Sometimes communication breaks down in families and conflicts develop. Each member of a family is invited to contribute

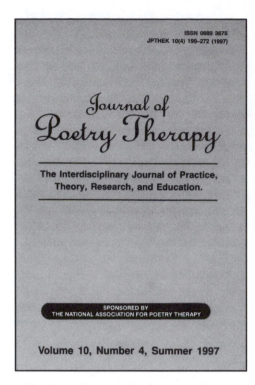

The National Association for Poetry Therapy sponsors a journal, in addition to annual conventions.

one or more lines to a family or group poem, thereby valuing each person's view. The task also allows the family to engage in problem solving (constructing the poem) and working together rather than pointing blame at each other.

- *Creative writing.* The writing could be free writing— that is, covering any topic and using any form—or it could consist of structured exercises. For example, an acrostic—where each line of the poem begins with a letter from a particular word, or the use of sentence stems like "If you knew me . . ."—could provide a structure to facilitate self-expression.
- *Journal writing.* Provides another outlet for an individual to express and sort out a variety of thoughts and feelings.
- *Letter writing.* Sometimes it is difficult or impossible to say things to important people in our life. Writing a letter to a deceased friend or family member

can be helpful in working through grief, anger, and frustration. It could also serve as a very positive memorial for a loved one.

- *Recommending specific readings for a particular problem.* In the tradition of bibliotherapy, certain fiction and nonfiction could be used for life guidance. For example, Judith Viorst's "The Tenth Good Thing About Barney" might be a good story to read to a child whose pet died.

Limitations of Poetry Therapy

Like any therapeutic tool, anything that has the power to heal also has the power to harm. Poetry therapy should be used by professionals with training in psychology and a good understanding of literature. It is very important that the individual using it stay within the boundaries of his or her profession. Care must be given to the selection and timing of a poem. Sharing a poem or song may bring up feelings one is not ready to deal with at the time. If a particular poem or song is not fully discussed, a destructive or unhealthy conclusion could be reached. Therapists should be sure to choose works that, while empathizing with the client's problem, ultimately express hope. The therapist should also know the problems and limitations of the clients. The use of poetry may be insulting, especially if there is a literacy problem and the person is asked to read. Sometimes, the poem may serve as a distraction for a client. A person might spend a great deal of time intellectualizing rather than dealing with a pressing problem. If a person focuses on journal writing at the exclusion of interpersonal relationships, his or her fear and isolation could increase, or conclusions could be reached without benefit of healthy discussion.

Advantages

Poetry therapy can serve as a non-threatening means for people to express their thoughts, feelings, and behaviors. It is respectful of different cultures and genders by trying to understand the personalized meanings of each person's language and story. Increasingly, more research is indicating that writing has a healing effect and can help people gain emotional strength. It has also been shown that in group counseling, the use of poetry therapy increases cohesion.

Poetry therapy is being used across the United States and around the world. It is used in a variety of settings, including hospitals, hospice facilities, correctional settings, homeless shelters, schools, runaway shelters, and mental health centers. In a time of pervasive social problems and rapidly increasing technology, poetry therapy touches and affirms our humanity.

—*Nicholas Mazza, Ph.D.*

Resources:

The *Journal of Poetry Therapy*
Human Sciences Press
233 Spring Street
New York, NY 10013-1578
The Journal of Poetry Therapy *is the official quarterly journal of the National Association for Poetry Therapy and is a membership benefit. The journal offers a wide variety of original articles, brief reports, dissertation abstracts, and poetry.*

The National Association for Poetry Therapy
   (NAPT)
P.O. Box 551
Port Washington, NY 11050
Tel: (516) 944-9791
The National Association for Poetry Therapy (NAPT) is an organization open to all persons interested in the healing capacities of the language arts. There are various levels of membership, including professional, regular, student, and retired. NAPT confers professional credentials— certified poetry therapist (CPT) and registered poetry therapist (RPT). It maintains a registry of practitioners and information regarding training.

Further Reading:

Hynes, Arleen McCarty, and Mary Hynes-Berry. *Biblio/Poetry Therapy–The Interactive Process: A Handbook.* St. Cloud, MN: North Star Press of St. Cloud, Inc., 1994.

PROBLEM	POEM
Decision Making	"The Road Not Taken" by Robert Frost
Anxiety	"If I Should Cast. . ." by Stephen Crane
Stress	"Can't Do It All" by Natasha Josefowitz
Family	Nikki Rosa" by Nikki Giovanni
Grief	"Good Night, Willie Lee. . ." by Alice Walker
Anger	"A Just Anger" by Marge Piercy
Despair	"Hope Is a Thing with Feathers" by Emily Dickinson
Alienation	"Alone/December night" by Victor Cruz
Communication	"Two Friends" by David Ignatow
Identity	"I'm nobody" by Emily Dickinson

Leedy, Jack J., ed. *Poetry as Healer: Mending the Troubled Mind.* New York: Vanguard Press, 1985. [Note: This book is a combination of two previous classics edited by Leedy, *Poetry Therapy* (1969) and *Poetry the Healer* (1973).]

Lerner, Arthur, ed. *Poetry in the Therapeutic Experience.* St. Louis: MMB Music, Inc., 1994.

Lerner, Arthur, and Ursula Mahlendorf, eds. *Life Guidance Through Literature.* Chicago: American Library Association, 1992.

Web Sites:
Internet Poetry Archive Home Page
www.sunsite.unc.edu/dykki/poetry/home.html

National Association for Poetry Therapy (NAPT)
www.poetrytherapy.org

National Coalition of Arts Therapies Associations (NCATA)
www.membrane.com/ncata

SANDPLAY THERAPY

Sandplay therapy is a form of psychological treatment that centers upon play with a vast collection of miniature figures and two sandboxes, one that contains damp sand, the other one dry. Unlike verbal therapies that deal directly with inner memories, sandplay involves the construction of scenes in which self-expression can be indirect and nonverbal. This therapeutic approach is considered particularly appropriate for children because it provides a safe way to act out troubling feelings that may be at the root of behavioral problems. Furthermore, the scenes themselves are thought to be a sensitive approach to determine the way mind and body come together in the totality of personal development. Sandplay therapy's most widely used theoretical model makes use of symbols and archetypes derived from the theories propounded by Swiss psychotherapist C. G. Jung. Though children are the usual clients of sandplay therapy, it is also used effectively with adults on their spiritual path to individuation.

The History of Sandplay Therapy

Sandplay therapy began with the research of Margaret Lowenfeld, a child psychiatrist active in England during the 1920s and 1930s—decades when the role of objects in child development attracted general interest among analysts who were working with children. The particular focus of Lowenfeld's work was the inner drama revealed in a child's use of his or her toys. The world technique, devised by Lowenfeld, transposed such play into structures that lent themselves to observation and analysis, yet did not force the child to adapt to adult logic. Lowenfeld asked the child to make pictures in the sandbox using the available miniatures. She found that a child would fashion intricate scenes that Lowenfeld regarded as representations of the child's world. Interpreting the pictures, she acknowledged, was difficult, in large part because of the ever-present danger of imposing adult norms on childhood experiences. Nonetheless, she believed that the world technique offered a means of gaining privileged access to the world of the child for both diagnostic and therapeutic purposes.

Dora Kalff, a Swiss therapist, brought Lowenfeld's work into the second half of the twentieth century, and she never doubted the healing powers of this technique. Kalff's training at the Jung Institute in Zurich led her to view the miniatures as a counterpart to Jungian archetypes. Kalff was influenced by German Jungian analyst Erich Neumann's studies of child development; she was able to correlate her observations of sandplay constructions with Neumann's theories. According to Kalff, the healing powers of sandplay therapy, as she termed her variant of world technique, are explained by its capacity to help

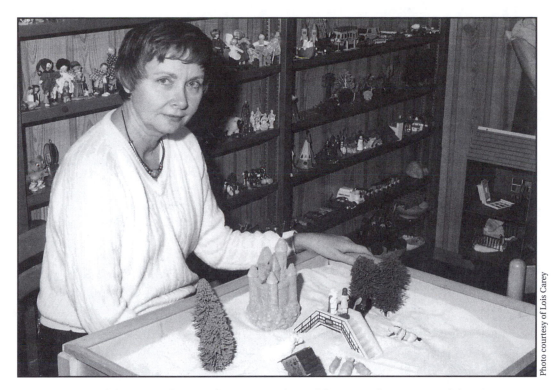

Photo courtesy of Lois Carey

Lois Carey with her vast collection of miniature archetypal figures used to create sandplay pictures.

traumatized children in their struggle toward internal ego support and full autonomy.

An understanding of Jungian archetypes and the archetypal level of the psyche is what differentiates this approach to sandplay from other theories. Jung's structure of the psyche proposes that the psyche is made up of three levels: the conscious, the personal unconscious, and the collective unconscious, which is the area wherein the archetypes are found. An archetype is simply a model or prototype of an idea, such as the "Great Mother," the "Wise Old Man," the "Hero," the "Anima/Animus," or the "Ego/Self." Archetypes are two-sided, having both positive and negative aspects. They are believed to be in the psyches of all people in all cultures. Knowledge of the archetypes allows the analyst to transmit his or her understanding of the client's struggle, most often nonverbally, in the interactive

field. For instance, the analyst is aware that a child's mother has died. It is to be assumed that the child in therapy will seek to connect with the lost mother in some way. If the analyst is aware of the archetypal level of the psyche, he or she will be able to observe, for example, when the Great Mother archetype (in both her positive and negative forms) emerges. This can enhance the analyst's unspoken understanding of this child's struggle and deepen the connection between child and therapist.

A System of Representation

As taught by Kalff, sandplay therapy is based on the belief that symbols and myth constitute a world history of, and psychological "guidebook" to, the ways by which human beings come to an understanding of themselves and their culture. By providing ready access to this system of representation, sandplay therapy enables clients to explore and expand their awareness of the dominant issues in their lives. The Kalffian/Jungian therapist approaches the child as a unique, complex being with an innate capacity for symbolic logic as revealed through an archetypal struggle witnessed in sandplay.

Making Pictures

Sandplay therapy employs sandboxes that are shallow, rectangular, and of a size (twenty by twenty-eight by four inches) that permits rapid, easy assembly of a picture. Two boxes—one with dry, the other with wet sand—are made available. The small size of the sandbox is important because it gives the client a sense of security and, at the same time, forces him or her to make choices since it can accommodate only a portion of the miniatures displayed on shelves around the sandplay room. After suggesting that the client make a picture, the therapist becomes more or less a silent observer of the process and has been taught to withhold interpretations until the therapy has progressed to the point where the ego is solid enough to accept interpretations. Premature interpretations usually impact the therapy quite negatively. In this technique, there is strong emphasis on the nonverbal ability of the psyche to seek its own healing, given the proper milieu.

The Benefits and Risks of Sandplay Therapy

While sandplay therapy poses no unusual risks to clients, it does require the help of a skilled analyst if the full range of its benefits is to be attained. One cautionary note: If there is any overt resistance to using sandplay, it is never pushed because the resistance may be serving a protective psychic function and must always be honored.

—*Lois Carey*

Resources:

Association for Play Therapy
California School of Professional Psychology
1350 M Street
Fresno, CA 93721
Holds conferences that include presentations on recent work with sandplay therapy.

Center for Sandplay Studies
252 South Boulevard
Upper Grandview, NY 10960
Tel: (914) 358-2318
Offers beginning and advanced courses in sandplay therapy.

Sandplay Therapists of America
P.O. Box 4847
Walnut Creek, CA 94596
Tel: (310) 607-8535
Organization that holds conferences and publishes a journal on sandplay therapy.

Further Reading:

Books:
Carey, Lois. *Sandplay with Children and Families.* Northvale, NJ: Jason Aronson, Inc., 1998.

Friedman, Harriet, and R. Mitchell. *Sandplay: Past, Present and Future.* London: Routledge, 1994.

Despite Dora Kalff's book *Sandplay* and many lectures, training in sandplay therapy has never been widely available. While some advocates remain committed to the Kalff-Jung legacy and offer a pure form of sandplay, a growing number of analysts and educators approach it on a pragmatic basis as a natural form of healing with strong affinities to art and play therapy.

Jung, C. G. *The Archetypes and the Collective Unconscious*. Princeton, NJ: Bollingen Paperback, 1980.

Kalff, Dora. *Sandplay: A Psychotherapeutic Approach to the Psyche*. Santa Monica: Sigo Press, 1980.

Lowenfeld, Margaret. *The World Technique*. London: George Allen and Unwin Ltd., 1979.

Neumann, Erich. *The Child*. Boston: Shambhala, 1990.

Stevens, Anthony. *Archetypes*. New York: Quill, 1982.

Wilmer, Harry. *Practical Jung*. Wilmette, IL: Chiron, 1991.

Journals:

Carey, Lois. "Sandplay Therapy with a Troubled Child." *Arts in Psychotherapy* 17, No. 3 (1990): 197–209.

——. "Family Sandplay Therapy." *Arts in Psychotherapy* 18 (1991): 231–39.

——. "A Child-Centered Approach to Family Sandplay Therapy." *Quaternio: Journal of the Brazilian Society of Jungian Psychotherapy* 1, No. 3 (1992): 6–11.

PART XVI: BODY-ORIENTED PSYCHOTHERAPIES

Bioenergetics • Bodynamic Analysis • Core Energetics • coreSomatics® • Emotional-Kinesthetic Psychotherapy • Focusing • Gestalt Therapy • Hakomi Integrative Somatics • Holotropic Breathwork™ • Medical Orgone Therapy • Organismic Body Psychotherapy • Pesso Boyden System Psychomotor • Process Oriented Psychology • Psychodrama • Psychosynthesis • Radix • Rebirthing • Rubenfeld Synergy Method • Unergi

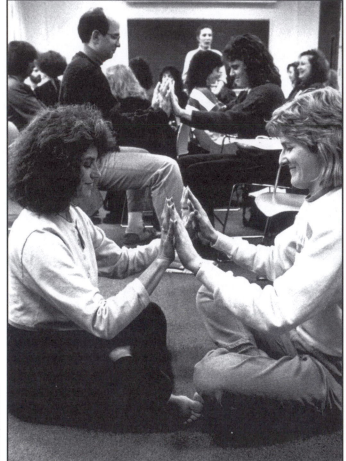

Photo: © Joel Gordon

Body-oriented psychotherapies combine physical activities with verbal analysis.

Body-oriented psychotherapies are healing modalities that use the body to help solve emotional problems. The term "body oriented psychotherapy" traditionally refers only to methods in which physical body postures or types and physical behavior patterns are used to diagnose and treat emotional disorders. However, this volume expands that definition to include many other methods that rely on a variety of physical activities to affect mental and emotional health. Although some people mistrust their unusual methods, many others credit a body-oriented psychotherapy as the only way they were able to change painful, limiting mental and emotional patterns and begin living a healthy and fulfilling life.

The Development of Body-Oriented Psychotherapy

Most body-oriented psychotherapies can trace their origins to the groundbreaking work of the Austrian neurologist and founder of psychoanalysis, Sigmund Freud (1856–1939). Through his work as a neurologist, Freud became aware that many of his neurotic patients' symptoms, including paralysis, headaches, fainting spells, and heart palpitations, were caused by something other than the physical working of their muscles, bones, and nerves. Working in tandem with his friend the physiologist Josef Breuer, Freud discovered that releasing repressed memories of childhood experiences or emotional conflicts, while in a hypnotic trance, alleviated his patients' physical symptoms. By combining clinical experience with deep insight into the nature of human behavior, Freud created a new model of the human mind that changed Western medical discourse forever.

Contrary to the popular belief that human beings are totally rational creatures, always aware of the causes of their actions, Freud saw the human mind as two parts—the conscious mind, which controls aspects of memory, speech, and logical thinking; and the unconscious mind, which contains the somatic reflexes such as breathing and heart rate, basic biological drives, dream imagery, and many other memories. Freud believed that when a memory or conflict was too painful for an individual to hold in his or her conscious mind, it would be repressed by a variety of defense mechanisms into the unconscious mind, where it affects the physical body and many aspects of behavior. Freud believed that many of these anxiety-producing conflicts were inherent to the human condition, especially in Victorian Europe, where one's basic biological drives contradicted the demands of civilized society.

Freud developed techniques to bring repressed memories to consciousness without the aid of hypnosis. This became the basis of psychoanalysis, a particular approach to psychotherapy consisting of many scheduled verbal encounters between the therapist and patient over a long period of time. The therapist guides the patient in dredging up and sorting through the repressed memories, emotions, impulses, or desires.

Although Freud's theories and practices were controversial, he drew many of the brightest doctors in Europe into his circle. However, as Freud became increasingly inflexible in his methods, and his theories about human nature became increasingly pessimistic, many of his students eventually departed. Among this group, the Austrian Wilhelm Reich (1897–1957) was the most influential in developing a body orientation to psychotherapy. Reich broke with Freud by asserting the primacy of the body and biological processes in the cause and treatment of physical and emotional symptoms. In his book *The Function of the Orgasm* (1942) Reich presented the idea that a psycho-physical energy exists that, if not released through sexual orgasm, becomes locked in muscular tensions in the body. From this basic premise he developed an entire model of human psychology in which conflicts were not only stored in the subconscious mind but were present in the physical body as a complex of muscular tensions he called "muscular armoring" and a complex of behavior patterns he called "character armoring." Reich's model of treatment, known today as medical orgonomy, uses hands-on manipulation of the body and breathing patterns to release the chronically tight muscles and repressed energy. It became the basis of many forms of body-oriented psychotherapies including bioenergetics, core energetics, hakomi integrative somatics, organismic body psychotherapy, and Radix.

Both Carl Jung (1875–1961) from Switzerland and Roberto Assagioli (1888–1974) from Italy departed from Freud because they believed he placed too much emphasis on the sexual drive in interpreting human behavior. The two approaches to psychotherapy they developed—analytical psychology and psychosynthesis, respectively—extended the range of Freud's model of human personality to include spiritual drives and goals. They introduced the West to the connection between spirituality and psychology, a connection that had dominated non-Western art, religion, and health practices for centuries. Jung and Assagioli's concepts of motivational drives had a huge impact on the development of techniques used in body-oriented psychotherapies, including core energetics, coreSomatics, emotional kinesthetic psychotherapy, Holotropic Breathwork, organismic body psychotherapy, and process oriented psychology.

As the twentieth century unfolded, psychotherapists continued to develop new models of personality and treatment methods. In the 1960s many approaches to psychotherapy, known collectively as humanistic psychology, developed by people such as Abraham Maslow and Carl Rogers, were based on observations of healthy people instead of neurotic ones, and on the human potential for growth and change. Especially important to the development of body-oriented psychotherapies was gestalt therapy, developed by Fritz and Laura Perls. In gestalt therapy many techniques, some borrowed from Jacob Moreno's psychodrama, are used to physically enact painful experiences and difficult relationships. Gestalt therapy, as well as all Humanistic psychology approaches, emphasizes developing a sense of wholeness, authenticity, and self-esteem through the conscious awareness of feelings and bodily expression in the present rather than by dredging up the past.

At the same time a new wave of spiritual teachers from non-Western religions came to the United States, filling the burgeoning "growth centers" across the country with the wisdom of ancient teachings regarding the connections between body, mind, and spirit. As a result, new approaches to psychotherapy evolved, including Leonard Orr's rebirthing, Stanislav Grof's Holotropic Breathwork, and Ilana Rubenfeld's Synergy. These psychotherapies offered new methods to discover psychic wholeness by combining physical, mental, emotional, and spiritual aspects of humanness in varying ways. Today literally hundreds of different body-oriented approaches to psychotherapy influenced by science, religion, or the arts offer individuals a choice from a plethora of paths of psychological healing or self-discovery.

Theories and Practices of Body-Oriented Psychotherapies

All body-oriented psychotherapies are based on the belief that the body, mind, and spirit are interdependent aspects of humanness. While Freud observed the mind's influence over the body, these disciplines reverse this relationship and study how the body affects the mind. They claim that creating a healthy, balanced body will help restore mental and emotional harmony. Body-oriented psychotherapists believe that the emotional and mental experiences of life, which in some methods include prenatal (before birth) or after-death experiences, are imprinted in the body as clearly as the words you are reading are printed on this page. To effect a real and lasting change in a human psyche, they believe, you must work through the physical body.

Unlike Freudian psychoanalysis, which relies exclusively on verbal exchange between therapist and patient, body-oriented psychotherapists believe the body to be primary in both reflecting emotional problems and working toward their cure. Therapists direct the patient's attention to the physical sensations of the body and the relationship of these sensations to other aspects of the whole self. The techniques used in body-oriented psychotherapies range from the direct, sometimes violent physical manipulation of Reichian–based methods to the barely physical guided imagery sessions of psychosynthesis. In some methods, such as Holotropic Breathwork, two patients will work together in a therapeutic process without the direct aid of the therapist. In others, such as Pesso Boyden system psychomotor, a group of people are needed to embody the healing process. Despite the differences in technique, all types of body-oriented psychotherapies use the body, rather than another individual, as the monitor of psychological well-being, the gauge of emotional truth.

Some Benefits and Limitations of Body-Oriented Psychotherapies

Body-oriented psychotherapies aim to give greater freedom and integration to the physical, mental, emotional, and spiritual aspects of human life. Most of the methods included here are based on a theoretical foundation that states that an individual's psychic development will ultimately lead to a spiritual unfolding, evidenced by a growing concern for and action toward the good of the entire community. Body-oriented psychotherapies have helped many people break painful physical or emotional addictions. Others report experiencing more pleasure, optimism, spontaneity, and a greater sense of participation in the process of living. Still others describe a stronger feeling of connection to other people and a clearer sense of purpose and value in their lives, as well as life in general.

These rewards are not easily gained. Body-oriented psychotherapies generally require a long-term commitment to a process that can require painful physical and emotional work. In addition, because these methods regard each individual as intrinsically whole, they are generally not appropriate for people suffering from psychoses or people whose self-esteem is so severely damaged that it cannot confront the truth of the body.

—Nancy Allison, CMA

Resources:

The United States Association for Body Psychotherapy
111 Bonifant Street, Suite 201
Silver Spring, MD 20910
Tel: (301) 587- 4011
Web site: www.usabp.com
Established in 1998, the USABP is a professional association of body psychotherapy professionals and students that holds conferences and publishes pro-fessional journals and newsletters that track research and development in the field of body psychotherapy.

Further Reading:

Brown, Dennis, and Jonathan Pedder. *An Introduction to Psychotherapy: An Outline of Psychodynamic Principles and Practice.* London and New York: Tavistock/Routledge. 1979.

BIOENERGETICS

Bioenergetics is a form of body-oriented psychotherapy developed by American doctor Alexander Lowen during the mid-twentieth century. Based on the groundbreaking work of Austrian psychotherapist Wilhelm Reich, bioenergetics views body, mind, and spirit as interdependent and reflective of each other. By combining active bodywork exercises with verbal therapy, Bioenergetics therapists aim to liberate both body and mind from restrictive holding patterns, helping people to live freer, more pleasurable, fulfilling lives.

Origins of Bioenergetics

Bioenergetics was developed by Alexander Lowen, M.D. (1910–), a student of Wilhelm Reich, M.D. (1897–1957). Reich, the founder of medical orgonomy and a colleague of the seminal psychoanalyst Sigmund Freud, is generally credited as the first person in modern Western psychotherapy to incorporate working directly with the body in psychotherapeutic treatment. He explored the body's involuntary responses to emotional situations to arrive at his own theoretical construct of human personality.

Reich believed that neuroses, or personality problems, are anchored in the body as chronic muscular tensions. He observed that chronic muscular tensions decreased a person's general energy level and ability to feel all emotions, particularly pleasurable ones. Reich believed that deepening a person's involuntary breathing process was key to releasing chronic muscular tension and opening muscular tissue to the full streaming of psychological and physical energy.

As a young man, Alexander Lowen noted that regular physical activity improved his physical and emotional state. He became interested in techniques that developed the body-mind relationship, such as Emile Jacques Dalcroze's eurythmics, Edmund Jacobson's progressive relaxation, and yoga. But it was not until 1940, when he heard Dr. Reich lecture at the New School for Social Research in New York, that he felt he found an answer to his own questions about the nature of the relationship between body and mind. Lowen studied with Reich from 1940 to 1952 and underwent therapy with him from 1942 to 1945. During these exciting and inspiring years he finished premedical studies and trained to become a Reichian therapist. Lowen saw his first patient in 1945. Disappointed with his progress with his early patients, Lowen spent the years from September 1947 to June 1951 studying medicine and earning his M.D. degree from Geneva University in Switzerland.

Although Lowen believed he had made substantial progress in his own therapy with Reich, he felt that many of his own conflicts had not been fully resolved. He perceived that the physical and emotional freedom gained in his therapy with Reich did not necessarily transfer to real-life situations. After his return from Europe, Lowen spoke with several other former patients of Reich, most notably John Pierrakos, M.D., who felt the same way.

In 1953, working together with Pierrakos, Lowen set out to develop the techniques of Reichian therapy so that deeper, more pervasive improvement could result. He believed a more active physical approach, as well as a deeper analytical approach, was needed. For three years Lowen experimented with Reich's bodywork techniques, using Pierrakos to apply pressure directly on Lowen's chronically tensed muscles. The exercises he developed form the basis of bioenergetics. During this time Lowen and Pierrakos met regularly with another Reichian associate, Dr. William Walling, M.D., in clinical seminars that enriched Lowen's theoretical understanding of Reich's approach as well.

Breaking Down Body Armor

Bioenergetics is based on a model of the human personality as comprised of biological impulses and conscious thought or will. According to Lowen, a healthy person follows his or her biological impulses completely, suppressing them only in response to a personal sense of desire. He believes neuroses develop when biological impulses are suppressed through conscious, willful control in response to fear.

Lowen believes this process begins very early in human development, for example, when a child consciously controls his or her impulse to cry in response to parental disapproval. According to Lowen, the child stops crying because it perceives his or her parents' disapproval as a threat to survival. The reflexive, physical act of restricting breathing that stops his or her crying is spontaneously developed, Lowen believes, as a survival mechanism. The child ceases to cry and parental affection and protection are secured. When a child alters its physical impulses by responding, as in this situation, to fear rather than pleasure, it creates a sense of personal power over its environment based on willful control of biological impulses. Lowen calls this psychological pattern the "neurotic character structure."

Lowen, like Reich, believes the neurotic character structure to be a survival defense, but it is also an imprisonment for the true nature of the human being. Following Reich, Lowen believes the neurotic character structure can be observed in the body, as well as the psyche, as a form of armor. Bioenergetic therapy strives to break down physical and emotional armoring by loosening rigid muscles and promoting the flow of psycho-physical energy, which Lowen calls bioenergy, through the body.

According to Lowen, "In Bioenergetic Therapy the breakdown of the neurotic character structure does not happen as a single event, but as a series of breakthroughs, each of which is experienced as an energetic release and transformation. With each release the patient begins to feel more alive and more open and has an awareness of an inner strength and force that he or she had not felt before." As the body becomes more alive, the will loosens its grip on feelings that come through more easily as physical sensations that act as catalysts for new responses to and interactions with others.

Throughout this process bioenergetic therapy includes talking about one's history and current life situation, relationships, and dreams. The verbal therapy enables the patient to integrate the new emotions and physical sensations into his or her whole personality. Without this conscious integration Lowen believes that muscular tension will simply recur because the mind has not incorporated the physical experiences into a new balanced personality structure.

Grounding Exercises

Individual bioenergetic therapy, which is the most common format, may begin with some initial conversation between therapist and client, but will generally proceed quickly to bodywork exercises. In all formats, group or individual, clients work in leotards, bathing suits, or more commonly their underwear, which allows the bioenergetic therapist to see the body and its changes more easily.

Most of the exercises involve lying, sitting, or standing in positions that actually increase the tension of chronically stressed muscles. It is believed that breathing deeply while in these positions pulls so much bioenergy into the muscles that it forces the client to release his or her willful hold on them, thereby allowing an involuntary stream of energy and sensation to flow through them. This stream of energy is experienced by the patient as a current, similar to an electrical current passing through a wire, and can be seen by therapist and client alike as actual physical vibrations in the muscle.

One of the most common series of postures used in bioenergetic therapy is called "grounding positions." These standing postures were developed by Lowen to help clients who feel out of touch with reality develop a firm sense of the connection between their feet and the ground. Practitioners of bioenergetics believe that allowing the breathing process to deepen while standing in the grounding positions helps pull bioenergy downward through the pelvis and legs. It increases a sense of rootedness and the ability to stand on one's own two feet, as well as literally being able to "stand" the increase in the amount of energy and emotion experienced.

Whichever body posture the client maintains, the bioenergetic therapist may use massage, forceful pressure, or gentle touch to encourage the release of contracted muscles. The client will also be advised to release sounds while holding the postures. The use of the voice increases vibration, sending more bioenergy through the system, thereby forcing the patient to surrender his or her hold on the body more quickly.

The breathing stool is another device, designed by Lowen to speed the releasing process, also called the surrender to the body. It is a padded wooden structure over which the client rests in a backward bending position. Supported by the stool in this position, clients may experience their current shallow breathing process and its connection to their fears. This position also stretches the torso, opening the entire pelvis and thorax to encourage deep involuntary breathing, the catalyst for releasing chronic muscular tension.

As the therapy progresses, "expressive exercises" will be added to the stationary lying, sitting, or standing poses. In these exercises clients perform actions such as kicking the legs alternately up and down while lying on a bed, or hitting a bed with fists or a tennis racket while standing in order to express anger and aggressive feelings. Bioenergetic therapists believe that experiencing aggression allows a patient to feel that he or she can defend (or stand up for) oneself. Releasing these aggressive feelings also means no longer having to keep them under conscious willful control, thereby releasing muscular tissue to experience pleasurable sensations.

Throughout the course of the therapy bodywork, sessions are interspersed with verbal therapy, allowing the patient to integrate the new sensations and emotions into his or her life with the support of the therapist. Over the course of an individual therapy, clients may also choose to participate in group intensive sessions that may last a weekend or longer. Bioenergetic group therapy sessions utilize many of the same exercises as individual therapy and may involve working with a partner to increase physical resistance in the positions.

A Long-Term Therapy

Bioenergetic therapy is not short-term therapy. It requires a commitment of time and energy to resolve deep conflicts and to free the body and mind from

---

Lowen's Therapy with Reich

Reich had his patients lie on a bed and do deep-breathing exercises. He applied pressure to chronically held muscles to help a person feel the pain of holding them tense and release the holding. He would direct a person to change the position of the body in some subtle way that allowed the energy and the feeling to flow out in an open channel. Lowen describes in his book *Bioenergetics* (1975) his first therapy session with Reich. Lowen lay on a bed in bathing trunks and began to breathe deeply; at the point he began to relax, Reich asked him to drop his head back and open his eyes wide. When he did this he screamed involuntarily, thus releasing a feeling he had unconsciously blocked for many years as well as freeing up the energy that had been used to hold it back.

neurotic, unproductive patterns. However, the bodywork seems to allow this deep healing process to proceed faster than it does with only verbal therapy. Bioenergetics seeks to integrate body and mind as it aims to help a person feel more relaxed, connected, spontaneous, and alive.

—Nancy Allison, CMA, with consultation by Nina Robinson, CMA

Resources:

International Institute for Bioenergetic Analysis
144 East 36th Street
New York, NY 10016
Tel: (212) 532-7742
Offers information about the discipline as well as qualified practitioners.

Further Reading:

Lowen, Alexander. *Bioenergetics.* New York: Penguin Books, 1975.

Lowen, Alexander, and Leslie Lowen. *The Way to Vibrant Health: A Manual of Bioenergetic Exercises.* New York: Harper & Row, 1977.

——. *Pleasure: A Creative Approach to Life.* New York: Penguin, 1987.

BODYNAMIC ANALYSIS

Bodynamic analysis helps people resolve life problems by building new coping skills, also known as "resources," in the body and psyche. Bodynamic analysis describes resources as the normal physical and psychological abilities that are learned during healthy childhood development. Developed principally by Scandinavian physical educator Lisbeth Marcher in the 1970s, bodynamic analysis is based on an intricate theory that links specific muscular actions to psychological abilities. Using Marcher's Bodymap™ as a guide, bodynamic analysis strives to help people develop retarded resources, empowering them to have new experiences and make new life choices.

The Development of Bodynamic Analysis

Bodynamic analysis was developed by Lisbeth Marcher and her colleagues in Denmark. It derived from the rich tradition of body therapy systems that emerged in Scandinavia early in the twentieth century. Bodynamic analysis has arrived recently in the United States, with the first U.S. program founded in Berkeley, California, in 1990.

Marcher was originally trained in the "relaxation method," an in-depth body education training system well known in Scandinavia. Dissatisfied with the treatment of psychological issues within the relaxation method, Marcher began to study theories of body-mind integration. Influenced by Lillimor Johnsen, a Norwegian physiotherapist, Marcher developed a theory connecting each muscle action to specific psychological issues. She also noticed how motor patterns and psychological abilities seem to develop according to a very specific timetable during childhood. For example, the muscle associated with saying no is the triceps, a muscle that extends the arm out in a pushing-away motion. The triceps first begins its "no" motion very early, before the child can even say no. Later, as the child begins to say no, the action and the word go together. Finally the no movement lessens or disappears and the word "no" stays. In this way Marcher believed the timetables for the evolution of motor patterns and psychological and social patterns are intimately linked.

Theory of Bodynamic Analysis

Bodynamic analysis is based on a fundamental way of thinking about the role the body plays in shaping who people are and how they think, feel, love, play, work, and grow. By observing the unfolding pattern of motor development in children, bodynamic analysts see how the child's motor system is intimately linked to core self-development. By linking a person's spontaneous movements to the underlying psychological expression, bodynamic analysts believe they are able to pinpoint the origins of the difficulties that people experience in their present lives.

Bodynamic analysis is based on the concept of seven overlapping stages of child development named by Marcher. These seven stages are related to the psychological characteristics of each particular stage. They are the existence stage (second trimester–3 months), when the child first develops a sense of secure existence; the need stage (0–18 months), when physical bonding and contact are established and core body rhythms of eating, sleeping, etc., are set; the autonomy stage (8–30 months), when the child begins to move directly out into the world through crawling, walking, and grasping; the will stage (2–4 years), when the child learns to manage power and master loving and angry feelings and begins to develop a structuring of the world through planning and role formation; the love/sexuality stage (3–5 years), when loving and sexual feelings emerge more intensely; the opinion stage (5–8 years), when the child learns to express ideas and compare them with the world around her or him; and finally the solidarity/performance stage (7–12 years), when the child masters her or his own abilities within the context of peer group activity. By determining the stage or age at which a person feels stuck, bodynamic analysis is able to help that person resolve past traumas and move him or her toward gaining new resources.

Bodynamic analysts believe that the thread that runs through all these stages is the child's intense desire and drive toward establishing deep, powerful connections to the outside world. Bodynamic analysts call this drive mutual connection, and believe it informs the basic movement of life energy. Ultimately what is most traumatic to the growing child is when the bond between the child and others is disturbed or broken.

What a Typical Session Is Like

A typical session of bodynamic analysis often begins with an agreement to focus on a specific issue, such as the ability to establish and maintain fulfilling relationships, or with an ongoing developmental issue or stage. Sessions may focus on body sensations, paying attention to any impulses, movements, images, or memories that emerge. The person's posture, movements, and language begin to tell a story. The story is developed by expanding the movements, and through supportive touch, role playing, or working with early historical experiences. Most healing is accomplished by an integration of sensing, experiencing, moving, and thinking, in the context of the supportive relationship with the practitioner.

Bodymap™

In bodynamic analysis, there is a way to see our body profile in a muscle test called the Bodymap™. This is a process in which each muscle is tested for four degrees of hyper- and four degrees of hypo-response as well as a healthy response. This is then charted visually on a map of the body, which becomes available for detailed interpretation of a person's early history. Therapists then look to see at what ages and in what ego aspects individuals may be most held or blocked, and in what areas they are the most developed and resourced. This information helps clients understand themselves and guides therapy.

To return to the earlier example of learning to say no, a person might have had difficulty during the will stage (2–4 years) with expressing her or his power. Therapy with such a person includes not only a verbal exploration of the experiences that led to this difficulty, but also teaching the body how to express no. Practitioners help the person by teaching the muscles to express no in a new way. In some situations this may be fairly straightforward, but often this teaching needs to engage the person in a deep and subtle, physical and verbal conversation.

Throughout the process the practitioner and recipient explore sensations and experiences located in the body, the fears and beliefs that hold back the expression of the no. There is a recognition that each person's defense system is unique and deserves respect and understanding before it can change. It is important to engage the person's sensory-motor system and wake up the developmental movements slowly and gently. Practitioner and recipient stay with a movement and the accompanying thoughts and feelings until it has a chance to resolve. A person is then ready to explore a new movement and its accompanying psychological state.

Benefits and Risks

What makes bodynamic analysis unique among body-oriented psychotherapies is its ability to work on specific developmental issues. With this capacity to work in sharp focus, people seem to achieve a more complete resolution in the body, developing what bodynamic therapists call a "new imprint." People typically report forming deeper, more intimate relationships after experiencing bodynamic analysis.

Because therapist and recipient are able to focus on specific issues, bodynamic analysis often works well as a short-term intensive therapy; however, it is more often seen as a long-term commitment. While bodynamic analysts try to work from people's innate strengths to help them build new resources, therapy can pose a personal challenge as deeper issues emerge and more profound changes are indicated.

—*Peter Bernhardt*

Resources:

Bodynamic Institute
PO Box 6008
Albany, CA 94706
Tel: (510) 524-8090
Offers information on national and international activities. The Bodynamic Institute provides a foundation training, a two-year practitioner training, and a two-year analytic training.

Further Reading:

Bernhardt, Peter. *Individuation: Mutual Connection and the Body's Resources.* An interview with Lisbeth Marcher. Alberta, Canada: Bodynamic Institute Monograph, 1992.

——. *The Art of Following Structure: An Interview with Lisbeth Marcher Exploring the Roots of the Bodynamic System.* Alberta, Canada: Bodynamic Institute Monograph, 1995.

Bernhardt, Peter, M. Bentzen, and J. Isaacs. *Waking the Body Ego: An Introduction to Lisbeth Marcher's Somatic Developmental Psychology, I and II.* Alberta, Canada: Bodynamics Institute Monograph, 1995.

CORE ENERGETICS

Core energetics is a mode of healing that combines bodywork, psychotherapy, and a spiritual process called the pathwork to activate the greater consciousness dwelling within every human soul to release and strengthen human energy at all levels—physical,

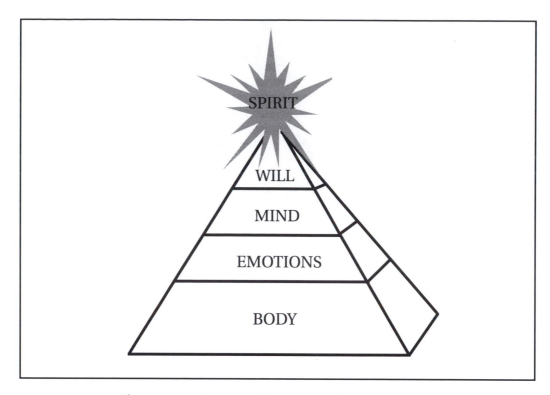

The core energetics model of the five levels of human existence.

emotional, mental, and spiritual. Unlike conventional psychiatric or medical therapies, core energetics views the spiritual dimension of life as an essential component in the process of recovery and growth. In fact, core energetics therapists believe that illness is a block in the life force said to be at the core of every individual. The core is called alternatively energy, love, or soul. According to core energetics theory, the unblocking of emotion promotes self-healing and benefits a variety of mental and physical disorders from depression to chronic fatigue syndrome.

The History of Core Energetics
Core energetics, sometimes called the core energetic evolutionary process, was developed by John Pierrakos, a Greek-American doctor who started his career as a follower of the innovative Austrian psychiatrist Wilhelm Reich. Reich had come to America after the Nazi rise to power and soon began to stir controversy in American medical

circles because of his unorthodox views on the fundamental nature of the human organism. He maintained that the body is infused with an invisible energy known as orgone, which also infuses all material aspects of the cosmos. What happens in the body affects what happens emotionally and mentally, therefore illness is to be understood as a dual body-mind phenomenon—a notion that was alien to a medical profession then organized around the separation of psychological and physical healing. Reich gave Pierrakos the framework for his life's work as a holistic physician committed to a search for effective body-mind treatments.

In the 1950s he and another physician, Alexander Lowen, made Reich's teachings the basis for bioenergetics, a body-oriented psychotherapy that uses the body to diagnose and heal emotional illness. Impressed by the parallels between Reich's notion of orgone and ancient Eastern ideas of human energy, Pierrakos began researching the nature of energy and human energy fields. By the early 1970s he had formulated a theory of the human organism, still Reichian in broad outline, but incorporating the conception of chakras (or energy centers). He developed an innovative system that looked at the chakras and correlated what he found to be their normal or abnormal functioning to the person's psychological and physical traits. Pierrakos became proficient at viewing the human energy field and chakras. He observed the energy of people in a medical setting and was able to tell what other physicians needed complex laboratory tests to show.

Eva Broch, a spiritual medium and eventually Pierrakos's wife, helped him complete his synthesis of Western and Eastern medical teachings. Her confidence in the existence of the spiritual, together with clinical observation that spiritual belief enhances patients' recuperative powers, inspired Pierrakos to risk going beyond the bounds of Western scientific reason in his definition of human energy. It is ultimately spiritual in nature, he concluded, and cannot be fully understood unless its relationship to the human capacity for love is recognized. The spiritual dimension, love, and the life force became synonymous in Pierrakos's thought during the late 1970s. He built core energetics on his work in bioenergetic analysis and the inspiration he obtained from the spiritual teachings of the pathwork, a spiritual process that consists of learning to activate the greater consciousness dwelling within every human soul.

In 1980 he founded an institute in New York City for study and training in the approach he called core energetics and regarded it as the culmination of his career. Most forms of body psychotherapy and transpersonal work in this country are informed by Dr. Pierrakos's work in bioenergetic analysis and core energetics. His work is unique because "the love force" is "the substance and movement of life." During the last decade interest in core energetics has grown rapidly in the United States and abroad. There are now branches of the Institute of Core Energetics in the United States, Canada, Mexico, Brazil, Germany, Switzerland, and Italy.

The Theory of Core Energetics

Core energetics is based on the belief that the individual has an innate capacity for love and a need to evolve and that these together constitute a life force of virtually unlimited creative potential. Further, it is believed that health is a dynamic state found only when the individual realizes his or her creative potential in a process of personal growth and change. Though the movement receives its impetus from the life force, it occurs in the body, the vehicle through which emotion, thought, and spirit are expressed.

Pierrakos is the first modern Western physician to connect the ancient knowledge of energy and spirituality to the science of new physics and to the current medical practice of psychiatry. He has created a holistic approach by combining work with all five levels of human existence in the human entity. These five levels are the physical body, feelings and emotions, mind and thought, will, and spirit.

Core energetics therapists believe that we are made up of layers of energy. At our center is the pulsing, moving energy of life that Pierrakos calls the core. This is our life force, which, following the laws of physics, seeks to expand and grow. When people are in touch with their life force, they feel love for themselves and their fellow creatures. The next layer is the lower self, which contains our wounded child and the dark side, or shadow part, of our nature. Core energetics theory contends that we block our life force when we are not allowed to express our emotional pain or negative emotions. This energy becomes stagnant and will produce a layer of defense, which becomes the physical armoring. Next we put on a social mask designed to protect ourselves. This mask, or false self, dampens the vibrancy and buoyancy of the life center—the core.

The process of this evolutionary work, therefore, is to unblock our defenses, move the stuck energy to create healthy flow, and transform the negative, distorted emotions back to the core self. This is done by first penetrating the mask, which uncovers the false self; second, by working with the physical body, the body armoring; third, by transforming the negative emotions of the dark side and allowing the primal wounds to be expressed; fourth, supporting the core to be experienced as loving, joyful, and connected to all life; and finally, this work organically leads to a deep understanding of a person's task and purpose in life.

According to core energetic theory, it is of primary importance to teach people to use their positive will, the will of the heart, to live in the present, and to be aware that people have choice in each moment to create their own lives.

Experiencing Core Energetics

A typical session in core energetics lasts approximately an hour. The receiver may wear a leotard or bathing suit so that the therapist can easily assess and treat the defenses built into the body. Initial work often involves breathing exercises to charge the system, bring awareness to the receiver, and start the process of release and transformation. There is always intensive work with bodily movement and exercise and emotional expression that unblock the flow of the life force. The therapist may use hands-on touch to help the receiver mobilize and direct energy through the body. All levels of the human entity—physical, emotional, mental, and spiritual—are addressed as appropriate for the individual.

Treatment will be adjusted to the particular needs of the receiver and be different at each stage of therapy, but is always approached as an evolutionary process that leads from unmasking of the shadow self to expression and transformation of pain to understanding and acceptance that opening the heart and feeling love is the healing agent. Transformation occurs when the client unmasks and expresses the energy of the wounded and lower self, which then allows connection to the core/spirit.

The Benefits of Core Energetics

Core energetics should not be confused with conventional psychotherapy. It teaches receivers about their capacity for self-healing and launches them on a process of transformation that is ultimately spiritual in nature. Proponents of core energetics credit it with providing a sense of well-being at all levels of human existence. It is also regarded as helpful for weight problems, panic attacks, unresolved anger, posttraumatic stress, sexual dysfunction, repairing troubled marital and familial relationships, making major personal and professional changes, and expanding spiritual awareness.

—*Pamela L. Chubbuck, Ph.D.*

Core Energetics Training

Training in core energetics requires four years of course work and extensive personal therapy at an Institute of Core Energetics. Generally prior involvement in another form of therapy such as chiropractic or osteopathy is required for admission. The curriculum features courses on anatomy, physiology, human energy theory, Reichian theory, bioenergetics, and pathwork spirituality. One year of postgraduate study is required for those who wish to become trainers of other core energetics therapists.

Resources:

Institute of Core Energetics International
115 East 23rd Street, 12th Floor
New York, NY 10010
Tel: (212) 982-9637
Fax: (212) 673-5939
Web site: www.core-energetics.org
A training and treatment center that organizes workshops and lectures, publishes a newsletter, and gives referrals to therapists trained in core energetics.

Institute of Core Energetics South
8733 Lake Drive
Lithonia, GA 30058
Tel: (770) 388-0086
Fax: (770) 388-0806
A training and treatment center for core energetics, organizes workshops, lectures, and publishes a newsletter.

Institute of Core Energetics West
P.O. Box 806
Mendocino, CA 95160
Tel: (707) 937-1825
Fax: (707) 937-3052
e-mail: lisycee@mcn.org
Offers treatment and training in core energetics.

Further Reading:

Books:
Pierrakos, Eva. *The Pathwork of Self-Transformation.* New York: Bantam, 1990.

Pierrakos, John. *Core Energetics: Developing the Capacity to Love and Heal.* Mendocino, CA: Life Rhythm, 1990.

——. *Eros, Love, and Sexuality.* Mendocino, CA: Life Rhythm, 1997.

Journals:
Energy and Consciousness: International Journal of Core Energetics. Jacqueline Carlton, Ph.D., ed.

Videotapes:

Chubbuck, Pamela. *Say Yes to Life: Grounding and Loving Your Body.* Lithonia, GA: The Institute of Core Energetics South, ND.

——. *Say Yes to Life: Expressing Your Emotions and Opening to Your Core.* Lithonia, GA: The Institute of Core Energetics South, ND.

CORESOMATICS®

CoreSomatics® is a discipline designed to increase awareness of the ways our childhood, emotions, and experiences influence the posture and alignment of our bodies. In coreSomatics, the habitual use of the body is seen as a mirror, reflecting all personal experience, creating a dynamic interdependence between the body and the mind. In the nonjudgmental environment of coreSomatics, individuals identify and change limiting habitual physical behaviors, leading to an improved state of mind and self-image. The discipline combines the Feldenkrais Method® and the Alexander technique with gestalt therapy, Jungian psychology, and the expressive arts therapies.

coreSomatics was developed in the 1970s by Kay Miller. During the early part of that decade, Miller created countless theater games and sound and movement exercises for the improvisational theater company she had founded in 1974. The exercises gained recognition for their success with at-risk young adults. By the late 1970s, Miller began to use theater exercises with the physical process therapies of the Feldenkrais Method and the Alexander technique. Integrating these with Jungian psychology and gestalt therapy, Kay Miller created coreSomatics. In 1983, the Somatic Institute, Pittsburgh, was founded as a not-for-profit organization to provide research and education in coreSomatics.

coreSomatics is founded on the premise that what the individual seeks, in order to bring about personal improvement and change, already exists in the unconscious. Negative aspects such as insecurity, self-doubt, fear, rigidity, and tension are seen as resulting from early trauma. coreSomatics practitioners believe that these early traumatizing experiences negatively impact an individual's nervous system, shaping the actions and postures used in adult life. Thus, a seemingly ineffectual or poor use of the body may actually be a highly complex reaction to childhood experience, a limiting muscular memory, that once brought into awareness can be released.

The first objective of the coreSomatics practitioner is to provide a safe environment in which the client is free to express past and current experiences. Having established trust, the coreSomatics practitioner employs touch, uses verbal expression, movement exercises, and works with breathing patterns and existing posture. Body tensions and pain are explored through imagery, sound, humor, and intuition.

In the process of the hands-on physical interventions and verbal expressions, individuals discover that their physical habits are connected to emotional and psychological memories, which are experienced as muscular armor, rigidity, tension, and pain. coreSomatics practitioners believe that it is through the physical and emotional releases of this process that individuals find more effective ways to manage their lives and experience the exuberance of having reclaimed their fluidity, flexibility, and spontaneity.

coreSomatics has been used to reduce stress, relieve tension, and allow individuals to experience their lives more fully. People have experienced significant improvements in intelligence, sensory acuity, memory, and concentration. Improvements in mood, interpersonal relationships, productivity, and general health and wellness follow naturally.

—*Kay Miller*

Resources:

Somatic Institute, Pittsburgh
8600 West Barkhurst Drive
Pittsburgh, PA 15237
Tel: (412) 366-5580

Fax: (412) 367-1026

Offers coreSomatics training through its two-year certification program, a mastery-level program, an associates program, and a variety of postgraduate internships. It sponsors research and education in coreSomatics and publishes a variety of materials, including the institute's journal, Touch®.

EMOTIONAL-KINESTHETIC PSYCHOTHERAPY

Emotional-kinesthetic psychotherapy (EKP) is a discipline that incorporates the body in psychotherapy, seeking to help clients integrate the physical, emotional, and spiritual aspects of their selves. It incorporates a variety of techniques, including touch, to facilitate this integrative process. Therapists attempt to create an environment of emotional safety and respect to allow clients to access and reveal their mind, body, heart, and soul.

EKP believes that there exist three levels of human intelligence: cognitive (consisting of knowledge), emotional, and somatic (consisting of body sensations). According to EKP, the heart is the place where somatic and emotional intelligence meet. Any life difficulty or body sensation can be accessed and explored by asking, "What's happening in your heart?" at a moment in time. Emotional and somatic sensations contain information and experience that inform a person's thought process, and without which a person often cannot move forward in his or her life.

Linda Marks developed EKP from her experience as a trauma survivor, which led her to study approaches to psychotherapy that study the body. EKP draws extensively from Ron Kurtz's Hakomi and incorporates aspects of Robert Assagioli's psychosynthesis and Eugene Gendlin's focusing. EKP responds to clients' particular needs by using character typology, the model of human personality conceived by Wilhelm Reich and developed by Alexander Lowen and John Pierrakos in Bioenergetics. Marks founded the Institute for Emotional-Kinesthetic Psychotherapy in 1990, but the principles of EKP had been applied in her private therapy practice and personal growth workshops since 1985.

An EKP therapist's goal is to help clients achieve a sense of integration that allows them to live meaningful and productive lives. The work aims to allow clients to heal their most wounded parts, meet their simplest unmet needs, and reclaim the deepest part of their selves. A typical session may include the following:

1. Leading the clients through a guided meditation, which EKP calls a heart meditation. In this process, clients explore the emotional and physical sensations they experience in their heart in relation to what is happening in important parts of their life, such as work, personal relationships, and self-esteem. A heart meditation begins each EKP session to help the client center himself or herself and create a safe, spiritually inclusive environment in which to do therapy.
2. Sharing aspects of the client's life to create a context for an ongoing therapy.
3. Calling attention to what is happening in the heart and body in the present moment, to help the client follow emotional and somatic processes.
4. Touching, when appropriate and with permission, to facilitate emotional processes.
5. Guiding a client toward perception of sensations, such as jitteriness, numbness, or tightness. These sensations, referred to as the emotional-kinesthetic charge, are considered the embodiment of the client's inner state. The EKP therapist helps the client follow the emotional-kinesthetic charge to its source, which may be a traumatic experience or unmet needs. This guiding is known as EKP process work.
6. Closing a session by calling attention to the emotions and somatic experiences that have emerged. This is often done with closed eyes so that the client can assimilate his or her inner experiences of the session. Finally, the client returns to an outer, open-eyed state of consciousness.

EKP has many benefits, the most simple of which can include stress reduction, developing a stronger sense of self, and alleviating pain. At a deeper level, EKP offers a healing context for trauma and neglect, allowing clients to bridge the split between body and mind that often follows traumatic experience. EKP can be used to help one find his or her voice, develop appropriate work and personal relationships from the core of one's being, and connect with a sense of spiritual purpose. For borderline clients and others in the midst of a serious psychotic crisis, other therapeutic approaches would be indicated.

—*Linda Marks*

Resources:

Institute for EKP
3 Central Avenue
Newton, MA 02160
Tel: (617) 965-7846
Fax and Office Line (617) 332-7262
Provides numerous seminars, workshops, and extended group therapeutic programs, in addition to running a three-year training program.

Further Reading:

Liedloff, Jean. *The Continuum Concept.* Reading, MA: Addison-Wesley, 1977.

Marks, Linda. *Living With Vision: Reclaiming the Power of the Heart.* Skokie, IL Knowledge Systems, Inc., 1989.

——. *The Emotional-Kinesthetic Study Guide* Newton, MA: Institute for EKP, 1991.

Small, Jacquelyn. *Becoming Naturally Therapeutic.* New York: Bantam, 1990.

FOCUSING

Focusing, developed by Dr. Eugene Gendlin, is a process that allows and encourages the mind and body to communicate in order to heed the wisdom that comes from our bodies. The focusing process can be used by itself, and it also makes all types of psychotherapy and counseling more effective. It facilitates problem solving, creative endeavors, stress reduction, and spirituality. The six steps of focusing invite people to unlock doors and move into dimensions that cannot be entered through intellect alone.

The Development of Focusing

Dr. Gendlin, a professor who is both a philosopher and psychologist, developed focusing while at the University of Chicago. The concepts of focusing evolved from his work in existential philosophy, which he wrote about in *The Creation of Meaning* (1962) and from his research in psychotherapy, which is described in an article entitled "Focusing" in *Psychotherapy: Theory, Research and Practice* (Vol. 6., No. 1, 1969).

Since 1969 Dr. Gendlin has been teaching focusing all over the world and writing about it in numerous articles and three books. There are certified focusing trainers located throughout North America, as well as in South America, Europe, and Asia. Training programs are available worldwide for those who want to become certified focusing trainers in order to teach or to apply it toward other disciplines.

The Basic Theory of Focusing

In his research on psychotherapy, Dr. Gendlin posed the question, "Why is some psychotherapy successful and some not?" From analyzing a large number of therapy sessions, he and his coworkers discovered that it is not *what* the client talks about, but rather *how* the client talks about an issue that determines whether a person gets better in therapy. Successful clients get in touch with what feels like a vague bodily experience, and then they keep their attention on it while it comes into focus. In essence, they attend to what they don't yet fully understand.

In the realm of focusing, the "body" means not only the physiological self, but also the storehouse of experience that is carried there. Dr. Gendlin called the body's version a "felt sense." By learning to tune in to the bodily "felt sense" of different experiences or difficulties, we can more easily resolve life issues and problems.

Another important assumption is that every problem has within it some wisdom about its next step, and some positive life energy that wants to move forward or to be released. When we accurately name how the body is carrying an experience, not only do we get new information and insights, but we get a physical release that feels good.

Currently, exciting work is being done to bring focusing into education, into the healing and creative arts, into medicine, and into spirituality. The potential of this simple yet powerful tool continues to unfold. As Dr. Gendlin says, "One step in the body is worth a thousand steps in the mind."

How to Practice Focusing

Focusing can be learned from a book, but is best learned from a person who guides one through the process. Many people begin by learning it in a class or workshop or from a focusing teacher, and then continue to practice with a focusing partner. Partners take turns so that each one has a chance to be the guide and the focuser.

Focusing Instructions

1. CLEAR A SPACE
   How are you? What's between you and feeling fine?
   Don't answer; let what comes in your body do the answering.
   Don't go into anything.
   Greet each concern that comes. Put each aside for a while, next to you.
   Except for that, are you fine?

2. USE FELT SENSE
   Pick one problem to focus on.
   Don't go into the problem. What do you sense in your body when you recall
   the whole of that problem?
   Sense all of that, the sense of the whole thing, the murky discomfort or the
   unclear body-sense of it.

3. GET A HANDLE
   What is the quality of the felt sense?
   What one word, phrase, or image comes out of this felt sense?
   What quality-word would fit it best?

4. RESONATE
   Go back and forth between word (or image) and the felt sense. Is that right?
   If they match, have the sensation of matching several times.
   If the felt sense changes, follow it with your attention.

   When you get a perfect match, the words (or images) being just right for this
   feeling, let yourself feel that for a minute.

5. ASK
   "What is it, about the whole problem, that makes me so_____?"

   When stuck, ask questions:
          What is the worst of this feeling?
          What's really so bad about this?
          What does it need?
          What should happen?
          Don't answer; wait for the feeling to stir and give you an answer.

   What would it feel like if it was all OK?
          Let the body answer:
          What is in the way of that?

6. RECEIVE
   Welcome what came. Be glad it spoke.
   It is only one step on this problem, not the last.
   Now that you know where it is, you can leave it and come back to it later.
   Protect it from critical voices that interrupt.

   Does your body want another round of focusing, or is this a good stopping place?

The focusing process involves six steps. In the first step, the Focuser is invited to "clear a space," which involves taking an inventory of the concerns or issues that the person can locate in his or her body at that time and placing each "down" or outside the body. After the simple act of putting the problems down, the person often feels a distinct release. Clearing a space often releases stress and creates a safe distance from the issues or feelings that are being carried around.

Next the focuser is asked to choose a problem that needs attention right now and to ask in a friendly way, "How does this whole issue feel in my body right now?" After a pause, the focuser checks to see if a word, phrase, or, perhaps, an image comes that feels like it matches the sensations inside. If there is a match, the focuser usually feels a "yes" inside, which is followed by a sense of bodily release. He or she then proceeds to the next step. If there isn't a match, the focuser tries other words or images until a good fit is found. Then the focuser sits with this body sense, just "keeping it company," or asking it open-ended questions such as "What's the crux of this?", "What does this problem need?", or "What's a step in the right direction?" In the pause after each question, the focuser is invited to let a fresh answer arise from the body sense. There is usually some physical relief or "felt shift," as well as new insight that results.

For example, a focuser might find on a given day that she is aware of three different and distinct unsettled feelings in her body: one from an uncomfortable conversation with her mother, one from an argument with her boyfriend, and one from worry about a test. After setting them all aside on an imaginary bench for a few moments, she chooses to work on the argument with her boyfriend. At first she thinks the word that best describes the tight feeling in her chest is "angry," but that doesn't quite fit. She finds that "hurt" better captures how she feels after their argument. When she says the word

"hurt" she heaves a sigh of acknowledgment. "Yes, that's how I really felt when I hung up the phone." She then senses into the whole thing about being "hurt," and finds that it has to do with feeling unrecognized and unseen. When she asks what this feeling of "hurt" needs, it becomes clear that the right step is to talk to her boyfriend about her hurt and disappointment, not about the anger, which has by now shifted.

Benefits of Focusing

The benefits of focusing include becoming aware that there is a realm of inner knowing that can be found in the body, reducing stress or tension in the body-mind, and increasing one's life energy. Focusing also offers a way to work through blocks, it facilitates effective problem solving and decision-making, it promotes creativity, it improves the effectiveness of psychotherapy, and it deepens spirituality.

—*Joan Klagsbrun, Ph.D.*

Resources:

The Focusing Institute
34 East Lane
Spring Valley, NY 10977
Tel: (914) 362-5222 or (800) 799-7418
e-mail: info@focusing.org
Web site: www.focusing.org
Provides training tapes, articles, and information about teachers and focusing-oriented psychotherapists around the world. Publishes the journal Focusing Folio.

Further Reading:

Boukydis, C. F. Z. "Client-Centered/Experiential Practice with Parents and Infants." In *Client-Centered and Experiential Psychotherapy in the Nineties,* edited by Lietar, G., et. al. Belgium: Leuven University Press, 1990.

Campbell, P., and G. McMahon. *Biospirituality: Focusing as a Way to Grow.* Chicago: Loyola University Press, 1985.

Cornell, A. Weiser. *The Power of Focusing*. San Francisco: New Harbinger, 1996.

Friedman, Neil. *On Focusing: How to Access Your Own and Other People's Direct Experience*. Self-Published (259 Massachusetts Ave., Arlington, MA, 02174).

Gendlin, E. T. "A Theory of Personality Change." In *Personality Change*, edited by Worchel and Byrne. New York: Wiley, 1964.

——. *Focusing*. New York: Bantam, 1981.

——. *Let Your Body Interpret Your Dreams*. Wilmette, IL: Chiron Publications, 1986.

——. *Focusing Oriented Psychotherapy: A Manual of the Experiential Method*. New York: Guilford Publications, 1996.

GESTALT THERAPY

Gestalt therapy is a form of humanistic psychology that attempts to help participants develop awareness of their unresolved needs and emotions. Gestalt therapy's notion of the mind is based on psychoanalysis, gestalt psychology, existentialism, and the theories of Wilhelm Reich. A person is thought to be psychologically healthy when he or she is aware of his or her needs and is able to resolve them in an effective way. Gestalt therapists try to identify when their clients are blocking emotions by observing their movements and postures. Instead of investigating the past, gestalt therapists address clients' problems and emotions as they manifest in the present moment, often using techniques that require the client to act out his or her emotions. By urging people to confront their emotions, gestalt therapy seeks to help them make choices, interact with others, and relieve the physical symptoms of anxiety and stress.

The History of Gestalt Therapy

The original theories and techniques of gestalt therapy were formed by Laura and Frederick "Fritz" Perls from the scientific and intellectual atmosphere of Germany in the 1920s. After receiving his medical training, Fritz Perls began working with brain-damaged soldiers at Frankfurt-am-Main in 1926. During this time he became interested in new theories of the mind conceived by the existential philosophy of Martin Heidigger and Martin Buber and gestalt psychology, developed by Max Wertheimer and Kurt Koffa. He became a psychoanalyst, studying with people such as Karen Horney and Wilhelm Reich, who were expanding Sigmund Freud's methods. In the 1930s Fritz Perls went into therapy with Reich, who led him to believe that the body was a critical aspect of psychological therapy. Laura Perls studied with the influential thinkers Martin Buber and Paul Tillich at the University of Frankfurt. Often writing under her husband's name, she incorporated the principles of existential philosophy and theology into a framework of psychological therapy.

In 1934 Fritz and Laura Perls fled Nazi Germany for South Africa, where they established the South African Institute for Psychoanalysis. *Ego, Hunger, and Aggression*, published in 1942, outlined the principles that were to become the foundation of gestalt therapy. In 1946 they moved to New York City, where they began conducting gestalt group therapy sessions in their apartment. The Gestalt Therapy Association of New York was established in 1952, followed by the Gestalt Institute of Cleveland in 1954. Through the 1960s, gestalt therapy's popularity grew. Fritz and Laura Perls moved to California in 1960 and conducted workshops throughout the West Coast. In his workshops, Fritz Perls established himself as a leader and a guru. Many participants accused him of abusing his power. He continued to promote gestalt therapy until his death in 1970. The variety of techniques developed throughout the history of gestalt therapy have become a resource for therapists in many other disciplines. At least sixty-two Gestalt Therapy Institutes currently exist throughout the world.

Gestalt Theory

The theory of gestalt therapy was inspired by the insights into human consciousness developed by gestalt psychology. This theory of mind originated in 1920s Berlin in reaction to the prevailing atomistic and analytical approaches to understanding perception. At that time, theorists believed that a person identifies a perceived object by mentally assembling each part. Gestalt psychology asserted that this model must be reversed. Instead, a person grasps the whole form of the object first. This whole, or gestalt, then determines the way that one recognizes the component parts. Thus, one's experiences are organized according to basic mental patterns, or gestalts. As gestalt psychologists believe that each person possesses a set of gestalt images, gestalt therapists claim that basic needs, drives, and beliefs are also gestalts. These gestalts impart value to the objects or people in a person's environment, affecting his or her view of a situation and motivating him or her to make certain choices. Like existential philosophy, this view emphasizes personal responsibility. To feel more in control of and satisfaction with one's choices, one must become aware of one's freedom instead of blaming external influences. The gestalt therapist's role is to help clients identify how their needs and beliefs shape the ways they see themselves and others.

According to this model, a healthy individual is able to manage his or her needs by acknowledging what he or she desires and identifying how to obtain it. Unfortunately, human needs are not always met, and gestalt therapy claims that these unfulfilled needs manifest as anxiety, frustration, muscular tension, and other disturbances. A person's needs may not be met because he or she is unaware of the needs or is unable to express or fulfill them. Adopting the essential framework of psychoanalysis, gestalt therapy seeks to reveal unexplored parts of a client's personality and allow him or her to resolve unfulfilled desires responsibly. However, gestalt therapy deviates from traditional Freudian psychoanalysis by replacing the therapist's search into a client's past with a dialogue and enactment techniques that reveal the client's feelings and opinions in the present moment. Gestalt therapy emphasizes the here-and-now to illuminate the ways that a person's current behaviors and attitudes influence the choices he or she makes. Despite this emphasis on the present, the client's past remains an important aspect of gestalt therapy. Since unresolved needs from the past are thought to persist in a person's mind, affecting his or her everyday functioning, important aspects of a client's history will directly or indirectly present themselves during the session. With this approach, the course of a session will be different for each person.

A Gestalt Therapy Session

Throughout a gestalt therapy session, a person's attention is always directed to the present. At any moment, a client may be asked to describe what he or she is feeling. The client and therapist must always speak in the first person and describe events in the present tense. For example, instead of telling the therapist "my back is tense" or "my father makes me angry," a client will be urged to describe his or her current feelings and behavior with a statement such as "I am tensing my back" or "I feel angry at my father." These statements are phrased to emphasize the person's responsibility. Gestalt therapy techniques are designed to force a client to confront and express his or her needs and emotions during the session. They are often intense emotional experiences. In one common technique, the client is asked to isolate an emotion or a part of his or her personality and address it as if it were sitting in an empty chair in the room. A client also may conduct an imaginary dialogue with a person from a dream or from his or her past.

Gestalt therapy is often practiced in groups, usually consisting of ten people, for two hours. The therapist attempts to create an environment in which each person must express what he or she feels and listen to others. For example, a person who has trouble expressing criticism may be instructed to make a critical statement about each other member of the group. Then the therapist may ask each person to describe his or her emotional reaction to this confrontation. Through this process, a person can identify and overcome his or her barriers to self-expression. The therapist mediates the group, giving instructions and setting boundaries. Through the process, participants investigate how their problems manifest in their interactions with the group.

Therapists ask their clients to monitor how they feel during each exercise, helping them to become aware of the different emotions that may surface. Therapists also will be able to observe how a client may be blocking emotions. Borrowing concepts from Reich, gestalt therapy claims that the body may be affected by blocked emotions. Thus, a therapist will look for signs of blocked emotion in a person's movement or posture. The therapist seeks to make clients more aware of how their bodies are affected by their blocked emotions. The goal of therapy is to equip an individual with the self-awareness to find effective and authentic ways to resolve his or her needs.

Benefits

Many individuals choose gestalt therapy to become more emotionally expressive and more confident in their ability to make decisions, and to develop greater self-awareness. An individual may attend a group session to improve the way he or she relates to others. Or a group of family members or coworkers may attend together to develop more successful ways of interacting. Gestalt

therapy traditionally appeals to people seeking help with anxiety, depression, or stress. Gestalt therapy is not designed to treat individuals with more severe psychological conditions, such as psychoses or schizophrenia. Since a typical session in gestalt therapy will require confronting one's emotions, it is possible that a participant will encounter a severe emotional experience. For this reason, people who are extremely unstable or vulnerable may choose to avoid gestalt therapy.

Resources:

Gestalt Center for Psychotherapy and Training
510 East 89th Street
New York, NY 10128
Tel: (212) 879-3669
Offers training and resources for those interested in gestalt therapy.

Gestalt Therapy Institute of Los Angeles
1460 Seventh Street
Suite 301
Santa Monica, CA 90410
Tel: (909) 629-9935
Promotes the study of gestalt therapy.

Further Reading:

Kogan, Gerald. *Gestalt Therapy Resources.* Berkeley, CA: Transformations Press, 1980.

O' Connell, Vincent, ed. *Gestalt Therapy Primer: Introductory Readings in Gestalt Therapy.* Springfield, IL: Thomas, 1975.

Van de Riet, Vernon. *Gestalt Therapy: An Introduction.* New York: Pergamon Press, 1980.

HAKOMI INTEGRATIVE SOMATICS

Hakomi integrative somatics is a form of therapy that combines bodywork with elements of psychological counseling. It grew out of the hakomi method of body-centered psychotherapy, founded by Ron Kurtz. Both forms of hakomi view the mind and body as a single integrated organism, in which past traumas, both mental and physical, are "somaticized," that is, manifested in the body as habitual tension and strain. Fixed attitudes and patterns of behavior are similarly formed. Hakomi integrative somatics seeks to teach students to bring these unconscious habits to conscious awareness, understand them, and change them.

The History of Hakomi

Kurtz based his original techniques of hakomi psychotherapy on his knowledge of Taoism, Buddhism, and various body-mind disciplines, including Reichian therapy and bioenergetics. His studies in these areas led him to observe that a person's psychological defenses arise from a desire to avoid pain; thus, Kurtz believed, they are more readily overcome when they are gently supported rather than opposed. He developed hakomi into a method of psychotherapy that strives to evoke and process inner experiences through techniques of "mindfulness," an Eastern meditative technique for becoming aware of one's feelings and sensations in the present moment.

In the mid-1970s, Pat Ogden, an apprentice to Kurtz and a student of various bodywork therapies, became intrigued with the pervasive pattern in her patients' dissociation of the mind from the body. She also noticed that bodywork therapies and psychotherapy were generally practiced independently of each other. Wanting to forge the two approaches into a tool for treating body-mind dissociation, Ogden began to include bodywork in psychotherapy sessions. She found that her patients negotiated the healing process in a more integrated way and with more lasting results. In addition, she found that by incorporating the psychological processing of emotional material during a bodywork session, a patient's

physical changes were more enduring. Ogden's efforts to join hands-on bodywork and movement work with psychotherapy resulted in the formation of Hakomi Integrative Somatics.

Increasing Self-Awareness

Hakomi is founded on the premise that human beings are self-organizing; we continually and creatively adapt our perceptions and behaviors in accordance with our environment. Eventually, however, we may form fixed attitudes about ourselves and these may become unconscious attitudes, or "core organizers," that can limit us to habitual, automatic styles of being and relating to the world. Further, they can restrict our creativity and capacity for personal fulfillment. Core organizers are held and expressed in belief systems and emotional habits, as well as in body structure and movement patterns. Hakomi recognizes two distinct types of wounds that affect the formation of core organizers: developmental and traumatic. Developmental wounds arise from the unsatisfactory completion of learning tasks. Such tasks include learning to get one's needs met and learning to be autonomous. Traumatic wounds occur in overwhelming situations in which actual survival is threatened, such as abuse, accidents, surgery, and war. When we suffer from either kind of wound, we may become habitually dissociated from one or more of our core organizers.

In hakomi integrative somatics, a healing relationship between therapist and patient is established, providing a crucial element in the creation of a context in which the cooperation of the patient's unconscious may be gained. Then, by means of exercises combining bodywork with verbalizations by the patient, core organizers are brought to consciousness and new information about them becomes available. In this experiential, rather than cognitive (analytical, thinking-based), process, the patient can explore new options—both physical and psychological—and spontaneously

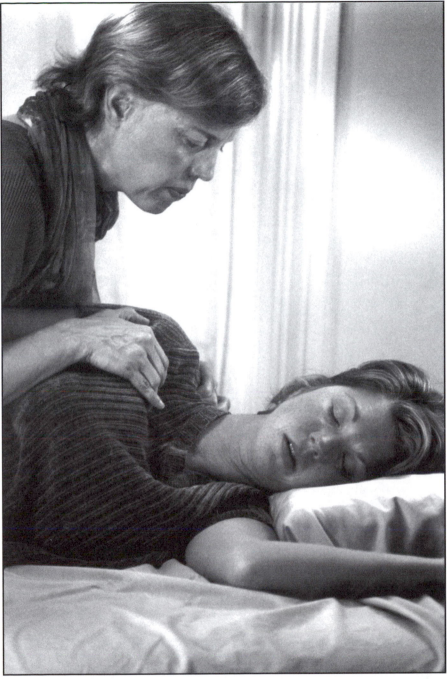

Photo by Susanna Drogsuold

Pat Ogden, developer of hakomi integrative somatics, building a healing relationship through gentle touch.

reorganize toward health. The patient also learns ways to deepen his or her awareness of the connection between the body and the mind. He or she becomes more attuned to the ever-changing flow of wordless information that is the language of the body. This awareness becomes a powerful healing tool for it naturally expands the patient's sense of a physical self—an essential step in correcting the dissociation of the mind from the body.

Achieving Mindfulness

The practitioner begins a session by talking with the patient to assess his or her situation and to establish a healing relationship in which the client feels safe and accepted. The client is helped to access a state of consciousness called mindfulness, a self-reflective state cultivated by gently focusing one's attention inward. Through mindfulness the client observes and describes present inner experience—specifically body patterns, emotions, images, memories, or thoughts. These facets of inner experience reflect basic attitudes such as "I'm not good enough," or "I am always alone." Core organizers are accessible through either body or mind; one level easily accesses the other. By means of verbal and physical experiments, a client begins to re-associate with previously dissociated core organizers. For example, a client is asked to attend to what happens as hands-on bodywork is performed on her shoulders. He or she may notice that a feeling of sadness arises as he or she is reminded of being alone as a child. The practitioner continues using such exercises to explore the places in the body that contain patterns of core organization—in this case, the one involved with feelings of loneliness. Throughout the process, the client actively participates and verbalizes his or her inner experiences and emotions.

A session also includes supporting a client's inner resources by developing an awareness of the strengths and potentials an individual already possesses. The therapist approaches the client in a manner that acknowledges that client's abilities, rather than adopting a stance that focuses exclusively on problems and supposed deficiencies.

Integrating the Body and Mind

Hakomi integrative somatics can enhance physical, psychological, and spiritual well-being. By working simultaneously with the body and the mind, Hakomi can often uncover information that remains unconscious in conventional therapies and can effect physical changes that are more lasting. Participants consistently report greater integration of the body and mind. While specific outcomes vary, results can include the reduction of pain and posttraumatic stress symptoms; improved physical alignment, capacity for intimacy, and creativity; and an overall feeling of being more in tune with oneself.

—*Pat Ogden, M.A.*

Resources:

Hakomi Integrative Somatics
P.O. Box 19438
Boulder, CO 80308
Tel: (303) 447-3290
e-mail: hakomisoma@aol.com
Offers workshops in Hakomi Integrative Somatics and training of practitioners.

Further Reading:

Kurtz, Ron. *Body-Centered Psychotherapy: The Hakomi Method.* Mendocino, CA: Life Rhythm, 1986.

HOLOTROPIC BREATHWORK™

Holotropic Breathwork™ is a recently developed method of self-exploration that combines rapid, deep breathing, evocative music, and focused bodywork. The term "holotropic" is derived from the Greek *holos*, meaning "whole" and *trepin*, meaning "to move in the direction of." Holotropic Breathwork aims to bring the mind and body together in a trance state, which furnishes access to buried memories and aspects of consciousness hidden under ordinary conditions.

While Holotropic Breathwork can be an effective treatment for mental and physical disorders, it is more often approached as shamanic activity for recovery of the deep past and entry into the spiritual realm.

The History of Holotropic Breathwork™

Holotropic Breathwork was developed by Stanislav Grof, a Czech psychiatrist trained in Prague during the 1950s, and his wife, Christine. A study of Jung's theories of the collective unconscious convinced Grof that faith in reason had led modern science to espouse a mechanistic model of the mind, incapable of assessing or utilizing its true range of powers. He was particularly interested in determining the scope and nature of experiences such as visions generally relegated to the category of parapsychological phenomena.

A breakthrough in the manufacture of psychedelic drugs gave Grof a way to experiment with altered states of consciousness. By his own account he soon realized that there were broad similarities between certain drug-induced states of mind and the experiences attained through meditative, mystic, and shamanic activity.

After emigrating to the United States in the early 1960s, Grof continued his research into altered consciousness and parapsychology at the Maryland Psychiatric Research Center, Johns Hopkins University, and eventually the Esalen Institute in Big Sur, California.

During the 1970s the Grofs emerged as leaders in the New Age healing and spiritual movement but kept strong ties with psychiatric theory and scholarship. Along with Kenneth Wilber, they are regarded as key figures in the formation of transpersonal psychology, a system integrating Jungian theory with contemporary physiological research and multicultural study of religion. Transpersonal psychology is sometimes the true basis for clinical treatment of mental disorders.

The Grofs incorporated its principles into Holotropic Breathwork, which they began to offer in workshop and training programs in 1976. Several books, most notably Stanislav Grof's *Realms of the Human Unconscious* of 1975 and *The Holotropic Mind* of 1992, have contributed to the steady rise of interest in the Holotropic Breathwork technique and transpersonal psychology.

A Transpersonal Theory of the Mind

Holotropic Breathwork is based on the premise that the psyche is a field of commingled personal and cosmic, or "transpersonal," energy. Breath is more than a metaphor of the fluid continuum of personal and transpersonal energy. According to the Grofs, breath acts as a conduit for the energy, sustaining the mind as well as the body. In ordinary "hylotropic" consciousness, one is aware of only a limited portion of the vast spectrum of energies being exchanged. The technique of Holotropic Breathwork is designed to accelerate breathing and at the same time greatly expand awareness of the transcendent forces pervading each moment of human life.

Faster and deeper breathing and music are used to bring about a trance state comparable to the state reached in Sufi dancing or Native American sweat-lodge rituals. The Grofs maintain that in this state it is possible to get access to kinds of consciousness experiences: sensory, biographical, perinatal (centered around the time of birth), and transpersonal.

In the sensory experience, sight and sound become richer and more compelling. In biographical experiences, the individual accesses buried memories and feeling known as coex systems. Coex systems are systems of condensed experience that have been stored up since childhood and are regarded by some alternative health care professionals as the source of many health problems. In perinatal experiences, the individual relives her or his birth. This is considered the doorway to the fourth, or transpersonal, category of experience, which corresponds to Jung's collective unconscious. Numinous experience floods the individual, boundaries of space and time are crossed, past life experiences reclaimed, myths and symbols may assume enhanced vitality, and visions of the future sometimes appear.

Grof refers to Holotropic Breathwork as "an adventure in self-discovery" rather than as a therapy or mystic rite. The therapeutic value of Holotropic Breathwork is thought to issue from the unblocking of conflicts and traumas stored in coex systems and from the enhancement of the individual's sense of inner potential.

Experiencing Holotropic Breathwork™

Holotropic Breathwork is presented at two-day workshops by facilitators certified by the Grofs. Participants are interviewed, then taught the principles and techniques of Breathwork. The sessions, which last from two to four hours, take place in a dimly lit room.

Participants work in pairs, alternating the roles of breather and sitter. As sitters, they watch over their companion, providing a sense of shelter and support and attending to any needs she or he may have. As breathers, they lie flat on the floor and undergo a process that leads from relaxation exercises to an extended period of accelerated, deep breathing. Music is played at a high volume throughout the session and generally features little-known classical pieces, film scores, New Age music, Gregorian chants, aboriginal drumming, and other types of music associated with ritual and trance experience. If requested or required, the facilitators provide hands-on touch for the breather, applying pressure to areas of resistance and tension in order to aid in their release.

The breathers soon enter a trance in which consciousness is altered, not lost. The effects vary from individual to individual. Some grow still as if in deep meditation. Others see vivid images and become active, rocking, moaning, weeping, crying out in anger, expressing a sensation or feeling. There may be a broad range of emotion from ecstatic rapture to abysmal despair within a single session. A breather does not necessarily experience all four categories of experience, and the experiences do not always progress in sequence from the sensory to the transpersonal. Each time the role of breather is assumed, a different response is likely to occur. Usually participants breathe and sit twice during the course of a workshop.

At the end of the session participants and facilitators work together, to release unresolved tensions. Mandala drawing, which involves graphic and symbolic figures, brings the session to conclusion. The typical workshop in Holotropic Breathwork includes meditation, lectures, and group sharing.

Benefits and Risks of Holotropic Breathwork™

Holotropic Breathwork is a highly charged, sometimes strenuous experience precluded during pregnancy and for anyone with glaucoma, heart disease, or a severe emotional disorder.

Participants in Holotropic Breathwork report that they receive intuitive insights and clarify troublesome areas

Training

Certification at the Grof Transpersonal Training center requires 150 hours of general experience in Holotropic Breathwork, 350 hours of training combining theory and practice, and a final two-week seminar. The instruction focuses upon breathwork techniques and correlated issues ranging from childhood sexual abuse to paranormal psychology and shamanism. The certification program takes at least two years to complete.

of their lives. Practitioners of the discipline believe that the technique promotes self-healing through the release of accumulated stress and trauma and greater connection with physical, emotional, and spiritual parts of oneself.

—*Kylea Taylor, M.S.*

Resources:

Association for Holotropic Breathwork International
P.O. Box 7169
Santa Cruz, CA 95061-7169
Web site: www.breathwork.com
Membership group that organizes conferences and publishes a quarterly newsletter, The Inner Door, *with articles on Holotropic Breathwork research and practice.*

East-West Retreats
P.O. Box 12
Philo, CA 95466
Tel: (707) 895-2856
Organizes Buddhist Vipassana/Holotropic Breathwork workshops.

Grof Transpersonal Training
20 Sunnyside, Suite A-253
Mill Valley, CA 94941
Tel: (415) 383-8779
Web site: www.holotropic.com
Trains and certifies practitioners of Holotropic Breathwork, provides referrals to certified practitioners, and publishes the Grofs' lecture and conference schedule.

Further Reading:

Grof, Christina. *The Thirst for Wholeness.* San Francisco: HarperCollins Publishers, 1993.

Grof, Stanislav. *The Adventure of Self-Discovery: Dimensions of Consciousness and New Perspectives in Psychotherapy and Inner Exploration.* Stonybrook: SUNY Press, 1988.

——. *Realms of the Human Unconscious.* London: Souvenir Press Ltd., 1975.

Grof, Stanislav, and Hal Bennett. *The Holotropic Mind.* San Francisco: Harper San Francisco, 1992.

Scotton, Bruce, Allan Chinen, and John Battista, eds. *Textbook of Transpersonal Psychiatry and Psychology.* New York: HarperCollins Publishers, 1996.

Taylor, Kylea. *The Breathwork Experience.* Santa Cruz, CA: Hanford Mead Publishers, 1994.

——. *The Ethics of Caring.* Santa Cruz, CA: Hanford Mead Publishers, 1995.

Wilber, Kenneth. *The Spectrum of Consciousness.* Wheaton, IL: Theosophical Publications, 1977.

MEDICAL ORGONE THERAPY

Medical orgone therapy is a unique approach to treating emotional and physical illness by reducing or eliminating those barriers that block the natural expression of emotion and healthy sexual feeling. This method of treatment was developed by Austrian psychiatrist and scientist Wilhelm Reich, M.D. (1897–1957). After years of clinical and experimental laboratory research, Reich concluded that emotions, sexual feelings, and all life processes are expressions of a biological energy in the body. He further concluded that this life energy is related to bioelectricity but is fundamentally different. He called this energy "orgone energy." Reich theorized that orgone energy fills the universe and pulsates in all living things. He believed that deep, genuine love and the ability to experience a gratifying orgasm mutually with one's partner are the fullest and deepest expressions of our being and are central to maintaining optimal health.

Reich contended that in almost all individuals, the flow and release of orgone energy are blocked by chronic

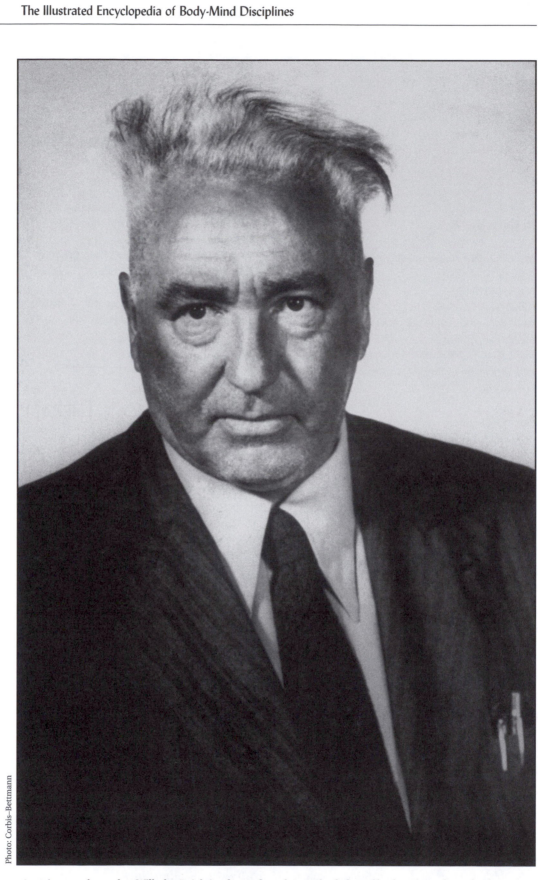

Austrian psychoanalyst Wilhelm Reich is often referred to as the father of body-oriented psychotherapies.

muscle contractions in various areas of the body and by emotional attitudes adopted early in life. The "nice little girl" who never gets angry, and the "strong, brave boy" who never shows fear and sadness are but two examples of such attitudes that prevent the full and rational expression of natural emotions. Blocked emotions interfere with pleasure in life and cause sexual feelings to become disconnected from tender emotions of love. Without emotional release, anxiety develops, which further increases physical and emotional contraction. This cycle results in a range of problems such as feelings of emptiness, depression, irrational fears, and self-destructive behavior. Medical orgone therapy employs direct work on the body, especially on spastic muscles, with verbal therapy to bring about a healthy state accompanied by satisfaction in one's work and love life.

The History of Medical Orgone Therapy

Dr. Wilhelm Reich began his career as a student and colleague of Sigmund Freud (1856–1939), the founder of psychoanalysis. During his work as a psychoanalyst, Reich discovered that the individual's deep emotions were bound up in defensive character attitudes, which he called "character armor." To treat these problems Reich developed a highly effective technique of character analysis, still used today by other psychotherapies, which focuses on the individual's attitudes and present-day concerns and less so on past relationships within the family.

While working with patients, Reich observed that only those who developed a satisfactory, healthy sexual life fully resolved their neurotic symptoms. Satisfaction was not determined by the mere presence of sexual activity. Rather, it required the ability to give in to both deep, tender love feelings and the intense sexual sensations that are experienced with a total body orgasm. Reich asserted that this all-encompassing

experience is possible only with a partner of the opposite sex, and concluded that only such a complete orgasm could regulate the energy metabolism.

Reich observed that defensive emotional attitudes are not just "in the mind" but are held in the body's muscles, and he called this the "muscular armor." He also found that inhibited feelings were accompanied by restrictions in respiration. These realizations led him to the groundbreaking conclusion that the successful treatment of emotional problems requires work on the body combined with verbal therapy.

Reich's theories about the link between sex, emotions, and the body, and his experimental work with orgone energy were very controversial. Legal action was taken against him by the United States Food and Drug Administration. He refused to defend his scientific work in a courtroom, believing the proper venue to challenge his research was the laboratory. He was found guilty of failing to obey an injunction and was jailed. He died in prison in 1957.

Reich's ideas about sexuality have often been misunderstood. This was especially true during the "sexual revolution" of the 1960s and 1970s, when his name and ideas were associated with the idea that one can become "free" by having sex. In fact, Reich clearly stated that loveless sexuality was neurotic and when harsh or mechanical was unhealthy.

Elsworth F. Baker, M.D. (1903–1985), Reich's associate, continued Reich's work in the late 1950s, overseeing the training of medical orgonomists and orgone research. He founded the *Journal of Orgonomy* in 1967 and established the American College of Orgonomy in 1968. The college actively continues the development of the science of orgonomy, and its journal publishes clinical and scientific research.

The Theory of Medical Orgone Therapy

Medical orgone therapy is based on Wilhelm Reich's theory of armoring. The method of treatment developed from observations on the movement and blockage of energy in the body. Infants and children naturally feel pleasure and reach out to the world. If these impulses are frustrated, the child contracts and develops methods to adapt to the stress. If frustrations continue, these defensive reactions become chronic and extend into adult life even when they are no longer needed. For example, a child may develop a submissive manner to deal with an angry parent and then as an adult react submissively to all authority figures, even when it would be better to be assertive. Other common examples of "character armor" are found in individuals who present themselves as aloof, superior, "cool," sophisticated, cute, or special. Medical orgonomists consider these character attitudes to be manifested in actual muscular rigidities (muscular armor), which hold back intolerable or unacceptable emotions such as anger, fear, or sadness. Individuals are usually unaware of their muscular armor or that their physical problems, such as headaches, stiff neck, or back pain, are often rooted in repressed emotions.

Armoring forms in infancy and early childhood as a defense against painful feelings, but it is not a satisfactory solution because it later interferes with healthy emotional life and energy discharge. Medical orgone therapy strives to eliminate chronic armor to restore the individual to more natural functioning in all aspects of his or her life.

Medical Orgone Therapy in Practice

The medical orgonomist is trained to understand the patient in all respects and diagnose the patterns of character and physical armor. Because all medical orgone therapists are physicians who also have specialized training in psychiatry, they are equipped to diagnose physical conditions and work directly on their patients. Treatment includes character analysis and the release of buried emotions facilitated by breathing and direct work on spastic muscles. The therapy

does not focus much on psychological causes or delve deeply into past relationships with parents. Therapy is also used to treat infants and children. The removal of early armoring allows the child to develop with a natural energy flow, emotional aliveness, and a sense of well-being. Treatment helps to prevent the development of chronic character and muscular armor in adult life.

It is important to note that the techniques used in this therapy are not the same as those in some other methods used to address physical tension such as acupressure, massage, and deep breathing. Character analysis also has its own specific techniques, which should not be confused with positive affirmations, guided self-examination, and similar therapeutic approaches.

In the *Journal of Orgonomy* (vol. 28, no. 1), Dr. Charles Konia describes a representative course of orgone therapy: "In medical orgone therapy, armor is intentionally dissolved. This invariably brings about anxiety, because the very function of the armor is to prevent the [individual] from experiencing such painful feelings. The medical orgonomist encourages the individual to experience and tolerate anxiety so that the underlying, contained emotions can be felt and then expressed. This brings about the desired, positive, therapeutic effect: anxiety is eliminated and replaced by a sense of pleasurable well-being."

The Benefits of Medical Orgone Therapy

Medical orgone therapy is a unique approach to the prevention and treatment of a wide range of mental and physical conditions. Medical orgonomists report successful treatment of the full range of emotional symptoms and relationship problems. Serious conditions such as depression, schizophrenia, panic disorder, and ADHD can often be treated without resorting to medications. Reich concluded—and present-day physicians who practice medical orgone therapy concur—that the elimination of armoring, in and of itself, restores natural, healthy functioning. Patients regain their natural capacities to enjoy satisfaction in love, work, and the pursuit of knowledge.

—*Peter A. Crist, M.D.,
and Richard Schwartzman, D.O.*

Resources:

The American College of Orgonomy
P.O. Box 490
Princeton, NJ 08542
Tel:(732) 821-1144
Fax:(732) 821-0174
Web site: www.orgonomy.org
Trains and certifies medical orgonomists. Provides referrals and offers seminars, conferences, and laboratory courses that are open to the general public. Orgonomic Publications, a division of the American College of Orgonomy, sells numerous in-print and out-of-print books on the subject of orgonomy and publishes the biannual Journal of Orgonomy.

Further Reading:

Books:
Baker, Elsworth F. *Man in the Trap*. New York: The Macmillan Co., 1967.

Reich, Wilhelm. *Character Analysis*. Translated by Theodore P. Wolfe. Third enlarged edition. New York: Noonday Press, 1949.

——.*Children of the Future: On the Prevention of Sexual Pathology*. New York: Farrar, Straus and Giroux, 1983.

——. *Cosmic Superimposition: Man's Orgonotic Roots in Nature*. Rangeley, ME: Wilhelm Reich Foundation, 1951.

——. *The Discovery of the Orgone:Vol. 1, The Function of the Orgasm: Sex-Economic Problems of Biological Energy*. Translated by Theodore P. Wolfe. 2nd edition. New York: Orgone Institute Press, 1948.

——.*The Discovery of the Orgone: Vol. 2, The Cancer Biopathy*. Translated by Theodore P. Wolfe. New York: Orgone Institute Press, 1948.

——. *The Emotional Plague of Mankind: Vol. 1. The Murder of Christ*. New York: Orgone Institute Press, 1953.

——. *Reich Speaks of Freud*. New York: Farrar, Straus and Giroux, 1967.

——. *Selected Writings: An Introduction to Orgonomy*. New York: Farrar, Straus and Cudahy, 1960.

Sharaf, Myron. *Fury on Earth: A Biography of Wilhelm Reich*. New York: St. Martin's Press/Marek, 1983.

Journals:
Konia, Charles. "Anxiety: Curse or Blessing?" *Journal of Orgonomy*, 28, No.1, 1994:1–3.

Numerous clinical and theoretical articles on medical orgone therapy have been published by various authors in the *Journal of Orgonomy* from 1967 to the present. A detailed and complete listing of these articles is available from the American College of Orgonomy.

ORGANISMIC BODY PSYCHOTHERAPY

Organismic body psychotherapy is a form of psychotherapy developed by Malcolm and Katherine Brown based on their belief that the body, mind, and spirit are interconnected, and that life-enhancing benefits can be realized using techniques that involve the body as well as the mind. Organismic body psychotherapy is termed neo-Reichian because it incorporates ideas put forth by Wilhelm Reich, such as the concept of body armoring, but makes significant modifications to Reich's ideas. One of the most important modifications is the belief that releasing body armor does not have to be strong and highly emotional; rather, organismic body psychotherapy theory recognizes the possibility of a gradual, quiet release. Physical exercise, verbal dialogue, and touch are combined to bring about release and eventual physical, emotional, and spiritual well-being.

The Development of Organismic Body Psychotherapy

Organismic body psychotherapy was created by Malcolm and Katherine Brown. Malcolm Brown is a clinical psychologist who has been strongly influenced by a variety of therapeutic models, including Fritz Perls and Kurt Goldstein's writings on gestalt therapy, Abraham Maslow's humanistic psychology, Carl Roger's client-centered therapy, and Jungian psychology as developed by Carl Jung and Erich Neumann. The writings of Alexander Lowen in biogenetics introduced Brown to the ideas of Wilhelm Reich and other body-oriented psychotherapists. Brown has worked with Alexander Lowen and European neo-Reichian psychotherapists, including Gerda Boyesan and David Boadella, who are known for developing a more subtle approach to Reich's work.

Katherine Brown is a therapist with a background in gestalt therapy, sensory awareness, and massage therapy. In 1972 she attended a lecture given by Malcolm Brown. She became very interested in his theories and eventually began collaborating with him. They subsequently married and started working as cotherapists with some of their respective clients. They found that practicing as a male-female therapist team was very effective. They coined the term organismic body psychotherapy for their work, and devoted the remainder of their professional pursuits exclusively to training psychotherapists in their methods. The Browns are now semi-retired.

A Body-Mind Discipline

Organismic body psychotherapy is designed to facilitate an increasing self-reliance on the human faculties, such as the abilities to sense, feel, think, and intuit that lie within a person's body. The internal flowering of these faculties enables a client to become relatively self-trusting and to lead a rich life. To awaken these self-healing resources, organismic body psychotherapy techniques seek to engage the mental, emotional, and spiritual aspects of a client.

A key tenet of organismic body psychotherapy is that the body as well as the mind must be engaged in the therapeutic process because a client's psychological defenses are also manifested at the body level. This physical manifestation of a client's defenses is called armoring and consists of physical tensions that block emotion, feeling, and the ability to satisfy fundamental emotional needs. According to organismic body psychotherapy, these needs include the ability to connect with others, the ability to connect to one's inner self, the ability to see the outer world and one's inner self objectively and make meaning of both, and the ability to fulfill personal goals.

According to the theoretical foundation of organismic body psychotherapy, there are three stages of growth in the therapeutic process. They are: loosening the armoring; resolving psychological conflicts; and finally, growth combined with self-actualization. Using these stages as a guide, the therapist attempts to identify a client's current state and to adjust the therapeutic modality accordingly. The process begins with more of a therapist-directed style and gradually becomes more patient-directed. Because organismic body psychotherapy is based on the belief that each individual is unique, it is believed that the unfolding and duration of each of these stages will be different for each individual.

Mobilization Exercises

Among the techniques used to dissolve the armoring are mobilization exercises and direct touch. Mobilization exercises are done with a client standing or lying on a padded mat. They are designed to release chronic armoring patterns, which consist primarily of tense muscles. Direct touch is given by the therapist in two forms: nurturing and catalytic. Nurturing is a very soft form of touch used to soften armoring by mobilizing energy within the body, causing the release of armoring. Catalytic touch is a harder, more aggressive form of touch that releases the armoring. While doing the exercises or receiving direct touch, the client may experience expressive emotional releases, such as crying or screaming, which are a result of loosening of the armoring.

While working with the body is an elemental aspect of organismic body psychotherapy, sessions are not entirely nonverbal. Verbal work, such as a discussion of emotional releases, dreams, or insight, also plays an important role in the organismic body psychotherapy process.

Feeling Connected

When applied properly, direct touch seems to increase a client's awareness of his or her primary need to feel connected and related that often has been unsatisfied since early childhood. Moreover, direct touch seems to accomplish this without creating overwhelming anxiety or hardening a client's defenses. Once the armoring has been loosened and healing has occurred through the resolution of psychological conflicts, practitioners of organismic body psychotherapy believe that a person's resources and faculties are accessible for development of the soul.

—*Elliot Greene*

Resources:

Washington Institute for Body Psychotherapy
Elliot Greene and Barbara Goodrich-Dunn, Directors
8830 Cameron Street, Suite 206
Silver Spring, MD 20910
Tel: (301) 588-9341
Offers a four-year training program in body psychotherapy and workshops on subjects related to body psychotherapy.

Further Reading:

Brown, Malcolm, Ph.D. *The Healing Touch*. Mendocino, CA: Life Rhythm Press.

PESSO BOYDEN SYSTEM PSYCHOMOTOR

Pesso Boyden system psychomotor (PBSP) therapy uses group therapy to help patients recall, encounter, and ultimately rebuild in a positive way their reactions to past events. The "psycho" in psychomotor refers to the psyche, or the mind. "Motor" refers to bodily sensations and movements, which include actions that may be blocked in the body by trauma. Through group role-playing activities called "structures," PBSP patients relive long-past memories and emotions that have saddled the patient with traumatizing feelings of dissatisfaction. With the guidance of the therapist and the assistance of the group, the patient undergoes emotional "reeducation": the truthful recollection of a painful event with a convincing reenactment of a happier conclusion.

An Innovative Movement Program

PBSP is based on the studies of Albert Pesso and Diane Boyden-Pesso, classically trained dancers and choreographers who, in the late 1950s, developed their own style of expressive dance. Much of their new style focused on the development of emotional and physical tools that could convincingly communicate internal feelings, visions, and ideas to an audience.

This research led Albert Pesso, in the early 1960s, to publish an essay that placed all movement into three categories: reflex, voluntary, and emotional. Reflex motion includes the reflex to keep our bodies upright. Voluntary movement is oriented to our environment, that is, those movements that we consciously initiate in order to manipulate and move through the world around us. By contrast, emotional movement includes any movement initiated by our reaction to our inner feelings and how we feel about the environment around us.

These three types of movement are inextricably interwoven. We can voluntarily alter or stop many reflex actions for a short period of time. Similarly, strong emotions can have a marked impact on our voluntary and reflex motions.

Albert and Diane were not the first researchers to envision such a breakdown of the patterns of movement. Their work built on the established system of French acting and singing teacher François Delsarte (1811–1871), who formulated specific principles of aesthetics based on a set of rules coordinating the voice with body gestures. As Albert and Diane continued to develop their style of expressive dance, they began to incorporate more and more exercises aimed at sharpening awareness of the three types of movement into their dance training programs. They found that a dance student, once made sensitive to these three types of movement, could eliminate unwanted and unpredictable motions from his or her performance by giving it its proper and therapeutic expression. Furthermore, the students reported that having full mastery of all three types of movement seemed to allow a more open and healthy expression of their needs in their everyday lives.

Recognizing Your Feelings

Diane and Albert soon theorized that these same exercises could help emotionally troubled people overcome their problems. To them, a person's emotions stored in the body represent the nearest thing to a true self. Most psychological problems, they believe, can be attributed to the absence and repression of the body's interactive needs that had

not been met by the participant's parents. These needs and hungers change the way people look at the world. Depending on the nature of the unfulfilled need, the effect from these unconscious hungers can range from occasional depression to total physical and emotional debilitation on the part of the sufferer.

PBSP tracks down clues to these hidden feelings and seeks to bring expression and healing to the damage they have caused. A patient first meets with a psychotherapist for an observation session, during which the therapist formulates some idea of what might be the underlying root cause of the patient's neuroses or problems. Diane Boyden-Pesso describes the agenda of the therapist at the meeting in this way: "My goal as a therapist is to make sure that the client works in [PBSP] from where he really is, what is really important and real, and not work on something that he or she may have decided in advance intellectually that it would be good to work on. We have to work on what is valid and spontaneous at the moment."

Structures

The primary tool of PBSP is a group role-playing activity, called "structures," comprised of a seamless series of steps (individually known as "a structure") within the total structure. Within a carefully controlled group session the therapist encourages the patient to share what is upsetting him or her in the present.

To this scene, however, two important characters are added: the "truth stater" and the "witness." The truth stater is used to eternalize and illustrate the participant's spoken thoughts and beliefs by stating out loud the "truths" by which the participant lives. If the participant says, "I have to take care of myself because there is no one in the world who will do that for me," the truth stater is instructed to announce, "You have to take care of yourself because there is no one in the world who will do that for you."

Meanwhile, the witness is used to track the emotional reactions of the participant as the therapist queries the participant on what they think they are feeling. Witnesses also validate the participant's emotional expressions, naming each emotion and the context of the emotion in a compassionate, accepting manner. A typical statement might be, "I see how bitter you feel as you hear that statement."

The input of the two special accommodators induces a participant to recognizing these current feelings as part of a pattern of behavior from his or her past. Participants can then see these patterns of dysfunction as a result of past life-shaping events. Memories evoked by these structures are powerful and experienced almost as if they were happening in the present. The participant is thus in the dual position of "reliving" a vivid memory while at the same time becoming aware of her- or himself from a therapeutic perspective. Finally, the patient can express the long-suppressed longings that were left unfulfilled, such as the isolation and self-loathing that can arise from desertion by a parent. Although absorbed with this memory, the participant is nonetheless able to use his or her new-found awareness of emotions, body sensations, and impulses to express what he or she is experiencing.

Once the patient feels thoroughly re-immersed in the recollection, he or she instructs the other members of the group, called accommodators, to positions and roles that reenact the event as it occurred. Accommodators play the antithesis role of whichever person has denied the patient his or her specific need. They are meant to provide the ideal role or figure in order for participants to meet the needs that were not met by history. In the above example, the ideal figure would play the role of a new, alternative parent who has deserted the patient. In this scenario, however, the new "ideal parent" offers clear, positive accommodation to the person, such as "If I had been there, I would not have left you."

Albert and Diane believe that although the activity occurs in the group session, the final and most meaningful locus of reconstruction takes place in the inner theater of the mind. Through this emotional reeducation,

---

In a safe, respectful setting, the PBSP therapist supplies the natural, comprehensive, and carefully crafted technology—discovered by Albert Pesso and Diane Boyden Pesso—which uses the resources of the body, mind, and soul to help people complete the five crucial life tasks necessary for intellectual, psychological, emotional, and spiritual well-being.

Those life tasks are:
1. Satisfy the basic developmental needs for:
   place
   nurture
   support
   protection
   limits
   experience needed by our human nature to fully mature and bear fruit.
2. Integrate and unify the polarities of our biological and psychological being—to own all parts of our body and mind.
3. Develop our consciousness—know that and why we are alive.
4. Develop our self-organizing center, or "pilot"—be in command of our own life.
5. Realize our personal uniqueness and potentiality—find our calling and become who we truly can be.

the participant has gotten in contact with his or her needs, feeling them again, and then has these needs met by this new positive figure in a way that leaves an imprint in the body-mind memory of the participant. The memory can then be recalled at will by the participant to reinforce the positive experience. This is a step toward final maturity. Through this, the participant has abandoned the hope of having his or her needs redressed by the original person. Instead, they have the need satisfied while they are in touch with the right age by someone representing the ideal mother or father, whichever is needed. The participant has taken an important step toward healing.

PBSP is considered a psychoanalytic process, a behavior modification process, a reparenting process, a gestalt process, a body therapy process, a family therapy process (without the family), and more. It contains so much that is fundamental to all forms of psychotherapy that it relates easily to all major techniques used to treat emotional and mental problems.

The Benefits of Emotional Maturation

PBSP gives participants a positive lens through which to see and experience the world. Following PBSP therapy they are less likely to be ruled by habitual, emotional reactions such as displaced anger, anxiety, depression, and emotionally immature desires. Through PBSP, clients can function more productively in the reality of present-day settings.

Therapists use PBSP, in groups and one-on-one, with a wide variety of populations. It is successfully used in psychiatric settings, drug and alcohol treatment centers, pain clinics, and obesity treatment programs. It is effective with victims of abuse, incest, and adolescents having trouble with their emotions, the law, and drugs. It has significant value in application to marriage and family problems and is now being used to alleviate executive stress

and to deal with other organizational problems.

PBSP is a safe procedure that puts a high emphasis on the comfort of its patients. Nevertheless, PBSP involves complex psychological evaluation that is best handled by professionals. Anyone interested in PBSP therapy should consult a trained PBSP psychotherapist or PBSP institution.

—*Albert Pesso*

Resources:

Pesso Boyden System/Psychomotor
Strolling Woods
Lake Shore Drive
Franklin, NH 03235
Tel: (603) 934-9809
Web site: www.pbsp.com
Provides information on practitioners as well as the discipline.

Further Reading:

Books:
Napier, Augustus Y., Ph.D. *The Fragile Bond: In Search of an Equal, Intimate and Enduring Marriage.* New York: HarperCollins, 1990.

Pesso, Albert. *Experience in Action.* New York: New York University Press, 1973.

——. *Movement in Psychotherapy.* New York: New York University Press, 1969.

——. *Moving Psychotherapy.* Cambridge, MA: Brookline Books, 1991.

Journals:
Foulds, Melvin, and Patricia S. Hannigan. "Effects of Psychomotor Group Therapy on Ratings of Self and Others." *Psychotherapy: Theory, Research and Practice,* Volume II, no. 4 (Winter 1974).

——. "Effects of Psychomotor Group Therapy on Locus of Control and Social Desirability," *Humanistic Psychology* 16, No. 2 (Spring 1975).

PROCESS ORIENTED PSYCHOLOGY

Process oriented psychology, or simply "process work," is a form of psychotherapy used to help a person become aware of and embrace all aspects of his or her experience, even those that at first seem too disturbing, strange, or socially unacceptable. According to process oriented psychology, the disturbing or traumatic experiences that we cannot accept tend to reappear as dreams, physical symptoms, relationship difficulties, or conflicts with society. A process oriented psychologist, believing that all experience is meaningful, helps a client approach the disturbing experience and explore its connection to current physical and emotional problems. Treating a disturbing experience with love and understanding may help one find a solution.

Process oriented psychology was developed by the American Jungian analyst Arnold Mindell. He developed methods to help couples and families explore disturbing experiences and worked with a wide variety of individuals not usually treated with psychotherapy. These techniques later became a part of Mindell's work with groups and organizations that were troubled by conflict. He found that groups, when faced with situations and individuals that challenge their purpose and unity, behave much like troubled individuals. By encouraging silent voices to speak, and allowing other members to experience what it feels like to occupy unpopular roles, he helped the majority of the group assimilate new points of view, often leading to unique solutions to the group's problems. Mindell developed these methods into "world work," a body of theory and practice for working with groups in conflict, even when they contain people from many ethnic and racial groups, socioeconomic classes, sexual orientations, and spiritual affiliations.

At the heart of Mindell's work is the belief that a mysterious, often irrational, and nonverbal current of subjective experience, which he calls "the dreaming process," flows alongside each person's conscious, objective, intentional activities of everyday life, often leading the person to experience things that conflict with his or her self-image. When a person puts aside such a disturbing experience, the dreaming process continues to express itself as physical symptoms, relationship difficulties, or conflicts with society. Mindell believes that the experiences with which a person least identifies consciously have the most power to produce change and restore the flow of the dreaming process. Because these experiences challenge our personal or collective identity, he believes that we stop them from completing themselves, fearing the inner or outer conflict they might produce. By focusing awareness on these experiences and encouraging them to unfold, process oriented psychology aims to help people find solutions to current problems and to tap into a source for continued personal growth.

Process work is most frequently practiced as a form of individual psychotherapy. A client typically visits his or her therapist for an hour-long session. A course of therapy may consist of one session, or may last for many years. The client may present a dream, a relationship difficulty, a physical symptom, or any other experience that he or she would like to explore. The process worker focuses on the client's subjective experiences of his or her concerns and problems, observing movement, body posture, and language. To help identify, clarify, and learn from aspects of the client's subjective experience, the process worker employs a wide array of techniques, some of which are drawn from psychodrama and art and dance therapy. A therapist may also employ bodywork techniques, including massaging or gently vibrating the client's body to help raise awareness of his or her physical sensations.

While process workers deal with a broad spectrum of human experiences, it is an adjunct, not a substitute, for medical or psychiatric treatment by a qualified physician or psychiatrist.

—*Dr. Joseph Goodbread*

Resources:

Process Work Center of Portland
2049 NW Hoyt
Portland, OR 97209
Tel: (503) 223 8188
Fax: (503) 227-7003
e-mail: pwcp@igc.apc.org
Web site: www.processwork.org
Provides information on process work therapy, seminars, and training.

Further Reading:

Books:

Goodbread, Joseph, *The Dreambody Toolkit: A Practical Introduction to the Philosophy, Goals and Practice of Process-Oriented Psychology.* Portland: Lao Tse Press, 1997.

Mindell, Arnold, and Amy Mindell. *Riding the Horse Backwards: Process Work in Theory and Practice.* London: Penguin Arkana, 1992.

Journals:

The Journal of Process Oriented Psychology, published since 1992 by the Lao Tse Press (Web site: www.lao-tse-press.com), keeps the reader up to date on the latest research and developments in process work.

PSYCHODRAMA

Psychodrama is a method for exploring problems by improvisationally enacting them as if in a play. In addition to its being a form of psychotherapy—the process of treating patients by psychological means—psychodrama is often applied in "role playing," one of psychodrama's derivatives, to deal with a wide range of situations in education, business, or community relations.

Psychodrama's Beginnings

Psychodrama was developed by psychiatrist Jacob Levi Moreno, M.D. (1889–1974). Moreno saw a need for spontaneity and creativity in social relations and began developing practical methods to address this need. In 1921, as an avocational interest, aside from his work as a family physician, he formed perhaps the first modern improvisational dramatic troupe, called the Theatre of Spontaneity. Through this group, Moreno discovered that the process of improvised role playing seemed to help the actors deal with personal problems; this was the beginnings of psychodrama. Moreno then emigrated to the United States in 1925, and later, in 1936, established a psychiatric sanitarium about sixty miles north of New York City. For the rest of his life, in addition to developing his method of psychodrama, Moreno was also a major pioneer of group psychotherapy, as well as of social role theory, and "sociometry," a method for applied social psychology.

The Theory of Psychodrama

All of Moreno's approaches to understanding and helping people are aimed at the goal of furthering people's creativity. Moreno believed that many of humanity's social and psychological problems arose out of people's tendencies to rely excessively on what others had previously created instead of themselves taking on the challenge of creating anew, to meet the needs of the present situation. He also declared that a truly holistic learning and experimental process required involvement through action, similar to the training of astronauts through the use of simulators. In his emphasis on dramatic, physical action, he ran counter to those tendencies in psychotherapy that constrain the process to verbal modes of interaction.

One of Moreno's major insights about creativity is that it emerges most effectively through spontaneity. According to Moreno, spontaneity isn't mere impulsivity, but rather improvisation where one gets gradually more involved and allows the insights to emerge. It involves some aim at finding a new solution or a fresh approach to problems, and includes a measure of rationality associated with intuition and feeling. Related to this was Moreno's view—based on his observations—that the best way to promote spontaneity and creativity in interpersonal problem-solving was through the use of improvised drama. Instead of engaging in the type of theater that requires actors to memorize and rehearse scripts, psychodrama involves the participants improvising scenes based on themes that they themselves feel are relevant to their lives.

At times, the term *psychodrama* has been used inaccurately to describe any psychologically laden piece of theater, literature, or news event. But people in those situations generally play out their parts without exploring other alternatives to the situation being enacted. Psychodrama involves consciously and intentionally pausing and reflecting on one's attitudes and behaviors toward situations or people rather than merely plunging ahead without reflection, which could compound the problem. It may be thought of as a kind of laboratory for examining psychological and social issues in depth. The primary goal of psychodrama is to help people become more creative in their lives. Psychodrama achieves this through structured improvisation, and by having the person whose problem is being enacted play the role not only of the main character, but also of other characters in the drama or of the director, to participate in discovering new understandings and more effective coping strategies.

Psychodrama offers a rich variety of techniques, many of which have been integrated into other forms of therapy. For example, the idea of talking to someone imagined to be sitting in an empty chair has been used in Fritz Perls's gestalt therapy. Family therapy transformed a psychodramatic technique of setting up family members as if they were a diorama representing the emotional relationships into what is known as "family sculpture." Role playing is now commonly used in assertiveness training or social skills classes. Other psychodrama warm-up techniques, with names such as "structured experiences," "action techniques," and "nonverbal games," have come to be used widely in group psychotherapy, personal-growth programs, and self-help groups.

How Does Psychodrama Work?

Psychodramas involve five elements:

1. The director (who often is also the therapist) who facilitates the process
2. The protagonist, the person whose problem is being explored
3. Auxiliaries, members of the group who play supporting roles in the enactment
4. The stage, a special area in which the scene is enacted
5. The audience, composed of the rest of the group.

The procedure begins with a warm-up, a five- to fifteen-minute general discussion in which issues are brought into focus and the level of trust in the group is strengthened. Sometimes structured exercises, like theater games, are used to stimulate the imagination, promote self-disclosure, and allow everyone to share an experience.

The protagonist is chosen and the problem is then presented, usually by having the protagonist show instead of explain the situation. The protagonist's underlying assumptions, which in part cause the problem, are brought into more explicit awareness using various dramatic devices, such as doubling, asides, or soliloquies. Also, in order to appreciate the predicament of the other roles in the enactment, the director has the protagonist change parts and then take on the challenge of responding to the interpersonal tension from that other person's viewpoint. This technique of role reversal is one of the most powerful ways to expand the imagination, cultivate empathy, and reduce tendencies toward egocentricity. The action proceeds often through a series of several scenes, including sub-scenes, in which the protagonist can step out of role and reflect on his or her attitudes and behavior. This phase generally requires about twenty to forty-five minutes.

Finally, the session closes with a period of "sharing," in which the members of the audience say how the enactment relates to their own lives. Because psychodramas are at times very emotional, the sharing itself often involves an opportunity for the expression of the evoked feelings in the audience, a catharsis that further supports and encourages the protagonist. A group that experiences a series of these psychodramas seems to build a trust that allows more unconscious material to emerge and be processed.

The Benefits and Limitations of Psychodrama

The benefits of psychodrama are manifold: shifting roles seem to help to develop empathy and greater flexibility in thinking. Improvisation appears to foster a trust of the healthy parts of the mind, especially the creative imagery flowing from the subconscious. The physical movement and direct encounter in enactments bypasses the mind's language-based avoidances and thus leads to a deep form of insight.

Psychodramatic methods seem to help improve participants' communication and problem-solving skills and enhance self-awareness. Thus, they may be applied in non-therapeutic contexts, such as schools, professional training, business, religious education, community building, and other settings.

However, the participants in a psychodrama must have some degree of mental coherency; they cannot be in states of intoxication, delirium, or psychotic confusion. But, in modified form, and applied with reasonable judgment, role-playing methods have been used with patients who are mentally retarded, suffering from delusions, and others who might be inaccessible to ordinary "talk" methods of therapy.

—*Adam Blatner, M.D.*

Resources:

The American Board of Examiners in Psychodrama, Sociometry, and Group Psychotherapy
P.O. Box 15572
Washington, DC 20003-0572
Tel: (202) 483-0514

To become a certified director, a psychodramatist must obtain both professional training as a psychotherapist and subspecialty training involving hundreds of hours of supervised personal involvement.

Psychodrama as a subspecialty of psychotherapy should be differentiated from "drama therapy." The latter is one of the creative arts therapies and involves more the use of theater itself as an aid to healing. However, in the last decade there have been increasing areas of overlap.

Information about training and names and addresses of certified directors may be obtained upon written request.

The American Society for Group Psychotherapy and Psychodrama (ASGPP)
301 North Harrison Street, Suite 508
Princeton, NJ 08540
Tel: (609) 452-1339
Fax: (609) 936-1659
Information about regional and national conferences, newsletters, and professional journals may be obtained upon written request.

National Coalition of Arts Therapies Association (NCATA)
2000 Century Plaza, Ste. 108
Columbia, MD 21044
Tel: (410) 997-4040
Fax: (410) 997-4048
This is an alliance of professional associations that promote the therapeutic nature of the arts.

Further Reading:

Books:
Blatner, Adam. *Acting-In: Practical Applications of Psychodramatic Methods.* 3rd ed. New York: Springer, 1996.

——. "Psychodrama." in *Current Psychotherapies.* R. J. Corsini and D. Wedding, eds. 5th ed. Itasca, IL: Peacock, 1995.

——. , and Allee Blatner. *The Art of Play: An Adult's Guide to Reclaiming Imagination and Spontaneity.* Bristol, PA: Brunner/Mazel, 1997.

——. , and Allee Blatner. *Foundations of Psychodrama: History, Theory, and Practice.* New York: Springer, 1988.

Corey, G. "Psychodrama." In *Theory and Practice of Group Counseling.* 4th ed. Pacific Grove, CA: Brooks/Cole, 1994.

Fox, J., ed. *The Essential Moreno: Writings on Psychodrama, Group Method, and Spontaneity.* New York: Springer, 1987.

Holmes, P., M. Karp, and M. Watson, eds. *Psychodrama Since Moreno: Innovations in Theory and Practice.* New York: Tavistock/Routledge, 1994.

Moreno, J. L. *Psychodrama,* Beacon, NY: Beacon House, Vol. 1., 1946, and, with Zerka T. Moreno, Vol. 2, 1959, and Vol. 3, 1969.

Journals:
Blatner, A. "Psychodrama: The State of the Art." *The Arts in Psychotherapy* 24, No. 1 (1997): 23–30.

Journal of Group Psychotherapy, Psychodrama and Sociometry. Heldref, 1318 18th St, Washington, DC 20006.

PSYCHOSYNTHESIS

Psychosynthesis is a theory of mind used to help a person realize his or her inner wisdom. According to this theory, there exists within each person a "higher self" that is a source of guidance, value, and creativity. It is the basis of a form of therapy that, through various methods, attempts to bring participants to a greater understanding of themselves. They are encouraged to access their higher selves to help solve problems and make decisions.

The Foundations of Psychosynthesis

Psychosynthesis was first developed by Roberto Assagioli (1888–1974). A colleague of Sigmund Freud and Carl Jung, Assagioli was the first person to practice psychoanalysis in Italy. In 1910, he left the psychoanalytic movement because he felt its view of human nature was too limited. He objected to the standardization of ideas and techniques, believing that there should be an individual method for each person.

He began to develop his own spiritual model of human development and opened an institute in 1927 in Rome. He chose the term "psychosynthesis" to give a name to the impulse in each person to develop, learn, and evolve. His early work ended in 1940, when he was arrested as a pacifist and jailed by Mussolini's fascist government. After his release, he lived under police surveillance. In 1943, he was persecuted by the Nazis and was forced into hiding. His institute was reopened in 1951 at his home in Florence. There he saw patients and trained professionals until his death in 1974. His work is now continued at more than 100 psychosynthesis institutes around the world.

What Is the Higher Self?

Assagioli's theory of the unconscious deviated from many of his contemporaries in psychoanalysis. While others saw unconscious motivation as a collection of base, biological needs, Assagioli claimed that the unconscious also encompasses nobler impulses, such as love, ethics, and creativity. He believed that repressing either impulse could be harmful. In his view, therapy should help foster these higher instincts.

The hidden source of wisdom and guidance within each person is considered his or her "higher self." The higher self, although part of a person's nature, is different from one's personality. While an individual's personality makes him or her unique, the higher self is concerned with universal values, such as compassion, truth, and life purpose. The higher self may be considered a part of the brain or mind, although it is just as often experienced in the body. The goal of psychosynthesis is to explore and utilize the concealed resources of human thought.

Psychosynthesis Therapy

A person may experience psychosynthesis therapy individually or within a group. At the start of each session, participants are encouraged to talk about their problems with a therapist or with the group. As a person proceeds to express his or her thoughts or emotions, the therapist may intervene to help a person clarify a particular image or

memory. According to psychosynthesis, people can overcome conventional ways of viewing their problems when they are able to access the insight within their imaginations. A therapist may draw from a variety of techniques to help a person enter his or her imagination. The therapist begins by helping a person to relax and withdraw his or her attention from the outer environment and concentrate inward. A therapist will then use guided imagery techniques to help a client enter his or her imagination and focus on a particular thought, feeling, or sensation. Finally the therapist will ask this person to express these images. Depending on what method works best, a therapist may help evoke these images through visual art, movement, music, analysis, personality study, traditional psychotherapeutic techniques, maps of consciousness, and many other methods. In accordance with Assagioli's theory, the techniques that a therapist may use in a session will vary with each person.

Benefits of Psychosynthesis

The higher self is a crucial part of psychosynthesis therapy. Therapy is not intended to develop the higher self, because it is thought to already exist in each person. Psychosynthesis therapy is used to acquaint people with the resources of their higher selves and equip them with the ability to approach problems imaginatively and to better understand themselves. The therapist's role is to help a person gain the inner skills to become aware of his of her higher self.

—*Richard Schaub, Ph.D.*

Resources:

International Association for Managerial and Organizational Psychosynthesis
3308 Radcliffe Road
Thousand Oaks, CA 91360
Tel: (805) 942-4815
Disseminates information on psychosynthesis.

New York Psychosynthesis Institute
2 Murray Court
Huntington, NY 11743
Tel: (516) 673-0293
Provides information and promotes the practice of psychosynthesis in the New York area.

Synthesis Center for Psychosynthesis Distributions
P.O. Box 575
Amherst, MA 01004
Tel: (413) 256-0772
Offers resources and information regarding psychosynthesis.

Further Reading:

Assagioli, Roberto. *Psychosynthesis: A Manual of Principles and Techniques.* New York: The Viking Press, 1971.

——. *Transpersonal Development.* New York: HarperCollins, 1991.

Ferrucci, Piero. *What We May Be.* Los Angeles: Tarcher, 1982.

Schaub, B., and R. Schaub. *Healing Addictions.* Albany, NY: Delmar, 1997.

Whitmore, Diana. *Psychosynthesis Counseling in Action.* London: SAGE Publications, 1991.

RADIX

Radix teaches students to become conscious of an invisible life force ("radix") and to restore its natural pulsation in their bodies. This requires confronting and changing acquired patterns of breathing and muscular tension that block a person's emotions. By getting in touch with the physical sensations flowing through their bodies and the emotions linked to those sensations, Radix students seek to gain better control over their life forces and physical defenses and to develop greater capacity for choice.

Dr. Charles R. (Chuck) Kelley founded the Interscience Research Institute in 1960. He changed its name to the Radix Institute in 1974 after he coined the term "radix" to describe his unique concept of the life force. He reserved the capitalized term "Radix" for the personal growth program that he developed with the help of his wife, Erica. He and Erica began their first bodywork programs in 1970 and ran worldwide training and teaching facilities from southern California until 1987, when Dr. Kelley retired and separated from the Radix Institute. The Kelleys now practice in Vancouver, Washington, and Dr. Kelley offers training tutorials and supervision by arrangement. Others now use the Radix name worldwide for their own work and training. They are not associated with Dr. Kelley or endorsed by him unless they display a certificate signed by him.

Dr. Kelley was influenced by the psychoanalyst and founder of medical orgonomy, Dr. Wilhelm Reich, who believed that people develop physical defenses against emotions they consider unacceptable. People build defenses early in life by selectively tightening muscles and holding their breath in different ways to inhibit the expression of particular emotions. This gradually forms the patterns of tension Reich called muscular armor. Over time, these inhibiting behaviors become anchored in the bodily structure. They block feelings, interfere with thinking, and may contribute to chronic disease and emotional difficulties. Nevertheless, Kelley believes that the muscular armor is not a negative attribute, because it is the mechanism of voluntary attention and basis of the will. We need it in order to function effectively as human beings. Radix work aims to help people learn how to use their muscular armor without unconsciously becoming its victim.

Radix teachers work with inhibitions to breathing, with the muscular armor, and with the mental attitudes that support them. They use suggestions, direct body contact, and exercises for loosening tensions and freeing feelings. Clients learn to develop a structure of muscular tensions that contain emotions and form personal boundaries. This results in a more effective, flexible type of muscular armor. Most sessions include work with the student lying supine on a mat, lightly clad in shorts or bathing suit, with the teacher kneeling alongside. This enables the teacher to observe skin color—an indicator of the degree of radix charge and flow in the body—and to observe breathing and patterns of muscle tension or flaccidity. A student may stand up for "grounding" exercises that are used to develop a sense of the relationship between the feet and the ground. A student may also stand to perform exercises that help him or her release anger. A student may also sit face-to-face with the teacher to discuss a problem or emotional issue.

There are a variety of Radix programs, reflecting the style of the teacher and needs of the student. Many students choose a mix of individual and group sessions. Group sessions are usually small and include periods of individual interaction with the teacher. A typical individual program lasts for fifty minutes on a weekly basis, but other arrangements are often made, including concentrated programs of up to ten sessions within five days.

—Erica Kelley

Resources:

Kelley/Radix
Chuck and Erica Kelley
13715 SE 36th Street
Vancouver, WA 98683-7770
Tel. & Fax: (360) 896-4004
e-mail: Kelley6@ix.netcom.com
Provides information on Radix, as well as promoting the practice.

Further Reading:

Bar-Levav, Reuven. *Thinking in the Shadow of Feelings.* New York: Simon & Schuster, 1988.

Branden, Nathaniel. *Taking Responsibility: Self-Reliance and the Accountable Life.* New York: Simon & Schuster, 1996.

Kelley, Charles R. *The Radix, Vol. I: Personal Growth Work,* and *Vol. II: The Science of Radix Processes.* (Compilation of articles from the 1960s to the 1990s. Also published in Spanish. Vancouver, WA: K/R Publications, 1992.)

Reich, Wilhelm, "The Expressive Language of Living in Orgone Therapy." Chapter 15 in *Character Analysis.* 3rd ed. New York: Orgone Institute Press, 1949. Reissued by Farrar, Straus & Giroux.

REBIRTHING

Rebirthing is a gentle, meditative breathing technique. Advocates of this therapy believe that it enables an individual to become more aware of thought and behavior patterns that may prevent him or her from enjoying life to the fullest. In this way, those who practice rebirthing reduce limiting psychological and emotional conditions, increase the vital transfer of oxygen to the organs and cells, and release deep-seated tensions from the body, thereby increasing physical comfort.

The Phenomenon of Rebirthing

Leonard Orr developed the process in California in the 1970s. Submerging himself in a hot tub, he achieved a relaxed mental and physical state that, he said, stimulated memories of being in the womb, prior to birth. Orr viewed rebirthing as a therapy for releasing the trauma associated with the birth process and our first breaths as infants. He believes that coming to terms with that trauma is the first step in resolving buried emotional and psychological issues. After a few years of introducing others to rebirthing, Orr observed that the pattern and quality of breathing attained during the sessions, characterized by a continuous cycle of inhalation and exhalation flowing deeply and fluidly through the mouth, remained constant, regardless of who participated. By comparison, normal breathing has a pause between one breath and the next. Orr also noted that the same quality of breathing could remain effective for individuals even out of the water. Currently, the most popular version of rebirthing is the "dry" method, which does not require being submerged in water.

The Importance of Breathing

Proper breathing can produce changes in a person's clarity of thinking and physical state. Controlled breathing has been used for centuries—often in conjunction with meditation—to achieve high levels of calmness and peace. Deep, even breathing has the natural tendency to slow the heartbeat as well as the flow of thoughts. Proper breathing also increases the flow of oxygen throughout the body, which is essential to the smooth function of cells and organs and the body as a whole. In fact, the body rids itself of 70 percent of its toxins and other body wastes through respiration.

Rebirthing utilizes breathing techniques to achieve maximum physical and emotional health. Rebirthers (rebirthing practitioners) use these techniques to shed tensions and foster a tranquil mental state. This in turn allows the body rest and recuperation and the mind a period of clear thinking to sort through complex or long-buried emotional issues. Rebirthing also relies on the use of positive affirmation, the planting of new thoughts in a person's consciousness to replace negative thought patterns that affect behavior. Rebirthing theory views many destructive patterns as stemming from the birth trauma and from later life experiences, all of which can be locked into the tissues/cells of the body and can prove harmful if not released. Rebirthing seeks to release trauma from the body and support increased well-being.

Rebirthing in Practice

Individuals are advised to seek the guidance of a rebirther who has enough rebirthing training and experience to provide safety and support during the first several sessions. A person should ask a prospective rebirther about the extent of his or her training and their number of rebirthing experiences. A series of ten sessions with the same rebirther is recommended. The continuity and trust generated by this relationship is believed to accelerate the progress of healing.

The rebirther begins by asking the individual about his or her life. Together they look for patterns and habits that the client seeks to change, or eliminate. They jointly identify positive thoughts that will help begin this change. This period of discussion is followed by a period of physical relaxation and breathing exercises, guided by the rebirther. The individual lies on a mat or pad on the floor. During this stage the breath slows, allowing tension to dissolve from the body. This results in a state of relaxation during which the individual consciously or subconsciously addresses his or her concerns. Review of traumatic life experiences may result in discomfort when feelings and long-suppressed thoughts resurface. At the end of a session, thoughts and feelings as well as questions can be shared with the rebirther. The rebirther may also offer some suggestions or affirmations to focus on until the next appointment. The recommended session length is one to two hours.

A Greater Quality of Life

People develop stress, frustration, anger, and worry, which, if not dispersed, can affect their physical and emotional health. Advocates of rebirthing say that

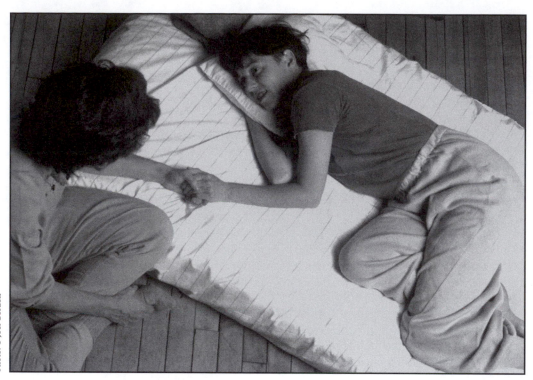

Photo: © Joel Gordon

A rebirther and client discuss the patterns and habits that he or she wishes to change.

their therapy allows the body to recuperate by teaching individuals to breathe in a way that promotes physical and emotional well-being. In addition, rebirthers assert that by upgrading the quality of thoughts while in a deep-breathing mode, quality of life also improves, thus producing greater health, improved relationships, self-esteem, and prosperity. Furthermore, by devoting time to the examination of buried emotional and psychological matters while in a relaxed physical and mental state, people are able to address deep-seated issues that affect behavior and thought patterns and make positive changes in their lives.

—*Maureen Malone*

Resources:

Inspiration University
P.O. Box 1026
Staunton, VA 24402
Source of rebirthing books, audio tapes, and videos.

Loving Relationships Training (LRT) International
c/o Clarity Productions
P.O. Box 160
Manhattan Beach, CA 90267
Tel: (800) 468-5578
Offers rebirthing seminars, training, certification, and books on related subjects.

The New York Rebirthing Center
205 East 95th Street, 23A
New York, NY 10128
Tel:(212) 534-2969
Fax: (212) 534-2969
Coordinates rebirthing seminars, group rebirths, and similar activities and provides a list of rebirthers in your area.

The Philadelphia Rebirthing Center
1027 69th Avenue
Philadelphia, PA 19126
Tel: (215) 424-4444
e-mail: tlomas@netreach.net
Web site: www.philadelphiarebirthing.com
Coordinates rebirthing seminars, group rebirths, and similar activities and provides a list of rebirthers in the area.

Further Reading:

Morningstar, Jim. *Breathing in Light and Love.* Milwaukee, WI: Transformations, 1994.

Orr, Leonard, and Sondra Ray. *Rebirthing in the New Age.* Berkeley, CA: Celestial Arts, 1977.

Ray, Sondra. *Celebration of Breath.* Berkeley, CA: Celestial Arts, 1983.

——. *Loving Relationships.* Berkeley, CA: Celestial Arts, 1983.

Sisson, Colin. *Rebirthing Made Easy.* New Zealand: Total Press, 1989.

Rubenfeld Synergy Method

The Rubenfeld synergy method is a holistic healing system for the integration of the body, mind, emotions, and spirit. It was developed in the 1960s by Ilana Rubenfeld, a psychotherapist and bodyworker who sought to teach people how to recognize, express, understand, and manage their emotions, feelings, and sensations. By combining gentle touch and verbalization, the Rubenfeld synergy method reportedly brings about beneficial changes in self-image, health, personal and family relationships, and spirit.

Rubenfeld's Vision

In the 1950s Rubenfeld was a conducting student at the Juilliard School of Music when she suffered a debilitating back spasm. Seeking help, she discovered Judith Leibowitz, a teacher of the Alexander technique, who taught her how to use her body efficiently and avoid re-injury. During these Alexander lessons, Rubenfeld sometimes expressed intense emotional feelings, but Leibowitz, untrained in treating emotions, suggested that she see a psychoanalyst. The analyst talked but wouldn't touch, and her feelings did not emerge.

Rubenfeld realized that the Alexander technique's specific methods of physical touch helped her access her memories, while verbal processing helped her understand them. She resolved to create a way of simultaneously integrating bodywork with psychotherapy. She became a master teacher of the Alexander technique and trained extensively with Moshe Feldenkrais in the Feldenkrais Method®, a technique for improving both physical and mental functioning through the learning of new body movements. For years, she taught these body-mind modalities but found that they missed what for her was the most vital element: processing the emotional material that emerged during lessons. She longed to know the emotional history, stresses, and life problems that created physical dysfunctions in the first place.

Rubenfeld's curiosity led her to train and collaborate with psychiatrist Dr. Peter Hogan and with Fritz and Laura Perls, cofounders of gestalt therapy, and to further combine body-oriented methods with psychotherapy. The addition of appropriate verbal processing to body-mind disciplines practiced in a safe, trusting, and nonjudgmental environment seemed to make the various modalities function synergistically, and remarkable results occurred in a short time.

Rubenfeld began the first professional Rubenfeld synergy training program in 1977 in New York City. This 1,600-hour, four-year training program includes lectures, demonstrations, discussion, and a great deal of supervised practice. Trainees learn self-care, maintain high standards of integrity and competency, and seek supervision, therapy, and continued education for themselves. The code of ethics for Rubenfeld synergists includes demonstrating respect for people, preserving their confidentiality, showing sensitivity to the difference in power between

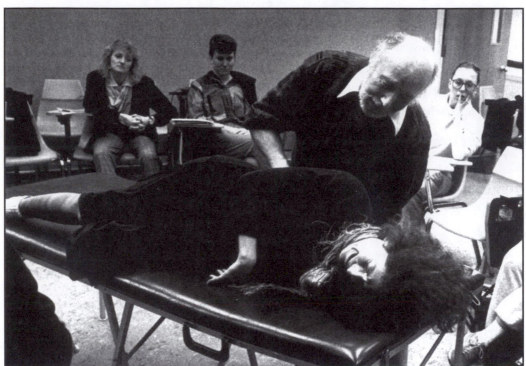

Photo: © Joel Gordon

A certified synergist demonstrates movement techniques used to unlock emotions from the body.

practitioners and help seekers, the avoidance of personal relationships with help seekers, and the maintaining of clear boundaries.

The Many Techniques of the Method

The goals of the Rubenfeld synergy method are to enhance people's natural capacity for self-healing and self-regulation, to teach them to recognize and learn from the truths their bodies tell, and to teach them to use their own resources for change, choice, and self-care. Synergists accomplish these goals by teaching people how to become aware of the messages, memories, and emotions locked in their bodies, causing energy blocks and imbalances.

Using a variety of techniques and elements—including verbal dialogue, movement training, imagination exercises, breathing techniques, and non-sexual, caring touch—synergists assist people in exploring the relationship between posture and emotions; discovering how body metaphors reveal life

patterns; healing their "inner child"; exploring somatic (regarding the body) dreams; and developing a sense of humor. Synergists believe that the combination of these techniques works to engage the help seeker in understanding the causes of discomfort and enables them to instruct the help seeker on how to alleviate physical pain and resolve emotional issues.

The establishment of a therapeutic relationship of safety and trust is essential, so that each person can journey inward, recognize and release traumas and dysfunctional memories, and reclaim his or her body, mind, and soul.

Rubenfeld Synergy Sessions

A typical session lasts about forty-five minutes and is conducted privately or in a group, with both synergist and help seeker(s) fully clothed. Help seekers are usually invited to lie on a padded table, but sessions may also be conducted with them sitting, standing, or moving. Sessions begin in the "here and now," then

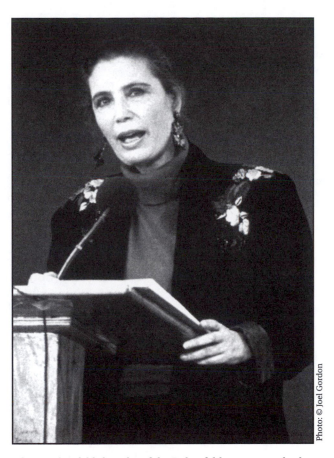

Ilana Rubenfeld, founder of the Rubenfeld synergy method.

move into the past and future within the context of each person's needs. No diagnoses are made, nor cures promised. Help seekers are in charge of the pace and direction of the sessions, and they may stop at any time. People interested in practicing the method may learn Rubenfeld bodymind exercises, which ease tensions, foster flexibility, develop strength, and teach "inner listening." These can be practiced anywhere. Although Rubenfeld synergy may bring insights in a short time, weekly sessions for a period of at least several months to several years are advised for fully integrated and lasting benefits.

Positive Aspects of Rubenfeld Synergy Sessions

People who experience Rubenfeld synergy sessions often report greater self-esteem and self-acceptance; a sense of clarity and purpose; increased energy, body awareness and body image; deep relaxation; and relief from pain. Trainees conduct pilot studies on such topics as body image, posttraumatic stress disorder, recovery from addictive behaviors, incest and abuse, and stress-related illnesses. There are no known contraindications to receiving Rubenfeld synergy sessions. Synergists are trained to recognize conditions requiring medical supervision and refer clients to appropriate professionals when necessary.

—*Ilana Rubenfeld*

Resources:

The Rubenfeld Synergy Center
115 Waverly Place

New York, NY 10011
Tel: (800) 747-6897
e-mail: rubenfeld@aol.com
Offers an introductory workshop.

National Association of Rubenfeld Synergists
1000 River Road, Suite 8H
Belmar, NJ 07719
Tel: (800) 484-3250, code 8516
Provides referrals to certified Rubenfeld synergists and distributes information about the synergists' code of ethics.

Canadian Association of Rubenfeld Synergists
112 Lund Street
Richmond Hill, ON L4C 5V9
Canada
Tel: (905) 883-3158
e-mail: aturner@yorku.ca
Supports members' professional growth and promotes high standards of professional ethics. Also seeks to educate the public about the Rubenfeld synergy method.

Further Reading:

Books:
Caldwell, Christine. *Getting in Touch: The Guide to New Body-Centered Therapies.* Wheaton IL: Quest Books, 1997.

Claire, Thomas. *Bodywork: What Type of Massage to Get—And How to Make the Most of It.* New York: William Morrow and Company, 1995.

——. "Gestalt Therapy and the Bodymind: An Overview of the Rubenfeld Synergy Method." In *Gestalt Therapy: Perspectives and Applications.* Edwin C. Nevis, ed. New York: Gardner Press, 1990.

Journals:
Lerkin, Jan Marie. "Sing the Body Electric." *Changes* June 1995.

Markowitz, Laura. "Therapists Explore Mind-Body Alternatives." *Family Therapy* 1996.

Rubenfeld, Ilana. "Ushering in a Century of Integration." *Somatics* Autumn-Winter 1990–91.

——. "Beginner's Hands: Twenty-Five Years of Simple Rubenfeld Synergy—The Birth of a Therapy." *Somatics* Spring-Summer 1988.

Simon, Richard. "Listening Hands." *Family Therapy Networker* September-October 1997.

UNERGI

Unergi is a holistic therapy method that aims to help participants integrate body, mind, emotions, spirit, creativity, and the healing forces of nature. Unergi was developed by Ute Arnold, combining healing forms derived from gestalt therapy, the Feldenkrais Method®, the Alexander technique, and Rubenfeld synergy.

Unergi combines the words *unity* and *energy,* reflecting Arnold's belief that all people originate in a state of unity and can restore their energy and prevent disease through self-care, self-expression, participation in community, and active involvement with the organic rhythms of nature. According to unergi there exists a vibrational energy, radiating from our natural environment, that is able to heal by restoring one's internal energy. Like all of the healing methods from which it draws, unergi considers physical and emotional problems to be a result of psychological patterns developed in early childhood. These patterns censor various aspects of our inner life and self-expression. When a person's body and psyche have been denied expression for a long time, unergi practitioners believe that his or her whole being will start to feel more and more ill at ease. One may feel this as aches, pains, or numbness, which over time become more acute. Healing is seen as a release of old ways of being and a return to wholeness.

During a unergi session, a client lies, sits, or moves on a bodywork table, fully clothed. The practitioner employs techniques such as body awareness, touch, movement exercises to balance the energy through the Hindu chakra system, creative expression, visualization, and dreamwork. The practitioner's techniques are used to invite a dialogue between a client's body and mind to access his or her deeply buried memories and emotions. They aim to allow a greater freedom of movement and create a safe environment for the expression and healing of a person's hidden qualities.

—Ute Arnold

Resources:

Unergi Training
P.O. Box 335
Point Pleasant, PA 18950
Tel: (215) 297-8006
Offers a three-year certification program in the unergi method. The training is conducted at retreat centers on the East Coast of the United States and in Europe.

Index

A

AAMT. See American Association of Music Therapy

AAPB. See Association for Applied Psychophysiology and Biofeedback

Abe-ryu, 293

absolute self, 319

abuse, 251, 400, 414
   recovery from, 139, 172, 190, 360, 427

academic performance, 248

Academy for Guided Imagery, 78

Academy of Science, 73

accidents, 6, 67, 111, 112, 149, 209, 221, 369, 400
   See also injury; trauma

Acorrido, 283

acrobatics, 297

action profiling, 338-339

actors, 211, 212, 216

acupoints, 178, 180, 182

acupressure, 24, 117, 118, 119, 126, 143, 144, 178, 180-183
   See also Jin Shin Do™; process acupressure

acupuncture, 9, 17, 23, 24, 81, 82, 119, 124, 126, 142, 143, 144, 163, 177-180, 183-187, 193
   colorpuncture and, 107
   See also traditional Chinese medicine

Acu-yoga, 182

Adams, Kathleen, 362

ADD. See Attention deficit disorder

addictions, 35, 39, 66, 358
   treatments for, 21, 65, 67, 70, 83, 99, 101, 103, 105, 106, 107, 139, 156, 172, 178, 184, 187, 311, 326, 356, 360, 363, 414, 427
   See also alcohol; drugs; smoking

adhesions, 42

Adler, Janet, 350

adrenal glands, 101

ADTA. See American Dance Therapy Association

AEDE. See Association des Eleves de Dr. Ehrenfried et des Practiciens en Gymnastique Holistique

affirmations, 423
   See also visualizations

Africa, 142, 275, 276, 280-281, 342

Age of Reason, 2

aggression, 276
   See also anger; emotions

aging, 365

agoraphobia, 270

AIDS, 66, 101, 146, 323, 358, 360

aiki-bujutsu, 278

aikido, 118, 250, 276, 278-280, 284, 293

Ainu people, 293

Akhilananda, Swami, 317

akiyama, 284

alcohol
   effect on health, 8, 46, 59, 139, 178, 184, 196
   See also addictions

Alexander, F.M., 157, 201, 204

Alexander the Great, 143

Alexander technique, 89, 157, 201, 204-207, 266, 391, 425, 428

alienation, 365, 371

alignment, 214, 237, 260, 264, 267, 391, 402

allergies, 97
   treatments for, 65, 101, 188, 194

allopathic medicine
   compared to alternative medicine, 1, 3, 46, 66
   costs and risks of, 57, 62
   naturopathy and, 17
   nutrition and, 61
   See also pharmaceutical drugs

aloe (Aloe vera), 59-60

alpha state, 68, 320

alternative health models, 1-4

Alzheimer's disease, 106, 356

American Association of Artist-Therapists, 364

American Association of Music Therapy (AAMT), 367

American Association of Professional Hypnotherapists, 76

American College of Orgonomy, 407

American Dance Therapy Association (ADTA), 354, 355

American Institute of Homeopathy, 12

American Journal of Dance Therapy, 354, 355

American Medical Association (AMA), 2, 47

American Music Therapy Association (AMTA), 367

American Polarity Therapy Association, 127, 128

American School of Osteopathy, 47

American Society of Clinical Hypnosis, 74, 76

AMMA, 180, 195

AMTA. See American Music Therapy Association

Anatomy of an Illness as Perceived by the Patient, 80

anesthesia, 73, 184

aneurysm, 162

anger, 96, 137, 226, 390, 414
   See also emotions

Angola, 281-282

animal magnetism, 73

ankylosing spondylitis, 79

anmo, 143, 198

anorexia
   treatments, 83, 139, 270, 358
   See also eating disorders

anthropology, 332, 337

Anthroposophical Society, 254

antibiotics, 2, 17, 54, 84, 104
    See also pharmaceutical drugs anti-inflam-
    matories, 87, 102
anxiety, 21, 95, 98, 152, 232, 379, 398, 399, 414
    effect on health, 8, 95
    treatments for, 14, 65, 67, 70, 73, 76, 106, 141,
    155, 187, 326
    See also emotions; stress
AOBTA. See American Oriental Bodywork
    Therapy Association
A-P. See Aston-Patterning
APP. See Audio-Psycho-Phonology
appendicitis, 14
appetite control, 19
APT. See Association for Poetry Therapy
archery, 284, 301
archetypes, 374, 375
Aristotle, 2, 65, 143
Armenia, 256
armoring, 189, 379, 382-383, 389-390, 407-408,
    409-411, 421
Arnold, Ute, 428-429
aromatherapy, 83, 85, 86-88
arrhythimia, 323
    See also heart conditions
arthritis, treatments for, 8, 14, 39, 67, 76, 86, 101,
    124, 125, 129, 151, 174, 182, 187, 199, 264
artists, 343
art sport, 249
art therapy, 347-350
asanas, 306, 314
ashokh, 256-257
ashrams, 309
Asia, 259, 317, 342
Asian bodywork, 34, 82, 143, 163, 177-180, 195
Assagioli, Roberto, 193, 379-380, 392, 419-421
assembly line work, 211
Association des Eleves de Dr. Ehrenfried et des
    Practiciens en Gymnastique Holistique
    (AEDE), 234
Association for Applied Psychophysiology and
    Biofeedback (AAPB), 68
Association for Poetry Therapy (APT), 370
asthma, 35, 260
    treatments for, 14, 37, 39, 67, 104, 129, 178,
    199, 344
    See also breathing difficulties
astigmatism, 231
Aston, Judith, 207-209, 222
Aston-Patterning® (A-P), 207-210, 222
astrology, 120
astronauts, 81
At a Journal Workshop, 361
athletics, 143, 153, 204, 206, 207, 209, 210, 211,
    216, 231, 317
    See also sports
at-risk youth, 391
atman, 319

attention deficit disorder (ADD), treatments for,
    67, 70, 93, 106, 113, 248, 408
attitude
    effect on health, 8, 67, 79, 226
    See also emotions
attunement, 135, 136
audio-psycho-phonology (APP), 111
aura, 48
Australia, 342
authentic movement, 350-352
autism, 113
Autobiography of a Yogi, 306
awareness through movement, 217-218
ayurvedic medicine, 2, 5-7, 54, 55, 116, 117, 126,
    143

B
Babylonia, 99
Bach, Dr. Edward, 83, 96-98
back pain, 204, 265-266
    treatment for, 39, 42, 125, 158, 159, 162, 164,
    182, 187, 194, 196, 209, 221, 262
bacteria, 54, 103
ba-gua, 122-123
Baker, Elsworth F., M.D., 407
balance, 270, 272
Baldwin, Christina, 361
balms, 86
Barnes, John F., PT, 158
Bartenieff Fundamentals, 210-212
Bartenieff, Irmgard, 201, 210-211, 336
"the basic six," 212
Bates method, 88-90, 229
Bates, William, 88-90
baths, 83, 99, 102, 143, 422
    See also hydrotherapy
Battle Creek Sanitorium, 100
Beatles, The 324
beauty, 366
bed sores, 125
bedwetting, 68
behavior
    effect on health, 204, 228
    See also lifestyle
behavioral vision therapy, 83, 90-93
behavior modification, 414
benign prostatic hyperplasia (BPH), 59
Benjamin, Dr. Ben, 157
Benjamin system of muscular therapy, 157
Benson, Dr. Herbert, 319, 322
beri-beri, 61
berimbau, 283
Berlowe, Dr. Jay, 332
Bernheim, Hyppolyte, 74
beta carotene, 55
Better Eyesight Without Glasses, 88-89
bhakti yoga, 309, 313
Bible, 116, 143, 366

Bimba, Mestre, 281
binde, 150
bindegewebsmassage, 150
bioenergetics, 382-385, 388-389, 393, 400, 410
biofeedback, 65, 66, 68-70, 72, 80, 89, 92
Biofeedback Research Society, 68
biofield, 137, 138
biomagnetic therapy, 125
biomorphism, 253
birth injury, 159
black diphtheria, 47
Black Plague, 144
bladder infection, 38
Bleuler, Eugen, 347, 353
blockages, 115-117, 174, 179, 191, 266, 269, 388,
    396, 407-408
    See also emotions; memories
blood, 35, 48, 107, 173, 174
    TCM view of, 26
blood clots, 147
    treatment cautions, 175, 242
blood flow enhancement, 174, 182
bloodletting, 10, 34, 46
blood pressure, 72, 85, 87, 311, 320, 322
    See also high blood pressure
Boadella, David, 410
Boas, Francizka, 354
Bodhidharma, 275, 289, 298
Bodies in Revolt: A Primer in Somatic Thinking,
    219
bodybuilding, 231, 260
body fluids, 26, 179
Bodymap™, 385, 386
body-memory, 169
Body-Mind Centering®, 212-215
bodynamic analysis, 385-387
body-oriented psychotherapies, 82, 378-381
body space, 269
bodywork, 55, 84, 177
    defined, 33, 115
    Oriental, 27, 177
    See also movement therapy
Bolesky, Karen L., 237
bone fracture, treatment cautions, 175
Bonnie Pruden School for Physical Fitness and
    Myotherapy, 160
botanical medicines, 15
Bothmer gymnastics, 268
boundaries, 399, 426
Bowen technique, 148-149
Bowen, Thomas A., 148-149
bowing, 278, 295, 303
boxing, 240, 260
Boyden-Pesso, Diane, 411, 412
Boyesan, Gerda, 410
BPH. See benign prostatic hyperplasia
Braid, James, 73
Braille, 228

brain, 41, 43, 48, 71, 94, 105, 169
    three-brain model, 237
    See also mind
Brain Gym®, 245, 247-249
brain waves, 320
Brazil, 275, 276, 280, 281
breast cancer, 55, 81
breathing, diaphragmatic, 264, 295
breathing difficulties, 35, 231, 408, 421, 423
    treatments for, 70, 218
    See also asthma
breathing exercises, 6, 118, 119, 168, 231, 253,
    298, 300, 311, 368, 382
breathing rate, 72, 85, 87, 320, 403
Bresler, David E., 77-78
Breuer, Josef, 379
brief strobic phototherapy (BSP), 106, 108
bright light therapy, 105, 106-107
    See also light therapy
British Columbia, 146
Broch, Eva, 389
Brockett, Sally, 91
bronchitis, 35
    treatments for, 14, 129, 187
Brooks, Peter, 259
Brown, Malcolm and Katherine, 409-411
bruises, 147
    treatments for, 88, 125
BSP. See brief strobic phototherapy
Buber, Martin, 397
Buddhism, 133, 134, 135, 275, 289, 298, 299, 301,
    306, 308, 317, 319, 400
Buelte, Dr. Arnhilte, 332
bulimia
    treatments, 83, 139, 270, 358
    See also eating disorders
Burmeister, Mary, 188, 191-192
burns, treatments for, 60, 88, 124, 125
bursitis, 39
bushi, 293
bushido, 295

C
Caesar, Julius, 143
caffeine, 8
Campbell, Don, 109
Canada, 146
cancer, 360
    conditions affecting, 55, 66, 147
    treatment cautions, 147, 175, 196
    treatments for, 14-15, 55, 61, 62, 71, 107, 129,
    264, 323
capoeira, 275, 276, 280-283
Capoeira Foundation, 282
capoeiristas, 281
cardiovascular disease, 58, 104
carpal tunnel syndrome, 125, 162
Cartesian Principle, 29

catalepsy, 75
cataracts, 228
    treatment cautions, 90
"cat stretch," 221
Center for Children and Parents, 333
Center for Enneagram Studies, 331
Center for Integral Studies, 330
Center for Journal Therapy, 362
Center for Self-Healing, 230
cerebral cortex, 105
cerebral palsy, 159, 344
certified infant massage instructor (CIMI), 153,
    155, 156
certified Laban movement analysts (CMAs),
    211
Chace, Marian, 353, 354
chakras, 127, 193, 389, 429
chamomile (*Matricaria recutita*), 54, 58, 60
Chang San-Feng, 270
Charcot, Jean-Martin, 353
Charing Cross Hospital, 83
chi, 23, 116, 120-123, 127, 177-178, 180, 183, 300
chi kung, 118
childbirth, 76
child care, 234
children, 102, 211
chills, 180
China, 7, 34, 37, 65, 83, 99, 118, 120, 124, 129,
    142, 143, 144, 163, 180, 187, 195, 244, 245, 275,
    284, 297, 319, 342
Chi Po, 118
chiropractic, 9, 33, 34, 36, 37-40, 48, 55, 126, 172,
    252, 261, 270
    See also network chiropractic
chit, 319
Cho Hong Hi, Gen., 301
cholecystitis, 14
cholera, 12, 104
    treatments for, 14, 104
cholesterol, 58-59
Christ, 116, 134, 171
Christianity, 65, 116, 134, 143, 245, 309, 317, 329,
    342
*Chronic Disease: Their Peculiar Nature and Their
    Homeopathic Treatment*, 12
chronic fatigue syndrome, 14, 42, 106, 159
Cicero, 143
CIMI. See certified infant massage instructor
cinchona, 10
circulatory system, 152, 162, 163, 164, 175, 196,
    270, 311
cirrhosis, 59
Clark, Barbara, 225
Classic of Difficult Issues (Nan Jing), 24
claustrophobia, 270
cleansing, 21
Cleveland Homeopathic College, 14
clinical guided imagery, 78

coex systems, 403-404
Cohen, Bonnie Bainbridge, 213, 214
colds, 57, 58, 61, 86, 88, 96, 194, 197
colon cancer, 55
colonics, 102
colors, feng shui and, 122
colorpuncture, 107-108
comedy, 79-80
communication, 338, 344, 356, 363, 418
complementation, 282
Complete Book of Yoga, The, 306
compresses, 99, 102
concentration, 111, 261, 263, 293, 300, 317, 320,
    325, 356, 392
Confucianism, 23, 24
congestion, 101
Connective Tissue Therapy℠, 145, 150-152, 166,
    167
Conrad-Da'oud, Emilie, 245, 252-253
Conscious Ear, The, 111
consciousness, 324, 325, 326, 369, 379, 398, 402-
    403
    See also mind; unconscious
constipation, 196
constitution, 5
contact improvisation, 245, 246, 249-252
Contact Newsletter/Quarterly, 249
contemplative dance, 350
continuum, 245, 246, 252-253
contraria contraris, 10
contrology, 245, 261
coordination, 344
core energetics, 380, 387-391
CORE structural integrative therapy, 152-153
coreSomatics, 380, 391-392
coronary artery disease, 55
    See also heart conditions
correctives, 211
cortisone, 146, 196
Coué, Émile, 74, 76
counseling, 126
Cousins, Norman, 79, 80
cranial osteopathy, 40
CranioSacral therapy, 34, 36, 40-42, 48
Creation of Meaning, The, 394
creative writing, 372
creativity, 84, 105, 111, 214, 237, 248, 326, 396,
    402, 417, 429
    See also expressive and creative arts thera-
    pies; imagination
cross-eye, 90
crying, 383
Cullen, Dr. William, 10
Cunningham, Merce, 249, 265
Cyriax, Dr. James, 157

D
Dalcroze, Emile Jacques, 258, 382

Damballah, 252, 253
dance, 119, 210, 212, 216, 226, 227, 234, 249-252, 254, 260, 263, 266, 281, 342, 343, 344
DanceAbility, 250
dance education, 201
dance therapy, 209, 210, 247, 328, 332, 350, 352-356
Dancer's Workshop Company, 360
dao-yin, 130
dar, 297
Darwin, Charles, 48
DC. See doctor of chiropractic
de Hartmann, Thomas, 258, 259
de Montgrillard, Guy, 287
de Salzmann, Alexandre, 258
de Salzmann, Jean, 258
deafness, 38
death, 98, 269
decision making, 338, 396
degenerative disorders, 151
Deguchi, Onisaburo, 278
dehydration, 102
Delsarte, François, 412
delta waves, 306
delusions, 124
Dennison, Gail, 245, 247
Dennison, Paul E., Ph.D., 245, 247
depression, 35, 399, 407, 414
    treatments for, 37, 55, 59, 61, 67, 70, 83, 103, 104, 106, 124, 139, 187, 326, 371, 408
    See also emotions
Desai, Amrit, 315
Descartes, René, 29, 65, 71
developmental disabilities, 42
Dharmapala, Anagarika, 317
diabetes, 55, 162
    treatment cautions, 60, 176
    treatments for, 125
Diagnostic Survey Manual (DSM), 329
Dialogue House, 362
diaphragmatic breathing, 264
diarrhea, 46
Dicke, Elizabeth, 150, 152
Dictionary of the Martial Arts, 293
dietary and nutritional practices, 53-56
Dietary Supplement Health and Education Act of 1994 (DSHEA), 57
diet, effect on health, 6, 8, 35, 36, 84, 100, 118, 126, 127, 128, 178, 196, 300
digestion, 72, 194
    See also indigestion
digestion aids, 57, 58
disabilities, 250, 358, 360, 365
disease
    homeopathic view of, 13
    osteopathic view of, 48
dissociative identity disorder, 106
D.O. See doctor of osteopathy

doctor of chiropractic (DC), 34, 39, 63, 162
doctor of naturopathy (ND), 15, 63
doctor of osteopathy (D.O.), 34, 48, 63, 162
do-in, 117, 118-119
dojang, 302
dojo, 278, 285-286, 287, 291, 295
dor-mor, 298
dos Reis Machado, Manoel, 281
doshas, 5-7
double gate theory of pain, 187
double vision, 92, 93
Downing, Dr. John, 105
drama, 417
drama therapy, 356-359
dreaming process, 415
dreams, 139, 429
    shamanism and, 19, 21
drugs
    effect on health, 8, 10, 34, 40, 46, 146, 344
    etymology of term, 57
    See also pharmaceutical drugs
drumming, 21
drumming circle, shamanism and, 22
DSM. See *Diagnostic Survey Manual*
Duncan, Isadora, 343
Durham, Else Henscke, 234
dynamis, homeopathic, 13
dyslexia, 113, 248

E
ear disorders, 111, 112
Ear and Language, The, 111
ear lavage, 102
eating disorders, 66, 76, 83, 106, 137, 139, 172, 215, 270, 356, 358, 360, 363, 380, 414
    See also anorexia; bulimia
echinacea (*Echinacea* spp.), 58, 60, 102
ecumenism, 313
eczema, 14
edema, 162
Edson, Dr. Susan, 14
education, 109, 258, 418
Education and Dyslexia, 111
Educational Kinesiology Foundation, 247
EEG. See electroencephalograph
effleurage, 174
effort phrasing, 338
Ego, Hunger, and Aggression, 397
Egypt, 34, 83, 86, 99, 124, 143, 163, 342
Ehrenfried, Dr. Lily, 234
Einstein, Albert, 268, 308
EKP. See Emotional Kinesthetic Psychotherapy
elderly, treatment cautions for, 102
electricity, feng shui and, 122
electroencephalograph (EEG), 68
electromagnetic energy, 103-109, 117
electromagnetism, 324
electronic ear, 111, 112, 113

Eliade, Mircea, 306, 307
Elizabeth Dicke Society, 152
Ellon, Inc., 98
EMDR. See Eye Movement Desensitization and Reprocessing
Emerson, Ralph Waldo, 317
emotional difficulties
    treatments for, 42, 44, 76, 81, 164, 378, 404, 414
    vision problems and, 89
emotional kaleidoscope, 188
emotional kinesthetic psychotherapy (EKP), 380, 392-394
emotional well-being, 289, 356, 357, 370
    defined, 29-31
emotions
    effect on health, 35, 48, 65, 67, 72, 73, 78-79, 96, 137, 139, 157, 204, 207, 343
    repressed, 8, 72, 106, 169, 189, 347, 398-399, 407
    shamanism and, 19, 21
    See also attitude; depression; memories
empathy, 355
emphysema, 8
endocrine system, 85, 101, 105, 196
endorphins, 66, 182
enema, 102
energetic forces, 2, 388-389
energy
    TCM view of, 26
    wellness and, 29, 263, 267
    Zero Balancing and, 50, 51
energy flows, 25, 35, 139, 224
energy vortex, 193
Enlightenment, the, 65
enneagram, 329-332
environment
    arrangement of, 119-124
    effect on health, 8, 207, 213, 221, 386, 392
    effect on vision, 90
    See also lifestyle, effect on health
ephedra (Ephedra sinia), 60
epilepsy, 143
Epsom salts, 102
Epstein, Dr. Donald, 43, 44, 238, 239
ergonomics, defined, 207
Erickson, Milton H., 74, 76
Esalen Institute, 209, 234, 240, 343, 403
Espenak, Liljan, 354
essence, TCM view of, 26
essential oils, 86, 87
etiquette, role of, 278, 280, 285, 291
eucalyptus, 87
Europe, 343
eurythmics, 258, 382
eurythmy, 245, 254-256
Evan, Blanch, 354
evolution, 48

exercise, 118, 126, 127, 128, 162, 225, 264
    effect on health, 36, 100, 178
    relation to wellness, 8, 16, 126, 196
expressive and creative arts therapies, 82, 341-346
eye disorders, 228-230
    treatments for, 42, 83, 93, 164, 188
eye exercises, 231, 295
eye gym, 91-93
eye movement desensitization and reprocessing (EMDR), 94-96
eye therapies
    Bates method, 88-90
    behavioral vision therapy, 90-93
    eye movement desensitization and reprocessing, 94-96

F
far-sightedness, 231
farming, 120
fascia, 150-151, 158-159, 165, 222, 223, 235-236
fasting, 53
fatigue
    treatments for, 97, 103, 106, 164, 172, 188, 226
    See also chronic fatigue syndrome
fats, 55
FDA. See Food and Drug Administration
fear, 67, 76, 96, 98, 137, 169, 231, 235, 286, 384, 391, 407
    coping mechanisms for, 14
Fehmi, Les, 68
Feldenkrais, Dr. Moshe, 201, 216, 219, 425
Feldenkrais Method®, 215-218, 391, 425, 428
fencing, 268
feng shui, 115-116, 117, 119-124
Fenichel, Clare, 234
fever, 145, 146, 196
    treatments for, 99
feverfew (Tanacetum parthenium), 58
fibromyalgia, 125, 159, 162, 264
Field, Tiffany, 155
fight-or-flight response, 247, 322
Finsen, Dr. Niels R., 103
fitness training, 207, 210
Fitsgerald, 163
five elements, 26, 184, 186
flexibility, enhancement of, 162, 206, 218, 224, 237, 240, 242, 263, 264, 267, 280, 291, 296
flower remedies, 84, 85, 96-99
flu, treatments, 57, 58, 88, 194
flushes, 99, 102
flying, 251
foam wedges, 208
focusing, 394-397
folk dancing, 211
folk medicine, 143, 195, 198
Food and Drug Administration (FDA), 57, 407
food, as medicine, 54, 62

435

foundation joints, 36
four methods of evaluation, 199
France, 258, 293
frankincense, 86
Franklin, Benjamin, 73
Frederic, Louis, 293
Freud, Sigmund, 66, 71, 74, 116, 343, 344, 347, 378-379, 382, 397, 398, 407, 419
friction, 174, 175
friction treatment, 157
Frigerio, Alejandro, 282
Fritz, Sandy, 143
Fromm, Erich, 234
Frost, Robert, 371
fulcra, 51
Fuller, Betty, 240
Function of the Orgasm, The, 379
Functional Integration®, 217-218
Fundamentals of Therapeutic Massage, 143

G
Gach, Michael Reed, 182
gait, 172, 173
Gandhi, Mahatma, 309
Gao Fu, Madame, 130
garlic (*Allium sativum*), 54, 58-59
gastrointestinal disorders, 204
    treatments for, 39, 67, 107, 164, 178, 199
    See also indigestion
Gattefosse, René Maurice, 86
Gautama, Siddhartha, 306
gekken, 293
gender equality, 251, 373
Gendlin, Dr. Eugene, 392, 394-397
genetic predispositions, effect on health, 6, 8, 16, 35, 39
geomancy, 120
geriatric problems, 159, 264
germ theory of disease, 7, 54
Gesell Institute of Child Development, 93
gestalt, homeopathic, 14
gestalt therapy, 234, 380, 391, 397-399, 410, 414, 417, 425, 428
Gi, 278, 291
Gichin, Funakoshi, 290, 291, 292
Gindler, Elsa, 169, 201, 226, 231, 232, 234
ginkgo (*Ginkgo biloba*), 59
glandular disorders, 164
glaucoma, treatment cautions, 60, 90, 404
Gnosticism, 116
goals, 363
God, 48, 65
Goethe, Johann Wolfgang von, 11
goldenseal, 102
Goldstein, Kurt, 410
golgi tendon reflex, 148
gonorrhea, 14
gout, 104, 125

Graham, Martha, 265, 350
Graham, Sylvester, 54
grave sites, 120
gravity, 165, 167, 219, 223, 231, 269, 272, 314, 324
Greece, 2, 37, 54, 65, 71, 83, 86, 99, 116, 143, 145, 163, 275, 329, 342, 363, 366, 370
Green, Drs. Elmer and Alyce, 66, 68
grief, effect on health, 79, 137, 139, 164, 363
Grof, Christine, 403
Grof, Stanislav, 380, 403
groundedness, 164, 383-384, 422
groups, 338, 399, 411-414, 415
Guest, Anne Hutchinson, 336
guided imagery, 65, 67, 71-73, 74, 80, 225
    ROM dance and, 265-267
    shamanism and, 21, 65
guilt, 137, 189
Gurdjieff Foundation, 258
Gurdjieff, George Ivanovitch, 245, 256-260, 257, 317, 329
Gurdjieff movements, 256-260
guruji, 314
gymnastics, 143, 260
gymnastik, 232
Gymnastique Holistique, 234

H
habits, 231, 259
Hahnemann, Samuel, 2, 10-12, 11, 116
Haiti, 252
hakama, 278, 295
hakomi integrative somatics, 392, 399-402
hakuda, 284
Hall, Edward T., 268
hallucinations, 124
Halprin, Anna, 360
Halprin life/art process, 359-361
hand therapy, 264
hands
    use in therapy, 37, 119, 128, 133
    See also touch
Hanna Somatic Education® (HSE), 218-222
Hanna Somatic educator, 221
Hanna, Thomas, 219, 220, 244
happiness, 326
hara, 295
Harlowe, Diane, M.S., 245, 263
hatha yoga, 65, 245, 305, 307-308
Hawkins, Alma, 354
Hayashi, Chijuro, 135
head, 204
Head, Henry, 150
head zones, 150
headaches, 97, 204
    treatments for, 70, 72, 93, 124, 129, 159, 162, 164, 178, 182, 187, 194, 199, 215, 221
    See also migraine headaches

436

healing crisis, alternative methods and, 4
Healing Massage Techniques, 142
healing process
   natural, 3, 9, 72, 349
   participation in, 17, 69, 141, 352
   self-healing, 3, 35, 38, 41, 88, 129, 140, 388,
   405
health
   behavioral model of, 89
   factors affecting, 8
Health Building, 126
health maintenance, compared to disease treatment, 3
Heard, Gerald, 317
hearing, defined, 112
hearing loss, 83
heart, 392
heart conditions, 35, 137, 404
   treatments for, 39, 61, 62, 67, 70, 175, 323
heart rate, 72, 85, 87, 311, 320, 322
Heidigger, Martin, 397
heiho, 293
Heller, Joseph, 202, 222
Hellerwork, 202, 222-224
hemorrhages
   treatment cautions, 175
   treatments for, 99
hepatitis, 14, 59
herbal medicine, 2, 17, 23, 25, 27, 53-54, 55, 57-
   60, 86, 126, 180
   types of herbs, 59
herpes, 86, 88
Herschel, John, 103
Hewitt, James, 306
Heyer, Lucy, 169
Hidden You, The, 225
high blood pressure, 55
   treatment cautions, 60, 196
   treatments for, 39, 67, 70, 129, 187, 215, 320,
   322, 323, 326
   See also blood pressure
higher self, 419, 420
Himalayan Institute, 306
Hinduism, 5, 135, 193, 305, 307, 308, 309
Hindu Vedanta, 317, 318, 319
hippies, 145
Hippocrates, 34, 37, 54, 62, 71, 83, 99, 116, 143
hip replacement, 264
Hisamaro, Takenouchi, 284
histiopathology, 39
Hoffer, Abram, 61, 63
Hogan, Dr. Peter, 425
holdings, 168, 170, 221
holism, 7, 29
holistic health, 3, 7-9, 46
Holotropic Breathwork™, 380, 402-405
Holotropic Mind, The, 403
homelessness, 358, 360, 373

homeopathy, 2, 5, 9, 10-15, 16, 116
homeostasis, 13, 173, 226
homeplay, 248
hormone levels, 85, 87, 105
Horney, Karen, 317, 397
hospices, 373
hospitals, 373
HSE. See Hanna Somatic Education
Hua Tuo, 129
*Huang-ti Nei Jing (Yellow Emperor's Internal
   Classic)*, 24, 118, 143, 184, 198, 297
Hull, Clark, 74
human beings, 154
   non-material aspects, 3, 213
   relation to environment, 25
Human Movement Potential, 225
human potential, 232
humanistic psychology, 380
Humanistic Psychology Institute, 219
Hunt, Dr. Valerie, 252
Huxley, Aldous, 89, 317
Hwarang, Code of, 301, 303
hydrotherapy, 15, 16, 83, 85, 99-103
hyodo, 293
hyperactivity, treatments for, 42
Hypericum perforatum (St. John's wort), 55
hypertension. See High blood pressure
hypnosis, 73, 322
Hypnosis and Suggestibility, 74
hypnotherapy, 19, 65, 66, 73-77
   self-hypnosis, 71
hysteria, 71
hyung, 303

I

IAIM. See International Association for Infant
   Massage
Ichazo, Oscar, 329
ideas, 355
ideokinesis, 201, 224-226
imagination, 71, 73, 78, 344, 350, 363, 370, 420
   See also creativity
immune system
   factors affecting, 78-81, 83, 88, 362
   strengthening, 99, 129, 136, 146, 196
immunity, 72
Imperial College of Medicine, 198
improvisation, 355
incense, 86
incest, 414, 427
   See also abuse; sexual dysfunction
incontinence, treatments for, 67
India, 5, 7, 73, 83, 118, 124, 126, 143, 153, 245,
   275, 298, 306, 317, 342
indigestion, 97, 128
   treatments for, 88, 139, 164, 188
   See also gastrointestinal disorders
infant, music therapy for, 366-370

Infant Massage: Handbook for Loving Parents, 153
infant massage, 153-157
infections, 79, 81, 97, 111, 112, 162
   treatment cautions, 175, 199
   treatments, 54, 73, 86, 104, 107, 141
infertility, 323
   treatment for, 164, 323
inflammation, treatment cautions, 175
influenza, 14, 146
infrared energy, 103
Ingham, Eunice, 163
inhibition, 169
injury
   See also accidents
   effect on health, 39, 111
   treatment for, 124, 151, 157, 172, 194, 199, 207, 212, 225, 337
innate intelligence, 38
inner child, 426
inner elixir qigong, 132
insect bites, 88, 125
insomnia, treatments for, 58, 67, 69, 70, 76, 103, 106-107, 124, 139, 178, 187, 188, 199, 323, 326
instincts, shamanism and, 19
Institute for Music, Health, and Education, 109
Institute for the Harmonious Development of Man, 258, 329
Institute of Noetic Sciences, 117
integral yoga, 313-314
Integral Yoga Institutes (IYIs), 313
integrated movement, 339
intelligence, 392
Interactive Guided Imagery, 72, 77-78
Intermodal Learning in Education and Therapy, 364
International Association for Infant Massage (IAIM), 153
International Kendo Federation, 293
International Medical and Dental Hypnotherapy Association, 76
International Somatic Movement Therapy and Education Association (ISMTEA), 202
Interscience Research Institute, 421
intimacy, 402
intuition, shamanism and, 19
irrigations, 99, 102
irritable bowel syndrome, 69, 70
ischemic compression, 160
Islam, 124, 144, 306
ISMTEA. See International Somatic Movement Therapy and Education Association
Iyengar, B.K.S., 314-315
Iyengar yoga, 314-315
IYIs. See Integral Yoga Institutes

J

Jacobson, Edmund, 382
Jacoby, Heinrich, 201, 232, 234

jam sessions, 249
James, William, 306
Japan, 118, 143, 163, 178, 191, 195, 285
Japanese Karate Association, 291
jaundice
   treatment cautions, 175
   treatments for, 103, 104, 107
Javal, Dr. Emile, 83, 90
jaw pain
   treatment for, 158, 159
   See also temporomandibular joint
jealousy, 96, 98
jet lag, 105, 106
jhana yoga, 308, 313
Jigoro, Kano, 216, 287, 288
Jin Shin Do®, 178, 180, 187-190
Jin Shin Jyutsu®, 180, 188, 190, 191-192
jin ye, 26
jing, 26
jogo, 282
jogo-de-capoeira, 283
Johnsen, Lillimor, 385
Johnsen, Linda, 306
Johnson, Lyndon B., 160
joint pain, treatments for, 188
jojoba, 88
Journal of Orgonomy, 407, 408
Journal of Practical Medicine, 10
Journal to the Self, 362
journal therapy, 361-363
journaling, 237, 372
journey, shamanistic, 21
Joy, Dr. Brugh, 222
joza, 295
ju-jutsu, 278, 283-286, 286, 287
Judaism, 116, 124, 143, 245, 329, 342
judo, 118, 216, 278, 284, 285, 286-289
judogi, 288
Judson Church Group, 249
Jung, Carl Gustav, 126, 169, 193, 343, 347, 350, 374, 379-380, 391, 404, 410, 419

K

Kabat-Zinn, Jon, 319
Kagan, Alfred, 157
Kalff, Dora, 374-377
Kamiya, Joe, 68
Kammertanzbuhne Laban, 335
Kanemon, Terada, 287
kapha, 5-7
karate, 118, 285, 289-292, 301
Karate/Kung-Fu Illustrated, 282
karateka, 289, 290, 291
karma yoga, 309, 313
kata, 292
keiko, 296
Kellogg, Dr. John Harvey, 100
Kelly, Dr. Charles R., 421-422

ken-jutsu, 293
kendo, 278, 293-297
kendoka, 293
Kennedy, John F., 144, 160
Kestenberg, Dr. Judith S., 332, 336
Kestenberg movement profile (KMP), 213, 328, 332-335
ki, 23, 116, 278, 286, 293, 295
ki-ai, 295, 296
kicking, 275, 276
kidney disorders, 152
kikentai-no-ichi, 296
kinesiopathology, 39
kinesphere, 251, 336
kinesthetic sense, 82, 231, 266
kinetic awareness, 226-228
Kinetography Laban, 335
kirlian photograph, 107
KMP. See Kestenberg Movement Profiler
Kneipp, Father Sebastian, 2, 15-16, 83, 99-100
Knill, Paolo, 364
Kodokan, 287
Koffa, Kurt, 397
Kogusoku, 284
kokodan judo, 278
Konia, Dr. Charles, 408
Korea, 118, 301, 319
Korean Taekwondo Federation, 301
Kousaleos, George P., 152
Kraeplin, Emil, 347
Kramer, Edith, 347
Krieger, Dolores, Ph.D., 140
kripalu yoga, 315-316
kripalvananda, 315
Krishna Consciousness Movement, 309
Krishnamacharya, Shree T., 314
Krishnamurti, Jidhu, 317
kriyas, 308
Kübler-Ross, Dr. Elizabeth, 29-30
kundalini yoga, 308, 315, 320
kung fu, 118
kung fu wu su, 297-301
kuntao, 275
Kunz, Dora, 140
Kurtz, Ron, 392, 400
Kushi, Michio, 54, 118

L
Laban Institute of Movement Studies, 211
Laban Lawrence industrial rhythm, 338
Laban movement analysis (LMA), 211, 213, 327, 328, 335-340
Laban personal effort assessment, 338
Laban, Rudolf, 210, 327, 333, 335, 338
Labanotation, 335
ladainha, 283
Lamb, Warren, 333, 336

Landau reflex, 219
Lao-tzu, 186
law of cure, 12
Lawrence, F. C., 338
lazy eye, 90, 93, 231
leadership, 329
learning, 84, 105, 329
learning disabilities, treatments for, 67, 70, 93, 103, 113, 215, 216, 247, 248, 369
Lee, Bruce, 285
Leedy, Jack J., 370
Leibowitz, Judith, 425
Lepkoff, Daniel, 249
Lerner, Arthur, 370
levity, 269
Lewis, Penny, 332
Liberman, Dr. Jacob, 106
licensing, 145-146
licking, 154
Liebault, Auguste Ambroise, 73-74
lifestyle, effect on health, 6, 7, 8, 16, 35, 36, 111, 112, 178, 196, 344
lifestyle counseling, 15
light, feng shui and, 122
light therapy, 83, 84, 85, 103-109, 320
Light of Truth Universal Services, 313
Light of Truth Universal Shrine (LOTUS), 313
limbic system, 85, 86-87, 105
Ling, Per Henrik, 144, 174
Ling System, the, 174
listening, 111, 248, 250
    defined, 111-112
    Sounding and, 109-111
liver disorders, 59, 147
LMA. See Laban Movement Analysis
lodestone, 124
logic, 2
Loman, Susan, 332
longevity, 118, 263
LOTUS. See Light of Truth Universal Shrine
love, 74, 407
love force, 389
Lowen, Dr. Alexander, 382-385, 388, 393, 410
Lowenfeld, Margaret, 374
lupus, 264
Lust, Benedict, 15-17, 83
lymphatic drainage, 148, 174
lymphocytes, 79

M
ma huang (*Ephedra sinia*), 60
MacArthur, Gen. Douglas, 290
macrobiotics, 54, 118
magic, 118, 257
magnesium, 249
magnet therapy, 115-116, 117, 124-126
magnetotherapy. See magnet therapy
makiwara, 302

malicia, 282
management, 329, 332
Mandel, Peter, 107
mandingas, 282
mantra yoga, 308, 313
mantras, 309, 326
manual lymph drainage, 145
Marcher, Lisbeth, 385-387
Marcus, Dr. Hershey, 332
Marks, Linda, 392-393
martial arts, 82, 118, 226, 249, 251, 274-277, 317
martial arts qigong, 131
Mary Starks Whitehouse Institute, 350
Maslow, Abraham, 345, 380, 410
massage therapy, 6, 9, 23, 74, 82, 84, 88, 118,
    119, 136, 142-147, 173, 174, 178, 195, 197-198,
    229, 231, 268, 328
materialism, 317
Maudsley, Henry, 353
Maury, Marguerite, 86
McClure, Vimala, 153-157
McMillan, Jaimen, 245, 268
M.D. See medical doctor
measles, 146
    treatments for, 14, 104
mechanistic paradigm, compared to wellness
    paradigm, 29
medical doctor (M.D.), 63, 162
medical orgone therapy, 405-409
medical orgonomy, 116, 382
medical qigong, 131
medicine men. See shamanism
medicine wheel, 22
meditation, 6, 64, 68, 69, 74, 117, 119, 131, 251, 298,
    300, 303, 315, 317-321, 403, 423
meditation in motion, 315-316
Meetings with Remarkable Men, 256, 257, 259
Meir Schneider's Miracle Eyesight Method, 230
Meir Schneider self-healing method, 228-231
melatonin, 105
Melzack and Wall, 187
memories
    effect on health, 79, 214
    emotional, 85, 106, 152, 169, 194, 248, 326,
        367, 379, 392, 402, 426
    vision and, 89, 94
    See also emotions
Menninger Foundation, 117
menopausal difficulties, 188
menstrual difficulties, 106, 139, 164, 188
mental disorders, 124, 187, 194, 403
mental health, 373
mental rejuvenation, 260
mental well-being, 276, 286, 289, 302, 311
    defined, 29-31
mentastics, 242
mercury, 40, 46
meridians, 24, 178, 180, 182, 184, 186, 189, 193, 195

Mesmer, Franz Anton, 64, 73
Mesmerism, 37, 48
miasms, 12
Middle Ages, the, 144
migraine headaches, 8
    treatments, 14, 39, 42, 58, 67, 70, 76, 139, 187
    See also headaches
milk thistle (*Silybum marianum*), 59
Miller, Kay, 391
Milton H. Erickson Institutes, 76
mime, 254, 356
mind
    effect on health, 65, 71, 77, 270, 325, 343, 379
    influence on health, 3
    See also brain; consciousness; unconscious
mind/body medicine, 64-67, 82
Mindanao, 275
Mindell, Arnold, 193, 415-416
mindfulness, 400, 402
mirroring, 354
mirrors, 207
Miss Sarah Farmer's Greenacre School of
    Comparative Religions, 317
mobility junction, 250
Modern Educational Dance, 336
monasticism, 143
Montague, Ashley, 154
Moreno, Jacob Levi, M.D., 380, 416
morphine, 46
Moshou, 198
motivation, 67, 84, 105, 113, 230, 332
motor-coordination, 42, 113, 226, 386-387
Mount Kuriyama, 135
movement, universal, 245-246
movement coaching, 207, 328
movement in depth, 350
movement dysfunction, 159, 207
movement pattern analysis, 328, 338-340
movement therapy, 82, 200-203, 247, 268, 270,
    332
    See also bodywork
moving imagination, 350
Mowrer, Hobart G., 68
moxibustion, 24, 186
Mrs. Ole Bull's Cambridge Conferences on
    Comparative Religions, 317
MTPT. See Myofascial Trigger Point Therapy
Mucope people, 281
mudras, 191
mugwort (*Artemesia vulgaris*), 186
Muktananda, Swami, 50
multi-modal expressive arts therapy, 363-366
multiple sclerosis, 14, 229
mummification, 86
Murai, Jiro, 180, 188, 189, 191
muscular dystrophy, 230, 240, 344
muscular pain, treatments for, 69, 86, 102, 124,
    125, 146, 148, 157, 182, 196, 236

muscular system, 36, 262, 311, 408

muscular therapy, 157-158

musculoskeletal system, 152-153, 204, 224, 225, 227

music, 72, 234, 254-255, 259, 280, 282-283, 403

music therapy, 366-370

musicians, 206, 211, 212, 216, 231, 267, 343

Myofascial Pain and Dysfunction, 160

myofascial release, 145, 158-160, 236

myofascial trigger point therapy (MTPT), 160-163

myopathology, 39

myrrh, 86

mysticism, 317, 403

My Water Cure, 100

N

nagi, 278, 280

NAMT. See National Association of Music Therapy

Nan Jing (Classic of Difficult Issues), 24

NAPT. See National Association for Poetry Therapy

Naranjo, Claudio, 329

NASA, 105, 222

National Association for Drama Therapy (NADT), 357, 359

National Association of Music Therapy (NAMT), 367

National Association for Poetry Therapy (NAPT), 362, 370

National Cancer Institute, 55

National Institutes of Health (NIH), 55, 57, 140

National Institute of Mental Health, 105

National Learning Foundation (NLF), 247

National Socialist Party, 335

Native Americans, 46, 83, 99, 142, 163, 342, 403

natural childbirth, 17

natural law, relation to health, 8, 118, 131

Natural Law Party, 324

nature, human beings and, 84, 245

naturopathic medicine, 15-17

naturopathy, 2, 9, 83

Naumburg, Margaret, 347

Nazism, 335, 397, 420

NCCAOM (National Commission for Certification of Acupuncture and Oriental Medicine), 28

ND. See doctor of naturopathy

nearsightedness, 83, 91, 231

neck, 204

neck pain, treatment for, 39, 42, 158, 159, 162, 206, 209, 236, 264

necromancy, 118

needs, 398, 412

nervous system, 35, 41, 42, 43, 48, 85, 99, 100, 102, 104-105, 146, 150, 152, 163, 172, 173-174, 175, 196, 203, 219, 392

autonomic, 148, 169

disorders of, 164

immune system and, 79

parasympathetic, 150

network chiropractic, 34-35, 43-45, 239

network spinal analysis. See network chiropractic

Neumann, Erich, 374, 410

neuralgia, treatment for, 125

neuro-hypnosis, 73

neurological disorders, 42, 216, 225

neurology, 173, 264

neuromuscular facilitation, 145, 150, 231

neuropathology, 39

neurosensory development, 105-106, 108

neurosis, 74, 116

neurotic character structure, 383

New Diary, The, 361

New School for Social Research, 234, 382

New York Academy of Science, 62

New Zealand, 248

Newton, Sir Isaac, 103

n'golo, 281

niacin, 55, 61

nibanna, 319

NIH. See National Institutes of Health

nine-pointed star, 329-330

nirvana, 319

Nixon, Richard, 144

NLF. See National Learning Foundation

Nolte, Marcia, 237

nonviolence, 313

norepinephrine, 105

Novato Institute for Somatic Research and Training, 219, 222

Nugent, John J., 37

numbness, 180

numerology, 120

nutrition, clinical, 15

nutritional counseling, 37

nutritional and dietary practices, 53-56

nutritional supplements, 16

O

O Sensei, 278-280

OAM. See Office of Alternative Medicine

obi, 288, 291

obsessive compulsive disorder, 106, 139

occupational health, 231

occupational therapy, 213, 245, 263

OEP. See Optometric Extension Program

Office of Alternative Medicine (OAM), 57

Ogden, Pat, 400, 401

Ohashi Institute, 195

Ohashi, Wataru, 195

Ohashiatsu, 195

Okinawa, 290

oM, 309

Omega Institute, 343
Omoto-Kyo, 278
On Vital Reserves, 306
oncology, 264
One to One: Self-Understanding Through Journal Writing, 361
opium, 46
Optiks (Newton), 103
Optometric Extension Program (OEP), 91
organismic body psychotherapy, 380, 409-411
Organon of Rational Medicine, 10
orgone, 388
   See also medical orgone therapy
Oriental medicine, 15, 17, 23
   See also traditional Chinese medicine
Orr, Leonard, 380, 422-425
orthomolecular medicine, 55, 56, 60-63
orthopedic disorders, 42
orthoptics, 90
Osmond, Humphrey, 61
osteoarthritis, 226
osteopathy, 33, 34, 36, 38, 40, 45-50, 55
osteoporosis, 221
otitis, 14
Ottenbacker, K. J., 154
Ouspensky, P. D., 258
overeating, 6
   See also eating disorders

P

PA. See Process Acupressure
PACE (Positive, Active, Clear, Energetic), 248
pain
   effect on health, 79, 133
   principles of, 173-174
   treatments for, 21, 33, 42, 57, 65, 67, 70, 72, 73, 76, 124, 129, 141, 145, 146, 158, 159, 160, 172-173, 182, 194, 196, 206, 209, 216, 218, 223, 227, 228, 229, 235, 240, 263, 264, 267, 323, 428
palliative treatment, homeopathic, 10
Palmer, Bartlett Joshua, 37
Palmer, Daniel David, 34, 35, 37, 38
Panchakarma, 6
pancreatitis, 14
panic attacks, 106, 139, 408
Paracelsus, 71
paralysis, 253
paranoia, 329
Paré, Ambroise, 144
parent-child interactions
   before/after birth, 334
   infant massage, 153-157
Parkinson's disease, 264
Parnell, Devakanya G., 315
Pasteur, Louis, 54
Pasteurization, 54
Pastinha, Mestre, 281
Pastinha, Vincente Ferreira, 281

Patanjali, 306
pathophysiology, 39
pathwork, 387-391
Pauling, Linus, 54-55, 61
Pavek, Dr. Richard R., 137, 138
Paxton, Steve, 245, 249, 250
pediatric problems, 159
pellagra, 61
penicillin, 2, 84
Pennebaker, Dr. James, 362
perceptual difficulties, 214
performing artists, 204, 206, 211, 227, 260, 267
perfumes, 86
Perls, Fritz, 234, 380, 397-399, 410, 417, 425
Perls, Laura, 380, 425
personal growth, 329, 357
personal kinesphere, 336
personality, 72, 96, 109, 330, 354, 359, 393, 398
   homeopathic view of, 14
Pesso, Albert, 411-414
Pesso Boyden system psychomotor (PBSP), 381, 411-414
petrissage, 174
pharmaceutical drugs, 2, 7, 16, 38, 54, 84, 144
   herbal medicine and, 57, 58
   See also Allopathic medicine
pharmacopiae, 27
Philippines, 275
phlebitis, 147
phobias, 35, 67, 73, 76, 270
photoluminesence, 107
photoreceptors, 105
photron ocular light stimulator, 105
phrenology, 48
physical education, 261, 268
physical fitness, 252, 276, 289
physical medicine, 15
physical reeducation, 234
physical therapy, 169, 210, 252, 261, 263, 268, 270
physical well-being, defined, 29-31
physiology, 144, 145-146
physiotherapy, 268
Picasso, Pablo, 343
Pierrakos, Dr. John, 382, 388-389, 393
Pilates, Joseph H., 245, 260, 261
Pilates Method of Body Conditioning®, 245, 246, 260-263
pitta, 5-7
placebo, 66-67
plantar fascitis, 162
plants, medicinal, 53-54, 119
   See also herbal medicine
Plato, 143, 342
playing, 261
pleasure, 195, 239, 240-242
PMS. See premenstrual syndrome
pneumonia, 46

treatments for, 14, 104
PNI. See psychoneuroimmunology
Poetry Cure, The, 370
poetry therapy, 370-374
Poetry Therapy Institute, 370
polarity therapy, 5, 116, 126-129, 145
Polarity Therapy, 126
polio, 210-211, 344
    treatments for, 14, 210-211
Polynesia, 342
poomse, 303
positive thinking, 79-80
post-traumatic stress disorder (PTSD)
    treatments for, 83, 94-95, 139, 194, 290, 356,
    402, 427
    See also stress; trauma
postural alignment, 264
posture, 113, 173, 174, 207, 209, 226, 231, 240,
    242, 262, 269, 306, 391
Power of Imagination Conference, 78
Practice of Aromatherapy, The, 86
prana, 116, 127, 311
pranayama, 308, 309, 310, 311, 314, 315
prayer, 74, 342
pregnancy, 267
    cautions in, 190, 196, 242, 404
premenstrual syndrome (PMS), treatments for,
    103, 139, 187, 196, 320
PressureStat Model, 41
preventative treatment
    homeopathic, 10
    naturopathic, 16
    physical, 172, 194
    spiritual, 198
Priessnitz, Vincent, 83, 99
primordial qigong, 132
Primum non nocere, 16
prisons, 358, 373
process acupressure (PA), 192-194
    See also acupressure
process oriented psychology, 380, 415-416
Progoff, Dr. Ida, 361-363
*Program Guide for Body-Mind Centering
    Certification Program*, 213
progressive relaxation, 382
prophesy, 118
prosperity, 424
prostate, 59
proving, homeopathic, 12-13
Prudden, Bonnie, 160, 161
psoriasis, 14, 103, 107, 320
    See also skin disorders
psyche, 256
psychiatric disorders, 61
psychiatry, 49, 264, 353
psycho-physical evaluation frameworks, 327-
    328
psychoactive drugs, 146

psychoanalysis, 343, 379, 398, 414, 419
psychodrama, 380, 416-419
psychology, 19, 111, 235, 332, 337
psychoneuroimmunology (PNI), 29, 65, 66, 67,
    78-81
psychopathology, 347, 353
psychosynthesis, 381, 392, 419-421
psychotherapy, 84, 95, 104, 106, 169, 172, 188,
    234, 317, 356
    See also body-oriented psychotherapies
pulses, 24
puppetry, 356
purging, 10, 34, 46
Pythagoras, 245

Q
qi, 23, 24, 25, 129, 132, 138, 183, 194, 195, 197,
    198
    TCM view of, 26, 27
qigong, 117, 129-133, 244-245, 320
quinine, 10

R
Radix, 421-422
Raheem, Dr. Aminah, 182, 192, 193
Rainer, Tristine, 361
raja yoga, 306, 307, 309
Rama, Swami, 306
Ramakrishna Vedanta, 317
Ramamani, 314
randori, 285, 288
rape, 94
rapid eye movement (REM), EMDR and, 95
Rational Hydrotherapy, 100
RDAs. See recommended daily allowances
RDT. See registered dance therapist
reading skills, 248
Realms of the Human Unconscious, 403
rebirthing, 380, 422-425
recommended daily allowances (RDAs), 62-63
recreation therapy, 263
reflexes, 219
reflexology, 163-165
registered dance therapist (RDT), 355, 358
Registered Movement Therapist, 202
rehabilitation medicine, 49
Reich, Dr. Wilhelm, 116, 157, 189, 379, 382, 384,
    393, 397, 400, 405-409, 406, 409-410, 421
reiki, 116, 133-137, 145
relationships
    effect on health, 35, 98, 107, 356, 363, 369,
    387, 390, 414, 424
    See also emotions
relaxation
    health and, 79, 99, 141, 200, 242, 368
    treatments for, 33, 69, 76, 77, 174, 175
relaxation response, 322-324
Relaxation Response Program, 319

religious persecution, 144, 317
religious rituals, 342, 353
REM. See rapid eye movement
remedy portrait, 14
Renaissance, the, 2, 71, 86, 144, 317, 343
Renaud, Jean-Joseph, 287
Rentsch, Oswald and Elaine, 148
reparenting, 414
resentment, 96, 98
resonance, 26
resources, 385
respiratory conditions, 81, 311
    treatments for, 67, 76, 107, 194
restorative observation, 201, 231
Return to Life, 261
rheumatism, treatments for, 101, 125, 144, 174,
    182, 264
rhythm, 269
rickets, 260
rigidity, 222, 391
Rilke, Rainer Maria, 343
Rishis, 5
Ritter, Johann, 103
rituals, 352
    shamanism and, 18, 19
"Road Not Taken, The", 371
Robin, Dr. Esther, 332
roda, 282
Rogers, Carl, 345, 380, 410
role play, 357-358, 412, 416, 418
Rolf, Dr. Ida, 50, 165-168, 166, 201, 209, 222, 235
Rolf Institute, 223
Rolfing®, 48, 50, 145, 165-168, 209, 222, 223, 235
ROM dance, 245, 263-265
    guided imagery and, 265-267
Rome, 83, 86, 143, 275, 342
Rosen, Marion, 169, 170
Rosen method, 168-172
Rosen method of bodywork, 169
Rosenthal, Norman, 105
Rosicrucians, 317
Rossman, Dr. Martin L., 77-78
Royal Gymnastic Central Institute, 144, 174
Rubenfeld, Illana, 380, 425-428, 427
Rubenfeld synergy method, 425-428

S
sabumnim, 303
sacred gymnastics, 258
SAD. See seasonal affective disorder
safety-energy locks, 190, 191-192
Salinger, J.D., 317
samadhi, 306, 311
samurai, 284-285, 293
sandplay therapy, 374-377
Sands Point Movement Study Group, 332, 333
Sanga, 281
Saraswati, Swami Brahamananda, 324

Saraswati, Swami Sivananda, 313
Satchidananda Ashram-Yogaville, 313
Satchidananda, Swami, 313
Saul, King, 366
saunas, 102
sauntering, 318
saw palmetto (*Serenoa repens*), 59
Scafifi, F.A., 154
scar tissue, 152
scarlet fever, 14, 104
Schauffler, Robert Haven, 370
schizophrenia, 55, 61, 399, 408
Schneider, Meir, Ph.D, 228
Schoenberg, Arnold, 343
School for Body-Mind Centering, 213
School of Nancy, 73
School for Self-Healing, 230
schools, 373, 418
Schoop, Trudi, 354
sciatica, 39, 162
scientific method, 2
scoliosis, 39, 42, 159, 188, 206
scurvy, 61
seasonal affective disorder (SAD), 105, 106-107
self-awareness, 169-171, 214, 215, 402
self-confidence, 96, 98, 235, 276, 285, 289, 291,
    302
self-defense, 260, 274, 300
    See also martial arts
self-discipline, 276, 286, 289, 293, 302
self-esteem, 8, 204, 218, 248, 326, 356, 363, 424
self-expression, 171, 224, 248, 267
Self-Healing: My Life and Vision, 230
self-image, 415
self-knowledge, 259
self-realization, 319
self-reliance, 203
self-study, 259
Selver, Charlotte, 233, 234
Selye, Hans, 66
Sen-Nin, 118
sensory awareness, 203, 231-235, 410
Sensory Awareness Foundation, 234
sensory-motor amnesia (SMA), 221
sensory recruitment, 72
sensory therapies, 82-85
sensory-motor amnesia (SMA), 221
sensuality, 195
sequences, 211
serotonin, 105
sexual activity, 309, 379-380
    effect on health, 8
sexual arousal, 72
sexual dysfunction, 97, 106, 390
shakti yoga, 50
Shaku, Rev. Soyen, 317
shamanism, 2, 18-23, 81, 65 129, 306, 403
    See also trance state

444

shamanistic counseling, 2, 21
shame, 137, 189
Shang Han Lun (Treatise on Harm Caused by Cold), 25
Shaolin Temple, 275, 289, 298
Shapiro, Francine, Ph.D., 94, 95
sharing, 418
shen, 26
SHEN, 116, 137-139
shiatsu, 117, 145, 146, 178, 180, 194-197
shinai, 293
shingles, 86
Shinto, 278
shoulder pain, 162
Shute, Evan and Wilfred, 61
Siberia, 306
Siegel, Bernie, 71
sign language, 254
similia similibus curentor, 10
Simons, David, M.D., 160
Simonton, Carl, 71
singers, 206
singing, 342
sinusitis, treatments for, 39, 164, 187, 188, 196
Skeffington, Dr. A.M., 91
skeletal manipulation methods, 33-36
skeletal system, 213
skeleton models, 207
skin
    hypersensitivity of, 162
    treatments for, 59-60, 102, 175
skin disorders
    treatments for, 88, 101
Skinner, Joan, 245, 265
Skinner releasing technique (SRT), 245, 246, 265-267
skull, 34, 36
slaves, 275, 281
sleep disorders. See insomnia
SMA. See sensory-motor amnesia
smallpox, treatments for, 104
Smith, Bruce Robertson, 296
Smith, Fritz Frederick, M.D., 50
Smith, Nancy Stark, 249, 250
Smith, William, M.D., 47
smoking, 6, 19, 73, 76, 178, 184
    effect on health, 8
    See also addictions
smudging ceremony, 21
Smuts, Jan Christiaan, 7
snake bite, 143
Snyder, Gary, 317
Society for Clinical and Experimental Hypnosis, 76
sociology, 337
sociometry, 416
Socrates, 143
sode, 288

sojutsu, 278
soma, 219, 244
SOMA Institute, 237
soma neuromuscular integration, 202, 235-238
somatic dysfunction, 49
somatic exercises, 221
Somatic Institute, 391
somatic practices, 82
somatics, 253
    defined, 219
somato respiratory integration (SRI), 238-239
Soodak, Dr. Martha, 332
Sossin, Mark, 332
soul, 96, 192, 389
sound, 119, 254-255, 308, 403
    feng shui and, 122
sounding, 109-111
South African Institute for Psychoanalysis, 397
Spatial Dynamics℠, 245, 246, 268-270
Speads, Carola, 226, 234
Specific Human Energy Nexus. See SHEN
speech, 109, 379
Spencer, Herbert, 48
spinal cord, 41, 43
spine
    illness and, 34, 38-39, 206, 231
    manipulation of, 36, 37, 48, 204, 295
spirits, 2, 3, 18, 19, 26, 65, 71
spiritual nature, 3, 315
spiritual qigong, 131
Spiritual Regeneration Movement, 324
spiritual well-being, 286, 380, 396
    defined, 29-31
spiritual world, 254
spiritualism, 48
Spitler, Harry, 84, 104
spontaneity, 417
sports, 73, 226, 247, 268
    See also athletics
sports injuries, 148, 165
sports training, 71, 328
sprains and strains, 178, 199
SRI. See Somato respiratory integration
SRT. See Skinner releasing technique
Ssu-ma Chien, 24
stamina, 270, 291
Stanislavsky, Konstantin, 343
startle response, 219, 221
Steiner, Rudolf, 245, 254-256, 268, 269
sterilization, 107
stiffness, 180
Still, Dr. Andrew Taylor, 33, 34, 35, 40, 45-50
stimulants, 60
St. John method of neuromuscular therapy, 172-174
St. John Neuromuscular Pain Relief Institute, 173
St. John, Paul, 172

St. John's wort (*Hypericum perforatum*), 55, 59
stomach. See gastrointestinal disorders
Stone, Randolph, 126
storytelling, 18, 370
strange flows, 189
strength conditioning, 262-263, 267, 280, 286,
    296, 311
    See also bodybuilding
stress
    coping mechanisms for, 14, 70, 77, 152, 155,
      356
    effect on health, 35, 39, 66, 68, 79, 83, 98, 111,
      112, 172, 221, 230, 427
    treatments for, 52, 65, 67, 101, 109, 124, 164,
      174, 178, 187, 194, 247, 267, 317, 326, 405
    See also tension
stress management, 17, 42, 89, 145, 264
Stress Reduction Clinic, 319
stroke, 55, 67
    treatment cautions, 176
    See also heart; high blood pressure
structural integration, 167
su bak, 301
subconscious, 95
subluxations, 37, 43
substance abuse. See addictions
subtle energy practices, 64, 82, 115-117, 163
    See also energy
Sufism, 306, 329, 403
sugar, 8
suggestive therapeutics, 73
Sullivan, Harry Stack, 354
Summers, Elaine, 226
sumo wrestling, 278
sun cure, 104
sun dance, 22
sun therapy, 6, 83
    See also light therapy
sunburn, treatments for, 60
sunyata, 319
support groups, 81
surgery, 76, 221, 323, 369, 400
    minor, 15, 17
suriashi, 295
Sutherland, Dr. William, 40
Suzuki, Daisetz T., 317
sweat lodge, shamanism and, 22
Swedish massage, 144, 146, 147, 148, 174-176
Sweigard, Lulu, 225
sword dance, 281
swordsmanship, 284, 293-297, 301
symbols, 71, 126, 328, 347, 354, 374
symptoms
    alternative vs. allopathic view of, 3, 9, 12, 46
    holistic view of, 9, 38
    homeopathic view of, 13
    naturopathic view of, 17
    suppression of, 54

synergy, 380
syntonic optometry, 104, 108
syphilis, 14

T
tachi-uchi, 293
tae kyon, 301
taekwondo, 301-304
t'ai chi ch'üan, 117, 118, 119, 211, 244-246, 250,
    263-264, 270-273, 276, 293, 297, 298, 320
tai-jutsu, 284
Takata, Hawayo, 135
Takenouchi Ryu, 284
talent, 232, 345
Tamalpa Institute, 360
Tameshiwara, 291
tanden, 295
tantra, 319
tantric yoga, 309
Tanzbuhne Laban, 335
Tao of the Body, 350
Tao Teh Ching, 184-186
Tao-Yin, 118
Taoism, 23, 24, 25, 65, 118, 120-121, 184, 198,
    245, 297, 299, 400
Taoist Canon, 131
tapotement, 174, 175
taste, 54
Taylor, Charles Faytte, 144
Taylor, George Henry, 144
TCM. See traditional Chinese medicine
teacher, shaman as, 18
teaching, 329, 332, 342
tee, 297
Teeguarden, Iona Marsaa, 180, 187-188
telepathy, 118
temperature, 322
    disease and, 145
temporomandibular joint (TMJ),
    treatments for, 42, 70, 162
    See also jaw pain
tendinitis, 162
Tenjin Shrine, 284
tennis elbow, 162
tension, 99, 190, 228, 230, 231, 379, 392, 398
    physiological, 46
    unconscious, 204
    See also stress
tension relief, treatments for, 39, 42, 43, 44, 182,
    223, 226, 228, 362
"Tenth Good Thing About Barney, The", 372
Teresa, Mother, 81, 309
Thai massage, 146
Theatre of Spontaneity, 416
Theosophical Society, 317
therapeutic touch (TT), 38, 116, 131, 139-141,
    145
Thinking Body, The, 225

thinking skills, 322
Thoreau, Henry David, 317
three-brain model, 237
thrombosis, treatment cautions, 175
thurmae, 143
thyroid problems, 106
Tibetan monks, 322-324
Tillich, Paul, 397
TM. See Transcendental Meditation
TMJ. See temporomandibular joint
to-jutsu, 293
Todd, Mabel Elsworth, 201, 225
toho, 293
tolle causam, 16
Tomatis, Dr. Alfred, 84, 111
Tomatis method, 84, 111-114
toning. See sounding
toothache, 125
Tori, 288
touch, 27, 115, 425
    use in therapy, 35-36, 115, 126, 135, 142, 192
touch communication, 153-154
Touch Research Institute (TRI), 146, 154-155
Touchdown, 250
Touching, 154
toxemia, 150
toxicity, factors affecting, 35, 59
toxins, elimination of, 6, 99, 152, 164, 179, 180, 182
traditional Chinese medicine (TCM), 177-178, 180, 183, 186, 189, 194, 195, 197
traditional massage. See Swedish massage
Trager, Dr. Milton, 201, 240
Trager Institute, The, 240
Trager psychophysical integration, 239-243
trance state, 21, 65, 73, 74, 106, 402, 404
    See also hypnotherapy; shamanism
Transcendental Meditation (TM), 308, 319, 324-326
transcendentalists, 318
transformations, 26, 359
transpersonal psychology, 193, 403
trauma, 42, 133, 153, 159, 172, 174, 224, 251, 253, 343, 358, 363, 392, 405, 423
    effect on health, 35, 66, 111, 112, 189-190, 194
trauma reflex, 219, 221
Travell, Dr. Janet, 160
Treatise on Harm Caused by Cold, 25
Treatise of Materia Medica, A, 10
TRI. See Touch Research Institute
trigger points, 160, 173
trigger-point myotherapy, 145
trust, 249, 250, 426
truth, 313, 366
Tschanpua, 143
tse, 297
tsubos, 194
TT. See Therapeutic Touch

tuberculosis, 14, 83, 100, 104, 201, 231
tui na, 143, 180, 197-199
types, 329, 330-331
typhoid, 46
typhus, 11

U
Ueshiba Academy, 278
Ueshiba, Kisshomaru, 280
Ueshiba, Morehei, 278-280
Ueshiba-ryu Aiki-bujutsu, 278
Uke, 278, 280, 288
ulcers, treatments for, 67, 76, 125, 129, 187
ultrasound, 16
ultraviolet energy, 103-104, 107
unconscious, 66, 74, 106, 343, 379
    See also consciousness; mind
unergi, 428-429
universal reformer, 262
universe, 245
University of California–Irvine, 43, 45
unruffling, 140
Upledger, Dr. John E., 40, 41, 42
Upledger Institute, The, 42
urogenital problems, treatments for, 188
U.S. Centers for Disease Control, 8
Usui, Mikao, 133-134
Usui System of Natural Healing, 135

V
valerian root (*Valeriana officinalis*), 58
Valnet, Jean, 86
varicose veins, 147
    treatment cautions, 175
vata, 5-7
Vazquez, Dr. Steven, 106
verbal unwinding, 163
verbalizations, 169
Veselko, Ruth, 234
vibration, 174, 175
Vietnam War, 47, 57, 94
violence, 358
Viorst, Judith, 372
Vis medicatrix naturae, 16
vision quests, shamanism and, 22
visualizations, 19-21, 119, 231, 429
    shamanism and, 19-21
vital life force, 34
vitamin B$_3$, 55, 61
vitamin C, 61, 79
vitamin D, 105
vitamin E, 61
vitamin therapy, 55, 60-62
Vivekananda, Swami, 317
vodoun religion, 18
voice, 254-255
    therapies for, 109-113, 201, 204-207, 213
vomiting, 10

W

Walden School, 347
Waldorf School, 245, 254, 269
wall-eye, 90
Walling, Dr. William, 382
water, 83, 99
   See also hydrotherapy
Watts, Alan, 234, 317
waza, 295
wellness, 3, 5, 8, 29-32
Wells, Dr. David, 90-91
Wertheimer, Max, 397
whiplash, treatment for, 39, 162, 209, 221
White House Task Force on Innovative
   Learning, 247, 248
Whitehouse, Mary, 350, 354
WHO. See World Health Organization
Wigman, Mary, 350
Wilber, Kenneth, 403
Williams, Drs. Bill and Ellen, 202, 235
Williams, Roger, Ph.D., 62
Winternitz, William, 100
wisdom, 258, 419
wisdom qigong, 132
women
   in homeopathy, 14
   in osteopathy, 47
World Health Organization (WHO), 57-58, 62,
   187
World Parliament of Religions, 317
World Taekwondo Federation, 301
world technique, 374
world work, 415
Worsley, Prof. J.R., 50
wound healing, 81, 104, 124, 141, 144, 152

wounds, 147, 1599
   emotional, 400
   treatments for, 60
writing skills, 248, 372

X

X ray, 323

Y

yantra yoga, 308
Yawara, 284
*Yellow Emperor's Internal Classic (Huang-ti Nei
   Jing)*, 24, 118, 143, 184, 195, 198
yin and yang, 26-27, 118, 120-121, 186, 272-273,
   309
Ying qi, 26
Yoga: Immortality and Freedom , 306
yoga, 64, 66, 82, 117, 118, 128, 250, 251, 305-312,
   317, 322, 324, 382
Yoga Journal International, 306
Yoga Sutras, 306
Yogananda, Paramahansa, 306, 317
Yogi, Marahishi Mahesh, 308, 319, 324, 325
Yoshin-Ryu, 284
Yu, Tricia, 263

Z

za-zen, 295-296, 319
ZB. See Zero Balancing
Zen Buddhism, 135, 285, 289, 291, 317, 319
Zero Balancing® (ZB), 35, 36, 50-52, 145, 192
Zhang Jie-Bin, 27
Zhang Zhong-Jing, 25
zone therapy, 163
zubon, 288